Pheochromocytoma (PHEO) and Paraganglioma (PGL)

Pheochromocytoma (PHEO) and Paraganglioma (PGL)

Special Issue Editors

Karel Pacak

David Taïeb

MDPI • Basel • Beijing • Wuhan • Barcelona • Belgrade

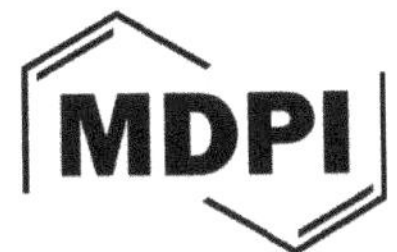

Special Issue Editors
Karel Pacak
Eunice Kennedy Shriver NICHD, NIH
USA

David Taïeb
La Timone University Hospital
France

Editorial Office
MDPI
St. Alban-Anlage 66
4052 Basel, Switzerland

This is a reprint of articles from the Special Issue published online in the open access journal *Cancers* (ISSN 2072-6694) from 2018 to 2019 (available at: https://www.mdpi.com/journal/cancers/special_issues/PHEO_PGL)

For citation purposes, cite each article independently as indicated on the article page online and as indicated below:

LastName, A.A.; LastName, B.B.; LastName, C.C. Article Title. *Journal Name* **Year**, *Article Number*, Page Range.

ISBN 978-3-03921-654-3 (Pbk)
ISBN 978-3-03921-655-0 (PDF)

Contents

About the Special Issue Editors ix

Karel Pacak and David Taïeb
Pheochromocytoma (PHEO) and Paraganglioma (PGL)
Reprinted from: *Cancers* **2019**, *11*, 1391, doi:10.3390/cancers11091391 1

Herui Wang, Jing Cui, Chunzhang Yang, Jared S. Rosenblum, Qi Zhang, Qi Song, Ying Pang, Francia Fang, Mitchell Sun, Pauline Dmitriev, Mark R. Gilbert, Graeme Eisenhofer, Karel Pacak and Zhengping Zhuang
A Transgenic Mouse Model of Pacak–Zhuang Syndrome with An *Epas1* Gain-of-Function Mutation
Reprinted from: *Cancers* **2019**, *11*, 667, doi:10.3390/cancers11050667 5

Mehdi Helali, Matthieu Moreau, Clara Le Fèvre, Céline Heimburger, Caroline Bund, Bernard Goichot, Francis Veillon, Fabrice Hubelé, Anne Charpiot, Georges Noel and Alessio Imperiale
^{18}F-FDOPA PET/CT Combined with MRI for Gross Tumor Volume Delineation in Patients with Skull Base Paraganglioma
Reprinted from: *Cancers* **2019**, *11*, 54, doi:10.3390/cancers11010054 17

Johannes A. Rijken, Leonie T. van Hulsteijn, Olaf M. Dekkers, Nicolasine D. Niemeijer, C. René Leemans, Karin Eijkelenkamp, Anouk N.A. van der Horst-Schrivers, Michiel N. Kerstens, Anouk van Berkel, Henri J.L.M. Timmers, Henricus P.M. Kunst, Peter H.L.T. Bisschop, Koen M.A. Dreijerink, Marieke F. van Dooren, Frederik J. Hes, Jeroen C. Jansen, Eleonora P.M. Corssmit and Erik F. Hensen
Increased Mortality in *SDHB* but Not in *SDHD* Pathogenic Variant Carriers
Reprinted from: *Cancers* **2019**, *11*, 103, doi:10.3390/cancers11010103 30

Achyut Ram Vyakaranam, Joakim Crona, Olov Norlén, Per Hellman and Anders Sundin
^{11}C-hydroxy-ephedrine-PET/CT in the Diagnosis of Pheochromocytoma and Paraganglioma
Reprinted from: *Cancers* **2019**, *11*, 847, doi:10.3390/cancers11060847 41

Divya Mamilla, Katherine Araque, Alessandra Brofferio, Melissa K. Gonzales, James N. Sullivan, Naris Nilubol and Karel Pacak
Postoperative Management in Patients with Pheochromocytoma and Paraganglioma
Reprinted from: *Cancers* **2019**, *11*, 936, doi:10.3390/cancers11070936 52

Judita Klímová, Tomáš Zelinka, Ján Rosa, Branislav Štrauch, Denisa Haluzíková, Martin Haluzík, Robert Holaj, Zuzana Krátká, Jan Kvasnička, Viktorie Ďurovcová, Martin Matoulek, Květoslav Novák, David Michalský, Jiří Widimský Jr. and Ondřej Petrák
FGF21 Levels in Pheochromocytoma/Functional Paraganglioma
Reprinted from: *Cancers* **2019**, *11*, 485, doi:10.3390/cancers11040485 79

Martin Ullrich, Susan Richter, Verena Seifert, Sandra Hauser, Bruna Calsina, Ángel M. Martínez-Montes, Marjolein ter Laak, Christian G. Ziegler, Henri Timmers, Graeme Eisenhofer, Mercedes Robledo and Jens Pietzsch
Targeting Cyclooxygenase-2 in Pheochromocytoma and Paraganglioma: Focus on Genetic Background
Reprinted from: *Cancers* **2019**, *11*, 743, doi:10.3390/cancers11060743 90

Lavinia Vittoria Lotti, Simone Vespa, Mattia Russel Pantalone, Silvia Perconti, Diana Liberata Esposito, Rosa Visone, Angelo Veronese, Carlo Terenzio Paties, Mario Sanna, Fabio Verginelli, Cecilia Soderberg Nauclér and Renato Mariani-Costantini
A Developmental Perspective on Paragangliar Tumorigenesis
Reprinted from: *Cancers* **2019**, *11*, 273, doi:10.3390/cancers11030273 . . . . **107**

Radovan Bílek, Petr Vlček, Libor Šafařík, David Michalský, Květoslav Novák, Jaroslava Dušková, Eliška Václavíková, Jiří Widimský Jr. and Tomáš Zelinka
Chromogranin A in the Laboratory Diagnosis of Pheochromocytoma and Paraganglioma
Reprinted from: *Cancers* **2019**, *11*, 586, doi:10.3390/cancers11040586 . . . . **128**

Nicole Bechmann, Isabel Poser, Verena Seifert, Christian Greunke, Martin Ullrich, Nan Qin, Axel Walch, Mirko Peitzsch, Mercedes Robledo, Karel Pacak, Jens Pietzsch, Susan Richter and Graeme Eisenhofer
Impact of Extrinsic and Intrinsic Hypoxia on Catecholamine Biosynthesis in Absence or Presence of Hif2α in Pheochromocytoma Cells
Reprinted from: *Cancers* **2019**, *11*, 594, doi:10.3390/cancers11050594 . . . . **143**

Esther Korpershoek, Daphne A.E.R. Dieduksman, Guy C.M. Grinwis, Michael J. Day, Claudia E. Reusch, Monika Hilbe, Federico Fracassi, Niels M.G. Krol, André G. Uitterlinden, Annelies de Klein, Bert Eussen, Hans Stoop, Ronald R. de Krijger, Sara Galac and Winand N.M. Dinjens
Molecular Alterations in Dog Pheochromocytomas and Paragangliomas
Reprinted from: *Cancers* **2019**, *11*, 607, doi:10.3390/cancers11050607 . . . . **161**

Valeria Bisogni, Luigi Petramala, Gaia Oliviero, Maria Bonvicini, Martina Mezzadri, Federica Olmati, Antonio Concistrè, Vincenza Saracino, Monia Celi, Gianfranco Tonnarini, Gino Iannucci, Giorgio De Toma, Antonio Ciardi, Giuseppe La Torre and Claudio Letizia
Analysis of Short-term Blood Pressure Variability in Pheochromocytoma/Paraganglioma Patients
Reprinted from: *Cancers* **2019**, *11*, 658, doi:10.3390/cancers11050658 . . . . **172**

Jacob Kohlenberg, Brian Welch, Oksana Hamidi, Matthew Callstrom, Jonathan Morris, Juraj Sprung, Irina Bancos and William Young Jr.
Efficacy and Safety of Ablative Therapy in the Treatment of Patients with Metastatic Pheochromocytoma and Paraganglioma
Reprinted from: *Cancers* **2019**, *11*, 195, doi:10.3390/cancers11020195 . . . . **186**

Joakim Crona, Samuel Backman, Staffan Welin, David Taïeb, Per Hellman, Peter Stålberg, Britt Skogseid and Karel Pacak
RNA-Sequencing Analysis of Adrenocortical Carcinoma, Pheochromocytoma and Paraganglioma from a Pan-Cancer Perspective
Reprinted from: *Cancers* **2018**, *10*, 518, doi:10.3390/cancers10120518 . . . . **199**

Anna Angelousi, Melpomeni Peppa, Alexandra Chrisoulidou, Krystallenia Alexandraki, Annabel Berthon, Fabio Rueda Faucz, Eva Kassi and Gregory Kaltsas
Malignant Pheochromocytomas/Paragangliomas and Ectopic Hormonal Secretion: A Case Series and Review of the Literature
Reprinted from: *Cancers* **2019**, *11*, 724, doi:10.3390/cancers11050724 . . . . **214**

Achyut Ram Vyakaranam, Joakim Crona, Olov Norlén, Dan Granberg, Ulrike Garske-Román, Mattias Sandström, Katarzyna Fröss-Baron, Espen Thiis-Evensen, Per Hellman and Anders Sundin
Favorable Outcome in Patients with Pheochromocytoma and Paraganglioma Treated with ^{177}Lu-DOTATATE
Reprinted from: *Cancers* **2019**, *11*, 909, doi:10.3390/cancers11070909 . . . . **230**

Annika M.A. Berends, Graeme Eisenhofer, Lauren Fishbein, Anouk N.A. van der Horst-Schrivers, Ido P. Kema, Thera P. Links, Jacques W.M. Lenders and Michiel N. Kerstens
Intricacies of the Molecular Machinery of Catecholamine Biosynthesis and Secretion by Chromaffin Cells of the Normal Adrenal Medulla and in Pheochromocytoma and Paraganglioma
Reprinted from: *Cancers* **2019**, *11*, 1121, doi:10.3390/cancers11081121 . . . . **245**

Alberto Cascón, Laura Remacha, Bruna Calsina and Mercedes Robledo
Pheochromocytomas and Paragangliomas: Bypassing Cellular Respiration
Reprinted from: *Cancers* **2019**, *11*, 683, doi:10.3390/cancers11050683 . . . . **278**

Laura Gieldon, Doreen William, Karl Hackmann, Winnie Jahn, Arne Jahn, Johannes Wagner, Andreas Rump, Nicole Bechmann, Svenja Nölting, Thomas Knösel, Volker Gudziol, Georgiana Constantinescu, Jimmy Masjkur, Felix Beuschlein, Henri JLM Timmers, Letizia Canu, Karel Pacak, Mercedes Robledo, Daniela Aust, Evelin Schröck, Graeme Eisenhofer, Susan Richter and Barbara Klink
Optimizing Genetic Workup in Pheochromocytoma and Paraganglioma by Integrating Diagnostic and Research Approaches
Reprinted from: *Cancers* **2019**, *11*, 809, doi:10.3390/cancers11060809 . . . . **300**

Jan Kvasnička, Tomáš Zelinka, Ondřej Petrák, Ján Rosa, Branislav Štrauch, Zuzana Krátká, Tomáš Indra, Alice Markvartová, Jiří Widimský Jr. and Robert Holaj
Catecholamines Induce Left Ventricular Subclinical Systolic Dysfunction: A Speckle-Tracking Echocardiography Study
Reprinted from: *Cancers* **2019**, *11*, 318, doi:10.3390/cancers11030318 . . . . **319**

Veronika Caisova, Liping Li, Garima Gupta, Ivana Jochmanova, Abhishek Jha, Ondrej Uher, Thanh-Truc Huynh, Markku Miettinen, Ying Pang, Luma Abunimer, Gang Niu, Xiaoyuan Chen, Hans Kumar Ghayee, David Taïeb, Zhengping Zhuang, Jan Zenka and Karel Pacak
The Significant Reduction or Complete Eradication of Subcutaneous and Metastatic Lesions in a Pheochromocytoma Mouse Model after Immunotherapy Using Mannan-BAM, TLR Ligands, and Anti-CD40
Reprinted from: *Cancers* **2019**, *11*, 654, doi:10.3390/cancers11050654 . . . . **332**

Ying Pang, Yang Liu, Karel Pacak and Chunzhang Yang
Pheochromocytomas and Paragangliomas: From Genetic Diversity to Targeted Therapies
Reprinted from: *Cancers* **2019**, *11*, 436, doi:10.3390/cancers11040436 . . . . **353**

About the Special Issue Editors

Karel Pacak is an endocrinologist and tenured Chief of the Section on Medical Neuroendocrinology at Eunice Kennedy Shriver National Institute of Child Health and Human Development (NICHD), NIH, Bethesda, MD. He is recognized nationally and internationally for patient-oriented pheochromocytoma (PHEO) and paraganglioma (PGL) research programs. He and his colleagues implemented the use of plasma metanephrines in the biochemical diagnosis of these tumors, the use of 68Ga-DOTATATE in their localization and several new therapeutic options, the latest one the use of PARP inhibitors together with temozolomide, particularly in succinate dehydrogenase mutated PHEO/PGL. He and his colleagues also described the role of *HIF2A, IRP1,* and *PHD1* mutations in the pathogenesis of paraganglioma, somatostatinoma, and polycythemia. This lead to the introduction of a new syndrome now known as the Pacak-Zhuang syndrome. Apart from but in line with his life's work, Dr. Pacak has skillfully applied his knowledge for the benefit of the greater good. He established a new series of international pheochromocytoma conferences (ISP), for which he has served as the president and principal organizer of the first conference in 2005. He has received distinguished awards from the International Association of Endocrine Surgeons, Australian Endocrine Society, Irish Endocrine Society, PheoPara Alliance, American Association of Clinical Endocrinologists, the Gold Jessenius Medal from the Slovak Academy of Sciences, the Gold Medal from the Slovak Medical Society, Purkyne Medal from the Czech Medical Society, and the Directors' award from the NIH and NICHD.

David Taïeb is full professor of Nuclear Medicine at Aix Marseille university, France. He is member of the EANM Oncology & Theranostics Committee. He holds numerous research grants and is co-editor of 2 textbooks dedicated to Nuclear Endocrinology. He has over 180 peer-reviewed publications. A major focus of his clinical research in collaboration with the NIH, has been to assess the relationship between imaging phenotypes and genotypes in pheochromocytoma and paraganglioma (PPGL). In addition, he is actively involved in radionuclide therapy with a major focus on endocrine neoplasms. He is also affiliated to INSERM (French Institute of Health and Medical Research) with several on-going basic research projects on castration-resistant prostate cancer and nanotheranostics. More recently, he has coordinated the EANM Practice Guideline/SNMMI Procedure Standard 2019 for radionuclide imaging of PPGL. He became the member of the International Advisory Board for the 6th international symposium on PPGL.

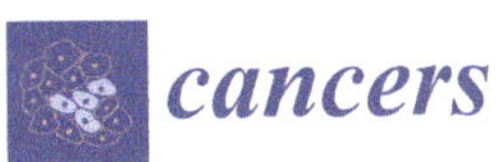 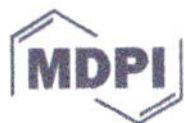

Editorial

Pheochromocytoma (PHEO) and Paraganglioma (PGL)

Karel Pacak [1,*] and David Taïeb [2,*]

1 Section on Medical Neuroendocrinology, Head, Developmental Endocrine Oncology and Genetics Affinity Group. Eunice Kennedy Shriver NICHD, NIH, Building 10, CRC, Room 1E-3140, 10 Center Drive MSC-1109, Bethesda, MD 20892-1109, USA

2 Department of Nuclear Medicine, La Timone University Hospital, European Center for Research in Medical Imaging, Aix-Marseille University, 13100 Marseille, France

* Correspondence: karel@mail.nih.gov (K.P.); David.TAIEB@ap-hm.fr (D.T.)

Received: 9 September 2019; Accepted: 16 September 2019; Published: 18 September 2019

This series of 23 articles (17 original articles, six reviews) is presented by international leaders in pheochromocytoma and paraganglioma (PPGL). PPGLs are rare neuroendocrine tumors originating from chromaffin cells in the adrenal medulla or paraganglia outside the adrenal medulla, respectively. Uniquely, these tumors produce and secrete catecholamines, mainly norepinephrine and epinephrine, that profoundly affect cardiovascular [1], gastrointestinal, and to lesser extents, other systems. One article shows that pheochromocytoma patients have a lower magnitude of global longitudinal strains (GLS) derived from speckle-tracking echocardiography compared to patients with essential hypertension, suggesting that catecholamines induce a subclinical decline in the left ventriclar systolic function [2]. Furthermore, if these tumors remain unrecognized, they pose a severe threat to patients by potentially causing sudden death due to lethal arrhythmias, myocardial infarction, and stroke. Therefore, all attempts should be made to diagnose and treat these tumors early before they strike a patient or become metastatic. Throughout the years, our knowledge and perception of these tumors have been greatly expanded and changed by new discoveries in genetics, metabolomics, proteomics, diagnostics, treatment, and follow-up of these tumors. Recently, there have been discoveries of new susceptible genes with either germline or somatic mutations [3]. Uniquely, metabolomic analysis has greatly improved the identification of these new genes and their pathogenicity, as well as the characterization of some variants of unknown significance. In this book, the spectrum of these new genes are described, as well as the implications on clinical management of patients. Recent studies have shown some gene-specific clinical risks that may warrant tailored management strategies [4]. The relevance of such mutations in tumorigenesis and catecholamine biosynthesis and secretion are also presented [5] with special emphasis on the role of hypoxia-inducible factors on the regulation of phosphorylation of tyrosine hydroxylase [6]. These findings, together with the excellent negative predictive value of histological PASS and GAPP algorithms [7], provide novel prognostic biomarkers and new therapeutic avenues [8–10]. Beyond catecholamines, PPGLs could also secrete a wide diversity of products which could serve as biomarkers, such as chromogranin A [11], and could be responsible in very exceptional situations of ectopic syndromes (mostly ACTH, IL6, PTH/PTHrp) [12]. A long-term overproduction of catecholamines by PPGL could also lead to the elevation of FGF21, especially in patients with secondary diabetes, that would require specific investigation to determine potential effects on metabolism and adipose tissue [13]. In recent years, molecular imaging has emerged at the forefront of personalized medicine. The use of molecular imaging, particularly with positron emission tomography compounds, in the localization of these tumors has been successfully expanded. Despite limited availability, [^{11}C]-hydroxyephedrine PET/CT has shown to be an accurate tool to diagnose and rule out pheochromocytoma in complex clinical scenarios and to characterize equivocal adrenal incidentalomas [14]. More specifically for head and neck PGL and metastatic cases, [^{68}Ga]-DOTATATE

PET/CT has become the best available imaging modality. These results prompted the introduction of peptide receptor radionuclide therapy using radiolabeled somatostatin analogs. At present, more than 200 PPGL patients have been treated on compassionate grounds with PRRT with promising results. Here, Vyakaranam et al. [15] report a series of patients with favorable outcomes and limited toxicity. PET/CT or PET/MR imaging using a specific tracer such as [^{18}F]-FDOPA might also allow improvement in treatment planning for external beam radiotherapy by allowing refinement of the gross tumor volume [16]. Kohlenberg et al. [17] also show excellent results of ablative therapy in the treatment of metastatic PPGL in order to achieve local control and decrease symptoms and signs from catecholamine excess. Given the potential for serious procedure-related complications, the balance-risk ratio should be discussed in each individual situation, and ablation procedures should be performed in high-volume centers. Throughout these therapies, as well as other situations (e.g., surgery), physicians must be aware of potential complications and be able to provide appropriate management to minimize morbidity and mortality associated with PPGLs, especially elevated catecholamine levels [18].

Although therapeutic and preventative options for PPGLs, especially metastatic disease, are still in their infancy, several new studies are now in progress or planned. To achieve these goals, preclinical models are needed, such as transgenic mice (e.g., Epas1 Gain-of-Function Mutation [19]), canine models that carry similar genomic alterations to humans [20], or patient-derived tumor xenografts (PDXs). This will accelerate our understanding on tumorigenesis, help to build original developmental models [21], and find new treatments. One promising approach in patients with metastatic PPGL relies on immunotherapy that initially activates innate immunity followed by an adaptive immune response. One original article shows a significant reduction or complete eradication of subcutaneous and metastatic lesions in a pheochromocytoma mouse model after immunotherapy using Mannan-BAM, TLR ligands, and anti-CD40 [22]. A pan-cancer RNA sequencing analysis also challenges the current classification of PPGL with clustering of PPGL with pancreatic neuroendocrine tumors or neuroblastomas, a finding that could open new therapeutic perspectives and help us understand the development of these tumors and their relationships [23]. The use of artificial intelligence, sophisticated computer algorithms, and modeling to classify information from a particular patient, as well as diagnostic and other methods done on that patient, will become a reality in the near future. This creates the potential to transform the lives of patients with these tumors, resulting in their prevention or even eradication. This series of unique articles represents a collaborative, international effort that reflects the scope and spirit of this issue by nicely blending current and future genetic, diagnostic, and therapeutic approaches to PPGLs. Understanding developmental, host, and environmental factors will also become very important to develop preventive strategies.

Let us conclude with a quotation from Dr. William Mayo: «The glory of medicine is that it is constantly moving forward, that there is always more to learn» Indeed, this issue provides new information not only to health care professionals but to basic scientists and others interested in learning something new about PPGL.

Conflicts of Interest: The authors declare no conflict of interest.

References

1. Bisogni, V.; Petramala, L.; Oliviero, G.; Bonvicini, M.; Mezzadri, M.; Olmati, F.; Concistrè, A.; Saracino, V.; Celi, M.; Tonnarini, G.; et al. Analysis of Short-term Blood Pressure Variability in Pheochromocytoma/Paraganglioma Patients. *Cancers* **2019**, *11*, 658. [CrossRef] [PubMed]
2. Kvasnička, J.; Zelinka, T.; Petrák, O.; Rosa, J.; Štrauch, B.; Krátká, Z.; Indra, T.; Markvartová, A.; Widimský, J.; Holaj, R. Catecholamines Induce Left Ventricular Subclinical Systolic Dysfunction: A Speckle-Tracking Echocardiography Study. *Cancers* **2019**, *11*, 318. [CrossRef] [PubMed]
3. Gieldon, L.; William, D.; Hackmann, K.; Jahn, W.; Jahn, A.; Wagner, J.; Rump, A.; Bechmann, N.; Nölting, S.; Knösel, T.; et al. Optimizing Genetic Workup in Pheochromocytoma and Paraganglioma by Integrating Diagnostic and Research Approaches. *Cancers* **2019**, *11*, 809. [CrossRef] [PubMed]

4. Rijken, J.; van Hulsteijn, L.; Dekkers, O.; Niemeijer, N.; Leemans, C.; Eijkelenkamp, K.; van der Horst-Schrivers, A.; Kerstens, M.; van Berkel, A.; Timmers, H.; et al. Increased Mortality in SDHB but Not in SDHD Pathogenic Variant Carriers. *Cancers* **2019**, *11*, 103. [CrossRef] [PubMed]
5. Berends, A.; Eisenhofer, G.; Fishbein, L.; Horst-Schrivers, A.; Kema, I.; Links, T.; Lenders, J.; Kerstens, M. Intricacies of the Molecular Machinery of Catecholamine Biosynthesis and Secretion by Chromaffin Cells of the Normal Adrenal Medulla and in Pheochromocytoma and Paraganglioma. *Cancers* **2019**, *11*, 1121. [CrossRef] [PubMed]
6. Bechmann, N.; Poser, I.; Seifert, V.; Greunke, C.; Ullrich, M.; Qin, N.; Walch, A.; Peitzsch, M.; Robledo, M.; Pacak, K.; et al. Impact of Extrinsic and Intrinsic Hypoxia on Catecholamine Biosynthesis in Absence or Presence of Hif2α in Pheochromocytoma Cells. *Cancers* **2019**, *11*, 594. [CrossRef] [PubMed]
7. Stenman, A.; Zedenius, J.; Juhlin, C. The Value of Histological Algorithms to Predict the Malignancy Potential of Pheochromocytomas and Abdominal Paragangliomas—A Meta-Analysis and Systematic Review of the Literature. *Cancers* **2019**, *11*, 225. [CrossRef]
8. Pang, Y.; Liu, Y.; Pacak, K.; Yang, C. Pheochromocytomas and Paragangliomas: From Genetic Diversity to Targeted Therapies. *Cancers* **2019**, *11*, 436. [CrossRef]
9. Cascón, A.; Remacha, L.; Calsina, B.; Robledo, M. Pheochromocytomas and Paragangliomas: Bypassing Cellular Respiration. *Cancers* **2019**, *11*, 683. [CrossRef]
10. Ullrich, M.; Richter, S.; Seifert, V.; Hauser, S.; Calsina, B.; Martínez-Montes, Á.; ter Laak, M.; Ziegler, C.; Timmers, H.; Eisenhofer, G.; et al. Targeting Cyclooxygenase-2 in Pheochromocytoma and Paraganglioma: Focus on Genetic Background. *Cancers* **2019**, *11*, 743. [CrossRef]
11. Bílek, R.; Vlček, P.; Šafařík, L.; Michalský, D.; Novák, K.; Dušková, J.; Václavíková, E.; Widimský, J.; Zelinka, T. Chromogranin A in the Laboratory Diagnosis of Pheochromocytoma and Paraganglioma. *Cancers* **2019**, *11*, 586. [CrossRef] [PubMed]
12. Angelousi, A.; Peppa, M.; Chrisoulidou, A.; Alexandraki, K.; Berthon, A.; Faucz, F.; Kassi, E.; Kaltsas, G. Malignant Pheochromocytomas/Paragangliomas and Ectopic Hormonal Secretion: A Case Series and Review of the Literature. *Cancers* **2019**, *11*, 724. [CrossRef] [PubMed]
13. Klímová, J.; Zelinka, T.; Rosa, J.; Štrauch, B.; Haluzíková, D.; Haluzík, M.; Holaj, R.; Krátká, Z.; Kvasnička, J.; Ďurovcová, V.; et al. FGF21 Levels in Pheochromocytoma/Functional Paraganglioma. *Cancers* **2019**, *11*, 485. [CrossRef] [PubMed]
14. Vyakaranam, A.; Crona, J.; Norlén, O.; Hellman, P.; Sundin, A. ^{11}C-hydroxy-ephedrine-PET/CT in the Diagnosis of Pheochromocytoma and Paraganglioma. *Cancers* **2019**, *11*, 847. [CrossRef] [PubMed]
15. Vyakaranam, A.; Crona, J.; Norlén, O.; Granberg, D.; Garske-Román, U.; Sandström, M.; Fröss-Baron, K.; Thiis-Evensen, E.; Hellman, P.; Sundin, A. Favorable Outcome in Patients with Pheochromocytoma and Paraganglioma Treated with 177Lu-DOTATATE. *Cancers* **2019**, *11*, 909. [CrossRef] [PubMed]
16. Helali, M.; Moreau, M.; Le Fèvre, C.; Heimburger, C.; Bund, C.; Goichot, B.; Veillon, F.; Hubelé, F.; Charpiot, A.; Noel, G.; et al. 18F-FDOPA PET/CT Combined with MRI for Gross Tumor Volume Delineation in Patients with Skull Base Paraganglioma. *Cancers* **2019**, *11*, 54. [CrossRef] [PubMed]
17. Kohlenberg, J.; Welch, B.; Hamidi, O.; Callstrom, M.; Morris, J.; Sprung, J.; Bancos, I.; Young, W. Efficacy and Safety of Ablative Therapy in the Treatment of Patients with Metastatic Pheochromocytoma and Paraganglioma. *Cancers* **2019**, *11*, 195. [CrossRef] [PubMed]
18. Mamilla, D.; Araque, K.; Brofferio, A.; Gonzales, M.; Sullivan, J.; Nilubol, N.; Pacak, K. Postoperative Management in Patients with Pheochromocytoma and Paraganglioma. *Cancers* **2019**, *11*, 936. [CrossRef] [PubMed]
19. Wang, H.; Cui, J.; Yang, C.; Rosenblum, J.; Zhang, Q.; Song, Q.; Pang, Y.; Fang, F.; Sun, M.; Dmitriev, P.; et al. A Transgenic Mouse Model of Pacak–Zhuang Syndrome with An Epas1 Gain-of-Function Mutation. *Cancers* **2019**, *11*, 667. [CrossRef]
20. Korpershoek, E.; Dieduksman, D.; Grinwis, G.; Day, M.; Reusch, C.; Hilbe, M.; Fracassi, F.; Krol, N.; Uitterlinden, A.; de Klein, A.; et al. Molecular Alterations in Dog Pheochromocytomas and Paragangliomas. *Cancers* **2019**, *11*, 607. [CrossRef] [PubMed]
21. Lotti, L.; Vespa, S.; Pantalone, M.; Perconti, S.; Esposito, D.; Visone, R.; Veronese, A.; Paties, C.; Sanna, M.; Verginelli, F.; et al. A Developmental Perspective on Paragangliar Tumorigenesis. *Cancers* **2019**, *11*, 273. [CrossRef] [PubMed]

22. Caisova, V.; Li, L.; Gupta, G.; Jochmanova, I.; Jha, A.; Uher, O.; Huynh, T.; Miettinen, M.; Pang, Y.; Abunimer, L.; et al. The Significant Reduction or Complete Eradication of Subcutaneous and Metastatic Lesions in a Pheochromocytoma Mouse Model after Immunotherapy Using Mannan-BAM, TLR Ligands, and Anti-CD40. *Cancers* **2019**, *11*, 654. [CrossRef] [PubMed]
23. Crona, J.; Backman, S.; Welin, S.; Taïeb, D.; Hellman, P.; Stålberg, P.; Skogseid, B.; Pacak, K. RNA-Sequencing Analysis of Adrenocortical Carcinoma, Pheochromocytoma and Paraganglioma from a Pan-Cancer Perspective. *Cancers* **2018**, *10*, 518. [CrossRef] [PubMed]

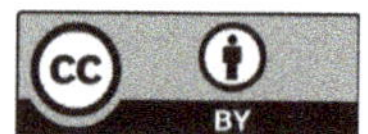

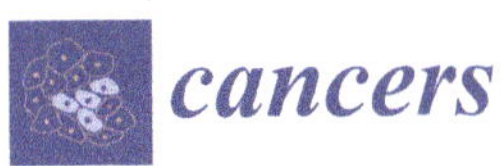
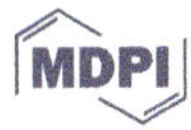

Article

A Transgenic Mouse Model of Pacak–Zhuang Syndrome with An *Epas1* Gain-of-Function Mutation

Herui Wang [1], Jing Cui [1], Chunzhang Yang [1], Jared S. Rosenblum [1], Qi Zhang [1], Qi Song [1], Ying Pang [2], Francia Fang [3], Mitchell Sun [3], Pauline Dmitriev [1], Mark R. Gilbert [1], Graeme Eisenhofer [4], Karel Pacak [2,*] and Zhengping Zhuang [1,3,*]

1. Neuro-Oncology Branch, Center for Cancer Research, National Cancer Institute, Bethesda, MD 20892, USA; herui.wang@nih.gov (H.W.); jing.cui@nih.gov (J.C.); chungzhang.yang@nih.gov (C.Y.); jared.rosenblum@nih.gov (J.S.R.); zhangqi86@gmail.com (Q.Z.); qisong725@gmail.com (Q.S.); pauline.dmitriev@nih.gov (P.D.); mark.gilbert@nih.gov (M.R.G.)
2. Eunice Kennedy Shriver National Institute of Child Health and Human Development, National Institutes of Health, Bethesda, MD 20892, USA; ying.pang@nih.gov
3. Surgical Neurology Branch, National Institute of Neurological Diseases and Stroke, National Institutes of Health, Bethesda, MD 20892, USA; franciafang@gmail.com (F.F.); mitchsun12@gmail.com (M.S.)
4. Institute of Clinical Chemistry and Laboratory Medicine and Department of Medicine III, University Hospital Carl Gustav Carus, Technische Universität Dresden, 01307 Dresden, Germany; Graeme.Eisenhofer@uniklinikum-dresden.de

* Correspondence: karel@mail.nih.gov (K.P.); zhengping.zhuang@nih.gov (Z.Z.); Tel.: +1-301-402-4594 (K.P.); +1-240-760-7055 (Z.Z.)

Received: 28 March 2019; Accepted: 10 May 2019; Published: 14 May 2019

Abstract: We previously identified a novel syndrome in patients characterized by paraganglioma, somatostatinoma, and polycythemia. In these patients, polycythemia occurs long before any tumor develops, and tumor removal only partially corrects polycythemia, with recurrence occurring shortly after surgery. Genetic mosaicism of gain-of-function mutations of the *EPAS1* gene (encoding HIF2α) located in the oxygen degradation domain (ODD), typically p.530–532, was shown as the etiology of this syndrome. The aim of the present investigation was to demonstrate that these mutations are necessary and sufficient for the development of the symptoms. We developed transgenic mice with a gain-of-function $Epas1^{A529V}$ mutation (corresponding to human $EPAS1^{A530V}$), which demonstrated elevated levels of erythropoietin and polycythemia, a decreased urinary metanephrine-to-normetanephrine ratio, and increased expression of somatostatin in the ampullary region of duodenum. Further, inhibition of HIF2α with its specific inhibitor PT2385 significantly reduced erythropoietin levels in the mutant mice. However, polycythemia persisted after PT2385 treatment, suggesting an alternative erythropoietin-independent mechanism of polycythemia. These findings demonstrate the vital roles of *EPAS1* mutations in the syndrome development and the great potential of the $Epas1^{A529V}$ animal model for further pathogenesis and therapeutics studies.

Keywords: paraganglioma; somatostatinoma; polycythemia; *EPAS1*; transgenic mice; erythropoietin

---

1. Introduction

We previously identified a novel syndrome (also known as Pacak–Zhuang Syndrome) characterized by the clinical constellation of paraganglioma, somatostatinoma, and polycythemia. Several features in this syndrome are unique and clustered [1,2]. First, the lack of family history of similar symptoms or pathologies suggests a non-hereditary pattern. Second, the syndrome demonstrates female sex predominance. Third, patients demonstrate early onset polycythemia, presenting at birth. Fourth, all patients develop several rare tumors, including paraganglioma (PGL) and somatostatinoma, which we suspected would be unlikely without a common underlying genetic pathogenesis [1,2].

We found that the patients share common postzygotic mutations, including p.A530T/V, P531S, Y532C, L529P, T519M, and P544S, in the oxygen degradation domain (ODD) of *EPAS1*, encoding hypoxia-inducible factor 2α (HIF2α) [1]. These mutations were found to disturb the hydroxylation of ODD of the HIF2α protein by prolyl hydroxylase 2 (PHD2), which impairs its binding with von Hippel–Lindau protein and subsequently increases HIF2α protein stability [1]. This leads to increased transcription of the genes downstream of the HIF2α/HIF1β dimer in the tumors, such as *EPO*, *VEGFA*, *SLC2A1*, and *VPS11* [2], which causes pseudohypoxia signaling and influences the developmental physiology and disease pathology of the syndrome.

PGLs are rare catecholamine-producing tumors that are derived from chromaffin cells of extra-adrenal paraganglia; somatostatinoma is also of neural crest origin. PGLs are classified into two expression clusters: (1) Cluster 1 with high *EPAS1* expression and immature phenotypic features, (2) Cluster 2 with low *EPAS1* expression and mature phenotypic features [3]. Patients with Pacak–Zhuang syndrome consistently fall into Cluster 1 and are found to have high levels of normetanephrine (NMN) and norepinephrine (NE) [1].

Polycythemia is an abnormal elevation of the hematocrit caused by either increased production or decreased destruction of red blood cells (RBCs). Secondary polycythemia occurs as a consequence of elevated circulating erythropoietin (EPO), while primary polycythemia is due to intrinsic factors (e.g., somatic $JAK2^{V617F}$ mutation and hereditary dominant *EPOR* mutations) of erythroid progenitors in the bone marrow and is EPO-independent [4]. Mixed polycythemia, such as Chuvash polycythemia caused by VHL^{R200W} mutation, has features of both primary and secondary polycythemias characterized by elevated EPO and erythroid progenitors hypersensitive to EPO [5]. Elevated plasma EPO confirmed secondary polycythemia in the syndrome patients, but it is still unclear whether primary polycythemia exists.

Hypoxia signaling pathways have been established as critical to disease pathogenesis as well as normal development [6–9]. *EPAS1* mutations were previously only found to cause familial polycythemia and pulmonary arterial hypertension [10–12]. This new syndrome of paraganglioma, somatostatinoma, and polycythemia provides a unique opportunity to study the impact of hypoxia signaling, specifically gain-of-function of HIF2α, on tumorigenesis.

In this study, we aimed to develop a transgenic mouse model to achieve the following aims: (1) to confirm *EPAS1* mutations are causative gene mutations for the syndrome and (2) to use this model for further pathogenesis and therapeutic studies of the syndrome.

2. Results

2.1. Establishment of A Somatic $Epas1^{A529V}$ Animal Model

The syndrome patients were found to carry somatic *EPAS1* mutations in the ODD without other germline mutations [2]. We thus generated a transgenic mouse model with a somatic heterozygous $Epas1^{A529V}$ mutation (corresponding to human $EPAS1^{A530V}$). Transcription activator-like effector nucleases (TALEN) were utilized to facilitate homologous recombination in the embryonic stem (ES) cells (Figure 1A). The targeting vector contained 1.3 kb 5′ and 1 kb 3′ homology arms, neomycin selection, and diphtheria toxin A negative selection cassettes. $Epas1^{A529V}$ point mutation is located in the 3′ homology arm. G418-resistant ES cell colonies were picked up after co-electroporation of TALEN expression vectors and *Epas1* A529V targeting vector into B6:129-mixed-background ES cells. Positive recombinant ES colonies were confirmed by PCR at both 5′ and 3′ ends (Figure 1B). Sanger sequencing also confirmed the presence of the A529V mutation (GCA>GTA) in the positive ES colonies before injection into the blastocysts (Figure 1C). Chimera and subsequent germline-transmitted mice ($Epas1^{neo/+}$) were derived. The neomycin cassette upstream of the A529V point mutation in exon 12 blocked the transcription of the mutant allele, and no obvious defects were observed in $Epas1^{neo/+}$ mice.

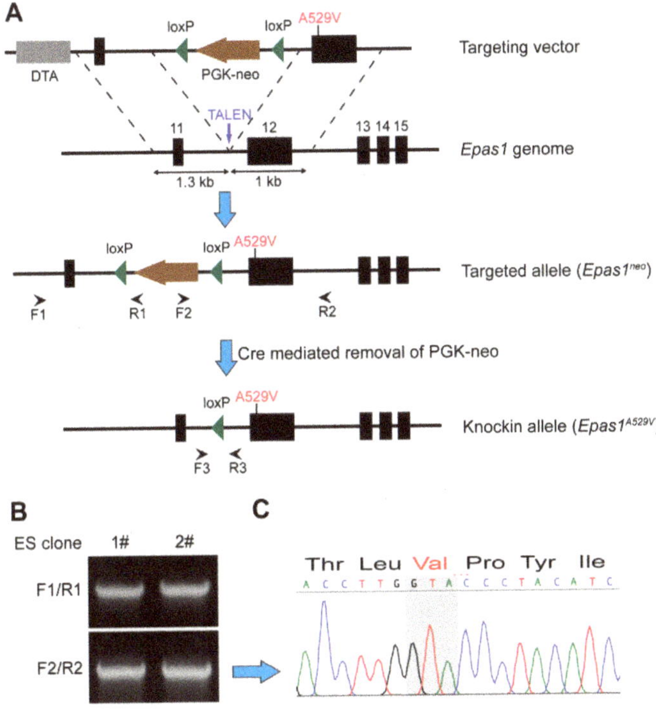

Figure 1. Establishment of the *Epas1*^{A529V} animal model. (**A**) Schematic strategy of the mutant mice generation. (**B**) Positive embryonic stem (ES) colonies were confirmed by PCR at both 5′ (F1/R1) and 3′ (F2/R2) ends. (**C**) Sanger sequencing result of the F2/R2 PCR band. The mutant codon is labeled in red.

To activate the expression of the A529V mutant allele, we mated *Epas1*$^{neo/+}$ mice with *E2a-Cre* transgenic mice in C57BL/6 background and generated somatic heterozygous *Epas1*^{A529V} mutant mice (*E2a-Cre; Epas1*$^{neo/+}$, in brief, *Epas1*^{A529V}) (Figure 2A). Genotyping PCR and Sanger sequencing confirmed the successful deletion of the neomycin cassette in tail DNA of *Epas1*^{A529V} mutant mice (Figure 2B). To confirm the expression of the *Epas1*^{A529V} mutant allele, we extracted RNA from multiple tissues of the *Epas1*^{A529V} mutant mice, including heart, lung, liver, kidney, duodenum, adrenal gland, spleen, and testis, and performed reverse transcription. Droplet digital PCR (ddPCR) with complementary DNA (cDNA) of each tissue confirmed high expression of *Epas1* in lung and heart (Figure 2C,D), consistent with a previous report [13]. The percentage of *Epas1*^{A529V} mutant allele in cDNA varied from 20.8% to 49.4% in different tissues (Figure 2E). These results confirmed Cre-mediated high expression of *Epas1*^{A529V} mutant allele in a wide range of tissues.

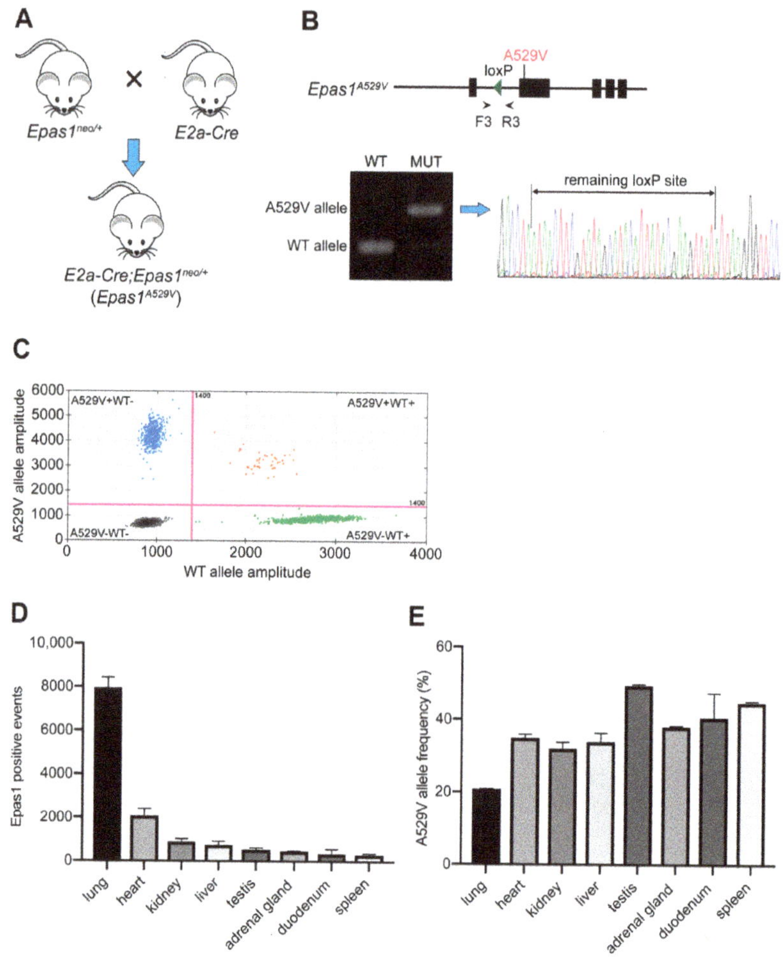

Figure 2. Successful expression of *Epas1*^{A529V} mutant allele in various tissues. (**A**) Mouse breeding strategy to generate the somatic mutant mice. (**B**) Genotyping PCR (F3/R3) and Sanger sequencing confirmed the successful deletion of the neomycin cassette by *E2a-Cre* in one-month-old *Epas1*^{A529V} mutant mice. (**C**) Representative image of *Epas1*^{A529V} droplet digital PCR (ddPCR). Green dots, droplets with PCR amplification of *Epas1* wild-type (WT) allele. Blue dots, droplets with PCR amplification of *Epas1* A529V mutant (MUT) allele. Orange dots, droplets with PCR amplification of both alleles. (**D**) Total *Epas1*-positive events of *Epas1* ddPCR from 100 ng cDNA of each tissue in two–three-month-old male mutant mice. $n = 3$. (**E**) *Epas1*^{A529V} allele frequency in the cDNA derived from each tissue.

2.2. Polycythemia and Elevated EPO in *Epas1*^{A529V} Mutant Mice

Red palms in *Epas1*^{A529V} mutant mice suggested an underlying polycythemia (Figure 3A). A complete blood count (CBC) test confirmed polycythemia by respective 39.9%, 60.7%, and 56.5% elevations in erythrocyte count, hemoglobin, and hematocrit of somatic *Epas1*^{A529V} mutant mice compared to littermate controls (Figure 3B). Minorly increased mean corpuscular volume (MCV) and significantly reduced platelets in the mutant mice were noted, and no change was observed for white blood cells (Figure 3B).

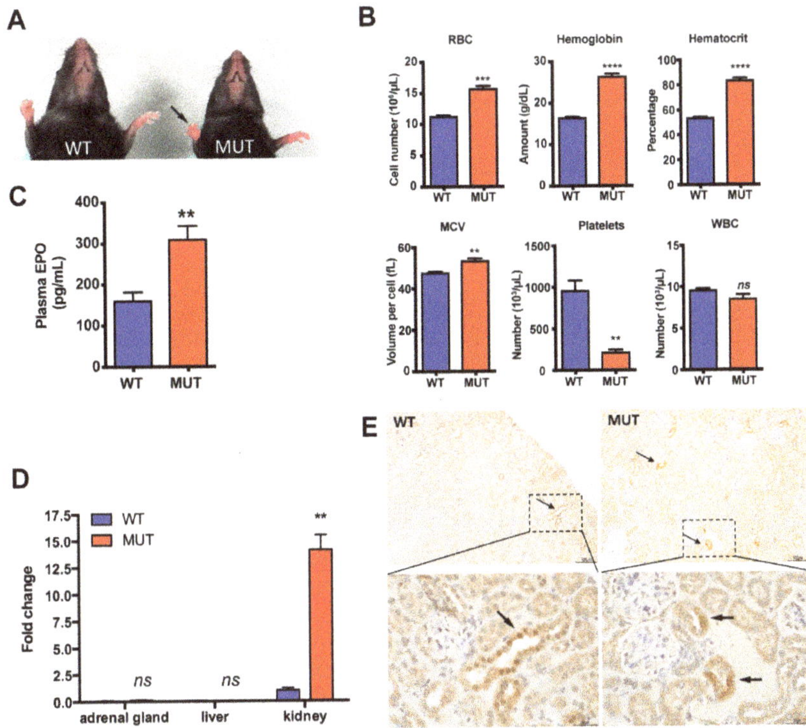

Figure 3. Polycythemia and elevated erythropoietin (EPO) in *Epas1*^{A529V} mutant mice. (**A**) Red palm (arrow) in three-month-old mutant mice. (**B**) Complete blood count (CBC) test confirmed polycythemia in two-month-old mutant mice. MUT, *Epas1*^{A529V} mutant mice. WT, littermate control mice. n(WT) = 4, n(MUT) = 3; ns, $p > 0.05$; ** $p < 0.01$; *** $p < 0.001$; **** $p < 0.0001$. (**C**) Elevated plasma EPO in *Epas1*^{A529V} mutant mice. ** $p < 0.01$. (**D**) *Epo* expression in different tissues of four-month-old mice; $n = 3$ for each group. (**E**) EPO immunohistochemistry (IHC) staining of control and mutant kidney. Arrows indicate EPO-positive cells. RBC: red blood cells, MCV: mean corpuscular volume, WBC: white blood cells. Scale bars: top, 100 μm, bottom, 30 μm.

We measured plasma EPO concentrations and observed significantly increased EPO levels in *Epas1*^{A529V} mice (Figure 3C). The EPO concentrations in mutant mice were about twice those in littermate control mice. Elevated plasma EPO level in mutant mice is expected because the *Epo* gene is a direct target of the HIF2α/HIF1β dimer [14,15]. We also performed real-time RT-PCR to compare *Epo* mRNA levels in different tissues and found that *Epo* expression was much higher in kidney than in other tissues of both control and mutant mice (Figure 3D). *Epo* expression level was dramatically enhanced in mutant kidney by about thirteen-fold compared to control kidney (Figure 3D). EPO immunohistochemistry (IHC) staining also confirmed increased EPO expression in the mutant kidney (Figure 3E). These results suggest that the *Epas1*^{A529V} mutation increased EPO expression in the kidney, leading to polycythemia.

2.3. Biochemistry Characteristics of *Epas1*^{A529V} Mutant Mice

There is no suitable animal model with spontaneous development of paraganglioma and somatostatinoma [16,17]. Thus, we sought to develop paraganglioma and somatostatinoma in *Epas1*^{A529V} mutant mice. Although no pheochromocytomas or paragangliomas were found in up to one-year-old mutant mice, lower ratios of urinary metanephrine (MN) to NMN were observed in

$Epas1^{A529V}$ mutant mice (Figure 4A). Expression of phenylethanolamine N-methyltransferase (PNMT), which converts norepinephrine (precursor of NMN) to epinephrine (precursor of MN) was similarly down-regulated in the adrenal glands of mutant mice (Figure 4B). These observations are consistent with previous findings that HIF2α negatively regulates PNMT expression and is thereby responsible for the immature noradrenergic features of chromaffin cell tumors with high *EPAS1* expression [3,18].

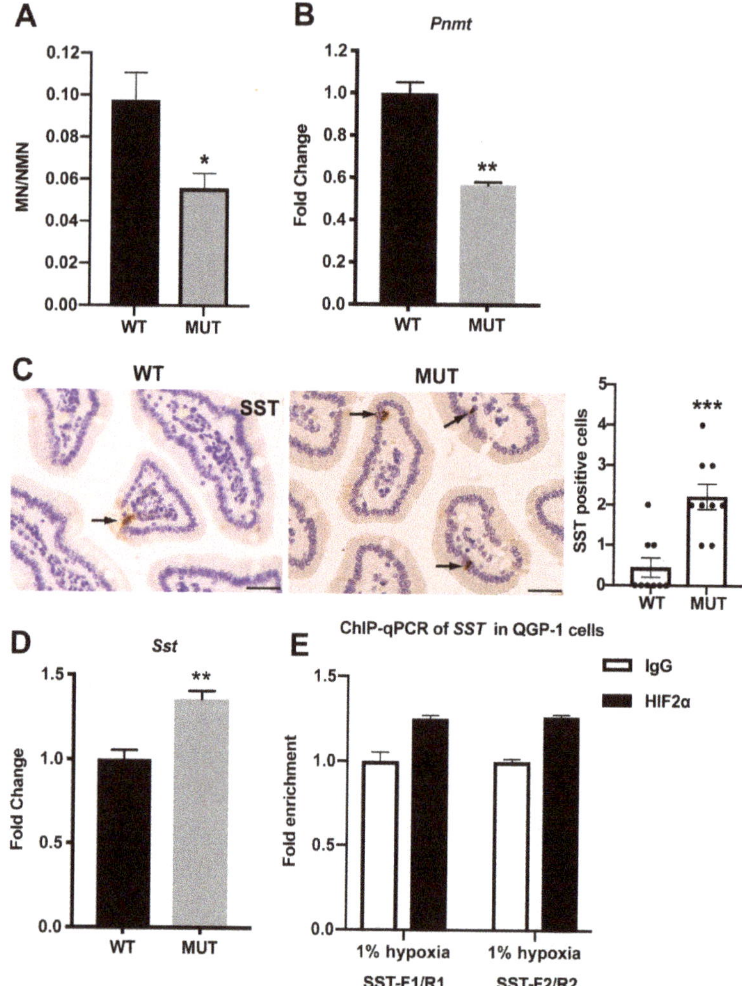

Figure 4. $Epas1^{A529V}$ mutant mice recaptured the biochemistry characteristics of the syndrome. (**A**) Decreased metanephrine (MN)/normetanephrine (NMN) ratio in three–five-month-old mutant mice. n(WT) = 6, n(MUT) = 7. * $p < 0.05$. (**B**) Decreased *Pnmt* mRNA in mutant adrenal gland. ** $p < 0.01$. (**C**) SST IHC staining of duodenum of control and mutant mice. Arrows indicate SST-positive cells. SST-positive cells were counted in nine random fields of view (400×) and summarized in the right column. *** $p = 0.0005$. Scale bars, 30 µm. (**D**) Increased *Sst* mRNA in mutant duodenum; $n = 3$ for each group. (**E**) ChIP qPCR with an HIF2α antibody or Rabbit IgG in QGP-1 cells.

In patients with this syndrome, somatostatinoma always appears in the ampullary region of the duodenum [2]. Somatostatin IHC staining confirmed more positive cells in the duodenum of mutant mice than in littermate control mice (Figure 4C). Although gross somatostatinoma was not found in our mice, enhanced expression of *Sst*, encoding somatostatin, was found in the duodenum tissue of *Epas1*^{A529V} mutant mice (Figure 4D). To check whether HIF2α binds to the promoter region of *SST*, we performed ChIP-qPCR with an HIF2α antibody in the human pancreatic islet cell carcinoma (somatostatinoma) cell line QGP-1. Both *SST* primer pairs in the *SST* promoter region confirmed that HIF2α can bind to the hypoxia response element (HRE) in the *SST* promoter (Figure 4E). These results suggest that *SST* may be a potential target of the HIF2α/HIF1β dimer.

2.4. Inhibition of HIF2α Reduced EPO but Not Polycythemia in *Epas1*^{A529V} Mutant Mice

Treatment of the mutant mice for one month with a specific antagonist of HIF2α, PT2385, demonstrated effective reduction of EPO levels in the mutant mice (Figure 5A). However, this antagonism of HIF2α did not resolve polycythemia even after treatment for two months (Figure 5B). We thus investigated an alternative mechanism causing polycythemia not responsive to EPO level reduction with transient treatment. The colony-forming unit (CFU) assay of bone marrow hematopoietic progenitors revealed increased erythroid colony number in mutant mice (Figure 5C,D), indicating that the gain-of-function mutant HIF2α increased the erythroid differentiation of the progenitor cells and further supporting an EPO-independent component of polycythemia in this syndrome [19].

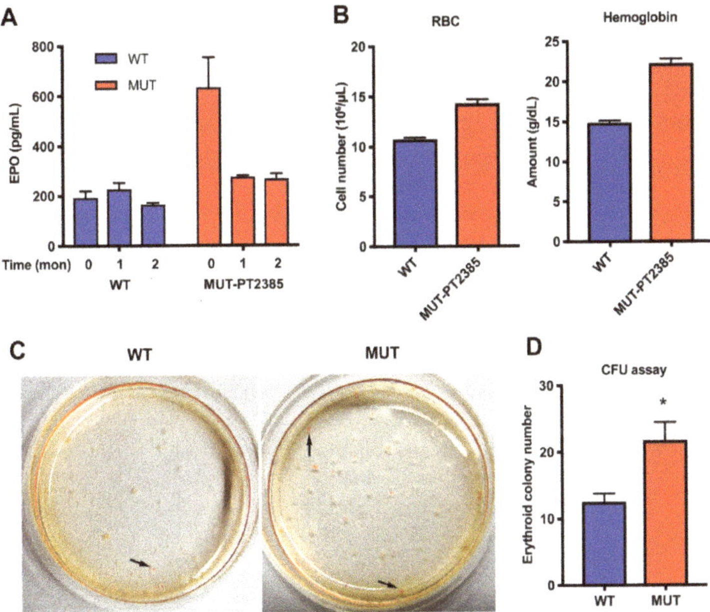

Figure 5. HIF2α inhibition in the mutant mice. (**A**,**B**) PT2385 reduced EPO (**A**) but not polycythemia (**B**) in three–four-month-old *Epas1*^{A529V} mutant mice; $n = 3$ for each group. (**C**) Representative image of the colony-forming unit (CFU) assay. Arrows indicate the erythroid colonies. (**D**) Summary of the erythroid colonies from bone marrow CFU assay; $n = 3$ for each group. * $p < 0.05$.

3. Discussion

In this study, we successfully generated a transgenic animal model mimicking postzygotic *EPAS1* mutations. These mice share polycythemia and biochemistry features of the Pacak–Zhuang syndrome. Inhibition of HIF2α with its specific inhibitor, PT2385, significantly reduced EPO. Increased erythroid colony number in the CFU assay in mutant mice indicates that somatic *Epas1*^{A529V} mutation in erythrocyte progenitor cells of the bone marrow may also contribute to primary polycythemia in the syndrome. Thus, the *Epas1*^{A529V} mutant animal model has great potential for further pathogenesis and therapeutic studies of the syndrome.

HIF2α plays an essential, tightly regulated role in development [20]. Stabilization of HIF2α due to gain-of-function mutations may impact organ systems of neural crest origin, according to the time point during early development. Somatostatin and adrenal medullary cells are of neural crest origin; early mutation of *Epas1* may impact the migration path of these cells and lead to tumors characterized by clusters of immature cells. The *Epas1*^{A529V} mouse model developed in the present study supports this mutation as the etiology of the Pacak–Zhuang syndrome. We have demonstrated that the mutation is sufficient for the development of polycythemia, increased EPO secretion, somatostatinoma-related manifestations, and immature chromaffin cell features consistent with the origins of the noradrenergic paragangliomas and pheochromocytomas characteristic of the affected patients. The developmental role of *Epas1* and its regulation by signaling cascades of neurulation provide a probable mechanistic rationale for the long duration of tumor development.

Notably, the overproduction of erythrocytes and decreased platelets in somatic heterozygous *Epas1*^{A529V} mice were more significant than what was observed in *Epas1*$^{G536W/G536W}$ mice [12]. This indicates that our model also mirrors human polycythemias with gain-of-function *EPAS1* mutations that are inherited in a dominant fashion (heterozygote). The proximity of A529 to P530, the hydroxylation site of PHD2, compared to G536, appears to result in a more severe phenotype, suggesting that severity is related to the degree of impact on the association of PHD2 with HIF2α.

PGL patients of Pacak–Zhuang syndrome consistently fall into Cluster 1 with very high plasma levels of NMN and NE and relatively normal levels of MN and epinephrine (EPI) [1,2]. These results suggest that stabilized HIF2α protein caused by gain-of-function mutations in the ODD domain is sufficient to block the differentiation of chromaffin progenitor cells and maintain their immature phenotype. In patients with this syndrome, the somatostatinoma always appears in the ampullary region of the duodenum and not in the pancreas. Although no discrete paraganglioma or somatostatinoma tumors were found in the mutant mice, we confirmed *Sst* increase in the duodenum but not in the pancreas, which supports cluster formation of immature cells with up-regulated *Sst* in the duodenum of the patients as the mechanism for this neuroendocrine tumor.

Unlike polycythemia, which is present from birth in both patients with the syndrome and mutant mice, Pacak–Zhuang syndrome patients develop paragangliomas and somatostatinoma in their early thirties. We believe that the development of discrete tumors may be more complicated and likely depends on multiple factors including acquiring additional driver gene mutations (e.g., copy number alterations of 1p *SDHB* and 3p *VHL*) and environment changes such as hypoxic stress [21]. Additional tests are necessary in the future to determine what factors are required to trigger tumor development in the *Epas1* gain-of-function mouse model.

4. Materials and Methods

4.1. Mouse Model and Genotyping

Briefly, two adjacent homologous arms were inserted into the Kpn1/Sal1 and Mlu1/Not1 sites of PGKneolox2DTA.2 (a gift from Philippe Soriano (Icahn School of Medicine at Mount Sinai, New York, NY, USA), Addgene plasmid #13449), respectively. The 5′ homologous recombination (HR) arm is a 1.3 kb PCR product (Kpn1-Forward: CGGGGTACCAGTAGATACTCAGGGACACCCAT, Sal1-Reverse: ACGCGTCGACAGTAGATACTCAGGGACACCCAT). The 3′ HR arm is adjacent to the 5′ HR arm sequence and is a 1 kb PCR product including exon 12 (Mlu1-Forward: CGACGCGTGGTGAGTGAGAACAGCAGTCCC, Not1-Reverse: AAGGAAAAAAGCGGCCGCATAAGCAGGTGTGTACATGTA). *Epas1* A529V point mutation was then introduced in the 3′ arm of the HR vector using QuikChange Lightning Site-Directed Mutagenesis Kit (Agilent, Santa Clara, CA, USA). TALEN vectors were assembled following ZiFiT instruction (http://zifit.partners.org/ZiFiT/Disclaimer.aspx). The HR vector and two TALEN vectors were electroporated into mouse ES cells at a ratio of 2:1:1. ES colonies were picked up after G418 selection (200 ug/mL) for 10 days and further identified by PCR and Sanger sequencing. Identification primers for the 5′ end: F1: CTACACCCAGTGCTTCAAG, R1: TGAGGCGGAAAGAACCA. Identification primers for the 3′ end: F2: CGAAGGAGCAAAGCTGCTA, R2: AAAGTGCCAGCTGCCTACACATAC. The ES colony with correct recombination was then micro-injected into mouse blastocysts to generate chimeric mice.

E2a-Cre transgenic mice with B6 background were kindly provided by Alex Grinberg of Eunice Kennedy Shriver National Institute of Child Health and Human Development. Progeny carrying the mutant genotype (*E2a-Cre; EPAS1*$^{neo/+}$, in brief, *Epas1*^{A529V}) was acquired. Littermate control mice were used for all experiments.

4.2. Complete Blood Count (CBC)

Mouse facial vein blood was collected in K2EDTA tubes (BD Microtainer, Franklin Lakes, NJ, USA). A total of 90 µL whole blood was diluted with 180 µL normal saline before sending to the Department of Laboratory Medicine at Clinical Center of NIH for complete blood count.

4.3. Enzyme-Linked Immunosorbent Assay (ELISA)

EPO in the mouse plasma was determined using an ELISA kit according to the manufacturer's instructions (R&D systems, Minneapolis, MN, USA). Briefly, facial vein blood was collected in heparin tubes, and plasma was collected by centrifuging at 10,000 g for 10 min at 4 °C and was frozen immediately at −80 °C. Plasma was thawed on ice when used and was diluted to 1:2–1:4 (depending on the volume of the plasma) for experiments. The samples were assayed in duplicates.

4.4. Quantitative Real-Time Polymerase Chain Reaction (qRT-PCR)

RNA of the indicated tissues was extracted with a Purelink RNA Mini Kit (Thermo Fisher Scientific, Waltham, MA, USA). Totally, 500 ng RNA was reverse-transcribed with iScript CDNA Synthesis kit (Bio-Rad, Hercules, CA, USA). The reactions were prepared with SsoAdvanced universal SYBR Green supermix (Bio-Rad) and were run on a CFX384 real-time system (Bio-Rad). Primers used for qRT-PCR included Epo (forward: ATGAAGACTTGCAGCGTGGA, reverse: TTCTGCACAACCCATCGTGA), Pnmt (forward: AAGTCAACCGTCAGGAGCTG, reverse: TCGAAGCTGGCGTTCTTTCT), Sst (forward: AGCTGGCTGCAAGAACTTCT, reverse: AGGGTCAAGTTGAGCATCGG), and Actb (forward: GACCTCTATGCCAACACAGT, reverse: AGTACTTGCGCTCAGGAGGA).

4.5. Immunohistochemistry (IHC) Staining

IHC staining was performed as previously described [2]. The primary antibodies used in this study were anti-EPO (Santa Cruz Biotechnology, Dallas, TX, USA; sc-7956, 1:100) and anti-SST (Abcam, Cambridge, MA, USA; ab30788, 1:100).

4.6. Droplet Digital PCR (ddPCR)

ddPCR was performed with the BioRad QX200 ddPCR system in the Genomics Core Facility of the NCI Center for Cancer Research (CCR), according to the manufacturer's instructions. ddPCR mutation assay of *Epas1*^{A529V} was designed on the basis of the mouse *Epas1* coding sequence with the Bio-Rad website tool. The unique assay ID is dMDS358400990. The probe for the wild-type allele was labelled with Hexachloro (HEX) fluorescence, and the probe for the A529V mutant allele was labelled with Fluorescein (FAM) fluorescence. In total, 100 ng cDNA of each tissue was used for ddPCR reaction, and the results were analyzed with the QuantaSoft software (Bio-Rad). *Epas1* gene expression level in different tissues was compared by combining positive events of both wild-type and mutant alleles. *Epas1*^{A529V} allele frequency was compared by the fractional abundance.

4.7. PT2385 Treatment

Three–four months old mice were selected for PT2385 treatment. Before treatment, plasma from facial vein blood of each mouse was collected as the basal level. PT2385 was dissolved in DMSO at 10 mM as stock solution. During treatment, the PT2385 stock solution was diluted with normal saline and intraperitoneally administrated to the mice every other day at a concentration of 400 μg/kg body weight. Plasma of facial vein blood was collected every month for the determination of EPO levels.

4.8. Determinations of Urinary Catecholamines and Metanephrines

Mouse urine was collected for measurements of catecholamines and metanephrines by liquid chromatography with mass spectrometry, as described previously [22].

4.9. ChIP-qPCR

ChIP assays were performed using SimpleCHIP Enzymatic Choromatin IP Kit (Magnetic beads) following the manufacturer's instructions (Cell Signaling Technology, Danvers, MA, USA; catalog 9003). Briefly, cross-linked protein-DNA complexes were precipitated by incubation with rabbit anti-HIF2α (Abcam; ab199) or rabbit IgG (negative control) overnight and then with magnetic beads for 2 hours. The purified DNA fragments including HIF-binding element (HRE) were quantitatively analyzed by real-time PCR with primers against the *SST* promoter (hSST-HRE-F1/B1 and F2/B1) following the standard-curve method. The standard curves were created by serial dilution of 2% input chromatin DNA. The values of chromatin DNA precipitated by HIF2α antibody were normalized to those precipitated by normal rabbit IgG, which was arbitrarily defined as 1. The primer sequences are: hSST-HRE-F1: ATCGTGGGGCATGTGGAATT; hSST-HRE-F2: AATCGTGGGGCATGTGGAAT; hSST-HRE-B1: TGTGTGCTCTCAACCGTCTC.

4.10. Colony-Forming Unit (CFU) Assay

The CFU assay was performed according to the manufacturer's instruction (R&D Systems, Minneapolis, MN, USA; HSC007). Briefly, 30,000 bone marrow cells of one-year-old $Epas1^{A529V}$ or control mice were plated in 35 mm cell culture dishes with methylcellulose-based media. Reddish colonies in each dish were counted after one week. Duplicate dishes were used for each mouse. Statistics was performed by the unpaired Student's *t*-tests.

4.11. Statistics

Data are shown by mean with SEM. The *p* values were calculated using Student's *t*-test; *p* values of less than 0.05 were considered statistically significant.

4.12. Study Approval

All in vivo experiments were performed under the animal protocol (NICHD 18-028) that was reviewed and approved by the Animal Care and Use Committee of NICHD.

5. Conclusions

Our somatic heterozygous $Epas1^{A529V}$ mutant mouse model is the first animal model of the syndrome of paraganglioma, somatostatinoma, and polycythemia. These mice share polycythemia and biochemistry features of the syndrome, demonstrating gain-of-function mutations of *EPAS1* in the ODD domain as the causative gene mutation of the syndrome development. This mutant animal model has great potential for further pathogenesis and therapeutics studies of the syndrome.

Author Contributions: Conceptualization, Z.Z., K.P., H.W. and C.Y.; methodology, H.W., J.C., C.Y., Q.Z., Q.S., Y.P. and G.E.; validation, H.W., F.F., M.S. and P.D.; formal analysis, H.W. and J.C.; resources, Y.P.; writing—original draft preparation, H.W.; writing—review and editing, Z.Z., K.P., M.R.G., J.C., Q.Z., P.D. and J.S.R.; supervision, Z.Z. and K.P.; project administration, Z.Z., M.R.G. and K.P.; funding acquisition, Z.Z., M.R.G. and K.P.

Funding: This research was funded by NCI, NICHD, NINDS Intramural Research Programs, the Deutsche Forschungsgemeinshaft (CRC/Trandregio 205/1) and the Paradifference foundation.

Acknowledgments: We thank Chuxia Deng (University of Macau) for his help with ES cell selection and establishment of the chimeric mice and Alex Grinberg (NICHD) for providing *E2a-Cre* transgenic mice with B6 background.

Conflicts of Interest: The authors declare no conflict of interest.

References

1. Zhuang, Z.; Yang, C.; Lorenzo, F.; Merino, M.; Fojo, T.; Kebebew, E.; Popovic, V.; Stratakis, C.A.; Prchal, J.T.; Pacak, K. Somatic HIF2A gain-of-function mutations in paraganglioma with polycythemia. *N. Engl. J. Med.* **2012**, *367*, 922–930. [CrossRef] [PubMed]
2. Pacak, K.; Jochmanova, I.; Prodanov, T.; Yang, C.; Merino, M.J.; Fojo, T.; Prchal, J.T.; Tischler, A.S.; Lechan, R.M.; Zhuang, Z. New syndrome of paraganglioma and somatostatinoma associated with polycythemia. *J. Clin. Oncol.* **2013**, *31*, 1690–1698. [CrossRef]
3. Qin, N.; de Cubas, A.A.; Garcia-Martin, R.; Richter, S.; Peitzsch, M.; Menschikowski, M.; Lenders, J.W.; Timmers, H.J.; Mannelli, M.; Opocher, G.; et al. Opposing effects of HIF1alpha and HIF2alpha on chromaffin cell phenotypic features and tumor cell proliferation: Insights from MYC-associated factor X. *Int. J. Cancer* **2014**, *135*, 2054–2064. [CrossRef] [PubMed]
4. Barba, T.; Boileau, J.C.; Pasquet, F.; Hot, A.; Pavic, M. [Inherited primitive and secondary polycythemia]. *Rev. Med. Interne.* **2016**, *37*, 460–465. [CrossRef] [PubMed]
5. Prchal, J.T. Secondary polycythemia (Erythrocytosis). In *Williams Hematology*, 9th ed.; Kaushansky, K., Lichtman, M.A., Prchal, J.T., Levi, M., Press, O.W., Burns, L.J., Caligiuri, M.A., Eds.; McGraw-Hill: New York, NY, USA, 2015; pp. 871–888.
6. Li, Z.; Bao, S.; Wu, Q.; Wang, H.; Eyler, C.; Sathornsumetee, S.; Shi, Q.; Cao, Y.; Lathia, J.; McLendon, R.E.; et al. Hypoxia-inducible factors regulate tumorigenic capacity of glioma stem cells. *Cancer Cell* **2009**, *15*, 501–513. [CrossRef]
7. Schonenberger, D.; Harlander, S.; Rajski, M.; Jacobs, R.A.; Lundby, A.K.; Adlesic, M.; Hejhal, T.; Wild, P.J.; Lundby, C.; Frew, I.J. Formation of Renal Cysts and Tumors in Vhl/Trp53-Deficient Mice Requires HIF1alpha and HIF2alpha. *Cancer Res.* **2016**, *76*, 2025–2036. [CrossRef] [PubMed]
8. Ryan, H.E.; Lo, J.; Johnson, R.S. HIF-1 alpha is required for solid tumor formation and embryonic vascularization. *EMBO J.* **1998**, *17*, 3005–3015. [CrossRef] [PubMed]
9. Tian, H.; Hammer, R.E.; Matsumoto, A.M.; Russell, D.W.; McKnight, S.L. The hypoxia-responsive transcription factor EPAS1 is essential for catecholamine homeostasis and protection against heart failure during embryonic development. *Genes Dev.* **1998**, *12*, 3320–3324.
10. Percy, M.J.; Furlow, P.W.; Lucas, G.S.; Li, X.; Lappin, T.R.; McMullin, M.F.; Lee, F.S. A gain-of-function mutation in the HIF2A gene in familial erythrocytosis. *N. Engl. J. Med.* **2008**, *358*, 162–168. [CrossRef]
11. Gale, D.P.; Harten, S.K.; Reid, C.D.; Tuddenham, E.G.; Maxwell, P.H. Autosomal dominant erythrocytosis and pulmonary arterial hypertension associated with an activating HIF2 alpha mutation. *Blood* **2008**, *112*, 919–921. [CrossRef]
12. Tan, Q.; Kerestes, H.; Percy, M.J.; Pietrofesa, R.; Chen, L.; Khurana, T.S.; Christofidou-Solomidou, M.; Lappin, T.R.; Lee, F.S. Erythrocytosis and pulmonary hypertension in a mouse model of human HIF2A gain of function mutation. *J. Biol. Chem.* **2013**, *288*, 17134–17144. [CrossRef]
13. Richter, S.; Qin, N.; Pacak, K.; Eisenhofer, G. Role of hypoxia and HIF2alpha in development of the sympathoadrenal cell lineage and chromaffin cell tumors with distinct catecholamine phenotypic features. *Adv. Pharmacol.* **2013**, *68*, 285–317. [CrossRef] [PubMed]
14. Jelkmann, W. Regulation of erythropoietin production. *J. Physiol.* **2011**, *589*, 1251–1258. [CrossRef] [PubMed]
15. Franke, K.; Gassmann, M.; Wielockx, B. Erythrocytosis: The HIF pathway in control. *Blood* **2013**, *122*, 1122–1128. [CrossRef]
16. Powers, J.F.; Pacak, K.; Tischler, A.S. Pathology of Human Pheochromocytoma and Paraganglioma Xenografts in NSG Mice. *Endocr. Pathol.* **2017**, *28*, 2–6. [CrossRef]

17. Lepoutre-Lussey, C.; Thibault, C.; Buffet, A.; Morin, A.; Badoual, C.; Benit, P.; Rustin, P.; Ottolenghi, C.; Janin, M.; Castro-Vega, L.J.; et al. From Nf1 to Sdhb knockout: Successes and failures in the quest for animal models of pheochromocytoma. *Mol. Cell. Endocrinol.* **2016**, *421*, 40–48. [CrossRef]
18. Eisenhofer, G.; Huynh, T.T.; Pacak, K.; Brouwers, F.M.; Walther, M.M.; Linehan, W.M.; Munson, P.J.; Mannelli, M.; Goldstein, D.S.; Elkahloun, A.G. Distinct gene expression profiles in norepinephrine- and epinephrine-producing hereditary and sporadic pheochromocytomas: Activation of hypoxia-driven angiogenic pathways in von Hippel-Lindau syndrome. *Endocr. Relat. Cancer* **2004**, *11*, 897–911. [CrossRef]
19. Jimenez, K.; Khare, V.; Evstatiev, R.; Kulnigg-Dabsch, S.; Jambrich, M.; Strobl, H.; Gasche, C. Increased expression of HIF2alpha during iron deficiency-associated megakaryocytic differentiation. *J. Thromb. Haemost.* **2015**, *13*, 1113–1127. [CrossRef] [PubMed]
20. Patel, S.A.; Simon, M.C. Biology of hypoxia-inducible factor-2alpha in development and disease. *Cell Death Differ.* **2008**, *15*, 628–634. [CrossRef]
21. Fishbein, L.; Leshchiner, I.; Walter, V.; Danilova, L.; Robertson, A.G.; Johnson, A.R.; Lichtenberg, T.M.; Murray, B.A.; Ghayee, H.K.; Else, T.; et al. Comprehensive Molecular Characterization of Pheochromocytoma and Paraganglioma. *Cancer Cell* **2017**, *31*, 181–193. [CrossRef]
22. Peitzsch, M.; Pelzel, D.; Glockner, S.; Prejbisz, A.; Fassnacht, M.; Beuschlein, F.; Januszewicz, A.; Siegert, G.; Eisenhofer, G. Simultaneous liquid chromatography tandem mass spectrometric determination of urinary free metanephrines and catecholamines, with comparisons of free and deconjugated metabolites. *Clin. Chim. Acta* **2013**, *418*, 50–58. [CrossRef] [PubMed]

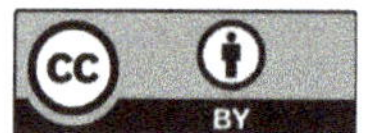

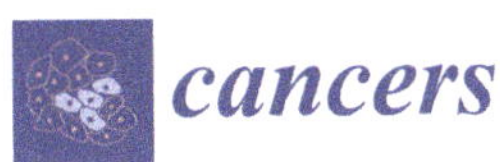
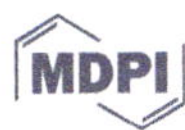

Article

^{18}F-FDOPA PET/CT Combined with MRI for Gross Tumor Volume Delineation in Patients with Skull Base Paraganglioma

Mehdi Helali [1], Matthieu Moreau [2], Clara Le Fèvre [3], Céline Heimburger [1,4], Caroline Bund [1,4], Bernard Goichot [5], Francis Veillon [6], Fabrice Hubelé [1,4], Anne Charpiot [7], Georges Noel [3,8] and Alessio Imperiale [1,4,*]

1 Biophysics and Nuclear Medicine, University Hospitals of Strasbourg, 67098 Strasbourg, France; mehdi.st.helali@gmail.com (M.H.); celine.heimburger@chru-strasbourg.fr (C.H.); caroline.bund@chru-strasbourg.fr (C.B.); Fabrice.HUBELE@chru-strasbourg.fr (F.H.)
2 Radiophysics, Centre Paul-Strauss, UNICANCER, 67065 Strasbourg, France; MMoreau@strasbourg.unicancer.fr
3 Radiotherapy, Centre Paul-Strauss, 67065 Strasbourg, France; c-lefevre56@hotmail.fr (C.L.F.); gnoel@strasbourg.unicancer.fr (G.N.)
4 ICube, University of Strasbourg/CNRS (UMR 7357) and FMTS, Faculty of Medicine, 67000 Strasbourg, France
5 Internal Medicine, University Hospitals of Strasbourg, Strasbourg University, 67098 Strasbourg, France; Bernard.Goichot@chru-strasbourg.fr
6 Radiology, University Hospitals of Strasbourg, Strasbourg University, 67098 Strasbourg, France; Francis.Veillon@chru-strasbourg.fr
7 Otolaryngology and Maxillofacial Surgery, University Hospitals of Strasbourg, 67098 Strasbourg, France; Anne.Charpiot@chru-strasbourg.fr
8 Université de Strasbourg, CNRS, IPHC UMR 7178, Centre Paul Strauss, UNICANCER, 67065 Strasbourg, France
* Correspondence: alessio.imperiale@chru-strasbourg.fr; Tel.: +33388127550; Fax: +33388128342

Received: 15 November 2018; Accepted: 2 January 2019; Published: 8 January 2019

Abstract: In this simulation study, we assessed differences in gross tumor volume (GTV) in a series of skull base paragangliomas (SBPGLs) using magnetic resonance imaging (MRI), ^{18}F-dihydroxyphenylalanine (^{18}F-FDOPA) combined positron emission tomography/computed tomography (PET/CT), and ^{18}F-FDOPA PET/MRI images obtained by rigid alignment of PET and MRI. GTV was delineated in 16 patients with SBPGLs on MRI (GTV_{MRI}), ^{18}F-FDOPA PET/CT (GTV_{PET}), and combined PET/MRI ($GTV_{PET/MRI}$). $GTV_{PET/MRI}$ was the union of GTV_{MRI} and GTV_{PET} after visual adjustment. Three observers delineated GTV_{MRI} and $GTV_{PET/MRI}$ independently. Excellent interobserver reproducibility was found for both GTV_{MRI} and $GTV_{PET/MRI}$. GTV_{PET} and GTV_{MRI} were not significantly different. However, there was some spatial difference between the locations of GTV_{MRI}, GTV_{PET}, and $GTV_{PET/MRI}$. The Dice similarity coefficient median value was 0.4 between PET/CT and MRI, and 0.8 between MRI and PET/MRI. The combined use of PET/MRI produced a larger GTV than MRI alone. Nevertheless, both the target-delivered dose and organs-at-risk conservancy were respected when treatment was planned on the PET/MRI-matched data set. Future integration of ^{18}F-FDOPA PET/CT into clinical practice will be necessary to evaluate the influence of this diagnostic modality on SBPGL therapeutic management. If the clinical utility of ^{18}F-FDOPA PET/CT and/or PET/MRI is confirmed, $GTV_{PET/MRI}$ should be considered for tailored radiotherapy planning in patients with SBPGL.

Keywords: paraganglioma; head and neck; radiotherapy; ^{18}F-FDOPA; PET; GTV

---

1. Introduction

Head and neck paragangliomas (HNPGLs) are rare and slow-growing tumors that result from paraganglia, neural crest-derived clusters of neuroendocrine cells. HNPGLs account for about 70% of extra-adrenal PGLs and develop from parasympathetic paraganglia of the jugular bulb and carotid body, or along the tympanic branch of the glossopharyngeal nerve, the vagus nerve, and its auricular branch [1]. About a third of HNPGLs are hereditary, mostly related to the mutation of the succinate dehydrogenase (*SDH*) complex genes [2]. When malignant, HNPGLs generally spread into the regional lymph nodes, lung, and bone [3]. Magnetic resonance imaging (MRI) and MR angiography are very accurate for tumor detection and local extension definition [4]. Combined positron emission tomography and computed tomography (PET/CT) with ^{18}F-dihydroxyphenylalanine (^{18}F-FDOPA) is highly sensitive (91%) and specific (95%) and is currently proposed as the first-line nuclear imaging modality in HNPGLs both at staging and during the post-treatment follow-up [5–7]. Once internalized, ^{18}F-FDOPA is decarboxylated to ^{18}F-dopamine, transported and stored in secretory vesicles. Indirectly, in PGLs, ^{18}F-FDOPA uptake reflects the pathological up-regulation of the catecholamine biosynthetic pathway [8].

Treatment of HNPGLs is often personalized and influenced by genetic status, lesion size and location, tumoral multifocality, patient age, and comorbidities [9]. Radiotherapy and stereotactic radiotherapy are proposed as valuable therapeutic options for HNPGLs as they are less invasive than surgery, especially for patients with skull-base paragangliomas (SBPGLs) [10–13]. Due to continuing technological advances, the role of such treatments has increased progressively in the last few decades, achieving excellent rates of local tumor control and patient outcome with few iatrogenic effects [14]. It is important to underline that PGLs are frequently characterized by slow cellular turnover rates, efficient DNA repair mechanisms, and consequently low radiosensitivity, requiring an elevated radiation dose to overcome radioresistance. On the other hand, the presence of surrounding critical neuroanatomical structures is an important factor to be taken into account, usually limiting the tumor's delivered dose [13]. The definition of gross tumor volume (GTV) is the first step of primary importance in planning external radiation therapy and is strictly related to the final irradiated volume. In the last few decades, continuous and successful technical improvements for external radiotherapy treatment have been seen, leading to the development of highly conformal intensity-modulated radiation therapy (IMRT) and personalized irradiation approaches. Consequently, remarkable efforts have been made to optimize GTV delineation. The current availability of hybrid multimodality imaging is gradually changing the paradigm for radiotherapy planning definition, which is classically based on CT or MRI imaging. Tumor morphological definition and functional characterization, combined in a single diagnostic exploration (i.e., PET/CT), could improve the definition of both GTV, which will receive the highest dose, and clinical target volume (CTV), which includes the subclinical tumor extension not visible on imaging modalities and subjective for many locations. Moreover, the recent availability of PET/MRI devices offers the potential advantages of high soft-tissue contrast and functional MRI capability to improve the diagnosis of cancer and its phenotype characterization. Several authors showed that the combination of MRI and PET potentially improves the accuracy of both the primary tumor and metastatic lymph node delineation in patients with HN malignancies, with consequent clinical advantages in disease control and toxicity reduction [15,16]. At present, radiotherapy planning for HNPGLs is defined utilizing contrast-enhanced CT and/or MRI. Metabolic information provided by PET/CT is only sporadically integrated. Moreover, no definitive consensus has been reached on the optimal modality for GTV definition on ^{18}F-FDOPA PET/CT in patients with HNPGLs. On the other hand, semi-quantitative uptake parameters such as the tumor-to-brain ratio (TBR) were successfully used to delineate gliomas on PET imaging with radiolabeled amino acids [17–21]. Overall, despite potential diagnostic advantages related to functional imaging [22], to our knowledge there are no reports concerning the use of ^{18}F-FDOPA PET/CT to delineate target volumes in patients with HNPGLs. In view of the above, the purpose of this simulation study was to assess the differences in GTV using contrast-enhanced MRI, ^{18}F-FDOPA PET/CT, and combined PET/MRI images in a series of SBPGLs.

We also evaluated the safety of irradiation therapy using PET/MRI fusion images, and in selected patients, compared the radiation treatment planning and dosimetry obtained from GTV assessed by MRI, which is the standard at several institutions, and PET/MRI-registered images.

2. Results

2.1. Patients

Sixteen consecutive patients with jugulotympanic SBPGLs were retrospectively included (nine men and seven women, mean age: 57 years, range: 37–84 years). Patient characteristics are detailed in Table 1. Seven and nine patients were evaluated at primary staging and during follow-up, respectively, because of clinical suspicion of tumor recurrence. Previous treatment included surgery, radiotherapy, and ^{90}Y-DOTATOC peptide receptor radionuclide therapy in seven, three, and three patients, respectively. Two patients were succinate dehydrogenase subunit B (*SDHB*) and *SDHC* mutation carriers. In the remaining 14 cases, the PGLs were apparently sporadic. No patient presented with regional lymph nodes or systemic metastases at the time of diagnostic imaging.

Table 1. Patient population characteristics.

Patient	Age, Sex (Man/Woman)	Symptoms	PGL Size (mm), Side (Left/Right)	Genetics	Primary Staging, Recurrence	Prior Treatment
1	62, M	Tinnitus	10, L	Sporadic	Primary Staging	-
2	57, W	Tinnitus Ear discharge	23, R	*SDHC* [3]	Recurrence	Surgery PRRT [2]
3	57, M	Tinnitus	8, R	Sporadic	Recurrence	Surgery
4	58, M	Tinnitus	8, R	Sporadic	Recurrence	Surgery IMRT [3]
5	43, W	Tinnitus Local pain	40, R	Sporadic	Recurrence	Surgery
6	84, W	Tinnitus	31, L	Sporadic	Recurrence	Surgery Gamma Knife
7	62, W	Asymptomatic	22, L	*SDHB* [1]	Recurrence	Surgery
8	67, W	Pulsatile tinnitus	8, L	Sporadic	Primary Staging	-
9	66, M	Dizziness	25, R	Sporadic	Primary Staging	-
10	70, W	Pulsatile tinnitus	21, L	Sporadic	Recurrence	PRRT [2]
11	47, M	Pulsatile tinnitus	7, L	Sporadic	Primary Staging	-
12	48, M	Pulsatile tinnitus	13, L	Sporadic	Recurrence	IMRT [3]
13	59, W	Asymptomatic	22, R	Sporadic	Recurrence	Surgery PRRT [2]
14	54, M	Tinnitus Ear discharge	12, L	Sporadic	Primary Staging	-
15	58, M	Pulsatile tinnitus	9, R	Sporadic	Primary Staging	-
16	37, M	Dizziness Hearing loss	30, R	Sporadic	Primary Staging	-

[1] *SDHB*: succinate dehydrogenase subunit B; [2] PRRT = peptide receptor tadionuclide therapy; [3] IMRT: intensity-modulated radiotherapy.

2.2. Tumor Volume Assessment

- MRI

The median lesion size was 17 mm (range: 7–40 mm). The median values of GTV_{MRI} were 1.4 cm^3 (range: 0.2–8.6 cm^3), 1.7 cm^3 (range: 0.3–9.6 cm^3), and 1.2 cm^3 (range: 0.2–8.7 cm^3) for the three observers. According to intraclass correlation coefficient (ICC) analysis, MRI was a highly reproducible method for GTV delineation (agreement coefficient: 0.95). The GTV_{MRI} assessed by the most experienced radiation oncologist (observer 1) was considered for the definition of both CTV_{MRI} (median value: 26.2 cm^3; range: 11.9–51.2 cm^3), and planning target volume (PTV_{MRI}) (median value: 54.1 cm^3; range: 21.8–79.1 cm^3).

- ^{18}F-FDOPA PET/CT and PET/MRI

Despite substantial heterogeneity of tumoral ^{18}F-FDOPA uptake among the patients studied, SBPGLs were distinctly detectable by PET/CT in all cases (median value of maximum standardized uptake value (SUV_{max}): 11.5; range: 1.4–82.8). The median value of GTV_{PET} was 0.9 cm^3 (range: 0.3–17.1 cm^3). In this series, although GTV_{PET} was lower than GTV_{MRI}, no significant difference was assessed when considering the entire population ($p = 0.09$), or only previously treated patients ($p = 0.12$), or only treatment-naïve patients ($p = 1$). GTV_{TBR} (median value: 5.1 cm^3; range: 0.3–26.1 cm^3) was significantly larger than both GTV_{PET} ($p = 0.01$) and GTV_{MRI} ($p = 0.006$). GTV_{TBR} largely exceeded tumoral boundaries on PET images, including several extratumoral voxels (with a similar activity to that of the background), often protruding in apparently healthy bone structures and an adjacent vasculonervous pedicle (Figure 1). Therefore, GTV_{TBR} has not been further considered and the $GTV_{PET/MRI}$ was assessed combining GTV_{MRI} and GTV_{PET} after visual adjustment by the radiation oncologist. The median values of $GTV_{PET/MRI}$ were 3.2 cm^3 (range: 0.5–18.8 cm^3), 2.7 cm^3 (range: 0.3–11.8 cm^3), and 2.3 cm^3 (range: 0.4–17.1 cm^3) for the three observers. ICC analysis showed excellent interobserver reproducibility with an agreement coefficient of 0.91. $GTV_{PET/MRI}$ assessed by the most experienced radiation therapist (observer 1) was used to estimate both $CTV_{PET/MRI}$ (median value: 33.8 cm^3; range: 15–82.7 cm^3) and $PTV_{PET/MRI}$ (median value: 62.7 cm^3; range: 26.5–112.7 cm^3). $GTV_{PET/MRI}$, $CTV_{PET/MRI}$, and $PTV_{PET/MRI}$ were significantly larger than GTV_{MRI} ($p = 0.00003$), CTV_{MRI} ($p = 0.003$), and PTV_{MRI} ($p = 0.003$), respectively. The details of GTV comparison between MRI and PET/CT, and between MRI and PET/MRI are reported in Table 2.

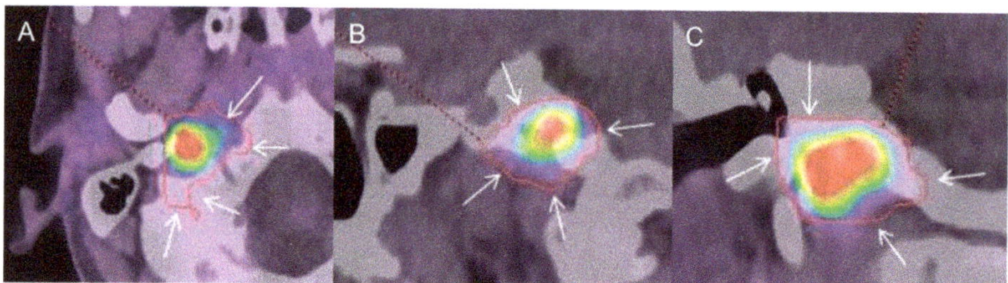

Figure 1. Typical example of gross tumor volume assessed by tumor-to-brain ratio (GTV_{TBR}) (red contour) evaluated on ^{18}F-dihydroxyphenylalanine (^{18}F-FDOPA) combined positron emission tomography/computed tomography (PET/CT) images (**A**: axial, **B**: sagittal, **C**: coronal) in a patient with a sporadic right skull base paraganglioma (SBPGL). A threshold value of 1.6 over the background uptake was used as the reference for semi-automatic definition of GTV. Note that GTV_{TBR} largely exceeds the metabolic tumoral edges (arrows).

Table 2. Volumetric and positional analysis of GTVs assessed by magnetic resonance imaging (MRI), ^{18}F-FDOPA PET/CT, and PET/MRI.

Patient	GTV [a] (cm^3)			DSC [b]	
	MRI	PET/CT	PET/MRI	MRI vs. PET/CT	MRI vs. PET/MRI
1	0.33	0.63	0.87	0.51	0.65
2	4.01	2.23	5.17	0.59	0.95
3	1.25	0.28	1.60	0.30	0.99
4	1.35	0.49	1.85	0.39	0.82
5	5.95	3.66	9.95	0.53	0.43
6	4.93	4.73	6.84	0.76	0.89
7	8.58	1.40	10.46	0.21	0.97
8	0.19	0.29	0.44	0.58	0.72
9	6.01	17.10	18.76	0.52	0.52
10	1.44	2.06	3.08	0.53	0.73
11	1.42	0.83	3.25	0.06	0.62
12	1.35	0.84	2.68	0.14	0.66
13	4.10	0.92	4.85	0.33	0.99

Table 2. *Cont.*

Patient	GTV [a] (cm^3)			DSC [b]	
	MRI	PET/CT	PET/MRI	MRI vs. PET/CT	MRI vs. PET/MRI
14	0.76	0.83	1.64	0.33	0.74
15	0.55	0.62	1.20	0.39	0.73
16	4.55	1.13	5.15	0.38	1.00
Median (range)	1.4 (0.19–8.58)	0.88 (0.28–17.1)	3.16 (0.44–18.76)	0.4 (0.06–0.76)	0.7 (0.43–1.0)
Mean (SD [c])	2.92 (2.54)	2.38 (4.12)	4.86 (4.79)	0.41 (0.18)	0.78 (0.18)

[a] GTV: gross tumor volume. [b] DSC: Dice similarity coefficient. [c] SD: standard deviation.

2.3. Positional GTV Assessment

There was some spatial difference between the locations of GTV delineated on MRI, PET/CT, and PET/MRI (Figures 2 and 3). According to the analysis of positional variability of GTVs, the median intersection volume between GTV_{PET} and GTV_{MRI} was 0.6 cm^3 (range: 0.1–6.0 cm^3), and between GTV_{MRI} and $GTV_{PET/MRI}$ it was 1.5 cm^3 (range: 0.3–9.3 cm^3). The median DSC was 0.4 (range: 0.1–0.8) between PET and MRI, and 0.8 (range: 0.4–1) between MRI and PET/MRI. The intersection volume between GTV_{PET} and GTV_{MRI} correlated positively with the size of the lesion (R = 0.84, p = 0.0001) and was significantly lower (p = 0.04) in patients with relapsing tumor (median: 0.9 cm^3; range: 0.3–12.1 cm^3) compared to newly diagnosed patients (median: 2.4 cm^3; range: 1.2–8.8 cm^3). Table 2 summarizes the results of positional GTV analysis and the DSC index.

Uniform expansions of the GTV_{MRI} contours were performed in increments of 1 mm until 100% of the $GTV_{PET/MRI}$ was covered. An average expansion of 7 mm (median: 7 mm; range: 2–9 mm) beyond contrast-enhanced T1-weighted MRI contours was necessary to cover 100% of the ^{18}F-FDOPA PET/MRI primary tumor volume. Finally, a mean contraction of 3.6 mm (median: 3 mm; range: 1–8 mm) of CTV_{MRI} made it possible to encompass the $GTV_{PET/MRI}$.

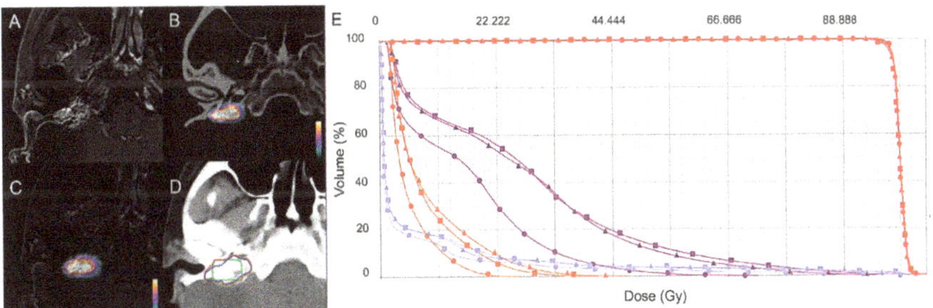

Figure 2. GTV delineation and dose-volume histogram (DVH) based on MRI (Δ), ^{18}F-FDOPA PET/CT (●), and ^{18}F-FDOPA PET/MRI (■) for a representative case. Contrast-enhanced T1-weighted MRI (**A**), ^{18}F-FDOPA PET/CT (**B**), and combined PET/MRI (**C**) axial images in a 57-year-old woman with a relapsing 23-mm right jugulotympanic *SDHC* PGL previously treated with surgery and peptide receptor radionuclide therapy (patient 2, Table 1). (**D**) GTV delineation for external radiation therapy based on MRI (blue contour), ^{18}F-FDOPA PET/CT (green contour), and combined ^{18}F-FDOPA PET/MRI images (orange contour). (**E**) Radiation treatment planning based on MRI, ^{18}F-FDOPA PET/CT, and combined ^{18}F-FDOPA PET and MRI data set assessed for volumetric-modulated arc therapy. Dose-volume histogram for PTV and organs at risk (OAR) are displayed. PTV: red curves; brainstem: purple curves; mandible: blue curves; parotid: orange curves. All the treatment plans were able to respect clinical objectives showing similar results concerning both target delivered dose and OAR conservancy.

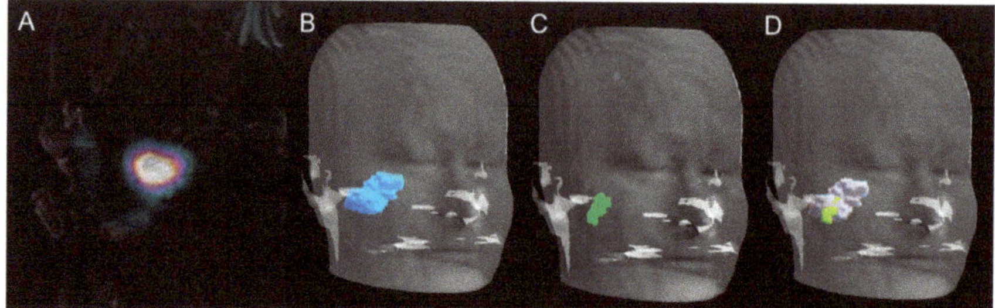

Figure 3. Volume rendering technique representations of GTV delineated on PET, MRI, and PET/MRI. Axial slice of combined ^{18}F-FDOPA PET/MRI imaging in a 43-year-old woman (patient 5, Table 1) with a relapsing 40-mm apparently sporadic right jugulotympanic PGL previously treated with surgery (**A**). Volume rendering technique representation of GTV delineated on MRI (**B**, blue volume), ^{18}F-FDOPA PET/CT (**C**, green volume), and combined ^{18}F-FDOPA PET/MRI imaging (**D**, green and gray volume).

2.4. Radiation Treatment Planning

MRI and PET/MRI-based radiation treatment planning was assessed in three patients with apparently sporadic relapsing jugulotympanic PGLs (Table 1, cases 2, 3, and 5). Patients were selected according to tumor size aiming to simulate treatment for tumors of different sizes, ranging from a few millimeters to several centimeters. Detailed results of the dosimetric evaluation in each patient are listed in Tables 3 and 4. Overall, all the plans generated on ^{18}F-FDOPA PET/MRI were able to respect clinical objectives despite the size discrepancy existing between GTV_{MRI} and $GTV_{PET/MRI}$. PTV_{MRI} and $PTV_{PET/MRI}$ plans were similar concerning both target delivered dose and OAR conservancy (deviation under 2.7% of prescription dose and 0.6% of OAR volume for dose and volume, respectively) without underdosing of $GTV_{PET/MRI}$ compared to target volumes generated on treatment plans using MRI alone (Table 3, Figure 3). Dosimetric details concerning tumoral target and OAR are reported in Table 4.

Table 3. Comparison of dosimetric results obtained from MRI- and PET/MRI-based radiation treatment planning in three patients with apparently sporadic relapsing jugulotympanic PGLs (patients 2, 3, 5, Table 1).

Patient	PGL Size (mm) [1]	V95% [2]		D98% [3]		D2% [4]	
		MRI	PET/MRI	MRI	PET/MRI	MRI	PET/MRI
1	23	99.8	99.5	97.1	96.7	101.9	102.2
2	8	99.5	99	96.9	96.3	102.5	103.1
3	40	99.2	99.1	96.4	96.3	102.4	102.5

[1] PGL size refers to MRI investigation; [2] V95%: volume of PTV (planning target volume) receiving 95% of prescription; [3] D98%: dose received by 98% of the PTV; [4] D2%: dose received by 2% of the PTV.

Table 4. Comparison of dosimetric results on organs at risk (OAR) obtained from MRI and PET/MRI-based radiation treatment planning in 3 patients with apparently sporadic relapsing jugulotympanic PGLs (patients no. 2, 3, and 5 of Table 1).

Table 1	SBPGL Size on MRI (mm) and Side (R/L [2])	OAR [3]	D_{max} [4] (Gy)		D_{mean} [5] (Gy)		V15Gy [6] (%)	
			MRI	PET/MRI	MRI	PET/MRI	MRI	PET/MRI
Pt [1] 2	23/R	Brainstem	42.9	45.8	11.7	12.3		
		R Parotid	21.2	18.8	4.1	3.7	1.5	1
		R IAC [7]	44.8	45.6	44.3	44.3		
		Mandible	45.6	45.3	3.1	3.3		
Pt 3	8/R	Brainstem	46.9	47.0	12.6	13.1		
		R Parotid	46.4	46.0	3.6	3.7	4.9	5.5
		L IAC *	2.5	2.8	2.2	2.7		
		L Cochlea *	3	3.3	2.3	2.5		

Table 4. *Cont.*

Table 1	SBPGL Size on MRI (mm) and Side (R/L [2])	OAR [3]	D_{max} [4] (Gy)		D_{mean} [5] (Gy)		V15Gy [6] (%)	
			MRI	PET/MRI	MRI	PET/MRI	MRI	PET/MRI
Pt 5	40/R	Brainstem	46.7	46.7	18.9	19.8		
		R Parotid	46.7	46.9	14.8	19.3	35.8	50.9
		R IAC	44.8	44.9	44.4	44.4		
		Mandible	45	45.8	2.6	3		

[1] Pt: patient; [2] R: right; L: left; [3] OAR: organ at risk; [4] D_{max}: dose maximum; [5] D_{mean}: mean dose; [6] V15Gy: the volume receiving doses above 15 Gy; [7] IAC: internal auditory canal. * R IAC and R Cochlea are included in PTV.

3. Discussion

To our knowledge, the present study evaluates for the first time the differences in GTV delineation using contrast-enhanced MRI, ^{18}F-FDOPA PET/CT, and combined PET/MRI images in patients with SBPGLs. We also compared the radiation treatment planning based on the MRI and PET/MRI data set, suggesting the safety of irradiation therapy using PET/MRI fusion images showing no differences in tumor-delivered dose and OAR conservancy between MRI- and PET/MRI-based radiation planning, regardless of the intermodality degree of volumetric agreement.

Although there were individual cases with greater volumetric disparities, GTV_{PET} and GTV_{MRI} were not significantly different. However, a trend toward significance was observed when considering the entire patient cohort, and the lack of statistical significance might be due to the limited number of patients studied. $GTV_{PET/MRI}$, which was defined as the union of GTV_{MRI} and GTV_{PET} after adjustment by a radiation oncologist, encompasses nearly all GTV regions. An average expansion of 7 mm beyond the MRI T1-gadolinum contours allowed 100% coverage of the ^{18}F-FDOPA PET/MRI volumes. Accordingly, as expected, the combined use of PET/MRI produced a larger GTV than MRI alone. In spite of this, both target delivered dose and OAR conservancy were respected when PTV was planned on MRI or the PET/MRI matched data set, probably due to the slight positional discordance as shown by the good DSC average value (0.8). V95 (i.e.: volume of PTV receiving 95% of prescription) was near the prescribed dose and was not significantly different between MRI- and PET/MRI-based GTVs for each patient and on average.

The integration of ^{18}F-FDOPA PET/CT to MRI was evaluated for radiotherapy planning of gliomas. In these patients, ^{18}F-FDOPA PET/CT generated larger target volumes compared to the standard-of-care MRI. The result was a customization of radiotherapy plans by the inclusion of "metabolic disease" without contrast enhancement [23–25]. Navarria et al. emphasized the idea of "biologic tumor volume" in a population of 69 patients with high-grade gliomas [26]. They showed that 50% of radiotherapy failures occurred outside the contrast-enhanced volume on T1-weighted MRI sequences and would have been included within the target volume generated according to ^{11}C-methionine PET.

DSC analysis revealed incongruences of GTV position between MRI and ^{18}F-FDOPA PET/CT in patients with SBPGL, warranting further investigations, longitudinal patient follow-up, and histopathology correlation. Overlap differences between GTV_{MRI} and GTV_{PET} could be attributable to several factors and needs to be discussed. First of all, no hybrid PET/MRI device was used for patient exploration. Indeed, for GTV delineation, the PET/CT and MRI data set were matched using a semi-automated volume-based registration algorithm with consequent potential spatial uncertainty in target volume identification induced by image misalignment. Secondly, a semi-automated SUV_{max}-based segmentation algorithm was used to outline the target volume on PET/CT images, taking into account the value of 40% of SUV_{max} according to ^{18}F-Fluorodeoxyglucose (^{18}F-FDG) PET/CT-related literature in general oncology. As reported, automated methods of image segmentation would be preferable to determine the metabolically active tumor volume (MATV) [27]. MATV delineation based on semi-quantitative uptake parameters such as the TBR has long been used for PET imaging of brain tumors with radiolabeled amino acids. In a biopsy-controlled study using ^{18}F-Fluoroethyl-L-tyrosine (^{18}F-FET) PET in patients with brain tumors [17], a threshold value of 1.6

over the background uptake was taken as the reference for a semi-automatic definition of tumor volume (GTV_{TBR}). Based on the assumption that the TBR contrast of ^{18}F-FDOPA uptake in brain tumor is similar to that of ^{18}F-FET [20,21], other authors successfully adopted the same approach in patients with gliomas investigated by ^{18}F-FDOPA PET/CT [18,19]. In our patients, GTV_{TBR} assessed in a similar manner was significantly larger than that obtained using 40% of tumor SUVmax or MRI. Moreover, GTV_{TBR} largely exceeded tumoral limits on PET images, covering apparently healthy bone or adjacent vasculonervous structures (Figure 1). Therefore, both the lack of biopsy-proven evidence of tumoral invasion (contrary to what Pauleit et al. have proven in gliomas [17]) and the potential high risk of radiation after-effects require further investigation before clinical utilization of this type of delineation method for SBPGLs. The heterogeneity of tumor size, ranging from 7 mm to 40 mm, and the high inter-tumor variability of ^{18}F-FDOPA uptake (range: 1.4–82.8) could contribute to explaining the difficulty in properly defining GTV_{TBR}, especially for lesions with metabolic activity as high as PGLs. Interestingly, in our population, the overall mean TBR was 16.3 (range: 1.4–83.4), approximately nine-fold higher than the TBR reported for brain tumors on ^{18}F-FDOPA PET studies (1.76 ± 0.60) [18]. Finally, optimal ^{18}F-FDOPA PET/CT segmentation algorithms for SBPGL GTV_{PET} contouring need to be optimized, also taking into account the lessons learned from patients with gliomas.

The third and last point to discuss concerns the population studied for GTV delineation, including patients naïve of treatment and subjects with relapsing tumors after surgery and/or radiotherapy. The iatrogenic distortion of regional anatomic architecture may lead to modification of vascular patterns and tissue enhancement on CT and MRI studies. Contrast medium arrival during the early arterial phases could be delayed and less pronounced, leading to erroneous image interpretations in patients with relapsing local disease [7,28]. Interestingly, overlap differences between GTV_{PET} and GTV_{MRI} were more pronounced for relapsing tumor compared to newly diagnosed lesions. In those patients, an average 46% of the ^{18}F-FDOPA PET/CT target volume extended outside GTV_{MRI} showing no pathological gadolinium enhancement. Integration of PET to MRI data could be advantageous for GTV delineation in previously treated patients due to a potentially challenging definition of tumoral infiltration [7]. In view of the above, the availability of PET/MRI hybrid devices will lead to radiotherapy planning based on spatially and temporally registered morphofunctional images [29].

It is important to underline that the majority of patients included in the present study presented with relatively small, benign and sporadic SBPGLs and that even the two cases of *SDH*-related PGLs did not have regional lymph node metastases. Consequently, to confirm our preliminary results, additional studies are required including patients with more aggressive and locally advanced tumors, in which modifications of GTV could have an important dosimetric impact and possibly clinical consequences. An additional attractive axis of clinical research, which would advance a further step towards the transition from the morphological tumor volume to the morphofunctional tumor volume concept, could be the comparison of ^{18}F-FDOPA, ^{18}F-FDG, and ^{68}Ga-DOTA-peptides for PET-based GTV delineation.

In a real clinical scenario, one more point of volumetric uncertainty is the definition of CTV usually made on CT or MRI. Ligtenberg et al. [30] recently determined the modality-specific CTV margins for CT, MRI, and ^{18}F-FDG PET in patients with laryngohypopharyngeal tumors. Although GTV overestimated the tumor volume in all modalities, CTV margins were needed to achieve complete tumor delineation. Interestingly, PET-based CTVs were the smallest and considered to be the most accurate, while MRI-based CTVs were larger than PET- and CT-based CTVs. In our patient population, by a mean contraction of 3.6 mm (median: 3 mm; range: 1–8 mm) of CTV_{MRI}, we encompassed every $GTV_{PET/MRI}$. This observation could contribute to the debate regarding the choice of CTV threshold, suggesting a role of hybrid PET/MRI imaging to modulate CTV margin expansion tailored to each clinical situation. It is possible that increased accuracy in GTV delineation with PET/MRI could allow the application of smaller CTV margins, possibly reducing toxicity while conserving reliability in tumor coverage and treatment efficacy.

Another advantage of multimodality imaging is likely the ability to specify a volume at high risk of relapse, which could be better controlled by the use of simultaneous integrated boost (SIB). This method has already been used in several tumors without deterioration of OAR protection [31,32].

4. Materials and Methods

4.1. Patients

The medical records of patients with clinical, radiological, and/or pathological diagnosis of HNPGLs referred to the Nuclear Medicine Department of Strasbourg University Hospitals from May 2012 to April 2017 for ^{18}F-FDOPA PET/CT were retrospectively reviewed. Only patients with confirmed SBPGLs, with positive ^{18}F-FDOPA PET/CT findings, and who underwent MRI within less than 3 months of ^{18}F-FDOPA PET/CT were retrospectively included. Conversely, patients without a final diagnosis of PGL, or patients with PGLs not arising from the skull base, or patients for whom MRI data were not fully available were not selected for the study.

Consistent with local institutional guidelines, all patients included gave free and informed consent for the use of anonymous personal medical data extracted from their file for scientific purposes. The local institutional review board approved this retrospective study (FC/dossier 2018-49).

4.2. Reference Diagnostic Imaging

HN MRI investigations were performed with a 1.5-T (Avanto, Siemens, Medical Systems, Erlangen, Germany) or a 3-T (Signa, General Electric Medical System, Milwaukee, WI, USA) scanner. Morphological T1-weighted contrast-enhanced axial and coronal images with a 1-mm slice thickness were used for diagnostic purposes and for radiotherapy volume delineation. ^{18}F-FDOPA PET/CT scans were performed using a combined PET/CT equipped by time of flight measurement capacity (Biograph mCT, Siemens Medical Systems, Erlangen, Germany). ^{18}F-FDOPA was used in the setting of approved marketing authorization. Patients fasted for at least 4 h before tracer injection. In all patients, 4 MBq/kg of ^{18}F-FDOPA was intravenously injected without carbidopa premedication. Whole-body ^{18}F-FDOPA PET/CT acquisition was performed about 30 min after radiotracer injection from the top of the skull to the upper thigh (4 min per step) starting from the head. CT studies for attenuation correction and anatomic registration were performed without administration of contrast medium. PET data were reconstructed iteratively. CT, PET (after attenuation correction), and PET/CT images were displayed on a dedicated workstation for analysis. A focal area of increased ^{18}F-FDOPA uptake in a usual anatomical site for paraganglia was considered as a positive finding. The tumor maximum standardized uptake value (SUV_{max}) was defined within a spherical volume of interest (VOI) centered on the tumor and including it completely. To obtain PET/MRI images, ^{18}F-FDOPA PET/CT were matched and registered with T1-weighted contrast-enhanced MRI including the whole SBPGL. MRI sequences were rigidly aligned to the CT data set of PET/CT using a semi-automated volume-based registration algorithm (Focal software, CMS-XIO).

4.3. Tumor Volume Assessment

Tumor volumes and radiation plans based on ^{18}F-FDOPA PET/CT, MRI, and matched PET/MRI images were delineated for research purposes only and were not used prospectively for radiation treatment planning in any patient. GTV encompasses the recognizable macroscopic tumor infiltration and defines both the extent and position of the primary tumor. In our series, GTV was assessed on the MRI (GTV_{MRI}), ^{18}F-FDOPA PET/CT (GTV_{PET}), and matched PET/MRI data set ($GTV_{PET/MRI}$). Two experienced radiation oncologists (observers 1 and 2) and one nuclear medicine physician (observer 3) independently performed the GTV delineation on MRI and fused PET/MRI data while aware of patient clinical history. To prevent biases, ^{18}F-FDOPA PET/CT results were not available before GTV_{MRI} definition. Similarly, GTV_{MRI} data were not accessible before $GTV_{PET/MRI}$ delineation. GTV_{MRI} was delineated using axial contrast-enhanced T1-weighted MRI images. GTV_{PET} was assessed on axial images using the automatic assistant arbitrarily calibrated at 40% of SUV_{max} of the primary tumor (Syngo.via VB10B, Siemens) according to the ^{18}F-FDG PET/CT-related literature in clinical oncology [33]. To delineate SBPGL on PET/CT imaging, the tumor-to-brain ratio (TBR) was also used. Based on previous studies on gliomas [17–21], a threshold value of 1.6 over the background uptake was taken as the reference for a semi-automatic definition of tumor volume (GTV_{TBR}). To measure background activity, a large region of interest above the upper ventricle and including both gray and white matter was used. Lastly, $GTV_{PET/MRI}$ was the union of GTV_{MRI} and GTV_{PET} and the final contour assessment was made based on visual adjustment of the images by the treating radiation oncologist. MRI- and PET/CT-related GTV and intersection volume were assessed using ARTIVIEW™ software (AQUILAB®, Lille, France). Concordance between GTV_{MRI} and GTV_{PET} contours and between GTV_{MRI} and $GTV_{PET/MRI}$ contours was evaluated according to the Dice similarity coefficient (DSC), a validated index measuring spatial overlap between two volumes. The DSC was calculated as follows: $2 \times (A \cap B)/(A + B)$, where A and B represent two volumes, $(A \cap B)$ represents the volume of intersection, and $(A + B)$ represents the sum of their volumes. A DSC ≥ 0.7 can be considered as a "good" overlap [34]. According to the standard of care of our institution, CTV and PTV of patients were defined by adding a 10-mm three-dimensional (3D) margin to GTV and a 3-mm 3D margin to CTV, respectively. Hence, starting from GTV, we assessed CTV and PTV on the MRI (CTV_{MRI}, PTV_{MRI}), ^{18}F-FDOPA PET/CT (CTV_{PET}, PTV_{PET}), and matched PET/MRI data set ($CTV_{PET/MRI}$, $PTV_{PET/MRI}$).

4.4. Radiation Treatment Planning

Dosimetric evaluation was performed for research purposes only aiming to assess the potential consequence of any volumetric differences between gold standard MRI and new PET/MRI-related GTV. In other words, we researched the eventual reduction of tumoral dose delivered when metabolic GTV_{PET} data were combined with GTV_{MRI}. Complete radiation treatment planning was assessed for volumetric-modulated arc therapy (VMAT). VMAT is a technique for IMRT that simultaneously combines varying dose rate, gantry speed, and the shape of the multileaf collimator aperture [35]. VMAT plans were generated using the Eclipse treatment planning system (version 11.0.31, Varian Medical Systems) on for a delivered dose of 45 Gy with 1.8-Gy fractions. The dose calculation was performed with the AAA algorithm and a 2.5-mm grid size; for the optimization, the PRO3 algorithm was used. Two co-planar double-arcs were generated for each PTV, where the collimator angle was set to 30° for counter-clockwise rotation and 330° for clockwise rotation. During the first optimizing process, the objectives (PTV and OAR) were the same for the two plans. During a second optimizing process, the penalties (dose-volume objective and/or weight) corresponding to the OAR were manually adapted to minimize the absorbed dose according to the clinical objectives. Dose to PTV was optimized and normalized to obtain the same V95% (volume of PTV receiving 95% of prescription dose), D98% (dose received by 98% of the PTV) and D2% (dose received by 2% of the PTV), with a maximum deviation of 1%. Radiotherapy planning was based on the MRI and PET/MRI GTV data set adding a standard 10-mm 3D margin to GTV to obtain CTV, and a 3-mm 3D margin to CTV for PTV definition.

4.5. Statistical Analysis

The results for continuous data were expressed as median and range, whereas categorical variables were presented as numbers and percentages. GTV, CTV, and PTV data were expressed in cubic centimeters. The intraclass correlation coefficient (ICC) was used for interobserver reproducibility assessment of both GTV_{MRI} and $GTV_{PET/MRI}$. ICC inter-rater agreement measurements were interpreted according to the following criteria: less than 0.40 = poor agreement; 0.40–0.59 = fair agreement; 0.60–0.74 = good agreement; 0.75–1 = excellent agreement [36]. A two-way mixed effect model with absolute agreement definition parameters was applied to the ICC. The nonparametric paired-sample Wilcoxon signed-rank test was used to evaluate differences between GTV_{MRI} and GTV_{PET}, and between GTV_{MRI} and $GTV_{PET/MRI}$, and to compare doses delivered according to GTV obtained from MRI and PET/MRI data. The nonparametric Mann–Whitney *U* test was used to test differences between patient groups. The Spearman rank correlation test was conducted to assess the relationship between variables. All statistical analyses were performed using R Studio (Version 1.0.153 2017, R Studio, Inc., Boston, MA, USA). A p-value less than 0.05 was considered significant.

5. Conclusions

In this era of multimodality imaging, we should consider that no single imaging modality encompasses an entire microscopic and macroscopic tumor, pointing out the difficulty selecting which imaging modality is superior for target volume delineation. In our opinion, the real question that at present remains without a definitive response is whether any difference in GTV delineation according to the available imaging modalities (MRI, PET/CT, and PET/MRI) is clinically significant in patients with SBPGL. For the moment, we can note that no differences exist in terms of tumor-delivered dose between MRI and PET/MRI-based radiation planning, regardless of the inter-modality degree of volumetric agreement. Future integration of ^{18}F-FDOPA PET/CT into clinical practice for SBPGL radiotherapy planning will be necessary to evaluate the influence of this combined diagnostic modality on tumor eradication or local control. If the clinical utility of ^{18}F-FDOPA PET/MRI is further confirmed in a large patient population, combined $GTV_{PET/MRI}$ should be considered for tailored SBPGL radiotherapy planning to identify positive disease not clearly detected by conventional MRI, to redefine CTV margins, or to give a radiation boost treatment.

Author Contributions: M.H.: manuscript writing, reviewing and approval, data analysis and interpretation. M.M.: manuscript writing, reviewing and approval; C.L.F.: GTV data analysis, manuscript reviewing and approval. C.H.: manuscript reviewing and approval. C.B.: manuscript reviewing and approval. F.H.: statistical analysis, manuscript reviewing and approval. C.H.: manuscript reviewing and approval. B.G.: patient clinical management, manuscript reviewing and approval. F.V.: MRI examinations, manuscript reviewing and approval. A.C.: patient surgical management, manuscript reviewing and approval. G.N.: GTV data analysis, manuscript reviewing and approval. A.I.: conception of the work, data analysis and interpretation, manuscript writing, reviewing and approval.

Funding: This research received no external funding.

Conflicts of Interest: The authors declare no conflict of interest.

References

1. Kumar, V.; Abbas, A.; Fausto, N.; Aster, J. *Robbins and Cotran: Pathological Basis of Disease*, 8th ed.; Saunders: Philadelphia, PA, USA, 2010.
2. Baysal, B.E.; Willett-Brozick, J.E.; Lawrence, E.C.; Drovdlic, C.M.; Savul, S.A.; McLeod, D.R.; Yee, H.A.; Brackmann, D.E.; Slattery, W.H.; Myers, E.N.; et al. Prevalence of SDHB, SDHC, and SDHD germline mutations in clinic patients with head and neck paragangliomas. *J. Med. Genet.* **2002**, *39*, 178–183. [CrossRef] [PubMed]
3. Lenders, J.W.M.; Duh, Q.-Y.; Eisenhofer, G.; Gimenez-Roqueplo, A.-P.; Grebe, S.K.G.; Murad, M.H.; Naruse, M.; Pacak, K.; Young, W.F.; et al. Pheochromocytoma and Paraganglioma: An Endocrine Society Clinical Practice Guideline. *J. Clin. Endocrinol. Metab.* **2014**, *99*, 1915–1942. [CrossRef] [PubMed]
4. Manolidis, S.; Shohet, J.A.; Jackson, C.G.; Glasscock, M.E., 3rd. Malignant glomus tumors. *Laryngoscope* **1999**, *109*, 30–34. [CrossRef] [PubMed]
5. Taïeb, D.; Timmers, H.J.; Hindié, E.; Guillet, B.A.; Neumann, H.P.; Walz, M.K.; Opocher, G.; Herder, W.W.; Boedeker, C.C.; Krijger, R.R.; et al. EANM 2012 guidelines for radionuclide imaging of phaeochromocytoma and paraganglioma. *Eur. J. Nucl. Med. Mol. Imaging* **2012**, *39*, 1977–1995. [CrossRef] [PubMed]
6. Treglia, G.; Cocciolillo, F.; De Waure, C.; Di Nardo, F.; Gualano, M.R.; Castaldi, P.; Rufini, V.; Giordano, A. Diagnostic performance of ^{18}F-dihydroxyphenylalanine positron emission tomography in patients with paraganglioma: A meta-analysis. *Eur. J. Nucl. Med. Mol. Imaging* **2012**, *39*, 1144–1153. [CrossRef] [PubMed]
7. Heimburger, C.; Veillon, F.; Taïeb, D.; Goichot, B.; Riehm, S.; Petit-Thomas, J.; Averous, G.; Cavalcanti, M.; Hubelé, F.; Chabrier, G.; et al. Head-to-head comparison between ^{18}F-FDOPA PET/CT and MR/CT angiography in clinically recurrent head and neck paragangliomas. *Eur. J. Nucl. Med. Mol. Imaging* **2017**, *44*, 979–987. [CrossRef] [PubMed]

8. Amodru, V.; Guerin, C.; Delcourt, S.; Romanet, P.; Loundou, A.; Viana, B.; Brue, T.; Castinetti, F.; Sebag, F.; Pacak, K.; et al. Quantitative ^{18}F-DOPA PET/CT in pheochromocytoma: The relationship between tumor secretion and its biochemical phenotype. *Eur. J. Nucl. Med. Mol. Imaging* **2018**, *45*, 278–282. [CrossRef]
9. Taïeb, D.; Kaliski, A.; Boedeker, C.C.; Martucci, V.; Fojo, T.; Adler, J.R.; Pacak, K. Current approaches and recent developments in the management of head and neck paragangliomas. *Endocr. Rev.* **2014**, *35*, 795–819. [CrossRef]
10. Wanna, G.B.; Sweeney, A.D.; Haynes, D.S.; Carlson, M.L. Contemporary management of jugular paragangliomas. *Otolaryngol. Clin. N. Am.* **2015**, *48*, 331–341. [CrossRef]
11. Moore, M.G.; Netterville, J.L.; Mendenhall, W.M.; Isaacson, B.; Nussenbaum, B. Head and Neck Paragangliomas: An Update on Evaluation and Management. *Otolaryngol. Head Neck Surg.* **2016**, *154*, 597–605. [CrossRef]
12. Marchetti, M.; Pinzi, V.; Tramacere, I.; Bianchi, L.C.; Ghielmetti, F.; Fariselli, L. Radiosurgery for paragangliomas of the head and neck: Another step for the validation of a treatment paradigm. *World Neurosurg.* **2017**, *98*, 281–287. [CrossRef] [PubMed]
13. Hu, K.; Persky, M.S. Treatment of head and neck paragangliomas. *Cancer Control* **2016**, *23*, 228–241. [CrossRef] [PubMed]
14. Huy, P.T.B. Radiotherapy for glomus jugulare paraganglioma. *Eur. Ann. Otorhinolaryngol. Head Neck Dis.* **2014**, *131*, 223–226. [CrossRef]
15. Queiroz, M.A.; Hüllner, M.; Kuhn, F.; Huber, G.; Meerwein, C.; Kollias, S.; Von Schulthess, G.; Veit-Haibach, P. PET/MRI and PET/CT in follow-up of head and neck cancer patients. *Eur. J. Nucl. Med. Mol. Imaging* **2014**, *41*, 1066–1075. [CrossRef] [PubMed]
16. Schaarschmidt, B.M.; Heusch, P.; Buchbender, C.; Ruhlmann, M.; Bergmann, C.; Ruhlmann, V.; Schlamann, M.; Antoch, G.; Forsting, M.; Wetter, A.; et al. Locoregional tumour evaluation of squamous cell carcinoma in the head and neck area: A comparison between MRI, PET/CT and integrated PET/MRI. *Eur. J. Nucl. Med. Mol. Imaging* **2016**, *43*, 92–102. [CrossRef] [PubMed]
17. Pauleit, D.; Floeth, F.; Hamacher, K.; Riemenschneider, M.J.; Reifenberger, G.; Müller, H.-W.; Zilles, K.; Coenen, H.H.; Langen, K.-J. *O*-(2-[^{18}F]fluoroethyl)-L-tyrosine PET combined with MRI improves the diagnostic assessment of cerebral gliomas. *Brain* **2005**, *128*, 678–687. [CrossRef] [PubMed]
18. Cicone, F.; Filss, C.P.; Minniti, G.; Rossi-Espagnet, C.; Papa, A.; Scaringi, C.; Galldiks, N.; Bozzao, A.; Shah, N.J.; Scopinaro, F.; et al. Volumetric assessment of recurrent or progressive gliomas: Comparison between F-DOPA PET and perfusion-weighted MRI. *Eur. J. Nucl. Med. Mol. Imaging* **2015**, *42*, 905–915. [CrossRef]
19. Carideo, L.; Minniti, G.; Mamede, M.; Scaringi, C.; Russo, I.; Scopinaro, F.; Cicone, F. ^{18}F-DOPA uptake parameters in glioma: Effects of patients' characteristics and prior treatment history. *Br. J. Radiol.* **2018**, *91*, 20170847. [CrossRef] [PubMed]
20. Kratochwil, C.; Combs, S.E.; Leotta, K.; Afshar-Oromieh, A.; Rieken, S.; Debus, J.; Haberkorn, U.; Giesel, F.L. Intra-individual comparison of ^{18}F-FET and ^{18}FDOPA in PET imaging of recurrent brain tumors. *Neuro Oncol.* **2014**, *16*, 434–440. [CrossRef] [PubMed]
21. Lapa, C.; Linsenmann, T.; Monoranu, C.M.; Samnick, S.; Buck, A.; Bluemel, C.; Czernin, J.; Kessler, A.F.; Homola, G.A.; Ernestus, R.-I.; et al. Comparison of the amino acid tracers ^{18}F-FET and ^{18}F-DOPA in high-grade glioma patients. *J. Nucl. Med.* **2014**, *55*, 1611–1616. [CrossRef] [PubMed]
22. Verma, V.; Choi, J.I.; Sawant, A.; Gullapalli, R.P.; Chen, W.; Alavi, A.; Simone, C.B. Use of PET and Other Functional Imaging to Guide Target Delineation in Radiation Oncology. *Semin. Radiat. Oncol.* **2018**, *28*, 171–177. [CrossRef] [PubMed]
23. Pafundi, D.H.; Laack, N.N.; Youland, R.S.; Parney, I.F.; Lowe, V.J.; Giannini, C.; Kemp, B.J.; Grams, M.P.; Morris, J.M.; Hoover, J.M.; et al. Biopsy validation of ^{18}F-DOPA PET and biodistribution in gliomas for neurosurgical planning and radiotherapy target delineation: Results of a prospective pilot study. *Neuro Oncol.* **2013**, *15*, 1058–1067. [CrossRef] [PubMed]
24. Pafundi, D.; Brinkmann, D.; Laack, N.; Sarkaria, J.; Yan, E.; Kemp, B.; Löwe, V. WE-G-214-02: Utility of ^{18}F-FDOPA PET for Radiotherapy Target Delineation in Glioma Patients. *Med. Phys.* **2011**, *38*, 3830. [CrossRef]

25. Kosztyla, R.; Chan, E.K.; Hsu, F.; Wilson, D.; Ma, R.; Cheung, A.; Zhang, S.; Moiseenko, V.; Bénard, F.; Nichol, A.; et al. High-grade glioma radiation therapy target volumes and patterns of failure obtained from magnetic resonance imaging and ^{18}F-FDOPA positron emission tomography delineations from multiple observers. *Int. J. Radiat. Oncol. Biol. Phys.* **2013**, *87*, 1100–1106. [CrossRef] [PubMed]
26. Navarria, P.; Reggiori, G.; Pessina, F.; Ascolese, A.M.; Tomatis, S.; Mancosu, P.; Lobefalo, F.; Clerici, E.; Lopci, E.; Bizzi, A.; et al. Investigation on the role of integrated PET/MRI for target volume definition and radiotherapy planning in patients with high grade glioma. *Radiother. Oncol.* **2014**, *112*, 425–429. [CrossRef] [PubMed]
27. Palaniappan, N.; Cole, N.; Jayaprakasam, V.; Rackley, T.; Spezi, E.; Berthon, B.; Evans, M. Head and neck target delineation using a novel PET automatic segmentation algorithm. *Radiother. Oncol.* **2017**, *122*, 242–247. [CrossRef]
28. Handel, S.F.; Miller, M.H.; Miller, L.S.; Goepfert, H.; Wallace, S. Angiographic changes of head and neck chemodectomas following radiotherapy. *Arch. Otolaryngol.* **1977**, *103*, 87–89. [CrossRef] [PubMed]
29. Wang, K.; Mullins, B.T.; Falchook, A.D.; Lian, J.; He, K.; Shen, D.; Dance, M.; Lin, W.; Sills, T.M.; Das, S.K.; et al. Evaluation of PET/MRI for Tumor Volume Delineation for Head and Neck Cancer. *Front. Oncol.* **2017**, *23*, 7–8. [CrossRef] [PubMed]
30. Ligtenberg, H.; Jager, E.A.; Caldas-Magalhaes, J.; Schakel, T.; Pameijer, F.A.; Kasperts, N.; Willems, S.M.; Terhaard, C.H.; Raaijmakers, C.P.; Philippens, M.E.; et al. Modality-specific target definition for laryngeal and hypopharyngeal cancer on FDG-PET, CT and MRI. *Radiother. Oncol.* **2017**, *123*, 63–70. [CrossRef] [PubMed]
31. Songthong, A.P.; Kannarunimit, D.; Chakkabat, C.; Lertbutsayanukul, C. A randomized phase II/III study of adverse events between sequential (SEQ) versus simultaneous integrated boost (SIB) intensity modulated radiation therapy (IMRT) in nasopharyngeal carcinoma; preliminary result on acute adverse events. *Radiat. Oncol.* **2015**, *10*, 166. [CrossRef] [PubMed]
32. Truc, G.; Bernier, V.; Mirjolet, C.; Dalban, C.; Mazoyer, F.; Bonnetain, F.; Blanchard, N.; Lagneau, É.; Maingon, P.; Noël, G.; et al. A phase I dose escalation study using simultaneous integrated-boost IMRT with temozolomide in patients with unifocal glioblastoma. *Cancer Radiother.* **2016**, *20*, 193–198. [CrossRef] [PubMed]
33. Erdi, Y.E.; Mawlawi, O.; Larson, S.M.; Imbriaco, M.; Yeung, H.; Finn, R.; Humm, J.L. Segmentation of lung lesion volume by adaptive positron emission tomography image thresholding. *Cancer* **1997**, *80*, 2505–2509. [CrossRef]
34. Zou, K.H.; Warfield, S.K.; Bharatha, A.; Tempany, C.M.; Kaus, M.R.; Haker, S.J.; Wells, W.M.; Jolesz, F.A.; Kikinis, R. Statistical validation of image segmentation quality based on a spatial overlap index. *Acad. Radiol.* **2004**, *11*, 178–189. [CrossRef]
35. Otto, K. Volumetric modulated arc therapy: IMRT in a single gantry arc. *Med. Phys.* **2008**, *35*, 310–317. [CrossRef] [PubMed]
36. Cicchetti, D.V. Guidelines, Criteria, and Rules of Thumb for Evaluating Normed and Standardized Assessment Instruments in Psychology. *Psychol. Assess.* **1994**, *6*, 284–290. [CrossRef]

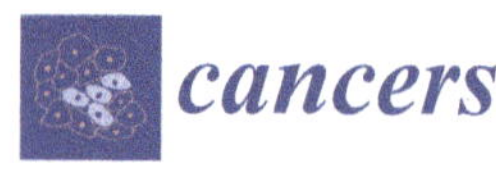

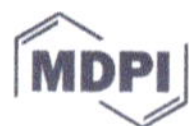

Article

Increased Mortality in *SDHB* but Not in *SDHD* Pathogenic Variant Carriers

Johannes A. Rijken [1,*], Leonie T. van Hulsteijn [2], Olaf M. Dekkers [2,3], Nicolasine D. Niemeijer [2], C. René Leemans [1], Karin Eijkelenkamp [4], Anouk N.A. van der Horst-Schrivers [4], Michiel N. Kerstens [4], Anouk van Berkel [5], Henri J.L.M. Timmers [5], Henricus P.M. Kunst [6], Peter H.L.T. Bisschop [7], Koen M.A. Dreijerink [8,9], Marieke F. van Dooren [10], Frederik J. Hes [11], Jeroen C. Jansen [12], Eleonora P.M. Corssmit [2] and Erik F. Hensen [1,12]

1 Department of Otolaryngology/Head and Neck Surgery, Amsterdam UMC, Vrije Universiteit Amsterdam, De Boelelaan 1117, 1081 HZ Amsterdam, The Netherlands; cr.leemans@vumc.nl (C.R.L.); E.F.Hensen@lumc.nl (E.F.H.)

2 Department of Endocrinology and Metabolic Diseases, Leiden University Medical Center, 2333 ZA Leiden, The Netherlands; lvanhulsteijn@hotmail.com (L.T.v.H.); O.M.Dekkers@lumc.nl (O.M.D.); nniemeijer@ysl.nl (N.D.N.); E.P.M.van_der_Kleij-Corssmit@lumc.nl (E.P.M.C.)

3 Departments of Epidemiology, Leiden University Medical Center, 2333 ZA Leiden, The Netherlands

4 Department of Endocrinology, University Medical Center Groningen, University of Groningen, Hanzeplein 1, 9713 GZ Groningen, The Netherlands; k.eijkelenkamp@umcg.nl (K.E.); a.n.a.van.der.horst@umcg.nl (A.N.A.v.d.H.-S.); m.n.kerstens@umcg.nl (M.N.K.)

5 Division of Endocrinology, Department of Internal Medicine, Radboud University Medical Center, Geert Grooteplein Zuid 10, 6525 GA Nijmegen, The Netherlands; anouk.vanberkel@radboudumc.nl (A.v.B.); henri.timmers@radboudumc.nl (H.J.L.M.T.)

6 Department of Otolaryngology/Head and Neck Surgery, Radboud University Medical Center, Geert Grooteplein Zuid 10, 6525 GA Nijmegen, The Netherlands; dirk.kunst@radboudumc.nl

7 Department of Endocrinology and Metabolism, Amsterdam UMC, University of Amsterdam, Meibergdreef 9, 1105 AZ Amsterdam, The Netherlands; p.h.bisschop@amc.uva.nl

8 Department of Endocrinology, University Medical Centre Utrecht, Heidelberglaan 100, 3584 CX Utrecht, The Netherlands; k.dreijerink@vumc.nl

9 Department of Endocrinology, Amsterdam UMC, Vrije Universiteit Amsterdam, De Boelelaan 1117, 1081 HZ Amsterdam, The Netherlands

10 Department of Clinical Genetics, Erasmus MC, University Medical Center Rotterdam, Doctor Molewaterplein 40, 3015 GD Rotterdam, The Netherlands; m.vandooren@erasmusmc.nl

11 Department of Clinical Genetics, Leiden University Medical Center, De Boelelaan 1117, 1081 HZ Leiden, The Netherlands; F.J.Hes@lumc.nl

12 Department of Otolaryngology/Head and Neck Surgery, Leiden University Medical Center, Albinusdreef 2, 2333 ZA Leiden, The Netherlands; j.c.jansen@lumc.nl

* Correspondence: j.rijken@vumc.nl; Tel.: +31-204443690; Fax: +31-204440314

Received: 17 December 2018; Accepted: 13 January 2019; Published: 17 January 2019

Abstract: Germline mutations in succinate dehydrogenase subunit B and D (*SDHB* and *SDHD*) are predisposed to hereditary paraganglioma (PGL) and pheochromocytoma (PHEO). The phenotype of pathogenic variants varies according to the causative gene. In this retrospective study, we estimate the mortality of a nationwide cohort of *SDHB* variant carriers and that of a large cohort of *SDHD* variant carriers and compare it to the mortality of a matched cohort of the general Dutch population. A total of 192 *SDHB* variant carriers and 232 *SDHD* variant carriers were included in this study. The Standard Mortality Ratio (SMR) for *SDHB* mutation carriers was 1.89, increasing to 2.88 in carriers affected by PGL. For *SDHD* variant carriers the SMR was 0.93 and 1.06 in affected carriers. Compared to the general population, mortality seems to be increased in *SDHB* variant carriers, especially in those affected by PGL. In *SDHD* variant carriers, the mortality is comparable to that of the general Dutch population, even if they are affected by PGL. This insight emphasizes the significance of

DNA-testing in all PGL and PHEO patients, since different clinical risks may warrant gene-specific management strategies.

Keywords: *SDHB*; *SDHD*; mortality; paraganglioma; pheochromocytoma

1. Introduction

Paragangliomas (PGL) are rare tumors that originate from cells of neural crest origin in the paraganglia associated with the autonomic nervous system. PGL can be subdivided into head and neck paragangliomas (HNPGL), pheochromocytomas (PHEO), and thoracic and abdominal extra-adrenal PGL (sympathetic PGL; sPGL). An increasing number of genes are associated with hereditary PGL/PHEO. Most frequently, hereditary PGL syndrome is caused by genes encoding subunits or cofactors of succinate dehydrogenase (SDH), such as *SDHA/B/C/D/AF2*. Other associated genes are *RET, NF1, VHL, HIF2A, FH, TMEM127*, and *MAX* [1,2]. In the Netherlands, pathogenic variants in *SDHD* are the most prevalent cause of PGL syndrome, followed by variants in *SDHB* and *SDHA* [3,4]. Although all SDHx genes encode subunits of the same SDH complex and pathogenic variants all disrupt its enzymatic function, different genes are associated with different phenotypes. The reported lifelong penetrance of pathogenic *SDHB* variants (22–42%) [5,6] is considerably lower than the penetrance of paternally inherited *SDHD* mutations (88–100%) [7–10].

When pathogenic *SDHB* variants cause disease, the clinical outcome is reported to be less favorable than that in *SDHD*-linked disease. *SDHB* mutation carriers are reported to develop metastatic PGL more frequently and patients with metastatic disease associated with *SDHB* variants are reported to have a poor 5-year survival rate compared to patients with metastatic disease associated with other causative genes [11]. The mortality of *SDHB* variant carriers is currently unknown [12]. In this study we estimate the mortality for a nationwide cohort of *SDHB* variant carriers and compare this risk with the mortality of *SDHD* variant carriers and that of the general Dutch population.

2. Subjects and Methods

2.1. Eligibility Criteria

The cohort of pathogenic germline variant carriers (hereafter variants) in *SDHB* included in this study has been described in detail previously [6,13]. The mortality of this nationwide *SDHB*-linked cohort was compared with the mortality of the general Dutch population and with the mortality of an updated cohort of *SDHD* variant carriers, which has been described previously [12]. Only *SDHD* variant carriers with paternal inheritance were included. Carriers of *SDHD* variants were identified using the database of the Laboratory for Diagnostic Genome Analysis (LDGA) at the Leiden University Medical Center (LUMC), a tertiary referral center for patients with PGL. Screening for *SDH* variants was performed in all persons diagnosed with PGL who agreed to genetic testing.

Screening for *SDHB* and *SDHD* variants was performed by direct sequencing of peripheral blood leucocytes using the Sanger method on an ABI 377 Genetic Analyzer (Applied Biosystems, Carlsbad, California) and by multiplex ligation-dependent probe amplification (MLPA) using the P226 MLPA kit (MRC Holland, Amsterdam, the Netherlands). Family members of index patients were tested for the family-specific variant. All variants described in this study were submitted to the Leiden Open (source) Variation Database LOVD database (http://chromium.liacs.nl/lovd_sdh). *SDHB* and *SDHD* germline variants were classified according to the international guidelines put forth by Plon et al. [14]. *SDHD* variants were described using the reference sequence NG_012340.1 covering SDHB transcript NM_003000.2, and NG_012337.1 covering SDHD transcript NM_003002.2, available from the TCA Cycle Gene Variant Database LOVD database. In this manuscript we report pathogenic or likely pathogenic variants, including missense mutations in highly conserved regions that are determined to be likely pathogenic as germline mutations based partly on mutation prediction analyses. Information on amino acid conservation can be found in the LOVD database (http://chromium.liacs.nl/lovd_sdh). Further information including mutation prediction analyses can be obtained on request.

The study was approved by the Medical Ethics Committee of the Leiden University Medical Center; participating centers complied with their local Medical Ethics Committee requirements. Written informed consent was obtained from the parents/guardians of individuals under 18 years of age.

2.2. Clinical Characteristics

Clinical data were retrieved from medical records. Pathogenic variant carriers were investigated for occurrences of PGL and/or PHEO according to the structured protocols used for standard care in the Netherlands for PGL or PHEO patients [15,16]. Patients were offered clinical surveillance for PGL/PHEO at the departments of otorhinolaryngology and endocrinology. For asymptomatic *SDHB* and *SDHD* variant carriers older than 18 years of age, surveillance consisted of magnetic resonance imaging (MRI) of the head and neck region once every 2–3 years, and MRI or computed tomography (CT) scans of the thorax, abdomen, and pelvis once every 1–2 years in *SDHB* variant carriers. Biochemical screening was performed annually on *SDHB* variant carriers, and every 1–2 years on *SDHD* variant carriers. This screening measured levels of (nor)epinephrine, vanillylmandelic acid, dopamine, (nor)metanephrine, and/or 3-methoxytyramine in two 24-hour urinary samples (depending on the Academic Center in which urinary measurement(s) were performed), and/or plasma free (nor)metanephrine and 3-methoxytyramine. In cases of excessive catecholamine secretion (i.e., any value above the upper reference limit), radiological assessment by MRI or CT scans of the thorax, abdomen, and pelvis, and/or 123I metaiodobenzylguanidine (MIBG) scans, positron emission tomography with 2-deoxy-2-[fluorine-18]fluoro-D-glucose (18F-FDG PET) scans, 18F-L-dihydroxyphenylalanine (18F-DOPA) PET-scans, or positron emission tomography with 1,4,7,10-tetraazacyclododecane-NI, NII, NIII, NIIII-tetraacetic acid (D)-Phe1-thy3-octreotide (68Ga-DOTATOC PET) scans were performed to identify potential sources of excessive catecholamine production. In cases without available tumor histology, tumors were classified as paraganglionic based on their specific characteristics in CT and/or MRI scans. When in doubt, additional nuclear medicine imaging studies were performed in order to confirm the diagnosis. At the time of this study, there were no national, structured protocols for surveillance in *SDHB* mutation carriers younger than 18 years of age. Therefore, the method and interval of surveillance in this age category varied between centers.

In case of a diagnosis of HNPGL, PHEO or sPGL, intensified surveillance or treatment was offered. Surgical resection was generally the preferred treatment option for PHEO or sPGL. In cases of HNPGL, the management strategy was guided by clinical symptoms, tumor characteristics such as localization, size, and growth rate, and patient characteristics such as age, comorbidity, and patient preferences. A wait and scan policy, radiotherapy, or surgical resection were possible treatment options.

2.3. Mortality and Survival

For this study, follow-up data from *SDHB* and *SDHD* variant carriers were included from the date of the DNA test. In cases where clinical follow-up was available for the period before the DNA test, this period was not considered in the mortality analysis because it would have introduced immortal time bias [17]. Follow-up was defined as the time between the DNA test and the last clinical follow-up date before the end of the study period. Patients who were alive at the last clinical follow-up were classified as alive. Follow-up ended at the end of the study period, at the date of death or, in case of emigration, at the date of emigration [13]. To compare mortality between *SDHB* and *SDHD* variant carriers and the general population, the standardized mortality ratio (SMR) was estimated. Mortality rates for the Dutch population were obtained from Statistics Netherlands (CBS, The Netherlands) [18], using rates stratified by sex, age (per 1 year) and date (1-year periods). The SMR was calculated by dividing the observed number of deaths in the *SDHB* and *SDHD* cohorts. The expected number of deaths was calculated as the sum of the stratified number of expected deaths (stratum-specific mortality rates from the general population times follow-up time at risk).

Survival was graphically displayed for *SDHB* and *SDHD* variant carriers by plotting survival in the carriers against the expected survival based on matched data from the general population. STATA 14.0 (Stata Corp, Texas, USA) was used for statistical analysis.

3. Results

In total, 192 *SDHB* variant carriers and 232 *SDHD* variant carriers were included in this study. The clinical characteristics are depicted in Table 1. The mean age at identification of the pathogenic gene variant was 46 years (range 9–77) in *SDHB* variant carriers and 44 years (range 16–73) in *SDHD* variant carriers. In total, 53 *SDHB* variant carriers (27.6%) and 198 *SDHD* variant carriers (85.3%) were diagnosed with HNPGL, either at time of presentation or during follow-up. Four *SDHB* patients (2.1%) and 16 *SDHD* patients (6.9%) developed PHEO and 26 *SDHB* patients (13.5%) and 18 (7.8%) *SDHD* patients developed sPGL. Malignant PGL, defined as metastatic PGL in non-paraganglionic tissue, were diagnosed in 14 *SDHB* (7.3%) and four *SDHD* patients (1.7%). Most *SDHB* variant carriers (110/193; 57.3%) were not affected at the time of DNA testing or during follow-up. In contrast, the majority of *SDHD* variant carriers was diagnosed with *SDHD*-associated disease (203/232; 87.5%). Details of the specific *SDHB* and *SDHD* variants are included in Appendix A.

Table 1. Clinical characteristics of carriers of pathogenic variants in succinate dehydrogenase subunits B and D (*SDHB* and *SDHD*).

Clinical Characteristics	*SDHB* $n = 192$	*SDHD* $n = 232$
Male (%)/female (%)	81 (42.2)/111 (57.8)	123 (53.0)/109 (47.0)
Mean age at genetic testing	46 years (range 9–77)	44 years (range 16–73)
HNPGL (%)	53 (27.6)	198 (85.3)
sPGL (%)	26 (13.5)	18 (7.8)
Pheochromocytoma (%)	4 (2.1)	16 (6.9)
Malignant PGL (%)	14 (7.3)	4 (1.7)
Unaffected (%)	110 (57.3)	30 (12.9)

HNPGL = head and neck paraganglioma, sPGL = sympathetic paraganglioma, PGL = paraganglioma.

Mortality and SMR

Mortality data were available for all *SDHB* and *SDHD* variant carriers. The mean follow-up period was 3.0 (range 0–14.5) and 5.1 (range 0–12.5) years, respectively, for *SDHB* and *SDHD* variant carriers. In total, 6/192 (3.1%) *SDHB* variant carriers died at age 32, 37, 49, 52, 62, and 63. In three patients the cause of death was directly related to progressive PGL disease. In contrast, 5/232 (2.2%) *SDHD* variant carriers died at age 41, 43, 71, 71, and 74. In two cases the cause of death was most likely associated with PGL disease. Clinical characteristics of the variant carriers who died during the study period are listed in Table 2.

A direct comparison between *SDHB* and *SDHD* variant carriers is hampered by the limited number of carriers and the heterogeneity between both groups. We performed an adjusted Poisson regression, adjusting for age, sex, and calendar time. The rate ratio comparing *SDHB* to *SDHD* variant carriers was 0.48 (95% confidence interval (CI) 0.15–1.62). However, the power for this analysis is low. As both groups have few events, we cannot draw conclusions from the non-significant p-value.

Table 2. Details of six *SDHB* and five *SDHD* variant carriers who died during follow-up.

Sex	Mutation	Predicted Protein Change	Location of PGL	Age at PGL Diagnosis (years)	Age at Diagnosis of Malignant Disease (years)	Age at Death (years)	Location of Metastases	Cause of Death
M	*SDHB* exon 3 deletion	p.?	Presacral	28	28	32	Bone	Progressive malignant PGL
F	*SDHB* c.654G > A	p.(Trp218*)	Bladder	19	58	62	Lymph nodes, bone	Progressive malignant PGL
F	*SDHB* exon 3 deletion	p.?	Para-vertebral abdominal	33	33	37	Lymph nodes, bone	Progressive malignant PGL
F	*SDHB* c.727T > A	p.(Cys243Ser)	Retroperitoneal (para-aortic)	52	55	63	Bone	Myocardial infarction, heart failure and acute respiratory distress syndrome
F	*SDHB* c.423 + 1G > A	p.?	n.a.	49	n.a.	52	n.a.	Respiratory insufficiency due to lung bleeding after chemoradiotherapy for lung cancer
F	*SDHB* c.423 + 1G > A	p.?	n.a.	42	n.a.	49	n.a.	Metastatic breast cancer
F	*SDHD* c.274G > T	p.(Asp92Tyr)	Bladder	42	42	43	Lymph nodes, bone marrow	Progressive malignant PGL
F	*SDHD* c.274G > T	p.(Asp92Tyr)	Mediastinal	67	67	74	Lymph nodes, bone	Unknown, however the patient was known to have progressive malignant PGL
F	*SDHD* c.274G > T	p.(Asp92Tyr)	Bilateral CBT, VBT	55	n.a.	71	n.a.	Cardiac arrest
F	*SDHD* c.242C > T	p.(Pro81Leu)	CBT	38	n.a.	41	n.a.	Breast cancer
M	*SDHD* c.274G > T	p.(Asp92Tyr)	CBT, jugular PGL, retroperitoneal	52	n.a.	71	n.a.	Prostate cancer

PGL = paraganglioma, CBT = carotid body tumor, VBT = vagal body tumor, n.a. = not applicable.

For the comparison of both the *SDHB*- and *SDHD*-linked cohorts with normative data of the Dutch population, a total of 1781 person-years were available (*SDHB* 590 and *SDHD* 1191 years, respectively). The SMR for *SDHB* mutation carriers was 1.89 (95% confidence interval (CI) 0.85–4.21) (Figure 1). A separate analysis including only symptomatic *SDHB* variant carriers—i.e., those with manifest disease—showed a higher SMR at 2.88 (95% CI 1.08–7.68). These results suggest an increased mortality risk for *SDHB* variant carriers compared to the general Dutch population, especially for carriers affected by *SDHB*-associated disease. For *SDHD* variant carriers, the SMR was 0.93 (95% CI 0.39–2.23), increasing only slightly to 1.06 (95% CI 0.44–2.54) in affected carriers, suggesting that mortality is not increased in *SDHD* variant carriers.

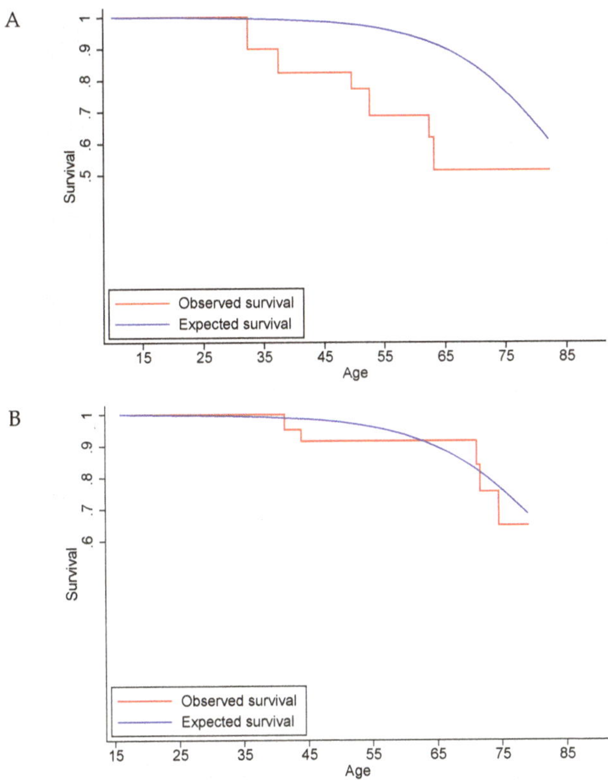

Figure 1. The Kaplan–Meier survival curve for *SDHB* variant carriers (**A**) and *SDHD* variant carriers (**B**) compared with the expected survival based on the general Dutch population.

4. Discussion

In this study we estimated the mortality for *SDHB* and *SDHD* pathogenic variant carriers. Whereas the mortality for *SDHD* variant carriers is comparable with a matched cohort of the general Dutch population (SMR = 0.93), *SDHB* variant carriers show a higher mortality (SMR = 1.89, meaning a 1.89 times higher risk of death than the matched cohort of the general Dutch population).

These mortality ratios should be interpreted with some caution. First, not all deaths in our cohort are directly attributable to PGL-linked disease. However, a comparison is made with the mortality of the general Dutch population. Therefore, eliminating other causes of death would be inappropriate.

Second, even though the *SDHB* variant carriers represent a nationwide cohort, PGL is a rare disease and patient numbers are inevitably limited. As a result, the study estimates have broad confidence intervals. In addition, the follow-up of the start of this study is defined as the time of DNA testing and not PGL/PHEO diagnosis. As the genetic causes of hereditary PGL syndromes have been determined only recently, follow-up is relatively limited. However, the differences between *SDHB* and *SDHD* variant carriers are remarkable, all the more so when considering that *SDHD* variants are characterized by a high penetrance of PGL (88–100%), and *SDHB* variants by a much lower lifelong PGL risk (22–42%) [5–10]. In *SDHD* variant carriers, the occurrence of often multiple associated (HN)PGL seems to have no clear impact on survival [12]. In contrast, *SDHB* variant carriers seem to face increased mortality even though they are under more intensive surveillance and, in our study, have a shorter follow-up. This decreased survival of *SDHB* variant carriers is attributable to the higher mortality of affected *SDHB* patients (SMR = 2.88). Moreover, the majority of deceased *SDHB*-linked patients suffered from progressive malignant PGL (Table 2). Unaffected *SDHB* variant carriers have a mortality ratio that is more in line with the general Dutch population (SMR = 1.12).

It is intriguing that the causative gene seems to determine variation in the prognoses for PGL/PHEO patients, even though pathogenic variants in *SDHB* and *SDHD* cause PGL/PHEO syndrome through defects in the same protein complex (succinate dehydrogenase, SDH). We speculate that this could be the result of intrinsic properties of the *SDHB*-associated PGL/PHEO syndrome, a deleterious effect of *SDHB* variants on other factors that influence survival, or differences between *SDHB* and *SDHD* variants in the potential to induce other types of malignancy. Interestingly, other types of malignancies (i.e. prostate cancer, lung cancer, breast cancer) are listed as causes of death both in the *SDHB*- and *SDHD*-linked cohorts (see Table 2). Although the *SDHx*-associated tumor spectrum is expanding, none of these malignancies have been directly linked to *SDHB* or *SDHD* variants. Even so, *SDHD* and/or *SDHB* variants could alter the susceptibility to certain types of malignancy other than PGL/PHEO. Indeed, 0.25% and 0.05% of breast cancer exomes carry somatic *SDHB* and *SDHD* variants, respectively [19,20].

The finding that all deceased *SDHB*-related PGL patients had metastatic PGL suggests that the occurrence of metastatic disease in *SDHB*-linked PGL syndrome particularly impacts survival, and that metastases may be either more prevalent in *SDHB*-linked cases, as suggested before [7,10,21–24], or more aggressive than metastatic diseases associated with other *SDHx* genes, a finding that is in line with the very poor 5-year survival rate of *SDHB*-linked metastatic disease reported by Amar et al. [11]. Another explanation might be that metastases from sPGL behave more aggressively than those of parasympathetic HNPGL, and that these sPGL are more prevalent in *SDHB*-linked disease [13,25]. Indeed, the PGL patients that died of progressive PGL disease both in the *SDHB*- and *SDHD*-linked cohorts all suffered from primary sPGL tumors.

The difference in the mortality between *SDHB* and *SDHD* variant carriers is another clear indication that causative genetic alteration is of critical importance to the outcome and risks of an individual PGL patient. This is important in counseling PGL/PHEO patients, but may also warrant gene-specific management strategies for PGL patients. In the present study, however, we did not evaluate the effect of PGL follow-up protocols or treatment on survival. From the patients that died of *SDHB*-related disease ($n = 3$), two already had proven metastatic disease at the time of diagnosis. Surgical resection with tumor-free margins seems to be a logical treatment strategy when trying to avoid progression of the disease, but there may be undetected metastases already present at the time of surgery [26,27]. The observation that the higher mortality associated with *SDHB* variant carriers seems to be attributable to patients that are affected by metastatic sPGL may warrant a more aggressive surgical strategy towards sPGL tumors in *SDHB*-linked patients. The risk of the malignant transformation of an sPGL tumor left untreated is, however, unknown. This unknown risk of disease progression must be weighed against the risk of surgical morbidity [28].

5. Conclusion

In conclusion, compared to a matched cohort of the general population, mortality is increased in *SDHB* variant carriers but not in *SDHD* variant carriers. This insight emphasizes the significance of DNA-testing; gene-specific clinical risks may warrant tailored management strategies. Further research is necessary to demonstrate the effect of (early) intervention of PGL/PHEO on mortality rates, especially in *SDHB* variant carriers.

Author Contributions: Conceptualization, J.A.R., L.T.v.H., O.M.D., F.J.H., J.C.J., E.P.M.C., and E.F.H.; Data curation, J.A.R., L.T.v.H., N.D.N., C.R.L., K.E., A.N.A.v.d.H.-S., M.N.K., A.v.B., H.J.L.M.T., H.P.M.K., P.H.L.T.B, K.M.A.D, M.F.D., F.J.H., J.C.J., E.P.M.C., and E.F.H.; Formal analysis, J.A.R., L.T.v.H., O.M.D., N.D.N., F.J.H., J.C.J., E.P.M.C., and E.F.H.; Investigation, K.M.A.D.; Methodology, J.A.R., L.T.v.H., O.M.D., A.v.B., F.J.H., E.P.M.C., and E.F.H.; Supervision, J.A.R., E.P.M.C., and E.F.H.; Visualization, J.C.J. and E.F.H.; Writing—original draft, J.A.R., L.T.v.H., O.M.D., N.D.N., C.R.L., K.E., A.N.A.v.d. H.-S., M.N.K., A.v.B., H.J.L.M.T., H.P.M.K., P.H.L.T.B., K.M.A.D., M.F.D., F.J.H., J.C.J., E.P.M.C., and E.F.H.; Writing—review and editing, J.A.R., L.T.v.H., E.P.M.C., and E.F.H.

Funding: This research received no external funding.

Conflicts of Interest: The authors declare no conflict of interest.

Appendix A. *SDHB* Variants and *SDHD* Variants

DNA Mutation	Predicted Protein Change	Number of Subjects (%)
Exon 3 deletion	p.?	59 (30.7)
c.423 + 1G > A	p.?	45 (23.4)
c.654G > A	p.(Trp218*)	19 (9.9)
c.653G > C	p.(Trp218Ser)	11 (5.7)
c.574T > C	p.(Cys192Arg)	8 (4.2)
c.200 + 1G > A	p.?	6 (3.1)
c.137G > A	p.(Arg46Gln)	4 (2.1)
c.328A > C	p.(Thr110Pro)	4 (2.1)
c.418G > T	p.(Val140Phe)	4 (2.1)
c.725G > A	p.(Arg242His)	3 (1.6)
c.649C > T	p.(Arg217Cys)	3 (1.6)
c.590C > G	p.(Pro197Arg)	3 (1.6)
c.686_725del	p.(Glu229fs)	3 (1.6)
c.343C > T	p.(Arg115*)	3 (1.6)
c.292T > C	p.(Cys98Arg)	2 (1.0)
Deletion promoter and exon 1	p.?	1 (0.5)
Deletion promoter till exon 8	p.0	2 (1.0)
Exon 2 deletion	p.?	2 (1.0)
Exon 1 deletion	p.?	2 (1.0)
c.713delT	p.(Phe238fs)	1 (0.5)
c.727T > A	p.(Cys243Ser)	1 (0.5)
c.761C > T	p.(Pro254Leu)	1 (0.5)
c.626C > T	p.(Pro209Leu)	1 (0.5)
c.380T > C	p.(Ile127Thr)	1 (0.5)

DNA Mutation	Predicted Protein Change	Number of Subjects (%)
c.325A > C	p.(Asn109His)	1 (0.5)
c.1A > G	p.?	1 (0.5)
c.119A > C	p.(Lys40Thr)	1 (0.5)
c.274G > T	p.(Asp92Tyr)	175 (74.7)
c.416T > C	p.(Leu139Pro)	34 (14.6)
c.284T > C	p.(Leu95Pro)	6 (2.6)
Deletion promoter, exon 1 and 2	p.?	4 (1.7)
c.242C > T	p.(Pro81Leu)	3 (1.3)
c.337_340delGACT	p.(Asp113fs)	2 (0.9)
c.122dupC	p.(Glu42fs)	2 (0.9)
Exon 1. c.3G > C	p.(Met1Ile)	1 (0.4)
Exon 2: c.169_169 + 9del10, splice donor mutation	p.?	1 (0.4)
Intron 2 c.169_169 + 9del	p.?	1 (0.4)
Specific *SDHD* variant unknown (tested elsewhere)	unknown	3 (1.3)

References

1. Cascon, A.; Comino-Mendez, I.; Curras-Freixes, M.; de Cubas, A.A.; Contreras, L.; Richter, S.; Peitzsch, M.; Mancikova, V.; Inglada-Perez, L.; Perez-Barrios, A.; et al. Whole-exome sequencing identifies MDH2 as a new familial paraganglioma gene. *J. Natl. Cancer Inst.* **2015**, *107*, djv053. [CrossRef] [PubMed]
2. Dahia, P.L. Pheochromocytoma and paraganglioma pathogenesis: Learning from genetic heterogeneity. *Nat. Rev. Cancer* **2014**, *14*, 108–119. [CrossRef] [PubMed]
3. Hensen, E.F.; van Duinen, N.; Jansen, J.C.; Corssmit, E.P.; Tops, C.M.; Romijn, J.A.; Vriends, A.H.; van der Mey, A.G.; Cornelisse, C.J.; Devilee, P.; et al. High prevalence of founder mutations of the succinate dehydrogenase genes in the Netherlands. *Clin. Genet.* **2012**, *81*, 284–288. [CrossRef] [PubMed]
4. Van der Tuin, K.; Mensenkamp, A.R.; Tops, C.M.J.; Corssmit, E.P.M.; Dinjens, W.N.; van de Horst-Schrivers, A.N.; Jansen, J.C.; de Jong, M.M.; Kunst, H.P.M.; Kusters, B.; et al. Clinical Aspects of SDHA-Related Pheochromocytoma and Paraganglioma: A Nationwide Study. *J. Clin. Endocrinol. Metab.* **2018**, *103*, 438–445. [CrossRef] [PubMed]
5. Andrews, K.A.; Ascher, D.B.; Pires, D.E.V.; Barnes, D.R.; Vialard, L.; Casey, R.T.; Bradshaw, N.; Adlard, J.; Aylwin, S.; Brennan, P.; et al. Tumour risks and genotype–phenotype correlations associated with germline variants in succinate dehydrogenase subunit genes SDHB, SDHC and SDHD. *J. Med. Genet.* **2018**, *55*, 384–394. [PubMed]
6. Rijken, J.A.; Niemeijer, N.D.; Jonker, M.A.; Eijkelenkamp, K.; Jansen, J.C.; van Berkel, A.; Timmers, H.J.L.M.; Kunst, H.P.M.; Bisschop, P.H.L.T.; Kerstens, M.N.; et al. The penetrance of paraganglioma and pheochromocytoma in SDHB germline mutation carriers. *Clin. Genet.* **2018**, *93*, 60–66. [CrossRef] [PubMed]
7. Neumann, H.P.; Pawlu, C.; Peczkowska, M.; Bausch, B.; McWhinney, S.R.; Muresan, M.; Buchta, M.; Franke, G.; Klisch, J.; Bley, T.A.; et al. Distinct clinical features of paraganglioma syndromes associated with SDHB and SDHD mutations. *JAMA* **2004**, *292*, 943–951. [CrossRef]
8. Kunst, H.P.; Rutten, M.H.; de Mönnink, J.P.; Hoefsloot, L.H.; Timmers, H.J.L.M.; Marres, H.A.M.; Jansen, J.C.; Kremer, H.; Bayley, J.-P.; Cremers, C.W.R.J. SDHAF2 (PGL2-SDH5) and hereditary head and neck paraganglioma. *Clin. Cancer Res.* **2011**, *17*, 247–254. [CrossRef]
9. Hensen, E.F.; Jansen, J.C.; Siemers, M.D.; Oosterwijk, J.C.; Vriends, A.H.; Corssmit, E.P.; Bayley, J.-P.; van der Mey, A.G.; Cornelisse, C.J.; Devilee, P. The Dutch founder mutation SDHD.D92Y shows a reduced penetrance for the development of paragangliomas in a large multigenerational family. *Eur. J. Hum. Genet.* **2010**, *18*, 62–66. [CrossRef]

10. Benn, D.E.; Gimenez-Roqueplo, A.P.; Reilly, J.R.; Bertherat, J.; Burgess, J.; Byth, K.; Croxson, M.; Dahia, P.L.; Elston, M.; Gimm, O.; et al. Clinical presentation and penetrance of pheochromocytoma/paraganglioma syndromes. *J. Clin. Endocrinol. Metab.* **2006**, *91*, 827–836. [CrossRef]
11. Amar, L.; Baudin, E.; Burnichon, N.; Peyrard, S.; Silvera, S.; Bertherat, J.; Bertagna, X.; Schlumberger, M.; Jeunemaitre, X.; Gimenez-Roqueplo, A.; et al. Succinate Dehydrogenase B Gene Mutations Predict Survival in Patients with Malignant Pheochromocytomas or Paragangliomas. *J. Clin. Endocrinol. Metab.* **2007**, *92*, 3822–3828. [CrossRef] [PubMed]
12. Van Hulsteijn, L.T.; Heesterman, B.; Jansen, J.C.; Bayley, J.P.; Hes, F.J.; Corssmit EPMDekkers, O.M. No evidence for increased mortality in SDHD variant carriers compared with the general population. *Eur. J. Hum. Genet.* **2015**, *23*, 1713–1716. [CrossRef] [PubMed]
13. Niemeijer, N.D.; Rijken, J.A.; Eijkelenkamp, K.; van der Horst-Schrivers, A.N.A.; Kerstens, M.N.; Tops, C.M.J.; van Berkel, A.; Timmers, H.J.L.M.; Kunst, H.P.M.; Leemans, C.R.; et al. The phenotype of SDHB germline mutation carriers; a nationwide study. *Eur. J. Endocrinol.* **2017**, *177*, 115–125. [CrossRef]
14. Plon, S.E.; Eccles, D.M.; Easton, D.; Foulkes, W.D.; Genuardi, M.; Greenblatt, M.S.; Hogervorst, F.B.L.; Hoogerbrugge, N.; Spurdle, A.B.; Tavtigian, S.V. Sequence variant classification and reporting: recommendations for improving the interpretation of cancer susceptibility genetic test results. *Hum. Mutat.* **2008**, *29*, 1282–1291. [CrossRef]
15. Dutch Guideline for Detecting Hereditary Tumors. 2010. Available online: https://www.stoet.nl (accessed on 17 March 2017).
16. Dutch Guidelines for Oncology Care. 2016. Available online: http://www.oncoline.nl/familiair-paraganglioom (accessed on 17 March 2017).
17. Suissa, S. Immortal time bias in pharmaco-epidemiology. *Am. J. Epidemiol.* **2008**, *167*, 492–499. [CrossRef]
18. Statistics Netherlands. Available online: https://www.cbs.nl/ (accessed on 17 March 2017).
19. Tate, J.G.; Bamford, S.; Jubb, H.C.; Sondka, Z.; Beare, D.M.; Bindal, N.; Boutselakis, H.; Cole, C.G.; Creatore, C.; Dawson, E.; et al. COSMIC: The Catalogue of Somatic Mutations in Cancer. *Nucleic Acids Res.* **2019**, *47*, D941–D947. [CrossRef] [PubMed]
20. Oudijk, L.; Gaal, J.; de Krijger, R.R. The Role of Immunohistochemistry and Molecular Analysis of Succinate Dehydrogenase in the Diagnosis of Endocrine and Non-Endocrine Tumors and Related Syndromes. *Endocr. Pathol.* **2018**. [CrossRef] [PubMed]
21. Timmers, H.J.; Kozupa, A.; Eisenhofer, G.; Raygada, M.; Adams, K.T.; Solis, D.; Lenders, J.W.; Pacak, K. Clinical presentations, biochemical phenotypes, and genotype-phenotype correlations in patients with succinate dehydrogenase subunit B-associated pheochromocytomas and paragangliomas. *J. Clin. Endocrinol. Metab.* **2007**, *92*, 779–786. [CrossRef] [PubMed]
22. Srirangalingam, U.; Walker, L.; Khoo, B.; MacDonald, F.; Gardner, D.; Wilkin, T.J.; Skelly, R.H.; George, E.; Spooner, D.; Monson, J.P.; et al. Clinical manifestations of familial paraganglioma and phaeochromocytomas in succinate dehydrogenase B (SDH-B) gene mutation carriers. *Clin. Endocrinol.* **2008**, *69*, 587–596. [CrossRef]
23. Amar, L.; Bertherat, J.; Baudin, E.; Ajzenberg, C.; Bressac-de Paillerets, B.; Chabre, O.; Chamontin, B.; Delemer, B.; Giraud, S.; Murat, A.; et al. Genetic testing in pheochromocytoma or functional paraganglioma. *J. Clin. Oncol.* **2005**, *23*, 8812–8818. [CrossRef]
24. Van Hulsteijn, L.T.; Dekkers, O.M.; Hes, F.J.; Smit, J.W.; Corssmit, E.P. Risk of malignant paraganglioma in SDHB-mutation and SDHD-mutation carriers: A systematic review and meta-analysis. *J. Med. Genet.* **2012**, *49*, 768–776. [CrossRef] [PubMed]
25. Hulsteijn, L.T.; den Dulk, A.C.; Hes, F.J.; Bayley, J.P.; Jansen, J.C.; Corssmit, E.P.M. No difference in phenotype of the main Dutch SDHD founder mutations. *Clin. Endocrinol.* **2013**, *79*, 824–831. [CrossRef] [PubMed]
26. Kapetanakis, S.; Chourmouzi, D.; Gkasdaris, G.; Katsaridis, V.; Eleftheriadis, E.; Givissis, P. Functional extra-adrenal paraganglioma of the retroperitoneum giving thoracolumbar spine metastases after a five-year disease-free follow-up: A rare malignant condition with challenging management. *Pan Afr. Med. J.* **2017**, *28*, 94. [CrossRef] [PubMed]

27. Valadea, S.; Chazeraina, P.; Khaninea, V.; Lazardb, T.; Baudinc, E.; Zizaa, J.M. Late bone metastases of a pheochromocytoma. *Rev. Med. Interne* **2010**, *31*, 772–775.
28. Papaspyrou, K.; Mann, W.J.; Amedee, R.G. Management of head and neck paragangliomas: Review of 120 patients. *Head Neck* **2009**, *31*, 381–387. [CrossRef] [PubMed]

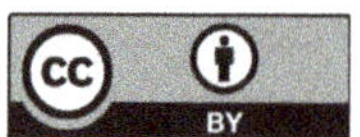

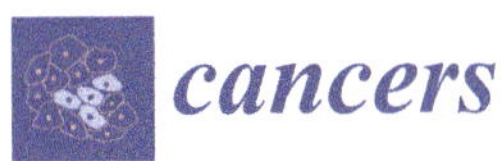
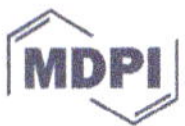
Article

^{11}C-hydroxy-ephedrine-PET/CT in the Diagnosis of Pheochromocytoma and Paraganglioma

Achyut Ram Vyakaranam [1,4,*], Joakim Crona [2,3], Olov Norlén [4], Per Hellman [4] and Anders Sundin [1,4]

1 Section of Radiology & Molecular Imaging, Department of Surgical Sciences, Uppsala University, Akademiska Sjukhuset, SE-751 85 Uppsala, Sweden; anders.sundin@radiol.uu.se
2 Department of Medical Sciences, Uppsala University, Akademiska Sjukhuset, SE-751 85 Uppsala, Sweden; joakim.crona@medsci.uu.se
3 Department of Immunology, Genetics and Pathology, Uppsala University, Akademiska Sjukhuset, SE-751 85 Uppsala, Sweden
4 Department of Surgical Sciences, Uppsala University, Akademiska Sjukhuset, SE-751 85 Uppsala, Sweden; olov.norlen@surgsci.uu.se (O.N.); per.hellman@surgsci.uu.se (P.H.)
* Correspondence: achyutram.vyakaranam@surgsci.uu.se

Received: 11 June 2019; Accepted: 16 June 2019; Published: 19 June 2019

Abstract: Pheochromocytomas (PCC) and paragangliomas (PGL) may be difficult to diagnose because of vague and uncharacteristic symptoms and equivocal biochemical and radiological findings. This was a retrospective cohort study in 102 patients undergoing ^{11}C-hydroxy-ephedrine (^{11}C-HED)-PET/CT because of symptoms and/or biochemistry suspicious for PCC/PGL and/or with radiologically equivocal adrenal incidentalomas. Correlations utilized CT/MRI, clinical, biochemical, surgical, histopathological and follow-up data. ^{11}C-HED-PET/CT correctly identified 19 patients with PCC and six with PGL, missed one PCC, attained one false positive result (nodular hyperplasia) and correctly excluded PCC/PGL in 75 patients. Sensitivity, specificity, positive and negative predictive values of ^{11}C-HED-PET/CT for PCC/PGL diagnosis was 96%, 99%, 96% and 99%, respectively. In 41 patients who underwent surgical resection and for whom correlation to histopathology was available, the corresponding figures were 96%, 93%, 96% and 93%, respectively. Tumor ^{11}C-HED-uptake measurements (standardized uptake value, tumor-to-normal-adrenal ratio) were unrelated to symptoms of catecholamine excess ($p > 0.05$) and to systolic blood pressure ($p > 0.05$). In PCC/PGL patients, norepinephrine and systolic blood pressure increased in parallel ($R^2 = 0.22$, $p = 0.016$). ^{11}C-HED-PET/CT was found to be an accurate tool to diagnose and rule out PCC/PGL in complex clinical scenarios and for the characterization of equivocal adrenal incidentalomas. PET measurements of tumor ^{11}C-HED uptake were not helpful for tumor characterization.

Keywords: pheochromocytoma; paraganglioma; PET-CT; ^{11}C-hydroxy-ephedrine; adrenal incidentaloma

1. Introduction

Pheochromocytoma (PCC) and paraganglioma (PGL) are rare, catecholamine-producing chromaffin cell tumors arising from the adrenal gland or extra-adrenal paraganglia, respectively [1–3]. These tumors may be difficult to recognize due to uncharacteristic symptomatology mimicking that of more common disorders. The diagnosis in patients with suspected PCC/PGL can be established by biochemical testing, revealing high levels of plasma/urinary catecholamines and/or catecholamine metabolites [4,5].

However, a vast majority of patients who require imaging work-up and hormonal testing to exclude PCC/PGL have so-called "adrenal incidentalomas," found on imaging that was performed because of reasons other than adrenal disease. Due to the rapid increase in the use of cross-sectional imaging and the fact that incidentalomas are found in approximately 5% of CT examinations, the characterization and follow-up of adrenal incidentalomas places increasing demands on healthcare resources [6,7]. Tumor attenuation measurements on non-contrast-enhanced CT or in/out-of-phase MRI, will in many patients allow for the characterization of lipid-rich adrenocortical adenomas, and the majority of the remaining uncharacterized incidentalomas can later be discarded based on the absence of tumor growth on follow-up imaging [8,9].

Another challenging scenario is when a primary tumor cannot be localized on CT/MRI in biochemically suspected PCC/PGL. In these situations, CT/MRI may be supplemented by functional imaging to depict and characterize the tumor and increase the imaging sensitivity and specificity [10]. Several nuclear medicine imaging tracers are available for positron emission tomography (PET)[11] and scintigraphy, including single-photon emission tomography (SPECT). The general PET-tracer ^{18}F-fluoro-deoxy-glucose (^{18}F-FDG) provides information on tumor metabolism [12], whereas more specialized tracers target specific pathways such as ^{123}I-meta-iodo-benzoguanidine (^{123}I-MIBG) [13] for scintigraphy,^{18}F-dihydroxy-fluoro-L-phenylalanine (^{18}F-DOPA) [14–19],^{18}F-Dopamine (^{18}F-DA) [20–23],^{68}Ga-DOTA-somatostatin analogs [15,24–27] and ^{11}C- hydroxy ephedrine (^{11}C-HED) [28–32] for PET/CT. ^{11}C-HED is a norepinephrine analog that binds to the norepinephrine transporter and has previously shown high diagnostic sensitivity and specificity in patients with PCC/PGL [28], including post-operative surveillance following PCC/PGL resection [29] as well as for other tumors such as neuroblastoma [33,34].

The aim of this study was to assess the value of ^{11}C-HED-PET/CT to diagnose or rule out PCC/PGL in complex clinical scenarios by allowing for tumor detection and/or characterization in patients with equivocal symptoms and/or biochemical and/or CT/MRI findings, in whom conventional work-up had failed to guide the clinical decision.

2. Results

2.1. Baseline Patient Characteristics

Median age in the 102 patients was 58 ± 2 years, with a male to female ratio of 1:1. Results from genetic testing was available in only eight patients; Multiple Endocrine Neoplasia type 2A was diagnosed in three patients (patients 10, 11, 12, Table 3), SDHB-related PGL in three patients (patients 21, 23, 25, Table 4), one had Neurofibromatosis type 1 and one had Multiple Endocrine Neoplasia type 2B (patients 7 and 9, respectively, Table 3). The patients presented with symptoms suspicious for PCC/PGL (n = 68), elevated biochemistry (n = 29) or borderline biochemistry (n = 57) and radiologically uncharacterized tumors (n = 26, out of which 16 presented as incidentalomas), or a combination thereof. The tumors in the latter 26 patients had not been possible to characterize on CT/MRI based on general radiological appearance in combination with attenuation measurements, contrast medium washout and results of in- and out-of-phase MRI. Also, several patients harbored bilateral tumors. Because the previous conventional work-up for adrenal disease had failed to provide the diagnosis, or to rule out PCC/PGL, they subsequently underwent ^{11}C-HED-PET/CT.

2.2. Diagnostic Performance

A flow chart of the study is presented in Figure 1. The results of ^{11}C-HED-PET/CT are shown in Tables 1 and 2. With correlation to a combined gold standard, comprising histopathology, biochemical diagnosis, findings at surgery and on radiological and clinical follow-up, ^{11}C-HED-PET/CT in the 102 patients showed 96% sensitivity, 99% specificity, 96% positive predictive value and 99% negative predictive value (Table 1). When the ^{11}C-HED-PET/CT results were strictly correlated to tumor histopathology, as the gold standard (n = 41), the sensitivity, specificity, positive predictive value and negative predictive value were 96%, 93%, 96% and 93%, respectively (Table 2).

Table 1. ^{11}C-HED-PET/CT results in all 102 patients with correlation to findings at surgery, histopathology, biochemistry, clinical and radiological follow-up (combined gold standard).

		Gold standard	
		Positive	Negative
^{11}C-HED-PET/CT	Positive	25	1
	Negative	1	75

Table 2. ^{11}C-HED-PET/CT results in the 41 patients operated on, with correlation to findings at surgery and histopathology (gold standard).

		Gold standard	
		Positive	Negative
^{11}C-HED-PET/CT	Positive	25	1
	Negative	1	14

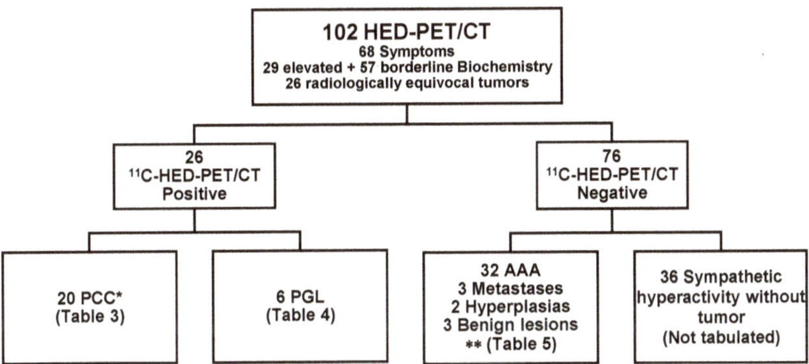

Figure 1. Flowchart of the 102 study patients. ^{11}C-HED-PET/CT visualized 20 PCC (Table 3) and six PGL (Table 4) and ruled out PCC/PGL in 76 patients, including 40 patients with adrenal tumors (Table S1) and 36 without tumors. * including one false negative ^{11}C-HED-PET/CT result, ** including one false positive PET/CT result. AAA; adrenocortical adenoma.

2.3. Tabulated Results

Table 3 shows the results for the patients with histopathologically confirmed PCC ($n = 20$). Table 4 displays the results for the patients with extra-adrenal tumors, which on subsequent histopathology were diagnosed as PGLs ($n = 6$). Table S1 (Supplementary Materials) gives the results for the 40 patients with ^{11}C-HED-negative adrenal tumors. The remaining 36/102 patients without an adrenal tumor on CT, and in whom ^{11}C-HED-PET/CT ruled out PCC/PGL, are not tabulated.

Out of the 20 PCC patients (Table 3), eight had symptoms indicating catecholamine excess and 12 presented with adrenal incidentaloma on CT/MRI. The PCC was bilateral in four patients and unilateral in 16, of whom one patient had a PCC (^{11}C-HED-positive) together with an adrenocortical adenoma (^{11}C-HED-negative) in the same adrenal (collision tumor). The only patient for whom ^{11}C-HED-PET/CT was false negative harbored a PCC in one adrenal gland and a hyperplasia in the other (Patient 19, Table 3). The PCCs measured 1–8 cm in size, with a mean of 2.9 cm.

Out of the six patients with histopathologically confirmed PGL (Table 4), four presented with symptoms and/or biochemistry indicating catecholamine excess and two with adrenal incidentaloma on CT/MRI. One patient (Patient 26, Table 4) with a ^{11}C-HED-negative tumor in the neck was diagnosed with a ^{11}C-HED positive metastasis to the right femur. The PGLs measured 4–7 cm in size, with a mean of 4.8 cm.

Table 3. CT characteristics and ^{11}C-HED-PET/CT parameters in the 20 patients with histopathologically confirmed pheochromocytoma (PCC) including 19 who were correctly characterized by ^{11}C-HED-PET/CT and one false negative ^{11}C-HED-PET/CT result (*). HT; hypertension, NET; neuroendocrine tumor, BP; blood pressure, CECT; contrast-enhanced CT, AAA; adrenocortical adenoma, L; left, R; right, A; epinephrine, NA; nor-epinephrine, A-Ref; ratio of value and upper normal reference range value, NA-Ref; ratio of value and upper normal reference range value.

Pat No.	Age	Sex	Clinical Information	Incidenta -loma	Systolic BP	Diagnosis (PAD)	NA -Ref	A-Ref	A/N Ratio
1	45	F	Sweating, palpitations anxiety	Y	220	L PCC R AAA	11.5	1.00	0.09
2	73	F	Palpitations, headache, HT, alpha blocker	Y	150	R PCC+AAA	2.00	3.50	1.75
3	67	F	Sweating, headache, alpha blocker	Y	150	R PCC L AAA	1.33	1.00	0.75
4	48	F	Anxiety, palpitations, muscle fasciculations, alpha blocker	Y	150	PCC	12.8	1.00	0.08
5	85	F	Rectal cancer Incidentaloma	Y	140	PCC with cystic areas	10.7	1.00	0.09
6	53	F	Polycystic kidney disease, HT	Y	180	PCC	1.00	5.00	5.00
7	52	M	No symptom	Y	190	PCC	2.00	1.44	0.72
8	71	F	Breast cancer, small-intestinal NET	Y	150	PCC	0.56	0.51	0.92
9	19	F	Bilateral incidentalomas	Y	180	PCC	1.83	3.50	1.91
10	58	F	Palpitations, alpha blocker	Y	130	PCC	1.33	1.00	0.75
11	28	F	No symptoms	Y	120	PCC	1.56	2.13	1.37
12	30	F	Palpitations, panic attack	N	110	PCC	1.33	3.02	2.27
13	72	F	Sweating, alpha blocker	N	220	PCC	3.74	1.67	0.45
14	50	F	Palpitations, headache, HT	N	215	PCC	61.7	95.0	1.54
15	59	M	Incidentaloma	Y	200	PCC	1.00	2.50	2.50
16	42	F	Palpitations, sweating, headache, tremor	N	130	PCC with cystic areas	2.68	9.80	3.66
17	58	F	Sweating, palpitations HT, alpha blocker	N	170	PCC with necrosis	8.83	39.5	4.47
18	64	M	HT, alpha blocker	N	220	PCC with necrosis	22.3	107	4.77
19	61	F	Headache, flushing, sweating, palpitations, alpha blocker	N	230	L PCC* R hyperplasia	11.4	3.89	0.34
20	65	F	Sweating, palpitations, alpha blocker	N	140	PCC	2	1	0.5

Table 4. CT characteristics and PET/CT parameters in six patients with ^{11}C-HED uptake in extra-adrenal sites that, after surgery, were histopathologically confirmed as paragangliomas (PGL). HT; hypertension, BP; blood pressure, ND; not done, HU; Hounsfield Units, CECT; contrast-enhanced CT, A; epinephrine, NA; norepinephrine.

Pat No.	Age	Sex	Clinical Information	Inci-denta -loma	Systolic BP	Location	Diagnosis (PAD)	P-met-tyramine (< 0.2)	NA	A	A/NARatio
21	60	F	Back pain	Y	145	Para-aortic	PGL	0.4	6.17	0.67	0.11
22	34	F	Headache, palpitations	N	220	Pre-aortic	PGL	ND	18.3	0.67	0.04
23	16	M	Palpitations, headache, HT	N	180	Pre-aortic	PGL	ND	1.67	2.00	1.20
24	71	M	Abdominal pain	N	130	Pre-aortic	PGL	1.1	0.50	0.67	1.33
25	56	M	Abdominal pain	Y	180	Pre-aortic	PGL	0.5	2.50	0.67	0.27
26	70	M	Unclear symptoms	N	135	Neck	PGL	0.8	2.33	0.67	0.29

Out of 40 patients with ^{11}C-HED-PET/CT-negative adrenal tumors (Table S1, Supplementary Materials), nine patients with symptoms of catecholamines excess and equivocal biochemistry underwent surgery and the histopathological examination showed adrenocortical adenomas. CT-guided biopsy in two patients revealed in both metastasis from lung adenocarcinoma. Bilateral ^{11}C-HED-positive adrenals were found in one patient who underwent surgery and multinodular hyperplasia was diagnosed an histopathology and constituted the only false positive ^{11}C-HED-PET/CT result (Patient 45, Table S1). The diagnoses in the remaining 28 patients were based on extended radiological and clinical follow-up.

2.4. ^{11}C-HED Accumulation and Uptake Measurements

^{11}C-HED was found to generally accumulate throughout the extent of the whole tumor, but in five patients showed heterogeneous, predominately peripheral ^{11}C-HED uptake, because of extended tumor necrosis (Figure 2).

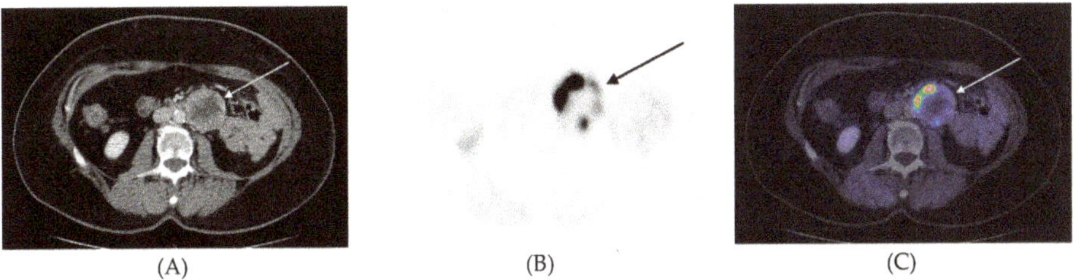

(A) (B) (C)

Figure 2. Transverse ^{11}C-HED-PET/CT images, (**A**) CT, (**B**) PET, (**C**) PET/CT fusion, of patient #21 (Table 4) with a retroperitoneal paraganglioma left of the descending aorta (arrows). In this paraganglioma there was extended necrosis and merely peripheral tracer accumulation in the tumor.

The ^{11}C-HED-PET measurements are shown in Tables S2 and S3 (Supplementary Materials). For the PCCs and PGLs ($n = 26$), no correlation was found between tumor SUVmax and tumor size ($R^2 = 0.05$, $p = 0.286$) The SUVmax and the tumor-to-liver ratio was significantly higher in tumors larger than 4 cm ($p = 0.045$, $p = 0.033$).

The systolic BP was less than 140 mmHg in 34 patients, between 140 and 180 mmHg in 39 subjects and exceeded 180 mmHg in 24 patients. The tumor SUVmax and the tumor-to-liver ratio were unrelated to the systolic BP, and also to symptoms of catecholamine excess.

In PCC & PGL patients with ^{11}C-HED-positive tumors, norepinephrine somewhat correlated with the systolic BP ($R^2 = 0.22$, $p = 0.016$) and increased in parallel. Patients with high norepinephrine had higher systolic BP (cutoff = twice the upper reference value, $p = 0.025$, cutoff = 10 times the upper reference value ($p = 0.013$). The tumor SUVmax and the tumor-to liver ratio was higher in patients with high norepinephrine (cutoff = 10 times the upper reference value, $p = 0.009$).

3. Discussion

In this study, ^{11}C-HED-PET/CT in a cohort of 102 patients with suspected PCC/PGL, based on equivocal clinical symptoms and/or biochemical and/or radiological findings, showed 96% sensitivity, 99% specificity, 96% positive predictive value and 99% negative predictive value. These data provide additional evidence that ^{11}C-HED-PET/CT can be used in the diagnostic work-up of patients with suspected PCC/PGL in whom the conventional clinical, biochemical and radiological work-up failed to provide diagnosis, or to exclude PCC/PGL.

Since 2005, our center has used ^{11}C-HED-PET/CT as a problem-solving tool in patients with suspected PCC/PGL, for postoperative surveillance, therapy monitoring and diagnosis of recurrent disease. A combined evaluation of ^{11}C-HED-PET and ^{11}C-HED-PET/CT, performed for several of these indications, has shown favorable diagnostic capacity [26]. In the present work, we instead concentrated on exclusively evaluating ^{11}C-HED-PET/CT performed for the sole purpose of primary diagnosis (or ruling out disease) in patients with suspected PCC/PGL.

In this retrospective setting, ^{11}C-HED was not compared with other PET tracers. ^{11}C-HED is not generally available and the 20 min half-life of ^{11}C is another inconveniency. PET tracers labeled with ^{18}F or ^{68}Ga (110 and 68 min half-life, respectively) are advantageous in this respect. The common metabolic PET tracer ^{18}F-FDG shows low specificity and lower diagnostic yield than ^{18}F-DOPA and ^{68}Ga-DOTA-somatostatin analogs [35].^{18}F-FDG has, however, been shown to be highly sensitive in the detection of *SDHB*-related PCCs/PGLs [36]. The sensitivity of ^{18}F-DOPA-PET/CT depends on the tumor type and, in a direct comparison, ^{68}Ga-DOTATATE has the advantage of fairly high availability and was better than ^{18}F-DOPA at visualizing PCCs but less sensitive for HNPGLs [15]. In 101 PCC/PGL patients, ^{18}F-DOPA showed 93% sensitivity and 88% specificity [37]. In a comparative PET/CT study in PCC/PGL patients, ^{18}F-DA was considered the preferred tracer, followed by ^{18}F-DOPA and ^{18}F-FDG [22].

CT/MRI characterization of PCC is a challenge because these tumors display a wide range of appearances [38]. PCC is therefore, in this sense, sometimes referred to as a chameleon among adrenal tumors. This was illustrated by the fact that the most abundant CT/MRI findings in our patients instead were tumor heterogeneity, necrosis and irregular margins. Interestingly, the CT/MRI findings were consistent with adrenocortical adenomas in nine patients (Tables 2 and 4). ^{11}C-HED-PET/CT was nevertheless performed because of equivocal biochemistry/symptoms to rule out PCC/PGL in other locations. An important example in this respect, is the ^{11}C-HED-positive patient (2, Table 2) harboring a PCC together with a benign adrenocortical adenoma ("collision tumor") (Figure 3).

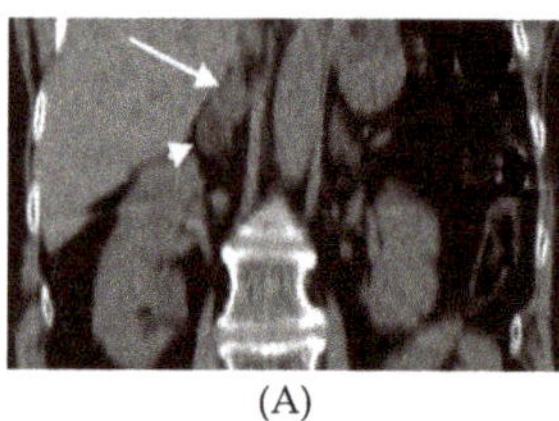
(A)

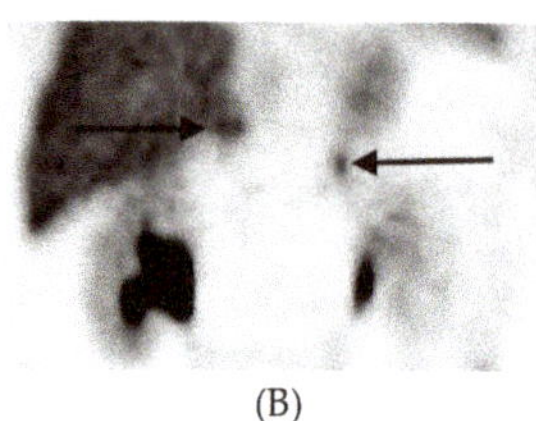
(B)

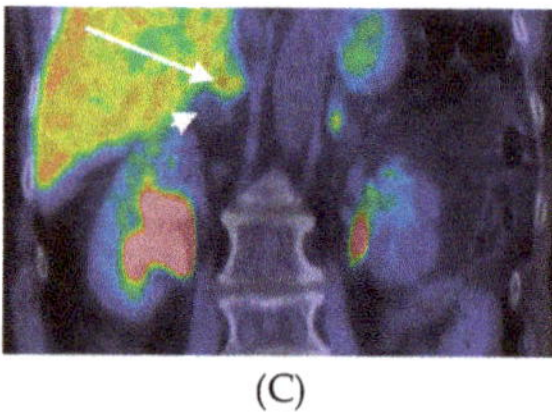
(C)

Figure 3. ^{11}C-HED-PET/CT, coronal mages, of patient #2 (Table 3) with a collision tumor in the right adrenal showing a cranial component with high tracer uptake comprising a PCC (arrows) and a caudal tumor portion representing an adrenocortical adenoma (arrow head). The normal contralateral adrenal is indicated with an arrow in the PET image. (**A**) CT, (**B**) PET, (**C**) PET/CT fusion.

Patients with biochemistry and/or symptoms consistent with PCC/PGL and the CT/MRI findings of an adrenal tumor usually undergo surgical resection. However, 16 such patients nevertheless underwent ^{11}C-HED-PET/CT, because of bilateral tumors, to localize possible extra-adrenal lesions and to assess the local tumor extent. When a tumor cannot be localized by CT/MRI, despite biochemistry and/or symptoms consistent with PCC/PGL, ^{11}C-HED-PET/CT can be useful to identify the PCC in cases of bilateral adrenal tumors and tumors of extra-adrenal origin. Further, ^{11}C-HED-PET/CT was found instrumental for ruling out PCC/PGL in 78 of our patients, in whom CT could not provide firm evidence on the origin of the tumor. Only PCC was missed (patient 19, Table 3), and the only false positive PET/CT result was represented by a nodular hyperplasia (patient 45, Table S1).

Interesting findings were encountered in a patient (26, Table 4) with a ^{11}C-HED negative primary HNPGL but with a ^{11}C-HED-positive metastasis in the left femur. Histopathology showed a parasympathetic paraganglioma with high proliferation (Ki-67 index 20%). Parasympathetic paraganglioma cannot be expected to be ^{11}C-HED-positive and the fact that the metastasis showed ^{11}C-HED uptake is intriguing and difficult to explain. Notably, ^{18}F-FDG-PET/CT in this patient showed both lesions to be ^{18}F-FDG avid. Sympathetic paragangliomas were, however, all visualized ^{11}C-HED, including metastases (Figure 4).

Some weaknesses in our study were its retrospective and single design and the fact that surgical and histopathological confirmation of the ^{11}C-HED-PET/CT findings was not provided for all patients. However, we believe that the extended clinical, biochemical and imaging follow-up of the patients provided us with unique material that may compensate for this absence of histopathological confirmation. We provide data from morphological imaging (CT) but no comparison with molecular imaging, and a prospective comparative PET/CT study primarily with ^{18}F-FDG and ^{68}Ga-DOTA-somatostatin analog is therefore warranted.

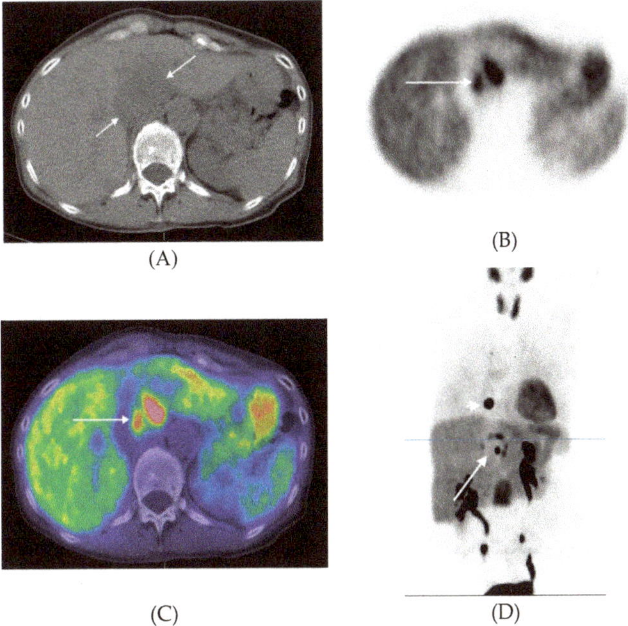

Figure 4. ^{11}C-HED-PET/CT of patient #24 (Table 4) with a retroperitoneal paraganglioma in front of the descending aorta with high heterogenous tracer uptake (long arrows) and a metastasis in the transverse process of the thoracic vertebra 10 shown in D (short arrow). In the coronal PET image an additional vertebral metastasis in the first lumbar vertebra is seen projected between the kidneys. (**A**) Transversal CT, (**B**) Transversal PET, (**C**) Transversal PET/CT fusion, (**D**) Coronal PET (Maximum Intensity Projection). The level of the transversal images are indicated in the coronal PET image (line).

4. Patients and Methods

4.1. Patients

This was a retrospective cohort study of 102 patients investigated at the Department of Nuclear Medicine, Uppsala University Hospital, Uppsala, Sweden. The study was approved by the Regional Ethics Committee (No. 2012/422). All patients that underwent ^{11}C-HED-PET/CT were screened for inclusion using information available through the digital radiological information and picture archive and retrieval systems (RIS-PACS). We selected those who underwent PET/CT examination between March 2005 to September 2017. Patients having undergone PET/CT for postoperative surveillance were excluded. Clinical, biochemical and radiological imaging follow-up data were retrieved from the RIS-PACS and from the hospital's digital patient record system.

4.2. ^{11}C-Hydroxy-ephedrine-PET/CT Examination

From March 2005, a GE Discovery ST PET/CT scanner was used (General Electric Medical Systems, Milwaukee, WI, USA). The PET scanner produced 47 slices with a 157 mm axial field of view (FOV) and 700 mm trans-axial FOV. Patients were injected with approximately 800 MBq of ^{11}C-HED and static whole-body images were obtained 20 min later, from the base of the skull to the upper thighs. The spatial resolution was equal to that of the individual crystal size in the block, approximately 5-6 mm. A non-contrast-enhanced, low-radiation-dose CT examination was performed before the PET acquisition for attenuation correction of the PET images and for anatomical correlation of the PET findings.

4.3. Image Analysis and Interpretation

Qualitative image interpretation and PET measurements were first performed by one of the authors (ARV) and then again in a second reading session together with a radiologist with 25 years of PET experience (AS) and a common consensus was reached regarding the image findings. Image reading and PET measurements were performed on a computer workstation connected to the hospital's PACS system. Any focal accumulation of ^{11}C-HED exceeding the normal physiological uptake was regarded as pathological. A tumor with a ^{11}C-HED uptake higher than that of the contralateral normal adrenal was considered ^{11}C-HED-positive and consistent with PCC/PGL. Moderate physiological tracer uptake in regions such as the salivary glands, myocardium, liver, spleen, pancreas and normal adrenal medulla was disregarded.

Quantification of ^{11}C-HED uptake in tumors utilized the standardized uptake value (SUV), which was calculated for each pixel by dividing its radioactivity concentration (Bq/mL) by the injected radioactivity (Bq) per gram of body-weight. Regions of interest (ROIs) were drawn manually to measure SUVmax (the maximum pixels in the ROI) in each lesion. Also, as a normal tissue reference, a 2-cm circular ROI was drawn in the posterior part of the right liver lobe and the SUVmean was registered. The tumor-to-liver ratio was calculated as tumor SUV_{max}/normal liver SUV_{mean}. In patients with adrenal tumors, the SUV_{max} of the contralateral normal adrenal was additionally assessed and the tumor-to normal-adrenal ratio was calculated.

Plasma and urinary epinephrine and norepinephrine samples were for matters of comparison normalized to the upper reference value and correlated to^{11}C-HED uptake measurements.

4.4. Statistical Analysis

Data were presented as mean ± standard deviation (SD). Differences in means between groups were evaluated using a *t*-test assuming unequal variances. Pearson's correlation test was performed to evaluate the relationship between variables. All statistical analyses were performed in IBM® SPSS® Statistics V.24 and JMP 13.1 (SAS Institute, Inc., Cary, NC, USA). $p < 0.05$ was regarded significant.

5. Conclusions

In conclusion, ^{11}C-HED-PET/CT is a valuable tool in complex clinical scenarios, with findings of biochemistry/symptoms/radiology suspicious of PCC/PGL, when conventional work-up fails to diagnose or rule out disease. ^{11}C-HED uptake measurements were, however, unable to assist with the tumor characterization.

Supplementary Materials: The following are available online at http://www.mdpi.com/2072-6694/11/6/847/s1, Table S1: CT and PET/CT parameters in 40 patients with 11C-HED-negative tumors, Table S2: Size and 11C-HED accumulation (standardized uptake value, SUV) in 11C-HED-PET/CT positive tumors, Table S3: Statistical analysis of various parameters using t-test assuming unequal variances.

Author Contributions: Conceptualization, A.S. and P.H.; Methodology, A.S.; Validation, A.R.V., A.S.; and J.C.; Formal Analysis, A.R.V.; and A.S.;. Investigation, A.R.V.; and A.S.;. Data Curation, A.R.V.; and A.S.; Writing—Original Draft Preparation, A.R.V.; Writing—A.R.V.; A.S.; P.H.; O.N.; J.C.; Review & Editing, J.C.; Supervision, A.S.; and P.H.

Funding: This research received no external funding.

Conflicts of Interest: Joakim Crona received lecture honoraria from Novartis and Educational Honoraria from NET Connect (funded by IPSEN). Anders Sundin received lecture honoraria from Ipsen. The other authors declare no potential conflicts of interest.

References

1. Kantorovich, V.; Pacak, K. Pheochromocytoma and Paraganglioma. In *Progress in Brain Research*; Elsevier: Amsterdam, The Netherlands, 2010; Volume 182, pp. 343–373. ISBN 978-0-444-53616-7.
2. Bravo, E.L. Evolving Concepts in the Pathophysiology, Diagnosis, and Treatment of Pheochromocytoma. *Endocr. Rev.* **1994**, *15*, 356–368. [CrossRef] [PubMed]

3. Lenders, J.W.; Eisenhofer, G.; Mannelli, M.; Pacak, K. Phaeochromocytoma. *Lancet* **2005**, *366*, 665–675. [CrossRef]
4. Lenders, J.W.M.; Pacak, K.; Walther, M.M.; Linehan, W.M.; Mannelli, M.; Friberg, P.; Keiser, H.R.; Goldstein, D.S.; Eisenhofer, G. Biochemical diagnosis of pheochromocytoma: Which test is best? *JAMA* **2002**, *287*, 1427–1434. [CrossRef] [PubMed]
5. Lenders, J.W.M.; Duh, Q.-Y.; Eisenhofer, G.; Gimenez-Roqueplo, A.-P.; Grebe, S.K.G.; Murad, M.H.; Naruse, M.; Pacak, K.; Young, W.F. Pheochromocytoma and Paraganglioma: An Endocrine Society Clinical Practice Guideline. *J. Clin. Endocrinol. Metab.* **2014**, *99*, 1915–1942. [CrossRef] [PubMed]
6. Song, J.H.; Chaudhry, F.S.; Mayo-Smith, W.W. The Incidental Adrenal Mass on CT: Prevalence of Adrenal Disease in 1,049 Consecutive Adrenal Masses in Patients with No Known Malignancy. *Am. J. Roentgenol.* **2008**, *190*, 1163–1168. [CrossRef] [PubMed]
7. Hammarstedt, L.; Muth, A.; Wängberg, B.; Björneld, L.; Sigurjónsdóttir, H.A.; Götherström, G.; Almqvist, E.; Widell, H.; Carlsson, S.; Ander, S.; et al. Adrenal lesion frequency: A prospective, cross-sectional CT study in a defined region, including systematic re-evaluation. *Acta Radiol.* **2010**, *51*, 1149–1156. [CrossRef]
8. Blake, M.A.; Cronin, C.G.; Boland, G.W. Adrenal Imaging. *Am. J. Roentgenol.* **2010**, *194*, 1450–1460. [CrossRef] [PubMed]
9. Morelli, V.; Scillitani, A.; Arosio, M.; Chiodini, I. Follow-up of patients with adrenal incidentaloma, in accordance with the European society of endocrinology guidelines: Could we be safe? *J. Endocrinol. Investig.* **2017**, *40*, 331–333. [CrossRef]
10. Brito, J.P.; Asi, N.; Gionfriddo, M.R.; Norman, C.; Leppin, A.L.; Zeballos-Palacios, C.; Undavalli, C.; Wang, Z.; Domecq, J.P.; Prustsky, G.; et al. The incremental benefit of functional imaging in pheochromocytoma/paraganglioma: A systematic review. *Endocrine* **2015**, *50*, 176–186. [CrossRef]
11. Taieb, D.; Neumann, H.; Rubello, D.; Al-Nahhas, A.; Guillet, B.; Hindie, E. Modern Nuclear Imaging for Paragangliomas: Beyond SPECT. *J. Nucl. Med.* **2012**, *53*, 264–274. [CrossRef]
12. Shulkin, B.L.; Thompson, N.W.; Shapiro, B.; Francis, I.R.; Sisson, J.C. Pheochromocytomas: Imaging with 2-[Fluorine-18]fluoro-2-deoxy-D-glucose PET. *Radiology* **1999**, *212*, 35–41. [CrossRef] [PubMed]
13. Berglund, A.S.; Hulthén, U.L.; Manhem, P.; Thorsson, O.; Wollmer, P.; Törnquist, C. Metaiodobenzylguanidine (MIBG) scintigraphy and computed tomography (CT) in clinical practice. Primary and secondary evaluation for localization of phaeochromocytomas. *J. Intern. Med.* **2001**, *249*, 247–251. [CrossRef] [PubMed]
14. Hoegerle, S.; Nitzsche, E.; Altehoefer, C.; Ghanem, N.; Manz, T.; Brink, I.; Reincke, M.; Moser, E.; Neumann, H.P.H. Pheochromocytomas: Detection with ^{18} F DOPA Whole-Body PET—Initial Results. *Radiology* **2002**, *222*, 507–512. [CrossRef] [PubMed]
15. Archier, A.; Varoquaux, A.; Garrigue, P.; Montava, M.; Guerin, C.; Gabriel, S.; Beschmout, E.; Morange, I.; Fakhry, N.; Castinetti, F.; et al. Prospective comparison of (68)Ga-DOTATATE and (18)F-FDOPA PET/CT in patients with various pheochromocytomas and paragangliomas with emphasis on sporadic cases. *Eur. J. Nucl. Med. Mol. Imaging* **2016**, *43*, 1248–1257. [CrossRef] [PubMed]
16. Moog, S.; Houy, S.; Chevalier, E.; Ory, S.; Weryha, G.; Rame, M.; Klein, M.; Brunaud, L.; Gasman, S.; Cuny, T. 18F-FDOPA PET/CT Uptake Parameters Correlate with Catecholamine Secretion in Human Pheochromocytomas. *Neuroendocrinology* **2018**, *107*, 228–236. [CrossRef] [PubMed]
17. Santhanam, P.; Taïeb, D. Role of (18) F-FDOPA PET/CT imaging in endocrinology. *Clin. Endocrinol. (Oxf.)* **2014**, *81*, 789–798. [CrossRef]
18. Timmers, H.J.L.M.; Chen, C.C.; Carrasquillo, J.A.; Whatley, M.; Ling, A.; Havekes, B.; Eisenhofer, G.; Martiniova, L.; Adams, K.T.; Pacak, K. Comparison of 18F-Fluoro-L-DOPA, 18F-Fluoro-Deoxyglucose, and 18F-Fluorodopamine PET and 123I-MIBG Scintigraphy in the Localization of Pheochromocytoma and Paraganglioma. *J. Clin. Endocrinol. Metab.* **2009**, *94*, 4757–4767. [CrossRef]
19. Amodru, V.; Guerin, C.; Delcourt, S.; Romanet, P.; Loundou, A.; Viana, B.; Brue, T.; Castinetti, F.; Sebag, F.; Pacak, K.; et al. Quantitative 18F-DOPA PET/CT in pheochromocytoma: The relationship between tumor secretion and its biochemical phenotype. *Eur. J. Nucl. Med. Mol. Imaging* **2018**, *45*, 278–282. [CrossRef]
20. Ilias, I.; Chen, C.C.; Carrasquillo, J.A.; Whatley, M.; Ling, A.; Lazúrová, I.; Adams, K.T.; Perera, S.; Pacak, K. Comparison of 6-18F-fluorodopamine PET with 123I-metaiodobenzylguanidine and 111in-pentetreotide scintigraphy in localization of nonmetastatic and metastatic pheochromocytoma. *J. Nucl. Med. Off. Publ. Soc. Nucl. Med.* **2008**, *49*, 1613–1619. [CrossRef]

21. Ilias, I.; Yu, J.; Carrasquillo, J.A.; Chen, C.C.; Eisenhofer, G.; Whatley, M.; McElroy, B.; Pacak, K. Superiority of 6-[18F]-Fluorodopamine Positron Emission Tomography *Versus* [131I]-Metaiodobenzylguanidine Scintigraphy in the Localization of Metastatic Pheochromocytoma. *J. Clin. Endocrinol. Metab.* **2003**, *88*, 4083–4087. [CrossRef]
22. Timmers, H.J.L.M.; Eisenhofer, G.; Carrasquillo, J.A.; Chen, C.C.; Whatley, M.; Ling, A.; Adams, K.T.; Pacak, K. Use of 6-[18F]-fluorodopamine positron emission tomography (PET) as first-line investigation for the diagnosis and localization of non-metastatic and metastatic phaeochromocytoma (PHEO). *Clin. Endocrinol. (Oxf.)* **2009**, *71*, 11–17. [CrossRef] [PubMed]
23. Kaji, P.; Carrasquillo, J.A.; Linehan, W.M.; Chen, C.C.; Eisenhofer, G.; Pinto, P.A.; Lai, E.W.; Pacak, K. The role of 6-[18F]fluorodopamine positron emission tomography in the localization of adrenal pheochromocytoma associated with von Hippel–Lindau syndrome. *Eur. J. Endocrinol.* **2007**, *156*, 483–487. [CrossRef] [PubMed]
24. Gild, M.L.; Naik, N.; Hoang, J.; Hsiao, E.; McGrath, R.T.; Sywak, M.; Sidhu, S.; Delbridge, L.W.; Robinson, B.G.; Schembri, G.; et al. Role of DOTATATE-PET/CT in preoperative assessment of phaeochromocytoma and paragangliomas. *Clin. Endocrinol. (Oxf.)* **2018**, *89*, 139–147. [CrossRef]
25. Janssen, I.; Chen, C.C.; Millo, C.M.; Ling, A.; Taieb, D.; Lin, F.I.; Adams, K.T.; Wolf, K.I.; Herscovitch, P.; Fojo, A.T.; et al. PET/CT comparing 68Ga-DOTATATE and other radiopharmaceuticals and in comparison with CT/MRI for the localization of sporadic metastatic pheochromocytoma and paraganglioma. *Eur. J. Nucl. Med. Mol. Imaging* **2016**, *43*, 1784–1791. [CrossRef] [PubMed]
26. Jha, A.; Ling, A.; Millo, C.; Gupta, G.; Viana, B.; Lin, F.I.; Herscovitch, P.; Adams, K.T.; Taïeb, D.; Metwalli, A.R.; et al. Superiority of 68Ga-DOTATATE over 18F-FDG and anatomic imaging in the detection of succinate dehydrogenase mutation (SDHx)-related pheochromocytoma and paraganglioma in the pediatric population. *Eur. J. Nucl. Med. Mol. Imaging* **2018**, *45*, 787–797. [CrossRef]
27. Janssen, I.; Blanchet, E.M.; Adams, K.; Chen, C.C.; Millo, C.M.; Herscovitch, P.; Taieb, D.; Kebebew, E.; Lehnert, H.; Fojo, A.T.; et al. Superiority of [68Ga]-DOTATATE PET/CT to Other Functional Imaging Modalities in the Localization of SDHB-Associated Metastatic Pheochromocytoma and Paraganglioma. *Clin. Cancer Res. Off. J. Am. Assoc. Cancer Res.* **2015**, *21*, 3888–3895. [CrossRef]
28. Yamamoto, S.; Hellman, P.; Wassberg, C.; Sundin, A. 11C-Hydroxyephedrine Positron Emission Tomography Imaging of Pheochromocytoma: A Single Center Experience over 11 Years. *J. Clin. Endocrinol. Metab.* **2012**, *97*, 2423–2432. [CrossRef]
29. Yamamoto, S.; Wassberg, C.; Hellman, P.; Sundin, A. (11)C-Hydroxyephedrine Positron Emission Tomography in the Postoperative Management of Pheochromocytoma and Paraganglioma. *Neuroendocrinology* **2014**, *100*, 60–70. [CrossRef]
30. Shulkin, B.L.; Wieland, D.M.; Schwaiger, M.; Thompson, N.W.; Francis, I.R.; Haka, M.S.; Rosenspire, K.C.; Shapiro, B.; Sisson, J.C.; Kuhl, D.E. PET scanning with hydroxyephedrine: An approach to the localization of pheochromocytoma. *J. Nucl. Med. Off. Publ. Soc. Nucl. Med.* **1992**, *33*, 1125–1131.
31. Trampal, C.; Engler, H.; Juhlin, C.; Bergström, M.; Långström, B. Pheochromocytomas: Detection with 11C Hydroxyephedrine PET. *Radiology* **2004**, *230*, 423–428. [CrossRef]
32. Franzius, C.; Hermann, K.; Weckesser, M.; Kopka, K.; Juergens, K.U.; Vormoor, J.; Schober, O. Whole-body PET/CT with 11C-meta-hydroxyephedrine in tumors of the sympathetic nervous system: Feasibility study and comparison with 123I-MIBG SPECT/CT. *J. Nucl. Med. Off. Publ. Soc. Nucl. Med.* **2006**, *47*, 1635–1642.
33. Rosenspire, K.C.; Haka, M.S.; Van Dort, M.E.; Jewett, D.M.; Gildersleeve, D.L.; Schwaiger, M.; Wieland, D.M. Synthesis and preliminary evaluation of carbon-11-meta-hydroxyephedrine: A false transmitter agent for heart neuronal imaging. *J. Nucl. Med. Off. Publ. Soc. Nucl. Med.* **1990**, *31*, 1328–1334.
34. Shulkin, B.L.; Wieland, D.M.; Baro, M.E.; Ungar, D.R.; Mitchell, D.S.; Dole, M.G.; Rawwas, J.B.; Castle, V.P.; Sisson, J.C.; Hutchinson, R.J. PET hydroxyephedrine imaging of neuroblastoma. *J. Nucl. Med. Off. Publ. Soc. Nucl. Med.* **1996**, *37*, 16–21.
35. Han, S.; Suh, C.H.; Woo, S.; Kim, Y.J.; Lee, J.J. Performance of 68Ga-DOTA–Conjugated Somatostatin Receptor–Targeting Peptide PET in Detection of Pheochromocytoma and Paraganglioma: A Systematic Review and Metaanalysis. *J. Nucl. Med.* **2019**, *60*, 369–376. [CrossRef] [PubMed]
36. Timmers, H.J.L.M.; Kozupa, A.; Chen, C.C.; Carrasquillo, J.A.; Ling, A.; Eisenhofer, G.; Adams, K.T.; Solis, D.; Lenders, J.W.M.; Pacak, K. Superiority of Fluorodeoxyglucose Positron Emission Tomography to Other Functional Imaging Techniques in the Evaluation of Metastatic *SDHB* -Associated Pheochromocytoma and Paraganglioma. *J. Clin. Oncol.* **2007**, *25*, 2262–2269. [CrossRef] [PubMed]

37. Rischke, H.C.; Benz, M.R.; Wild, D.; Mix, M.; Dumont, R.A.; Campbell, D.; Seufert, J.; Wiech, T.; Rossler, J.; Weber, W.A.; et al. Correlation of the Genotype of Paragangliomas and Pheochromocytomas with Their Metabolic Phenotype on 3,4-Dihydroxy-6-18F-Fluoro-L-Phenylalanin PET. *J. Nucl. Med.* **2012**, *53*, 1352–1358. [CrossRef]
38. Blake, M.A.; Kalra, M.K.; Maher, M.M.; Sahani, D.V.; Sweeney, A.T.; Mueller, P.R.; Hahn, P.F.; Boland, G.W. Pheochromocytoma: An Imaging Chameleon. *RadioGraphics* **2004**, *24*, S87–S99. [CrossRef]

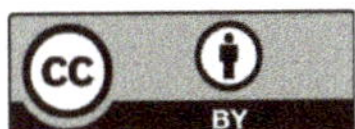

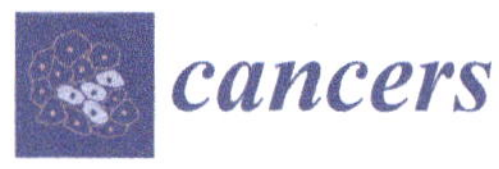

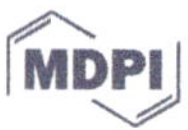

Review

Postoperative Management in Patients with Pheochromocytoma and Paraganglioma

Divya Mamilla [1], Katherine A. Araque [2], Alessandra Brofferio [3], Melissa K. Gonzales [1], James N. Sullivan [4], Naris Nilubol [5] and Karel Pacak [1,*]

1. Section on Medical Neuroendocrinology, *Eunice Kennedy Shriver*, National Institute of Child Health and Human Development, National Institutes of Health, Bethesda, MD 20892, USA
2. Adult Endocrinology Department, National Institute of Diabetes and Digestive and Kidney Diseases, National Institutes of Health, Bethesda, MD 20892, USA
3. Cardiovascular and Pulmonary Branch, National Heart, Lung, and Blood Institute, National Institutes of Health, Bethesda, MD 20892, USA
4. Department of Anesthesiology, University of Nebraska Medical Center, Omaha, NE 68198, USA
5. Endocrine Oncology Branch, National Cancer Institute, National Institutes of Health, Bethesda, MD 20892, USA

* Correspondence: karel@mail.nih.gov; Tel.: +1-301-402-4594; Fax: +1-301-402-0884

Received: 13 June 2019; Accepted: 1 July 2019; Published: 3 July 2019

Abstract: Pheochromocytomas and paragangliomas (PPGLs) are rare catecholamine-secreting neuroendocrine tumors of the adrenal medulla and sympathetic/parasympathetic ganglion cells, respectively. Excessive release of catecholamines leads to episodic symptoms and signs of PPGL, which include hypertension, headache, palpitations, and diaphoresis. Intraoperatively, large amounts of catecholamines are released into the bloodstream through handling and manipulation of the tumor(s). In contrast, there could also be an abrupt decline in catecholamine levels after tumor resection. Because of such binary manifestations of PPGL, patients may develop perplexing and substantially devastating cardiovascular complications during the perioperative period. These complications include hypertension, hypotension, arrhythmias, myocardial infarction, heart failure, and cerebrovascular accident. Other complications seen in the postoperative period include fever, hypoglycemia, cortisol deficiency, urinary retention, etc. In the interest of safe patient care, such emergencies require precise diagnosis and treatment. Surgeons, anesthesiologists, and intensivists must be aware of the clinical manifestations and complications associated with a sudden increase or decrease in catecholamine levels and should work closely together to be able to provide appropriate management to minimize morbidity and mortality associated with PPGLs.

Keywords: postoperative; pheochromocytoma; hypertension; hypotension; arrhythmia

1. Introduction

Pheochromocytomas (PHEOs) are rare catecholamine-secreting neuroendocrine tumors derived from chromaffin cells of the adrenal medulla (80–85%). Paragangliomas (PGLs) are extra-adrenal tumors, originating from similar cells present in both sympathetic and parasympathetic ganglion cells (15–20%) [1]. Catecholamines, i.e., epinephrine (EPI), norepinephrine (NE) and dopamine (DA), are synthesized and secreted from almost all pheochromocytomas and paragangliomas (PPGLs) [2,3]. They are either released in large amounts during tumor manipulation or may suddenly drop after tumor resection causing wide swings in hemodynamics [4]. Clinical manifestations of fluctuating perioperative and postoperative hemodynamics are hypertensive crisis, arrhythmias (most commonly tachyarrhythmias), headache, sweating, constipation and anxiety. Therefore, attention should be focused on minimizing tumor manipulation by careful handling of tumor tissue, limiting intra-abdominal pressure, providing adequate anesthesia and maximizing the use of vasoactive agents to achieve intraoperative hemodynamic stability, hence improving outcomes during the postoperative period [4,5]. The use of an appropriate preoperative antihypertensive regimen can be counterproductive when effects continue after surgical tumor removal, i.e., a rapid decline of catecholamine levels may lead to hypotension [6,7]. As such, administration of volume expanders and vasopressor management would be critical in reversing vascular collapse [8]. Reports have shown that patients with higher preoperative metanephrines and catecholamines have higher postoperative complications including organ ischemia, bowel obstruction, hypoglycemia, etc. [9–11].

Since the pioneering work by Gagner et al. of the first laparoscopic resection of PHEO in 1992, surgical management of PHEO has considerably improved owing to the advancement in pre, intra, and postoperative care of these patients [12]. Postoperatively, patients are closely monitored in the intensive care unit for hemodynamic fluctuations along with a careful assessment of electrolyte and endocrine abnormalities.

To our best knowledge, most of the published articles focus primarily on preoperative and intraoperative care of PPGL patients, whereas studies detailing postoperative management are only available from individual case reports. It is extremely important for physicians of PPGL patients to provide not only appropriate preoperative evaluation and treatment but also adequate postoperative care.

In this article, we describe the medical approaches to treat these patients after tumor resection based on our unique, long-standing experience with these patients at the National Institutes of Health. Additionally, we present the notable complications physicians should become aware of, including those emergencies that require immediate attention by a well-trained and experienced endocrinologist working alongside intensivists. Finally, this article provides clinical caveats to practicing clinicians regarding postoperative management of these patients.

2. Catecholamines and Adrenoceptors

PPGLs secrete catecholamines with substantial variation in their content based on the expression of various biosynthetic enzymes. Typically, adrenal PHEOs produce either EPI or NE while extra-adrenal and metastatic PHEOs mainly produce NE. Rarely, these tumor cells produce DA. Adrenoceptors (α_1, α_2, β_1, β_2) are the final target site of action for these catecholamines. Therefore, it is essential to recognize the impact of catecholamines from PPGL on specific organs (Tables 1 and 2).

Table 1. Characteristics of subtypes of adrenergic receptors.

Adrenoceptor Subtype	Agonists	Tissue	Responses
α_1 *	EPI≥NE>>Iso Phenylephrine	Vascular smooth muscle	Vasoconstriction
		Liver [Ŧ]	Glycogenolysis, gluconeogenesis
		Intestinal smooth muscle	Hyperpolarization and relaxation
		Heart	Chronotropic, arrhythmias
α_2 *	EPI≥NE>>Iso Clonidine	Pancreatic islets (/cells)	Decreased insulin secretion
		Platelets	Aggregation
		Nerve terminals	Decreased release of NE
		Vascular smooth muscle	Vasoconstriction
β_1	Iso>EPI=NE Dobutamine	Heart	Chronotropic and inotropic

Table 1. *Cont.*

Adrenoceptor Subtype	Agonists	Tissue	Responses
β_2	Iso>EPI>>NE Terbutaline	Juxtaglomerular cells Smooth muscle (vascular, bronchial, and gastrointestinal) Skeletal muscle Liver ‡	Increased renin secretion Relaxation
β_3 †	Iso=NE>EPI	Adipose tissue	Glycogenolysis, uptake of K^+ Glycogenolysis, gluconeogenesis lipolysis

* At least three subtypes each of α_1– and α_2–adrenoceptor are known, but distinctions in their mechanisms of action and tissue locations have not been clearly defined. ‡ In some species (e.g., rat), metabolic responses in the liver are mediated by α_1–adrenoceptor, whereas in others (e.g., dog), β_2–adrenoceptor are predominantly involved. Both types of receptors appear to contribute to responses in humans. † Metabolic responses in adipocytes and certain other tissues with atypical pharmacologic characteristics may be mediated by this subtype of receptor. Most β_2–adrenoceptor antagonists (including propranolol) do not block these responses. EPI, epinephrine; NE, norepinephrine; Iso, isoproterenol; AV, atrioventricular. Adapted from Goodman and Gillman's The Pharmacological Basis of Therapeutics [13].

Table 2. Responses of effector organs to autonomic nerve impulses.

Effector Organs	Adrenergic Impulses		Cholinergic Impulses
	Receptor Type *	Responses ‡	Responses ‡
		Heart †	
SA node	β_1, β_2	Chronotropic ++	Chronotrophy −−, vagal arrest +++
Atria	β_1, β_2	Inotropic and chronotropic ++	Inotropic −−, shortened AP duration ++
AV node	β_1, β_2	Increase in automaticity and chronotropic ++	Chronotropic −−, AV block +++
His-Purkinje system	β_1, β_2	Increase in automaticity and chronotropic +++	Little effect
Ventricles	β_1, β_2	inotropic, chronotropic automaticity, and rate of idioventricular pacemakers +++	Slight decrease in contractility
		Arterioles	
Coronary	$\alpha_1, \alpha_2, \beta_2$	Constriction +, dilations § ++	Constriction +
Skin and mucosa	α_1, α_2	Constriction +++	Dilation ‖
Skeletal muscle	α_1, β_2	Constriction +, dilation § ++, $ ++	Dilation ** +
Cerebral	α_1	Constriction (slight)	Dilation ‖
Pulmonary	α_1, β_2	Constriction +, dilations §	Dilation ‖
Abdominal viscera	$\alpha_1; \beta_2$	Constriction +++, dilation $ +	–
Salivary glands	α_1, α_2	Constriction +++,	Dilation++
Renal	$\alpha_1, \alpha_2, \beta_1, \beta_2$	Constriction +++, dilation $ +	–
		Veins (systemic)	
Veins	$\alpha_1, \alpha_2, \beta_2$	Constriction ++, dilation++	–
		Lung	
Tracheal and bronchial muscle	β_2	Relaxation +	Contraction ++
Bronchial glands	α_1, β_2	Decreased secretion, increased secretion	Stimulation +++
		Stomach	
Mobility and tone	$\alpha_1, \alpha_2, \beta_2$	Decrease (usually) ‡‡ +	Increase +++

Table 2. *Cont.*

Effector Organs	Adrenergic Impulses		Cholinergic Impulses
	Receptor Type *	**Responses** ‡	**Responses** ‡
Sphincters	α_1	Contraction (usually) +	Relaxation (usually) +
Secretion		Inhibition	Stimulation +++
		Intestine	
Mobility and tone	α_1, α_2, β_1, β_2	Decrease (usually)+	Increase +++
Sphincters	α_1	Contraction (usually) +	Relaxation (usually) +
Secretion	α_2	Inhibition	Stimulation ++
		Gallbladder and ducts	
	β_2	Relaxation +	Contraction +
		Kidney	
Renin Secretion	α_1, β_1	Decrease +, increase ++	–
		Urinary bladder	
Detrusor	β_2	Relaxation (usually) +	Contraction +++
Trigone and sphincter	α_1	Contraction ++	Relaxation ++
		Ureter	
Mobility and tone	α_1	Increase	Increase (+)
		Adrenal medulla	
		–	Secretion of epinephrine and norepinephrine (primarily nicotinic and secondarily muscarinic)
		Skeletal muscle	
	β_2	Increased contractility, glycogenolysis, K^+ uptake	–
		Liver	
	α_1, β_2	Glycogenolysis and gluconeogenesis $$ +++	–
		Pancreas	
Acini	α	Decreased secretion +	Secretion ++
Islets (β cells)	α_2	Decreased secretion +++	–
	β_2	Increased secretion +	–

* Where a designation of subtype is not provided, the nature of the subtype has not been determined unequivocally. ‡ Responses are designated highest (+++ and −−) to lowest (+ and −) to provide an approximate indication of the importance of adrenergic and cholinergic nerve activity in the control of the various organs and functions listed. † Although it had been thought that β_1–adrenoceptor predominates in the human heart. Recent evidence indicates some involvement of β_2–adrenoceptor. § Dilation predominates in situ due to metabolic autoregulatory phenomena. ‖ Cholinergic vasodilation as these sites is of questionable physiologic significance. $ Over the usual concentration range of physiologically released, circulating epinephrine, β–adrenoceptor response (vasodilation) predominates in blood vessels of skeletal muscle and liver, α–receptor response (vasoconstriction), in blood vessels of other abdominal viscera. The renal and mesenteric vessels also contain specific dopaminergic receptors, activation of which causes dilation. ** Sympathetic cholinergic system causes vasodilation in skeletal muscle, but this is not involved in most physiologic responses. ‡‡ It has been proposed that adrenergic fibers terminate at inhibitory β–adrenoceptors on smooth muscle fibers and at inhibitory α–adrenoceptors on parasympathetic cholinergic (excitatory) ganglion cells of Auerbach's plexus. $$ There is significant variation among species in the type of receptors that mediates certain metabolic responses. α- and β-adrenoceptor responses have not been determined in human beings. A β_3–adrenoceptor has been cloned and may mediate lipolysis or thermogenesis or both in fat cells in some species; SA, sinoatrial; AV, atrioventricular. Adapted from Goodman and Gillman's The Pharmacological Basis of Therapeutics [13].

EPI and NE have some overlapping but distinct effects on α- and β-adrenoceptors. EPI has more potent effects on β_2-adrenoceptors than NE, but equivalent effects on β_1-adrenoceptor, along with dominant effects on α-adrenoceptors in comparison to NE (Table 1). More than 95% of EPI is released from the adrenal medulla, which acts on the β_2-adrenoceptors of skeletal muscle vasculature causing vasodilation leading to hypotension. In contrast, NE released from sympathetic nerve endings within the effector sites causes α_1-adrenoceptor mediated vasoconstriction, leading to hypertension and its profound action on β_1-adrenoceptors causes increased ionotropic and chronotropic effects in the heart [14]. Eventually, the resulting concentration of catecholamines at effector sites are significant determinants of adrenoceptor mediated responses [14,15].

Persistently high catecholamine levels may lead to adrenoceptor desensitization due to receptors' internalization, reduction of their numbers on the cell surface, or decreased binding affinity of catecholamines to receptors [16,17]. These mechanisms may partially explain why some patients with PPGL are only moderately hypertensive, despite high plasma catecholamine levels. Decreased or desensitized adrenoceptors, perioperative α-adrenoceptor blockade, and abruptly decreased catecholamine production contributes to postoperative hypotension.

Differences in receptor binding, affinity, and downstream effects explain the spectrum of clinical signs that patients with PPGL develop. Patients with predominantly EPI secreting PPGL have episodic symptoms and signs of palpitation, lightheadedness or syncope, anxiety, and hyperglycemia. Conversely, patients with primarily NE secreting tumors have continuous symptoms and signs of hypertension, sweating, and headache [18–20]. These effects could extend to peri and postoperative periods due to excessive catecholamines release while handling the tumor during surgical resection. Thus, it is mandatory that these patients are followed by a multidisciplinary team in a close monitoring setting like the intensive care unit during the postoperative period.

3. Cardiovascular Complications Related to PPGLs

3.1. Hypertension

According to the American College of Cardiology/American Heart Association (ACC/AHA) 2017, hypertension is defined as blood pressure > 130/80 mmHg [21]. Risk factors associated with postoperative hypertension following PPGL resection include incompletely removed/metastatic tumor, additional tumor at an unknown location, underlying essential hypertension, excessive intravenous fluid administration, pain, and excessive use of vasopressors (management of transient hypotension resulting from a significant drop in catecholamine levels).

One possible mechanism behind hypertensive crisis during PPGL resection includes massive catecholamine release secondary to tumor manipulation. Watchful and precise resection, appropriate vasodilator use, and clear communication between the surgeons and anesthesiologists are helpful in minimizing intraoperative hemodynamic fluctuation [22–24]. Other tumor-related factors resulting in hemodynamic instability include large tumor size (>4 cm), urinary catecholamines >2000 μg/24 h, large postural drop in blood pressure (>10 mmHg) after α-adrenoceptor blockade, preoperative mean arterial blood pressure (MAP) > 100 mmHg and prolonged duration of anesthesia [25–27]. Therefore, hypertension should be treated promptly with quickly titratable and shorter-acting agents. Below we summarize the most important therapeutic options available to treat perioperative hypertension among patients with PPGL (Figure 1) (Table 3).

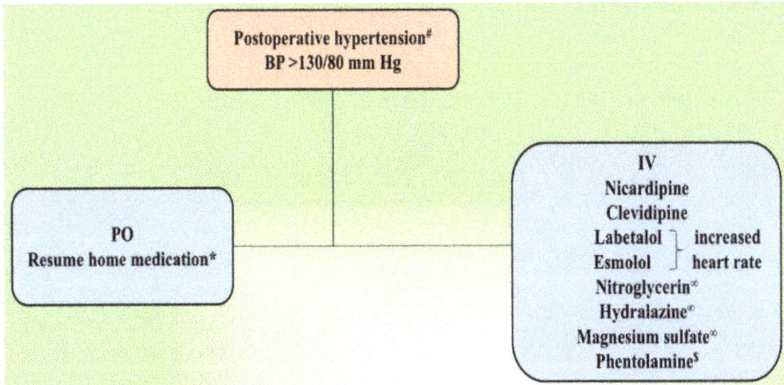

Figure 1. Postoperative management of hypertension following tumor resection. # Residual or metastatic disease causing an increased blood pressure is treated using α–adrenoceptor blocker. If necessary, β-adrenoceptor blocker and/or calcium channel blocker is added. β-adrenoceptor blocker might be used at first for epinephrine-secreting tumors. ∞ Management of hypertensive emergency. * Underlying essential hypertension is treated according to currently accepted guidelines. $ Phentolamine is used to manage hypertensive crisis or in cases of resistant hypertension. BP, blood pressure; IV, intravenous; PO, per oral.

Table 3. Anti-hypertensive medications used in hypertensive crisis after pheochromocytoma and paraganglioma (PPGL) resection.

Anti-Hypertensive Medication	Mechanism of Action	Route of Administration	Dose
	α- and β-adrenoceptor blockers		
Phentolamine	Competitive α_1- and α_2-adrenoceptor blocker	IV	Bolus dose 5 g Maintenance dose 0.5 mg/min
Esmolol	β_1-adrenoceptor antagonist	IV	Starting dose 0.5 ml/kg Maintenance dose 50–300 μg/kg/min
Metoprolol	β_1-adrenoceptor antagonist	IV	5 mg every 5 mins as tolerated up to 15 mg total dose
Labetalol	Selective α_1- and nonselective β-adrenoceptor antagonist	IV	Loading dose 10–20 mg, double initial dose every 10 mins until target blood pressure is attained
	Calcium channel blockers		
Nicardipine	NE mediated transmembrane calcium influx into vascular smooth muscles	IV	Starting dose 5 mg/h, dose increased by 2.5 mg/h every 5mins to a maximum of 15 mg/h
Clevidepine	Increase cardiac output Decrease afterload	IV	Starting dose 1–2 mg/h Maintenance dose 4–6 mg/h
	Others		
Nitroglycerin	Venous dilator Decrease preload	IV	Starting dose 5–10 μg/min (increase the dose by 5 μg/min every 5 mins until desired effect is achieved)
Hydralazine	Decrease arterial vascular resistance	IV	10 mg over 2 mins, additional doses as needed
Magnesium sulfate	•Inhibition of release catecholamines •Direct inhibition of catecholamines receptors •Endogenous calcium antagonist	IV	Bolus dose 2–4 g over 2 mins Maintenance dose 1–2 g/h, dose adjusted on magnesium blood levels

Abbreviations: IV, intravenous; NE, norepinephrine.

3.1.1. α- and β-Adrenoceptor Antagonist

α-adrenoceptor antagonists are categorized according to specific receptor activity: Non-selective antagonists such as phenoxybenzamine and phentolamine and selective α_1-adrenoceptor antagonists such as doxazosin, prazosin, and terazosin. These are predominantly used to manage perioperative hypertension following PPGL resection [2,28]. However, hypertensive crisis in the intra and postoperative period is managed by using phentolamine (Regitine) given as a 5 mg bolus intravenously with additional bolus doses given as needed [29]. The most common side effect is reflex tachycardia caused by baroreceptor reflex after α_2-adrenoceptor blockade. Therefore, it is recommended to be used in combination with esmolol (Brevibloc), a rapidly acting cardio-selective β_1-adrenoceptor antagonist [30]. The negative inotropic and chronotropic effect with no direct vasodilatory action of esmolol makes a good pair with direct acting α-adrenoceptor antagonists [30]. It is given intravenously at a loading dose of 0.5–1.0 mg/kg over 30 s or one minute followed by 50–150 µg/kg/min infusion (lower dose and slower infusion for more gradual control, higher dose and faster infusion for immediate control) and, if necessary, the dose may be increased up to a maximum of 300 µg/kg/min [31,32]. At higher doses, esmolol inhibits β_2-adrenoceptors located in the musculature of bronchi and blood vessels. Moreover, as patients' oral intake improves, cardio-selective β_1-adrenoceptor blockers such as metoprolol (Lopressor) 25–50 mg three to four times a day or atenolol (Tenormin) 12.5–25 mg once a day (occasionally twice daily) orally are also administered to control catecholamines or α-adrenoceptor blocker induced tachyarrhythmia [33,34].

Labetalol (Normodyne or Trandate) is a combined selective α_1- and non-selective β-adrenoceptor blocker with α to β blocking ratio of 1:4–7 [35]. Prolonged duration of action (2–4 h) of labetalol makes it challenging to titrate as a continuous infusion [36]. Poopalalingam et al. reported the use of continuous infusion of labetalol during PHEO resection, thus, providing sufficient α- and β-adrenoceptor blockade for the duration of surgery including the immediate postoperative period. Additionally, labetalol also minimizes the risk of postoperative hypotension and somnolence associated with preoperative use of phenoxybenzamine for the surgical preparation of a patient [37]. Labetalol is given intravenously at a loading dose of 10–20 mg followed by doubling of the initial dose every 10 mins until target blood pressure is achieved. If continuous infusion is planned, the dose is started at 2 mg/min and the drip rate is adjusted depending on blood pressure response with a total dose of up to 300 mg (FDA dosage). Labetalol and the other β-adrenoceptor blockers are used with caution in patients with bradycardia, atrio-ventricular block, and it may potentiate the action of other drugs such as calcium channel blockers [38,39].

3.1.2. Calcium Channel Blockers

Although calcium channel blockers (CCBs) are less effective than α- and β-adrenoceptor blockers, it is an important class of drug used to manage hypertension following PPGL resection. They minimize complications related to catecholamines overload, such as coronary vasospasm [40]. CCBs inhibit NE mediated transmembrane calcium influx into vascular smooth muscle, resulting in arterial vasodilation [41]. In a clinical setting, nicardipine (Cardene) is most commonly used either alone or in combination with α- and β-adrenoceptor blockers in the postoperative period. However, we might also consider using those CCBs such as amlodipine or nifedipine, when already used in the preoperative period to control blood pressure. Nicardipine is started at a dose of 5 mg/h and dose is increased by 2.5 mg/h every five minutes to a maximum of 15 mg/h until target blood pressure is achieved. Recently, the use of Clevidipine (Cleviprex), an ultrashort-acting third-generation dihydropyridine CCB, has become popular. It acts by selective arteriolar dilatation which helps in decreasing peripheral vascular resistance [42]. Clevidipine starting dose is 1–2 mg/h intravenously and doubled every 90 s with a maximal dose up to 32 mg/h for a maximum duration of 72 h. Once the target blood pressure is reached, infusion is titrated based on therapeutic response and usually, maintained at a rate of 4–6 mg/h [43]. Multiple clinical trials have demonstrated promising effects of Clevidipine to control both pre and postoperative hypertension [44,45].

3.1.3. Nitroglycerin

Nitroglycerin is an antianginal drug and a more potent venous dilator than arterial dilator. However, arterial dilation occurs at higher doses [46]. It has a rapid onset of action, and the dose is easily titratable, thus, often used to manage hypertensive emergency [4]. Nitroglycerin is most commonly used to manage intraoperative hypertensive crisis due to its effective safety profile [8]. The initial dose of intravenous nitroglycerin is 5 μg/min, which can be increased to a maximum of 100 μg/min. Nitroglycerin should be administered cautiously among patients undergoing PPGL resection as it is associated with hypotension, reflex tachycardia, and headache.

3.1.4. Hydralazine

Hydralazine (Apresoline) use is very limited in the management of postoperative hypertension following PPGL resection due to its long duration of action resulting in hypotension and reflex tachycardia [47]. Hydralazine is preferably used among those patients who have underlying essential hypertension. The initial dose of hydralazine for an acute hypertensive episode is 10 mg intravenously (not exceeding 40 mg) given over two minutes with additional doses given every four to six hours as needed [30]. If patient's oral intake is improved, hydralazine can be given at a dose of 100–200 mg orally two to three times a day. Adverse effects include tachycardia, negative effect on myocardial metabolism precipitating acute myocardial ischemia or infarction, and cerebral vasodilation leading to increased intracranial pressure [47]. Thus, hydralazine is not considered a first-line agent to treat acute postoperative hypertension.

3.1.5. Magnesium Sulfate

Magnesium (Sulfamag) is considered safe and potent supplemental medication to block catecholamine action, bringing hemodynamic control in adults and children undergoing PPGL resection [24]. Multiple case reports have verified the use of magnesium in pediatric age with PHEO [48–50]. The vasodilator property of magnesium is evoked by direct inhibition of catecholamine receptors and release of catecholamines from the adrenal medulla and adrenergic nerve terminals which act as endogenous calcium antagonists [51,52]. Given its safety profile and efficient blockade, it is considered a first-line agent in the intraoperative management of PPGL resection during pregnancy [53,54]. It is usually given at a dose of four grams in 250 mL of 5% Dextrose injection at a rate not exceeding 3 mL/min. Magnesium sulfate is also beneficial in the management of cardiac arrhythmias due to its stabilizing effect on cardiac electrical conduction [55]. Therefore, continuous infusion of magnesium is given under close monitoring due to its associated neuromuscular and cardiovascular toxicities especially among patients with renal insufficiency. These toxic complications can be reversed with the intravenous calcium administration.

3.1.6. Treatment of Underlying Hypertension

Persistent hypertension following PPGL resection might be related to coexistence of essential hypertension. Oral antihypertensive medications, preferably a preoperative antihypertensive medication regimen, should be used under close monitoring to make any necessary adjustments in dosage. After discharge, a patient is followed by his or her primary care provider. Approximately six weeks later, laboratory evaluation is performed to evaluate for the presence of catecholamines and metanephrines in blood and urine, thus, identifying the presence of residual tumor, tumor at an unknown location, or metastatic tumor. However, if laboratory results are negative, a diagnosis of underlying essential hypertension is established, and antihypertensive medications are given as necessary.

3.2. *Hypotension*

Hypotension is defined as blood pressure below 90/60 mmHg or any degree of low blood pressure leading to organ hypoperfusion or end-organ damage. Potential risk factors attributed to postoperative hypotension following PPGL resection include chronically low circulating plasma volume, an abrupt decrease in serum catecholamine levels, down-regulation of adrenoceptors, increased blood loss, and cardiogenic or septic shock [56]. Independent tumor-related risk factors are open procedures, high preoperative plasma NE and EPI levels and increased urinary fractionated catecholamines excretion [25,26,57,58]. EPI secreting PPGLs cause decreased cardiac contractility owing to downregulation of β-adrenoceptors on the heart, resulting in left heart failure, thus precipitating hypotensive state and collapse after resection [59–61]. However, NE secreting PPGLs cause a decrease in circulating plasma volume secondary to α_1-adrenoceptor mediated vasoconstriction [2]. Moreover, profound irreversible α-adrenoceptor blockade by phenoxybenzamine triggers recalcitrant postoperative hypotension by: (1) Prolonged half-life of the drug and (2) permanent covalent binding to adrenoceptors which are curtailed only after de novo synthesis [2,62]. Nevertheless, this effect is comparatively less with selective α_1-adrenoceptor blockers.

First line management for postoperative hypotension following PPGL resection includes vigorous intravenous fluid administration [40]. If fluid therapy fails, vasopressor use is justified to restore normal blood pressure. Vasopressors used to manage hypotension include NE, EPI (rarely), and vasopressin. However, pure α-adrenoceptor agonists such as phenylephrine are not used because of remnant effects of preoperative α-adrenoceptor blockade. Finally, the ultimate goal of managing hypotension is both restoration of adequate and prevention of inadequate tissue perfusion (Figure 2).

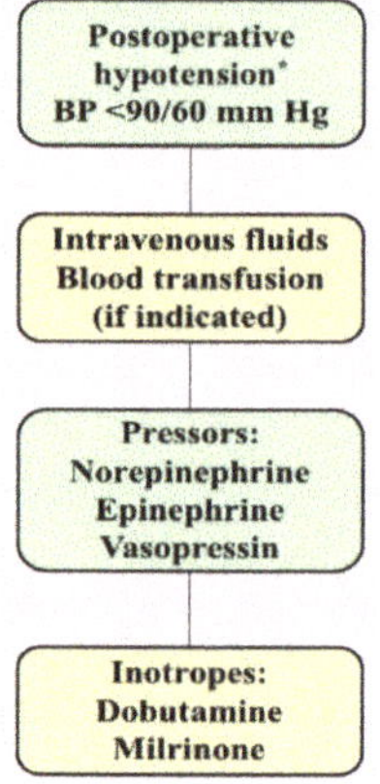

Figure 2. Postoperative management of hypotension following tumor resection. * In the differential diagnosis of hypotension consider downregulation of adrenoceptors, cardiogenic shock, sepsis, and medication-induced. BP, blood pressure.

3.2.1. Intravenous Fluid

Fluid loss during the postoperative period results from: (1) Surgical site bleeding or occult bleeding, (2) suction drainage (nasogastric tube, chest tube for pleural fluid, ascites from abdominal drains and urinary system), (3) third spacing of fluid, i.e., capillary leak and extravasation of protein-rich serum into the interstitial spaces of the soft tissues, organs, deep space cavities (chest, abdomen), or retroperitoneum, (4) insensible or evaporative losses, and (5) loss of systemic vascular resistance after sudden withdrawal of catecholamines following tumor resection [63]. First line management for hypotension is giving adequate amounts of intravenous fluid to restore blood volume, blood pressure, and adequate tissue perfusion, by filling the large acute increase in volume of distribution thus, reducing morbidities associated with hypotension [64]. Blood transfusion is reserved for those patients who present with excessive operative site bleeding while monitoring serum hemoglobin levels at regular intervals and in patients with known coronary disease. Knowledge of both systolic and diastolic left ventricular function is essential to anticipate the possibility of volume overload and associated complications. Every patient should be monitored carefully for signs of volume overload since this may lead to postoperative hypertension and pulmonary edema leading to respiratory compromise. The use of vasopressors is justified only when there is persistent hypotension despite administration of adequate amounts of intravenous fluids. Patients who are hemodynamically at risk, i.e., low ejection fraction or known coronary disease can be monitored by echocardiography, pulmonary artery catheters or other non-invasive devices.

3.2.2. Norepinephrine

NE (Levophed) is an α- and β-adrenoceptor agonist with stronger affinity towards α_1-adrenoceptor and mild to moderate β_1-adrenoceptor and minimal β_2-adrenoceptor agonist effects [65]. It is considered a first-line agent if intravenous fluid therapy fails to correct hypotension. The loading dose of NE is 8–12 μg/min intravenously with flow rate adjusted to maintain low normal blood pressure with mean arterial pressure >65 mm Hg. Maintenance dose is adjusted to 2–4 μg/min with daily doses as high as 68 mg. NE increases mean arterial pressure, effective circulating volume, venous return, and preload with minimal increase in heart rate [66]. As the dose of NE is increased within safety limits, improved fluid responsiveness can be seen due to β_1-adrenoceptor mediated augmentation of venous return [67]. NE infusion is used in patients with adequate volume resuscitation, otherwise this may cause profound ischemia leading to serious adverse effects. Therefore, judicious use of NE is carefully monitored in postoperative PPGL patients due to altered hemodynamics caused by excessive release of catecholamines from tumor cells.

3.2.3. Epinephrine

EPI (adrenalin) is an α- and β-adrenoceptor agonist with dose-dependent actions. Mixed actions of epinephrine cause an increase in both mean arterial blood pressure by vasoconstriction (α_1-adrenoceptor effect) and cardiac output (β_1-adrenoceptor effect) [68,69]. The starting dose of infusion is 1–4 μg/min and can be titrated up by 1–2 μg/min every 20 min until the desired effect is achieved. Total infusion dose should not exceed >10 μg/min [70]. It is considered a second-line agent in the treatment of refractory hypotension [71,72]. Adverse effects associated with the use of EPI include pulmonary hypertension, tachyarrhythmia, myocardial ischemia, lactic acidosis, and hyperglycemia. Henceforth, EPI is cautiously used in PPGL resected patients since it can prolong the effects of catecholamines released from the tumor cells.

3.2.4. Vasopressin

Vasopressin (pitressin, pressin), a nonapeptide hormone, is released from the posterior pituitary gland in response to increased plasma osmolality, decreased intravascular volume and low blood pressure. Vasopressin restores water balance and blood pressure by acting on vasopressin 1 (V_1), and V_2 receptors in the following ways: (1) Increased systemic vascular resistance by V_1 receptor stimulation on arterial smooth muscle cells and (2) water reabsorption at collecting ducts by stimulation of V_2 receptors in kidney. Additionally, vasopressin may increase responsiveness of catecholamines allowing lower doses of adrenergic drugs to be used [73]. Few patients develop catecholamine-resistant vasoplegia through severe catecholamine deficiency induced by tumor removal. In some cases, aggressive catecholamine and fluid replacement therapy might not be helpful to restore vascular tone. Augoustides et al. proposed that a chronic increase in NE levels can inhibit vasopressin release through downregulation of the neurohypophyseal vasopressin synthesis [74]. Vasopressin has no action on adrenergic receptors and is thus useful to treat refractory hypotension after PPGL resection [24]. In clinical practice, vasopressin is most often used at 0.03 to 0.04 units/min. Higher doses have been used but with a higher risk of adverse events.

3.3. *Arrhythmia*

Broadly, arrhythmias are classified as tachyarrhythmias (>100 beats/min) and bradyarrhythmias (<60 beats/min). Tachyarrhythmia is commonly documented following PPGL resection from either increased catecholamine levels or inotropes used to correct postoperative hypotension [75]. Other important risk factors include rebound effect of β-adrenoceptor blocker discontinuation and residual effect of α-adrenoceptor blockade used in preoperative preparation, postoperative hypotension, anemia and pain that also may cause an increase in sympathetic activity. Sinus tachycardia is the most commonly observed tachyarrhythmia after PPGL resection as a compensatory response to an underlying condition. Therefore, treatment is focused on addressing underlying causes, such as relieving pain or anxiety and replacing volume deficit. If heart rate is persistently elevated for a prolonged period of time, rate-controlling medications may be indicated. Other tachyarrhythmias observed following PPGL resection may include atrial fibrillation, atrial flutter, and occasionally life-threatening ventricular fibrillation. Management of tachyarrhythmia is based on a patient's hemodynamic stability, presence or absence of narrow or wide complex QRS, and regular or irregular rhythm.

Residual anesthetic effects and opioids and analgesics used in the postoperative period makes it difficult to identify the signs and symptoms of unstable tachyarrhythmia. Therefore, a multidisciplinary team of physicians, including intensivists, surgeons, anesthetists, cardiologists, and endocrinologists are required to manage these patients.

In stable patients with narrow, regular (<0.12 sec) QRS complex that is not sinus tachycardia (non-sinus tachycardia), vagal maneuvers such as Valsalva or carotid sinus massage can be executed. If rhythm is regular, adenosine 6 mg rapid intravenous push is injected followed by a bolus dose of 12 mg when no response is observed within one to two minutes. An additional dose of 12 mg is given in resistant cases. Usually, adenosine is helpful to effectively terminate and/or diagnose tachyarrhythmia. If tachycardia resumes or is not responsive to adenosine, treatment with longer-acting atrioventricular (AV) nodal blocking agents such as diltiazem or β-adrenoceptor blocker is required. Stable patients with irregular narrow complex tachycardia usually have either atrial fibrillation or atrial flutter requiring an expert consultation and use of rate-controlling agents such as diltiazem, β-adrenoceptor blockers or antiarrhythmics such as amiodarone. Diltiazem (Cardizem) is given intravenously at a starting dose of 0.25 mg/kg over two minutes followed by a maintenance dose with an infusion at 5–15 mg/h. Commonly used β-adrenoceptor blockers to control tachyarrhythmia include metoprolol (intravenous and oral forms) and esmolol (very short half-life, existing in drip form). Esmolol (Brevibloc) is loaded initially as 500 μg/kg over one minute with maintenance doses of 50–200 μg/kg/min and repeat bolus doses between each dose increase. However, a major drawback of using esmolol is that arrhythmias may recur after discontinuation. Therefore, longer acting β-adrenoceptor blocker, metoprolol tartrate (Lopressor), is used and given at a bolus dose of 2.5–5.0 mg intravenously over two minutes with repeated doses every 10 min up to a maximum three times before using longer intervals (every six to eight hours) [76]. These medications must be given under careful supervision as they can cause a significant drop in blood pressure, resulting in decreased perfusion to vital organs. Once a patient's oral intake improves, these medications can be changed to oral formulations such as metoprolol tartrate, given orally at a dose of 25–100 mg twice daily accordingly. Rhythm controlling agent such as amiodarone, an iodinated benzofuran antiarrhythmic may be considered. It is easily titratable and is used to treat both supraventricular and ventricular tachyarrhythmia with limited negative inotropic effects. Typical doses in stable patients includes a bolus of 150 mg intravenously over 10 min followed by an infusion of 1 mg/min over six hours which is titrated to 0.5 mg/h after the first six hours with a maximum dose of up to 2.2 g in the first 24 h. One large metanalysis done on the effect of amiodarone on recent-onset atrial fibrillation showed a similar efficacy and safety profile to other antiarrhythmics [77].

For hemodynamically stable patients with wide complex tachycardia, 12-lead electrocardiogram (EKG) and expert consultation are obtained. Amiodarone is often the first medication used if there are no contraindications (hypersensitivity, history of severe bradycardia) are observed [78]. Recommended doses are described earlier in this section. Other antiarrhythmics frequently used after obtaining appropriate expert consultation include propafenone, flecainide, and procainamide.

For prolonged, refractory or hemodynamically compromising tachyarrhythmias, electrical cardioversion is considered in combination with antiarrhythmics. If a patient has pulseless electrical activity [2], immediately follow the ACC/AHA treatment guidelines for pulseless electrical activity (PEA) algorithm to manage appropriately (Figure 3).

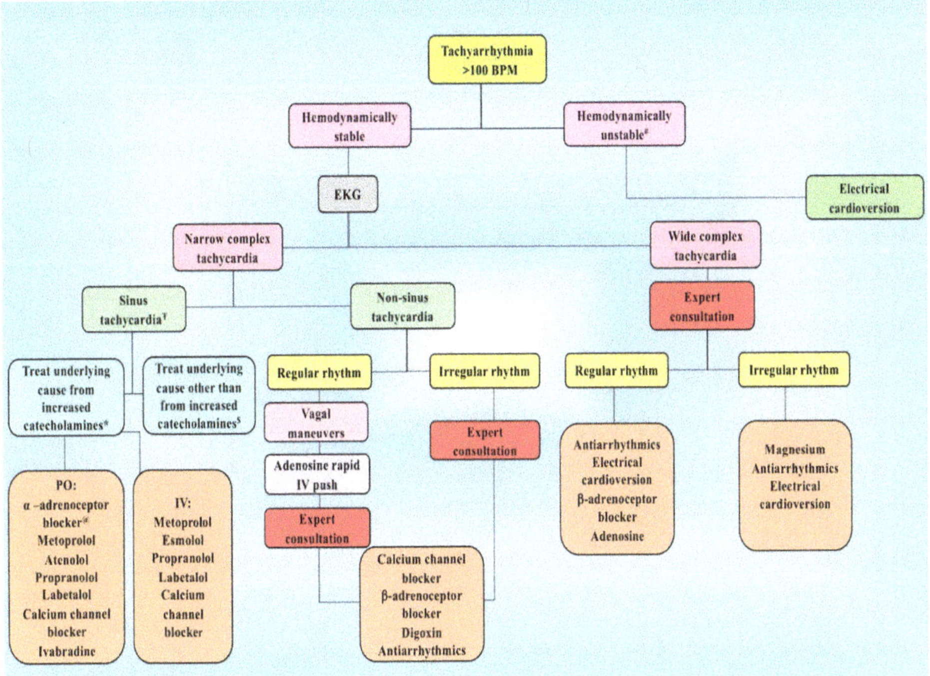

Figure 3. Management of tachyarrhythmia following PPGL resection in the postoperative period. # Unstable tachyarrhythmia implies patient has tachyarrhythmia along with hemodynamic instability or concerning symptoms. Ŧ Treatment in intensive care unit usually begins with calcium channel blockers. If heart rate is not well controlled, β-adrenoceptor blockers such as esmolol or metoprolol is added. In patients with increased blood pressure along with increased heart rate, use of combined α– and β-adrenoceptor blocker such as labetalol is recommended. Moreover, β-adrenoceptor blocker might be used at first for epinephrine-secreting tumors. * Underlying causes for increased catecholamines include their release during manipulation / resection of tumor and residual/ metastatic disease (patient must be on appropriate adrenoceptor blockade). $ Other causes include inotropes used to correct postoperative hypotension, rebound tachycardia by discontinuation of β-adrenoceptor blockers used preoperatively as well as anemia, hypovolemia, pain, and anxiety. @ α-adrenoceptor blocker are used in the presence of residual or metastatic disease. BPM, beats per minute; EKG, electrocardiogram; IV, intravenous; PO, per oral.

It is not unusual for sinus tachycardia to remain uncontrolled despite using all drugs including esmolol, metoprolol, and diltiazem. Therefore, another therapeutic approach may be considered. Recently, ivabradine has been introduced to treat patients with heart failure and sinus tachycardia who failed or were intolerant to β-adrenoceptor blockers. Ivabradine selectively inhibits I_f current in the sinus node, resulting in decreased heart rate without compromising myocardial contractility and cardiovascular hemodynamic status [79]. Thus, Ivabradine is prescribed at a dose of 2.5–7.5 mg two times a day orally to PPGL patients with medication-resistant sinus tachycardia, providing excellent control of tachycardia (personal observations). It is recommended to start Ivabradine at low doses and titrate to achieve heart rate control [80,81].

In contrast, bradyarrhythmia's after PPGL resection might result from sinus node or atrioventricular node dysfunction caused by progression of native conduction disease, overdose of rate controlling agents, i.e., β-adrenoceptor blocker, and metabolic or electrolyte disturbances. Bradycardia is defined in postoperative PPGL patients as heart rate below 60 beats/min. Therapeutic intervention is unnecessary for cases of transient bradycardia with no hemodynamic instability [82]. Detrimental effects of sustained bradycardia in the postoperative period include hypotension and inadequate cardiac output (decreased coronary circulation leading to myocardial infarction). Thus, atropine or β-adrenoceptor agonists may be indicated [75,82]. Atropine is administered at a dose of 0.5 mg intravenously, repeated every three to five minutes to a total dose of 3 mg intravenous until target heart rate of >60 beats/min is achieved. If bradycardia remains uncontrolled, consider using DA or EPI. DA actions are mediated either directly or by conversion and release of NE, leading to the stimulation of β-adrenoceptors on the heart while EPI increases heart rate by directly stimulating β-adrenoceptors on the heart [83]. DA has a dose range of 2–20 μg/kg/min whereas EPI is given at a dose of 2–20 μg/min until the desired heart rate >60 beats/min is sustained. Other agents which can be utilized to chemically pace are isoproterenol and dobutamine.

Unusually, bradyarrhythmias are unresponsive to atropine, DA, and EPI. Henceforth, transcutaneous or transvenous pacing becomes necessary.

3.4. Myocardial Infarction

It is not uncommon to recognize myocardial injury following PPGLs resection. The mechanism behind injury to myocytes by increased catecholamines includes hemodynamic compromise (increased afterload), tachycardia, increased oxygen consumption, and coronary arterial vasoconstriction [84]. Moreover, myocardium is rich in paraganglionic fibers with higher NE affinity which might produce structural and functional remodeling in the heart [85]. Direct actions of increased EPI and NE levels may result in myocarditis or cardiomyopathy causing leakage of cardiac enzymes [86]. Perhaps, hypotension, hypertension, anemia, hypoxemia, systolic, and/or diastolic dysfunction are common risk factors associated with myocardial infarction in the postoperative period. Clinical presentation of myocardial infarction in the postoperative period is commonly asymptomatic or non-specific, thus, relying on classic symptoms alone might lead to missed diagnoses [87]. Moreover, ischemic electrocardiographic signs may be subtle, and angina is masked by residual anesthetic effect and use of stronger analgesics concealing the diagnosis of myocardial injury [88]. Therefore, a higher index of suspicion of acute myocardial infarction is necessary in the absence of classic coronary risk factors [89]. According to ACC/AHA 2014 perioperative clinical practice guidelines, may consider comprehensive risk assessment with 12-lead EKG, 2D-echocardiography, and exercise or non-pharmacological stress testing to allocate them to low-risk or high-risk groups [90,91]. Measurement of troponin levels and obtaining a 12-lead EKG is recommended among patients with signs and symptoms of myocardial ischemia or infarction in the postoperative period [91]. To manage patients appropriately, myocardial infarction in the postoperative period is classified similarly as in the non-surgical setting: (1) Non-ST-elevation myocardial infarction (NSTEMI) (Figure 4) (Table 4) and (2) ST-elevation myocardial infarction (STEMI), management is dependent on expert consultation.

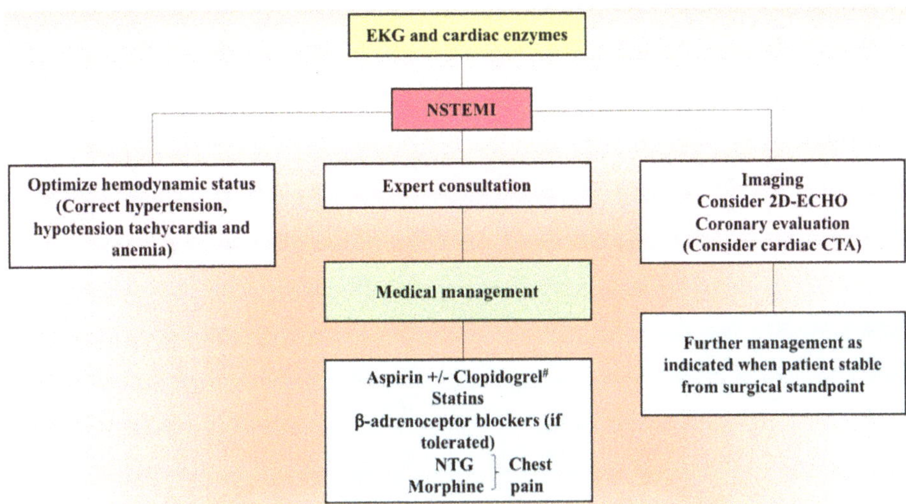

Figure 4. Management algorithm of postoperative NSTEMI. # Aspirin and clopidogrel is given in the postoperative period only when it is safe from surgical point of view. CTA, computed tomography angiography; 2D-ECHO, two-dimensional echocardiography; EKG, electrocardiography; NSTEMI, non-ST-elevation myocardial infarction; NTG, nitroglycerin.

Table 4. Medical Therapy for NSTEMI following PPGL resection.

Medications	Dosage	Goal of Treatment
Aspirin	325 mg PO	Inhibition of platelet aggregation and activation
High-intensity Statin		Lowers LDL cholesterol levels in blood by approximately ≥ 50%, atherosclerotic plaque stabilization
Atorvastatin	40–80 mg PO	
Rosuvastatin	20–40 mg PO	
β-adrenoceptor blocker		Lowering heart rate, pain resolution, ST-segment normalization
Metoprolol	1–5 mg IV, incrementally repeat as needed up to 15 mg total dose 25–50 mg PO three to four times a day	
Esmolol	10–50 mg IV bolus, infusion up to 200 µg/kg/min	
Morphine sulfate	2–5 mg IV, repeat as needed	Pain control
Nitroglycerin	0.4 mg sublingual every five minutes up to a total of three doses. Transdermal patch starting at 0.2 mg/h and increasing to 0.6 mg/h with drug-free period from 6 to 8 PM 50 µg/min IV, titrate upwards as mean arterial pressure tolerates	Pain elimination by coronary vasodilation and ST-segment normalization

Abbreviations: BPM, beats per minute; IV, intravenous; LDL, low density lipoprotein; PO, per oral.

3.5. Heart Failure

Heart failure may also be seen as one of the rare complications seen following PPGL resection. Myocardium may have been dependent on the excess catecholamines prior to resection due to desensitized adrenoceptors, possible catecholamine-induced cardiomyopathy or non-ischemic cardiomyopathy. Reduced circulatory volume may also play a significant role in the development of heart failure following tumor resection [92]. Therefore, patients in the postoperative period following PPGL resection might develop either heart failure with preserved ejection fraction (HFpEF) or heart failure with reduced ejection fraction (HFrEF). HFpEF is usually seen in the setting of hypertensive damage with diastolic dysfunction resulting in increased susceptibility to volume overload and resulting pulmonary edema. In contrast, HFrEF may be observed in patients with significant myocardial ischemia secondary to postoperative instability. Heart failure may also develop in the setting of stress-induced cardiomyopathy called Takotsubo cardiomyopathy or broken-heart syndrome, that has been frequently described in patients with PPGL. Diuretics and inotropes may be utilized to treat heart failure. However, when medical therapy fails, mechanical devices such as intra-aortic balloon pump, impella, extracorporeal membrane oxygenation may need to be utilized. It is appropriate to promptly obtain cardiology consultation when there is a suspicion of heart failure to apply the most relevant diagnostic and therapeutic tools.

3.6. Cerebrovascular Accident

Clinical course of patients with PPGL can be complicated by ischemic or hemorrhagic stroke. The main mechanisms include: (1) Thrombotic or embolic occlusion of cerebral artery secondary to increased platelet aggregation [93], (2) cerebral hypoperfusion secondary to tissue hypoxia causing increased susceptibility in the watershed regions [94,95], and (3) rupture of intracranial artery causing intracerebral or subarachnoid hemorrhage secondary to catecholamine-induced hypertension [96].

Patients with PPGL have a higher rate of ischemic stroke in comparison to hemorrhagic events in the postoperative period [97,98]. The potential risk factors for catecholamine-induced ischemic stroke include uncontrolled hypertension (failure of cerebrovascular autoregulation), vascular spasm, dilated cardiomyopathy with risk of left ventricular thrombus (embolic) or atrial fibrillation (embolic).

Symptoms may range from headaches to motor and/or sensory deficits, to confusion and seizures. Recognition of these symptoms is challenging due to the concomitant use of anesthetic or sedative therapy in the postoperative period [99]. The modified National Institute of Health Stroke Scale (mNIHSS) has improved reliability benefits and, therefore, should be used for detailed neurological examination of patients with increased risk of postoperative stroke [100].

For patients that develop ischemic or hemorrhagic stroke following PPGL resection, it is advisable to provide a multidisciplinary patient-centered treatment plan including neurology, critical care, surgery, interventional neuroradiology, and anesthesiology.

4. Other Complications

4.1. Adrenocortical Insufficiency

Surgical approaches for PHEO resection can lead to primary adrenal insufficiency (PAI) in order of ascending frequency: Cortical sparing vs. unilateral vs. bilateral adrenalectomy. Glucocorticoids supplementation is not routinely prescribed for patients undergoing unilateral adrenalectomy because the contralateral adrenal gland can maintain eucortisolemia [101]. An individualized preoperative evaluation to identify risk factors for primary or secondary adrenal insufficiency (AI) is recommended, which includes but are not limited to identification of exposure to exogenous glucocorticoids or other medications that inhibit steroidogenesis, suppression of hypothalamic pituitary adrenal (HPA) axis secondary to endogenous cortisol co-secretion, or patient-related comorbidities. Currently, cortical sparing surgical approach for PHEOs with germline mutations and low risk for metastasis have increased. Adrenal sparing surgery is also preferred in patients with either solitary adrenal gland or bilateral adrenal involvement, as chronic glucocorticoid replacement is associated with decreased quality of life, increased cardiovascular risk, fatigue, infections and decreased resistance to stress [102,103].

When adrenal insufficiency is clinically suspected among patients undergoing bilateral adrenalectomy or in cases of subclinical or overt cortisol co-secretion, hydrocortisone 50 mg intravenous bolus is administered before anesthesia induction followed by 25–50 mg intravenously every eight hours thereafter, with tapering over the next 24–48 h. If no immediate postoperative complications develop, and patient can tolerate oral intake, transition to physiological oral maintenance dose with hydrocortisone 10–12 mg x body surface area (BSA) is recommended [104,105]. The proposed dosages can be individualized based on the patient's history and length of surgery. If immediate complications develop, patients should remain on supraphysiologic doses of steroids as per clinical judgment.

Clinical surveillance for symptoms suggestive of AI during the postoperative period is paramount. In addition, morning serum cortisol measurements with adrenocorticotropic hormone (ACTH) levels and Cosyntropin stimulation test are routinely used to confirm the diagnosis of AI [106]. Cosyntropin stimulation test can be performed as early as postoperative day 1 (unless precluded by clinical instability) to three to six weeks later to identify those non-critically ill patients who will benefit with glucocorticoid replacement therapy [107]. Once the diagnosis of AI is established, continuation of physiological glucocorticoid replacement is indicated. In cases of cortisol co-secretion or underlying central AI, HPA axis should be evaluated every six months to annually to assess for recovery. In contrast, after bilateral adrenalectomy, lifelong glucocorticoid and mineralocorticoid supplementation without further HPA axis testing is recommended [101,108,109].

Mineralocorticoid replacement therapy is indicated among patients with evidence of primary AI or after bilateral adrenalectomy. In these cases, fludrocortisone should be initiated when hydrocortisone dosages fall below 50 mg/day. Fludrocortisone is usually administered at dosages of 50–100 µg/day. Mineralocorticoid replacement is monitored based on the development of clinical symptoms like salt cravings, volume depletion, and orthostatic hypotension, followed by measurement of renin activity levels to a target goal in the upper end of the reference range without development of side effects [106].

Preceding discharge of patients with a confirmed diagnosis of AI, education should be provided for early recognition of adrenal crisis and sick day rules. Patients should be equipped with a steroid emergency card to be placed in wallets, set up on smartphones, and a medical alert bracelet [106].

4.2. Renal Failure

Renal injury is a rare complication associated with PPGL resection. The mechanism of renal injury is due to massive catecholamine release in the postoperative period that can potentially lead to: (1) Stimulatory effects on renin activity and (2) hypertensive crisis from severe vasoconstriction leading to hypoperfusion at the renal bed, ischemia, and necrosis of skeletal muscles provoking rhabdomyolysis [110,111]. In contrast, hypotension due to a rapid drop in catecholamine levels, or intravascular volume depletion, can lead to acute tubular necrosis [111].

Occasionally, "mass effect" from tumor may lead to renal ischemia causing direct compression of the renal artery or vasospasm secondary to catecholamines excess [112–114]. Renal artery stenosis has been reported only during a hypertensive crisis. Diagnosis can be established by the use of Doppler ultrasonography, gadolinium-enhanced 3D magnetic resonance angiography, and contrast-enhanced arteriography. Stenosis tends to be transient and reversible after tumor resection. Failure to correct the mass effect on the renal artery may lead to postoperative renal artery thrombosis, resulting in permanent kidney damage. A second surgery to correct renal artery stenosis is risky and might result in secondary nephrectomy [115]. In cases of persistent renal artery stenosis, percutaneous balloon angioplasty is recommended [116]. When angioplasty fails, open surgical revascularization should be attempted [117].

In scenarios of hypertension leading to acute kidney injury, antihypertensive therapy must be initiated as mentioned earlier in this review. In cases of severe rhabdomyolysis-related acute kidney injury, hemodialysis is recommended. Intravenous fluids must be used judiciously. Colloids, such as albumin 4%, are recommended in patients at risk or with pre-existent renal failure and low albumin levels. Nephrotoxic agents should be discontinued, and supportive care should be provided under nephrology guidance.

4.3. Hypoglycemia

PPGL patients can have glucose homeostasis abnormalities mediated by elevated catecholamine secretion leading to increased liver glycogenolysis, inhibited insulin secretion from pancreatic β-cells, and increased insulin resistance in the skeletal muscle. These pathological changes can lead to preoperative hyperglycemia [118]. Sudden withdrawal of plasma catecholamines and pre-existence of preoperative hyperglycemia may result in postoperative hypoglycemia [119]. Chen et al. reported other risk factors associated with postoperative hypoglycemia following PPGL resection including tumor size, higher pre-operative 24-hour urine metanephrine levels, and prolonged operative time. Similarly, preoperative β-adrenoceptor blockers exposure leads to increased liver glycogenolysis subsequently contributing to hypoglycemia development [9].

Classic symptoms of hypoglycemia (anxiety, sweating, chills, irritability, lightheadedness, nausea, etc.) may be masked in the postoperative period due to residual effects of anesthesia, opioid, or β-adrenoceptor blocker use. If untreated, hypoglycemia may result in neuronal cell death and brain damage [120]. Consequently, serum glucose levels should be monitored at regular intervals for at least 24 h postoperatively following a PPGL resection [121]. If a patient develops hypoglycemia, evaluation of related risk factors (for example, associated medications, critical illness, sepsis, renal or hepatic failure, or adrenal insufficiency, etc.) and identification of reversible culprits are recommended, independent of the catecholamine levels and the surgical approach [122].

Treatment considerations include administration of glucose tablets, glucose gels, or carbohydrate containing juices to provide 15–50 g of glucose. Moreover, if the patient is unable to tolerate oral intake, treatment with Dextrose 5% infusion should be started and titrated to a glucose goal of >100 mg/dL. In emergent situations, where treatment with oral or intravenous dextrose is not feasible, administration of 1 mg intramuscular glucagon should be considered [123–125]. Institutional hypoglycemia treatment guidelines and hospital policies should be promptly enforced, depending on individual patient needs and access to available resources [121,126–129].

4.4. Intestinal Pseudo-Obstruction

Increased catecholamine levels in the postoperative period following PPGL resection affects gastrointestinal smooth muscle cells and inhibits acetylcholine release from the parasympathetic nervous system, resulting in complications ranging from transient intestinal motility abnormalities to constipation, pseudo-obstruction, bowel infarction and perforation [130,131]. Moreover, commonly used medications in the postoperative period like analgesics and CCBs might demonstrate these symptoms. Moreover, α-adrenoceptor stimulation induces vasoconstriction of mesenteric arteries leading to ischemic colitis, ulceration, necrosis, and intestinal perforation, particularly in patients with risk factors for atherosclerotic or microvascular disease such as diabetes mellitus [132,133]. Ischemic colitis may be transient and reversible or associated with increased morbidity involving full thickness of the bowel wall, causing infarction and irreversible stricture requiring segmental resection. Paralytic ileus presents as constipation, abdominal distension, and discomfort for more than two to three days postoperatively. Therefore, patients are encouraged to be mobile, constantly change position, and recommended to be in sitting posture soon after surgery. Additionally, pain tolerance should be monitored to reduce analgesic dosage and avoid opioid drugs as soon as possible. Oral intake is slowly advanced starting from liquids to semi-solid and finally solid diet. High fiber diet is supplemented as the patient tolerates an oral diet. However, the use of liquid laxatives (milk of magnesium, magnesium citrate, Miralax) or rectal suppositories (bisacodyl, docusate sodium, polyethylene glycol) is advisable in some patients to relieve discomfort. Conservative management is preferred for patients with colonic distension measured on a plain radiograph as <12 cm, which includes fasting, nasogastric suction, intravenous fluid and electrolytes replacement, and discontinuation of drugs affecting colonic motility (narcotics) [134]. If conservative treatment is inefficient, endoscopic desufflation and pharmacologic treatment are initiated, especially for those who are confirmed to have increased catecholamine levels due to widespread metastatic disease [135]. α-adrenoceptor blockers such as phenoxybenzamine or doxazosin are initially considered as the pharmacological management among those with widespread metastatic disease, due to their additional beneficial effect on the smooth muscle cells of the intestine and blood vessels. Moreover, Metyrosine, a tyrosine analog competitively inhibiting tyrosine hydroxylase (enzyme catalyzing rate-limiting step of conversion of tyrosine to dihydroxyphenylalanine DOPA in catecholamine synthesis) causes significant catecholamine store depletion inside tumor cells. Therefore, it is our strong recommendation to start metyrosine at 250 mg orally twice daily and, if necessary, increase the dose every 48 h. Occasionally, pseudo-obstruction is extremely severe with no improvement, despite using conservative and pharmacologic management. At this point of time, the use of phentolamine (short-acting, competitive α_1- and α_2-adrenoceptor antagonist) at a dose of 1–5 mg intravenously is justified. Additionally, phentolamine is also helpful in controlling elevated blood pressure following PPGL resection [134,136]. Nevertheless, major drawbacks associated with its use are: (1) Recurrence of pseudo-obstruction following discontinuation of drug and (2) intravenous administration requiring continuous intensive care monitoring to avoid a precipitous drop in blood pressure [137–140] (Table 5).

Table 5. Postoperative complications following PPGL resection.

Complication	Reason	Recommended First Line Management
Hypertension	•Incomplete tumor removal •Tumor present at unknown location •Metastatic tumor •Excessive vasopressor use •Surplus IV fluids administration •Pain medication •Underlying essential hypertension	Nicardipine Labetalol
Hypotension	•Chronically low circulating plasma volume •Prolonged (preoperative) α-adrenoceptor blockade action •Abrupt decrease in serum catecholamines levels •Downregulation of adrenoceptors •Blood loss	IV fluids #
Arrhythmia	Tachyarrhythmia: •Elevated sympathetic activity from increased catecholamines levels and pain •Use of inotropes for postoperative hypotension •Rebound effect of preoperative discontinuation of β-adrenoceptor blockers	*Stable narrow complex sinus tachycardia:* Treat underlying cause *Stable regular narrow complex non-sinus tachycardia*: Vagal maneuvers- adenosine, expert consultation *Stable irregular narrow complex tachycardia*: Expert consultation. *Stable wide complex tachycardia*: Expert consultation *Hemodynamically unstable tachycardia*: Electrical cardioversion
	Bradyarrhythmia: •Progression of native conduction disease •Electrolyte disturbance •Sinus node dysfunction •Heart block •Excessive medication used such as β-adrenoceptor blockers	Treatment of underlying abnormalities Atropine Dopamine Epinephrine
Myocardial infarction	Increased catecholamines causes myocyte injury by: •Hemodynamic compromise •Tachycardia •Increased oxygen consumption •Coronary artery vasoconstriction	12-lead EKG Expert consultation
Heart failure	•Desensitized adrenoceptors on myocardium •Cardiomyopathy	Expert consultation
Cerebrovascular accident	•Uncontrolled hypertension •Thrombotic or embolic occlusion of cerebral artery •Rupture of intracranial artery leading to hemorrhage	Expert consultation

Table 5. *Cont.*

Complication	Reason	Recommended First Line Management
Adrenocortical insufficiency	•PHEO resection with concomitant cortisol hypersecretion	Hydrocortisone Fludrocortisone
	•Bilateral adrenalectomy	
Renal Failure	•Hypoperfusion of renal bed (hypotension, hypertension and massive bleeding) •Secondary to rhabdomyolysis	Antihypertensive medication (if hypertension exits) IV fluid therapy based on electrolytes Hemodialysis
Hypoglycemia	•Hyperinsulinemia from increased catecholamine secretion (predominantly β-adrenergic) •Sudden withdrawal of catecholamines	50% Dextrose (0.5 ml ampules) Maintenance fluid must include 5–20% dextrose.
Intestinal pseudo-obstruction	•Hypomotility from increased catecholamines •Mesenteric vasoconstriction (predominantly α-adrenergic) •Use of opioid analgesics	Laxatives diet with high fiber content, enema

Blood transfusion if indicated. Abbreviations: BSA, body surface area; EKG, electrocardiogram; IV, intravenous; PHEO, pheochromocytoma.

5. Other Common Surgical Complications

Complications observed after any surgical procedure which were not mentioned earlier include nausea, vomiting, urinary retention, hemorrhage, and wound infection. These complications are not elaborately described here as they can be managed similarly to any other surgical procedures. Meticulous monitoring along with the skills of a multidisciplinary team of physicians and appropriate nursing care, together with patient cooperation are helpful for faster recovery with no or minimal complications in the postoperative period.

PPGL patients are at a significant risk of bleeding, which is difficult to be identified as hypotension. It is not uncommon after tumor resection. Elevated blood pressure as a result of higher catecholamines causes hemorrhage either intra or postoperatively. Precise surgical technique is crucial to avoid redundant blood loss intraoperatively. Therefore, an experienced surgeon is preferred to resect PPGL, minimize blood loss, and make use of meticulous surgical techniques to accurately scissor out tumor from a complex site. However, in the incidence of major hemorrhage, hemodynamic stability of the patient is assessed, and appropriate transfusion is given as per the needs of the patient and clinical judgment of the surgeon and anesthetist. Depending on the risk to benefit ratio, necessary medications would be stopped or continued during the perioperative period and if in doubt, a consult specialist opinion is considered.

Surgical site/wound infection is a potential cause of morbidity and mortality in the postoperative period. Risk factors depend on location, nature of surgical wound/incision, and the procedure performed [141]. Postoperatively, regular wound inspection, infection control, and strict hygiene (specifically hand hygiene and early removal of clips, sutures, drains, and foreign materials) minimize the risk of wound infection. However, patients with surgical site infection present with pain, swelling, redness, warmth, purulent wound discharge, or dehiscence. Such patients are managed with appropriate laboratory work and targeted empiric antibiotic therapy is initiated as soon as possible.

Urinary retention, commonly regarded as a minor and trivial complication by surgeons, might cause increased restlessness, confusion, and delirium [142]. A catecholamine surge in the postoperative period from PPGL resection inhibits detrusor contraction via α-adrenoceptor mediated increase in bladder outlet and proximal urethral tone. Moreover, residual anesthetic effects cause bladder atony by acting as smooth muscle relaxants and interfering with autonomic regulation of detrusor muscle tone. Furthermore, vasopressors used to treat postoperative hypotension promote urinary retention by their effects on β-adrenoceptor in bladder and α-adrenoceptor in the bladder neck and proximal urethra. Moreover, aggressive fluid administration to correct hypotension might cause overdistension of the urinary bladder resulting in urinary retention. Diagnosis is based on the patient complaining of discomfort, palpable bladder on examination, and ultrasound bladder scanning for rapid and accurate assessment of bladder volume [143,144]. Therefore, the first step in the management of urinary retention in the postoperative period is urethral catheterization. If a prolonged period of urinary retention is observed, the use of indwelling catheter is not advised as it may result in infection. Henceforth, pharmacotherapy with α-adrenoceptor blockers such as tamsulosin, alfuzosin, or long-acting doxazosin is recommended.

Splenectomy is required among those patients who are undergoing unilateral adrenalectomy on the left side due to the presence of a large-sized PHEO. Such patients need to be vaccinated preoperatively against pneumococcus, *Hemophilus influenzae*, and Meningococcus [2].

6. Conclusions

Patients with PPGL resection must be managed appropriately in the intensive care setting during the postoperative period. Detailed physical examination and complete laboratory workup must be conducted at regular intervals to identify a patient at risk and provide treatment at the right point of time.

Funding: This article was supported by the *Eunice Kennedy Shriver* National Institute of Child Health and Human Development, National Institutes of Health.

Conflicts of Interest: The authors declare no conflict of interest.

References

1. Martucci, V.L.; Pacak, K. Pheochromocytoma and paraganglioma: Diagnosis, genetics, management, and treatment. *Curr. Probl. Cancer* **2014**, *38*, 7–41. [CrossRef] [PubMed]
2. Pacak, K. Preoperative management of the pheochromocytoma patient. *J. Clin. Endocrinol. Metab.* **2007**, *92*, 4069–4079. [CrossRef] [PubMed]
3. Eisenhofer, G.; Peitzsch, M. Laboratory evaluation of pheochromocytoma and paraganglioma. *Clin. Chem.* **2014**, *60*, 1486–1499. [CrossRef] [PubMed]
4. Ramakrishna, H. Pheochromocytoma resection: Current concepts in anesthetic management. *J. Anaesthesiol. Clin. Pharmacol.* **2015**, *31*, 317–323. [CrossRef] [PubMed]
5. Pisarska, M.; Pedziwiatr, M.; Budzynski, A. Perioperative hemodynamic instability in patients undergoing laparoscopic adrenalectomy for pheochromocytoma. *Gland. Surg.* **2016**, *5*, 506–511. [CrossRef] [PubMed]
6. Kiernan, C.M.; Du, L.; Chen, X.; Broome, J.T.; Shi, C.; Peters, M.F.; Solorzano, C.C. Predictors of hemodynamic instability during surgery for pheochromocytoma. *Ann. Surg. Oncol.* **2014**, *21*, 3865–3871. [CrossRef] [PubMed]
7. Domi, R.; Laho, H. Management of pheochromocytoma: Old ideas and new drugs. *Niger. J. Clin. Pract.* **2012**, *15*, 253–257. [CrossRef] [PubMed]
8. Ramachandran, R.; Rewari, V. Current perioperative management of pheochromocytomas. *Indian. J. Urol.* **2017**, *33*, 19–25. [CrossRef]
9. Chen, Y.; Hodin, R.A.; Pandolfi, C.; Ruan, D.T.; McKenzie, T.J. Hypoglycemia after resection of pheochromocytoma. *Surgery* **2014**, *156*, 1404–1408. [CrossRef]
10. Cruz, S.R.; Colwell, J.A. Pheochromocytoma and ileus. *JAMA* **1972**, *219*, 1050–1051. [CrossRef]
11. Fee, H.J.; Fonkalsrud, E.W.; Ament, M.E.; Bergstein, J. Enterocolitis with peritonitis in a child with pheochromocytoma. *Ann. Surg.* **1977**, *185*, 448–450. [CrossRef] [PubMed]
12. Gagner, M.; Lacroix, A.; Bolte, E. Laparoscopic adrenalectomy in Cushing's syndrome and pheochromocytoma. *N. Engl. J. Med.* **1992**, *327*, 1033. [CrossRef] [PubMed]
13. Brunton, L.L.; Hilal-Dandan, R.; Knollmann, B.C. *Goodman & Gilman's: The Pharmacological Basis of Therapeutics*, 13th ed.; Mcgraw-Hill: New York, NY, USA, 2018.
14. Ito, Y.; Fujimoto, Y.; Obara, T. The role of epinephrine, norepinephrine, and dopamine in blood pressure disturbances in patients with pheochromocytoma. *World J. Surg.* **1992**, *16*, 759–763. [CrossRef] [PubMed]
15. Eisenhofer, G.; Kopin, I.J.; Goldstein, D.S. Catecholamine metabolism: A contemporary view with implications for physiology and medicine. *Pharmacol. Rev.* **2004**, *56*, 331–349. [CrossRef] [PubMed]
16. Tsujimoto, G.; Manger, W.M.; Hoffman, B.B. Desensitization of beta-adrenergic receptors by pheochromocytoma. *Endocrinology* **1984**, *114*, 1272–1278. [CrossRef] [PubMed]

17. Tsujimoto, G.; Honda, K.; Hoffman, B.B.; Hashimoto, K. Desensitization of postjunctional alpha 1- and alpha 2-adrenergic receptor-mediated vasopressor responses in rat harboring pheochromocytoma. *Circ. Res.* **1987**, *61*, 86–98. [CrossRef] [PubMed]
18. Eisenhofer, G.; Walther, M.M.; Huynh, T.T.; Li, S.T.; Bornstein, S.R.; Vortmeyer, A.; Mannelli, M.; Goldstein, D.S.; Linehan, W.M.; Lenders, J.W.; et al. Pheochromocytomas in von Hippel-Lindau syndrome and multiple endocrine neoplasia type 2 display distinct biochemical and clinical phenotypes. *J. Clin. Endocrinol. Metab.* **2001**, *86*, 1999–2008. [CrossRef] [PubMed]
19. Bravo, E.L.; Tarazi, R.C.; Fouad, F.M.; Textor, S.C.; Gifford, R.W., Jr.; Vidt, D.G. Blood pressure regulation in pheochromocytoma. *Hypertension* **1982**, *4*, 193–199. [PubMed]
20. Ueda, T.; Oka, N.; Matsumoto, A.; Miyazaki, H.; Ohmura, H.; Kikuchi, T.; Nakayama, M.; Kato, S.; Imaizumi, T. Pheochromocytoma presenting as recurrent hypotension and syncope. *Intern. Med.* **2005**, *44*, 222–227. [CrossRef]
21. Whelton, P.K.; Carey, R.M.; Aronow, W.S.; Casey, D.E., Jr.; Collins, K.J.; Dennison Himmelfarb, C.; DePalma, S.M.; Gidding, S.; Jamerson, K.A.; Jones, D.W.; et al. 2017 ACC/AHA/AAPA/ABC/ACPM/AGS/APhA/ASH/ASPC/NMA/PCNA Guideline for the Prevention, Detection, Evaluation, and Management of High Blood Pressure in Adults: Executive Summary: A Report of the American College of Cardiology/American Heart Association Task Force on Clinical Practice Guidelines. *Hypertension* **2018**, *71*, 1269–1324. [CrossRef] [PubMed]
22. Livingstone, M.; Duttchen, K.; Thompson, J.; Sunderani, Z.; Hawboldt, G.; Sarah Rose, M.; Pasieka, J. Hemodynamic Stability During Pheochromocytoma Resection: Lessons Learned Over the Last Two Decades. *Ann. Surg. Oncol.* **2015**, *22*, 4175–4180. [CrossRef] [PubMed]
23. Weingarten, T.N.; Cata, J.P.; O'Hara, J.F.; Prybilla, D.J.; Pike, T.L.; Thompson, G.B.; Grant, C.S.; Warner, D.O.; Bravo, E.; Sprung, J. Comparison of two preoperative medical management strategies for laparoscopic resection of pheochromocytoma. *Urology* **2010**, *76*, 508.e6–508.e11. [CrossRef] [PubMed]
24. Lord, M.S.; Augoustides, J.G. Perioperative management of pheochromocytoma: Focus on magnesium, clevidipine, and vasopressin. *J. Cardiothorac. Vasc. Anesth.* **2012**, *26*, 526–531. [CrossRef] [PubMed]
25. Kinney, M.A.; Warner, M.E.; vanHeerden, J.A.; Horlocker, T.T.; Young, W.F., Jr.; Schroeder, D.R.; Maxson, P.M.; Warner, M.A. Perianesthetic risks and outcomes of pheochromocytoma and paraganglioma resection. *Anesth. Analg.* **2000**, *91*, 1118–1123. [PubMed]
26. Bruynzeel, H.; Feelders, R.A.; Groenland, T.H.; van den Meiracker, A.H.; van Eijck, C.H.; Lange, J.F.; de Herder, W.W.; Kazemier, G. Risk Factors for Hemodynamic Instability during Surgery for Pheochromocytoma. *J. Clin. Endocrinol. Metab.* **2010**, *95*, 678–685. [CrossRef]
27. Aksakal, N.; Agcaoglu, O.; Sahbaz, N.A.; Albuz, O.; Saracoglu, A.; Yavru, A.; Barbaros, U.; Erbil, Y. Predictive Factors of Operative Hemodynamic Instability for Pheochromocytoma. *Am. Surg.* **2018**, *84*, 920–923. [PubMed]
28. Zelinka, T.; Eisenhofer, G.; Pacak, K. Pheochromocytoma as a catecholamine producing tumor: Implications for clinical practice. *Stress* **2007**, *10*, 195–203. [CrossRef] [PubMed]
29. Aronow, W.S. Treatment of hypertensive emergencies. *Ann. Transl. Med.* **2017**, *5*, S5. [CrossRef]
30. Rhoney, D.; Peacock, W.F. Intravenous therapy for hypertensive emergencies, part 1. *Am. J. Health Syst. Pharm.* **2009**, *66*, 1343–1352. [CrossRef]
31. Gray, R.J. Managing critically ill patients with esmolol. An ultra short-acting beta-adrenergic blocker. *Chest* **1988**, *93*, 398–403. [CrossRef]
32. Varon, J.; Marik, P.E. Clinical review: The management of hypertensive crises. *Crit. Care* **2003**, *7*, 374–384. [CrossRef] [PubMed]
33. Sibal, L.; Jovanovic, A.; Agarwal, S.C.; Peaston, R.T.; James, R.A.; Lennard, T.W.; Bliss, R.; Batchelor, A.; Perros, P. Phaeochromocytomas presenting as acute crises after beta blockade therapy. *Clin. Endocrinol.* **2006**, *65*, 186–190. [CrossRef] [PubMed]
34. Bravo, E.L. Pheochromocytoma: An approach to antihypertensive management. *Ann. N. Y. Acad. Sci.* **2002**, *970*, 1–10. [CrossRef] [PubMed]
35. Lund-Johansen, P. Pharmacology of combined alpha-beta-blockade. II. Haemodynamic effects of labetalol. *Drugs* **1984**, *28*, 35–50. [CrossRef] [PubMed]
36. Kanto, J.; Allonen, H.; Kleimola, T.; Mantyla, R. Pharmacokinetics of labetalol in healthy volunteers. *Int. J. Clin. Pharmacol. Ther. Toxicol.* **1981**, *19*, 41–44. [PubMed]

37. Poopalalingam, R.; Chin, E.Y. Rapid preparation of a patient with pheochromocytoma with labetolol and magnesium sulfate. *Can. J. Anaesth.* **2001**, *48*, 876–880. [CrossRef] [PubMed]
38. Cressman, M.D.; Vidt, D.G.; Gifford, R.W., Jr.; Moore, W.S.; Wilson, D.J. Intravenous labetalol in the management of severe hypertension and hypertensive emergencies. *Am. Heart J.* **1984**, *107*, 980–985. [CrossRef]
39. Hecht, J.P.; Mahmood, S.M.; Brandt, M.M. Safety of high-dose intravenous labetalol in hypertensive crisis. *Am. J. Health Syst. Pharm.* **2019**, *76*, 286–292. [CrossRef]
40. Bravo, E.L. Pheochromocytoma. *Cardiol. Rev.* **2002**, *10*, 44–50. [CrossRef]
41. Lehmann, H.U.; Hochrein, H.; Witt, E.; Mies, H.W. Hemodynamic effects of calcium antagonists. Review. *Hypertension* **1983**, *5*, II66–II73. [CrossRef]
42. Nordlander, M.; Sjoquist, P.O.; Ericsson, H.; Ryden, L. Pharmacodynamic, pharmacokinetic and clinical effects of clevidipine, an ultrashort-acting calcium antagonist for rapid blood pressure control. *Cardiovasc. Drug. Rev.* **2004**, *22*, 227–250. [CrossRef]
43. Awad, A.S.; Goldberg, M.E. Role of clevidipine butyrate in the treatment of acute hypertension in the critical care setting: A review. *Vasc. Health Risk Manag.* **2010**, *6*, 457–464.
44. Kieler-Jensen, N.; Jolin-Mellgard, A.; Nordlander, M.; Ricksten, S.E. Coronary and systemic hemodynamic effects of clevidipine, an ultra-short-acting calcium antagonist, for treatment of hypertension after coronary artery surgery. *Acta. Anaesthesiol. Scand.* **2000**, *44*, 186–193. [CrossRef]
45. Powroznyk, A.V.; Vuylsteke, A.; Naughton, C.; Misso, S.L.; Holloway, J.; Jolin-Mellgard, A.; Latimer, R.D.; Nordlander, M.; Feneck, R.O. Comparison of clevidipine with sodium nitroprusside in the control of blood pressure after coronary artery surgery. *Eur. J. Anaesthesiol.* **2003**, *20*, 697–703. [CrossRef]
46. Bussmann, W.D.; Kenedi, P.; von Mengden, H.J.; Nast, H.P.; Rachor, N. Comparison of nitroglycerin with nifedipine in patients with hypertensive crisis or severe hypertension. *Clin. Investig.* **1992**, *70*, 1085–1088. [CrossRef] [PubMed]
47. Varon, J.; Marik, P.E. Perioperative hypertension management. *Vasc. Health Risk Manag.* **2008**, *4*, 615–627. [CrossRef]
48. Bryskin, R.; Weldon, B.C. Dexmedetomidine and magnesium sulfate in the perioperative management of a child undergoing laparoscopic resection of bilateral pheochromocytomas. *J. Clin. Anesth.* **2010**, *22*, 126–129. [CrossRef] [PubMed]
49. Kaufman, B.H.; Telander, R.L.; van Heerden, J.A.; Zimmerman, D.; Sheps, S.G.; Dawson, B. Pheochromocytoma in the pediatric age group: Current status. *J. Pediatr. Surg.* **1983**, *18*, 879–884. [CrossRef]
50. Minami, T.; Adachi, T.; Fukuda, K. An effective use of magnesium sulfate for intraoperative management of laparoscopic adrenalectomy for pheochromocytoma in a pediatric patient. *Anesth. Analg.* **2002**, *95*, 1243–1244, table of contents. [CrossRef]
51. Iseri, L.T.; French, J.H. Magnesium: nature's physiologic calcium blocker. *Am. Heart J.* **1984**, *108*, 188–193. [CrossRef]
52. Shimosawa, T.; Takano, K.; Ando, K.; Fujita, T. Magnesium inhibits norepinephrine release by blocking N-type calcium channels at peripheral sympathetic nerve endings. *Hypertension* **2004**, *44*, 897–902. [CrossRef] [PubMed]
53. Bierlaire, D.; Pea, D.; Monnier, F.; Delbreil, J.P.; Bessout, L. Phaeochromocytoma and pregnancy: Anaesthetic management about two cases. *Ann. Fr. Anesth. Reanim.* **2009**, *28*, 988–993. [CrossRef] [PubMed]
54. Golshevsky, J.R.; Karel, K.; Teale, G. Phaeochromocytoma causing acute pulmonary oedema during emergency caesarean section. *Anaesth. Intensive Care* **2007**, *35*, 423–427. [CrossRef] [PubMed]
55. Kasaoka, S.; Tsuruta, R.; Nakashima, K.; Soejima, Y.; Miura, T.; Sadamitsu, D.; Tateishi, A.; Maekawa, T. Effect of intravenous magnesium sulfate on cardiac arrhythmias in critically ill patients with low serum ionized magnesium. *Jpn. Circ. J.* **1996**, *60*, 871–875. [CrossRef] [PubMed]
56. Namekawa, T.; Utsumi, T.; Kawamura, K.; Kamiya, N.; Imamoto, T.; Takiguchi, T.; Hashimoto, N.; Tanaka, T.; Naya, Y.; Suzuki, H.; et al. Clinical predictors of prolonged postresection hypotension after laparoscopic adrenalectomy for pheochromocytoma. *Surgery* **2016**, *159*, 763–770. [CrossRef] [PubMed]
57. Kercher, K.W.; Novitsky, Y.W.; Park, A.; Matthews, B.D.; Litwin, D.E.; Heniford, B.T. Laparoscopic curative resection of pheochromocytomas. *Ann. Surg.* **2005**, *241*, 919–926. [CrossRef] [PubMed]
58. Chang, R.Y.; Lang, B.H.; Wong, K.P.; Lo, C.Y. High pre-operative urinary norepinephrine is an independent determinant of peri-operative hemodynamic instability in unilateral pheochromocytoma/paraganglioma removal. *World J. Surg.* **2014**, *38*, 2317–2323. [CrossRef] [PubMed]

59. Cryer, P.E. Physiology and pathophysiology of the human sympathoadrenal neuroendocrine system. *N. Engl. J. Med.* **1980**, *303*, 436–444. [CrossRef] [PubMed]
60. Olson, S.W.; Deal, L.E.; Piesman, M. Epinephrine-secreting pheochromocytoma presenting with cardiogenic shock and profound hypocalcemia. *Ann. Intern. Med.* **2004**, *140*, 849–851. [CrossRef]
61. Bartels, E.C.; Cattell, R.B. Pheochromocytoma; its diagnosis and treatment. *Ann. Surg.* **1950**, *131*, 903–916. [CrossRef]
62. Frang, H.; Cockcroft, V.; Karskela, T.; Scheinin, M.; Marjamaki, A. Phenoxybenzamine binding reveals the helical orientation of the third transmembrane domain of adrenergic receptors. *J. Biol. Chem.* **2001**, *276*, 31279–31284. [CrossRef] [PubMed]
63. Mannelli, M. Management and treatment of pheochromocytomas and paragangliomas. *Ann. N. Y. Acad. Sci.* **2006**, *1073*, 405–416. [CrossRef] [PubMed]
64. Kayilioglu, S.I.; Dinc, T.; Sozen, I.; Bostanoglu, A.; Cete, M.; Coskun, F. Postoperative fluid management. *World J. Crit. Care Med.* **2015**, *4*, 192–201. [CrossRef] [PubMed]
65. Bangash, M.N.; Kong, M.L.; Pearse, R.M. Use of inotropes and vasopressor agents in critically ill patients. *Br. J. Pharmacol.* **2012**, *165*, 2015–2033. [CrossRef] [PubMed]
66. Herget-Rosenthal, S.; Saner, F.; Chawla, L.S. Approach to hemodynamic shock and vasopressors. *Clin. J. Am. Soc. Nephrol.* **2008**, *3*, 546–553. [CrossRef] [PubMed]
67. Maas, J.J.; Pinsky, M.R.; de Wilde, R.B.; de Jonge, E.; Jansen, J.R. Cardiac output response to norepinephrine in postoperative cardiac surgery patients: Interpretation with venous return and cardiac function curves. *Crit. Care Med.* **2013**, *41*, 143–150. [CrossRef] [PubMed]
68. ECC Committee, Subcommittees and Task Forces of the American Heart Association. 2005 American Heart Association Guidelines for Cardiopulmonary Resuscitation and Emergency Cardiovascular Care. *Circulation* **2005**, *112*, IV1–IV203. [CrossRef]
69. Sato, Y.; Matsuzawa, H.; Eguchi, S. Comparative study of effects of adrenaline, dobutamine and dopamine on systemic hemodynamics and renal blood flow in patients following open heart surgery. *Jpn. Circ. J.* **1982**, *46*, 1059–1072. [CrossRef] [PubMed]
70. De Backer, D.; Creteur, J.; Silva, E.; Vincent, J.L. Effects of dopamine, norepinephrine, and epinephrine on the splanchnic circulation in septic shock: Which is best? *Crit. Care Med.* **2003**, *31*, 1659–1667. [CrossRef]
71. Dellinger, R.P.; Levy, M.M.; Rhodes, A.; Annane, D.; Gerlach, H.; Opal, S.M.; Sevransky, J.E.; Sprung, C.L.; Douglas, I.S.; Jaeschke, R.; et al. Surviving Sepsis Campaign: International guidelines for management of severe sepsis and septic shock, 2012. *Intensive Care Med.* **2013**, *39*, 165–228. [CrossRef]
72. Myburgh, J.A.; Higgins, A.; Jovanovska, A.; Lipman, J.; Ramakrishnan, N.; Santamaria, J.; CAT Study Investigators. A comparison of epinephrine and norepinephrine in critically ill patients. *Intensive Care Med.* **2008**, *34*, 2226–2234. [CrossRef] [PubMed]
73. Overgaard, C.B.; Dzavik, V. Inotropes and vasopressors: Review of physiology and clinical use in cardiovascular disease. *Circulation* **2008**, *118*, 1047–1056. [CrossRef] [PubMed]
74. Augoustides, J.G.; Abrams, M.; Berkowitz, D.; Fraker, D. Vasopressin for hemodynamic rescue in catecholamine-resistant vasoplegic shock after resection of massive pheochromocytoma. *Anesthesiology* **2004**, *101*, 1022–1024. [CrossRef] [PubMed]
75. Hollenberg, S.M.; Dellinger, R.P. Noncardiac surgery: Postoperative arrhythmias. *Crit. Care Med.* **2000**, *28*, N145–N150. [CrossRef] [PubMed]
76. Fenster, P.E.; Quan, S.F.; Hanson, C.D.; Coaker, L.A. Suppression of ventricular ectopy with intravenous metoprolol in patients with chronic obstructive pulmonary disease. *Crit. Care Med.* **1984**, *12*, 29–32. [CrossRef] [PubMed]
77. Hilleman, D.E.; Spinler, S.A. Conversion of recent-onset atrial fibrillation with intravenous amiodarone: A meta-analysis of randomized controlled trials. *Pharmacotherapy* **2002**, *22*, 66–74. [CrossRef] [PubMed]
78. Neumar, R.W.; Otto, C.W.; Link, M.S.; Kronick, S.L.; Shuster, M.; Callaway, C.W.; Kudenchuk, P.J.; Ornato, J.P.; McNally, B.; Silvers, S.M.; et al. Part 8: Adult advanced cardiovascular life support: 2010 American Heart Association Guidelines for Cardiopulmonary Resuscitation and Emergency Cardiovascular Care. *Circulation* **2010**, *122*, S729–S767. [CrossRef] [PubMed]
79. Savelieva, I.; Camm, A.J. If inhibition with ivabradine: Electrophysiological effects and safety. *Drug Saf.* **2008**, *31*, 95–107. [CrossRef]

80. Swedberg, K.; Komajda, M.; Bohm, M.; Borer, J.S.; Ford, I.; Dubost-Brama, A.; Lerebours, G.; Tavazzi, L.; Investigators, S. Ivabradine and outcomes in chronic heart failure (SHIFT): A randomised placebo-controlled study. *Lancet* **2010**, *376*, 875–885. [CrossRef]
81. Fox, K.; Ford, I.; Steg, P.G.; Tendera, M.; Ferrari, R.; Investigators, B. Ivabradine for patients with stable coronary artery disease and left-ventricular systolic dysfunction (BEAUTIFUL): A randomised, double-blind, placebo-controlled trial. *Lancet* **2008**, *372*, 807–816. [CrossRef]
82. Costa, G.A.; Tannuri, U.; Delgado, A.F. Bradycardia in the early postoperative period of liver transplantation in children. *Transplant. Proc.* **2010**, *42*, 1774–1776. [CrossRef] [PubMed]
83. Habuchi, Y.; Tanaka, H.; Nishio, M.; Yamamoto, T.; Komori, T.; Morikawa, J.; Yoshimura, M. Dopamine stimulation of cardiac beta-adrenoceptors: The involvement of sympathetic amine transporters and the effect of SKF38393. *Br. J. Pharmacol.* **1997**, *122*, 1669–1678. [CrossRef] [PubMed]
84. Brown, H.; Goldberg, P.A.; Selter, J.G.; Cabin, H.S.; Marieb, N.J.; Udelsman, R.; Setaro, J.F. Hemorrhagic pheochromocytoma associated with systemic corticosteroid therapy and presenting as myocardial infarction with severe hypertension. *J. Clin. Endocrinol. Metab.* **2005**, *90*, 563–569. [CrossRef] [PubMed]
85. Galetta, F.; Franzoni, F.; Bernini, G.; Poupak, F.; Carpi, A.; Cini, G.; Tocchini, L.; Antonelli, A.; Santoro, G. Cardiovascular complications in patients with pheochromocytoma: A mini-review. *Biomed. Pharmacother.* **2010**, *64*, 505–509. [CrossRef] [PubMed]
86. Cheng, T.O. Pheochromocytoma as an MI mimic. *Hosp. Pract. (Off. Ed.)* **1990**, *25*, 16.
87. Devereaux, P.J.; Goldman, L.; Yusuf, S.; Gilbert, K.; Leslie, K.; Guyatt, G.H. Surveillance and prevention of major perioperative ischemic cardiac events in patients undergoing noncardiac surgery: A review. *CMAJ* **2005**, *173*, 779–788. [CrossRef]
88. Adams, J.E., 3rd; Sicard, G.A.; Allen, B.T.; Bridwell, K.H.; Lenke, L.G.; Davila-Roman, V.G.; Bodor, G.S.; Ladenson, J.H.; Jaffe, A.S. Diagnosis of perioperative myocardial infarction with measurement of cardiac troponin I. *N. Engl. J. Med.* **1994**, *330*, 670–674. [CrossRef]
89. Landesberg, G.; Beattie, W.S.; Mosseri, M.; Jaffe, A.S.; Alpert, J.S. Perioperative myocardial infarction. *Circulation* **2009**, *119*, 2936–2944. [CrossRef]
90. Adesanya, A.O.; de Lemos, J.A.; Greilich, N.B.; Whitten, C.W. Management of perioperative myocardial infarction in noncardiac surgical patients. *Chest* **2006**, *130*, 584–596. [CrossRef]
91. Fleisher, L.A.; Fleischmann, K.E.; Auerbach, A.D.; Barnason, S.A.; Beckman, J.A.; Bozkurt, B.; Davila-Roman, V.G.; Gerhard-Herman, M.D.; Holly, T.A.; Kane, G.C.; et al. 2014 ACC/AHA guideline on perioperative cardiovascular evaluation and management of patients undergoing noncardiac surgery: Executive summary: A report of the American College of Cardiology/American Heart Association Task Force on Practice Guidelines. *Circulation* **2014**, *130*, 2215–2245. [CrossRef]
92. Mulla, C.M.; Marik, P.E. Pheochromocytoma presenting as acute decompensated heart failure reversed with medical therapy. *BMJ Case Rep.* **2012**, *2012*. [CrossRef] [PubMed]
93. Cohen, J.K.; Cisco, R.M.; Scholten, A.; Mitmaker, E.; Duh, Q.Y. Pheochromocytoma crisis resulting in acute heart failure and cardioembolic stroke in a 37-year-old man. *Surgery* **2014**, *155*, 726–727. [CrossRef] [PubMed]
94. Lee, Y.; Tan, L.Y.R.; Ho, Y.H.; Leow, M.K.S. Giant phaeochromocytoma presenting with an acute stroke: Reappraising phaeochromocytoma surveillance for the neurofibromatosis type 1 phakomatosis. *BMJ Case Rep.* **2017**, *2017*. [CrossRef] [PubMed]
95. Lin, P.C.; Hsu, J.T.; Chung, C.M.; Chang, S.T. Pheochromocytoma underlying hypertension, stroke, and dilated cardiomyopathy. *Tex. Heart Inst. J.* **2007**, *34*, 244–246. [PubMed]
96. Kam, P.C.; Calcroft, R.M. Peri-operative stroke in general surgical patients. *Anaesthesia* **1997**, *52*, 879–883. [CrossRef] [PubMed]
97. Mashour, G.A.; Sharifpour, M.; Freundlich, R.E.; Tremper, K.K.; Shanks, A.; Nallamothu, B.K.; Vlisides, P.E.; Weightman, A.; Matlen, L.; Merte, J.; et al. Perioperative metoprolol and risk of stroke after noncardiac surgery. *Anesthesiology* **2013**, *119*, 1340–1346. [CrossRef] [PubMed]
98. Ng, J.L.; Chan, M.T.; Gelb, A.W. Perioperative stroke in noncardiac, nonneurosurgical surgery. *Anesthesiology* **2011**, *115*, 879–890. [CrossRef]
99. Norris, J.W.; Hachinski, V.C. Misdiagnosis of stroke. *Lancet* **1982**, *1*, 328–331. [CrossRef]

100. Adams, H.P., Jr.; del Zoppo, G.; Alberts, M.J.; Bhatt, D.L.; Brass, L.; Furlan, A.; Grubb, R.L.; Higashida, R.T.; Jauch, E.C.; Kidwell, C.; et al. Guidelines for the early management of adults with ischemic stroke: A guideline from the American Heart Association/American Stroke Association Stroke Council, Clinical Cardiology Council, Cardiovascular Radiology and Intervention Council, and the Atherosclerotic Peripheral Vascular Disease and Quality of Care Outcomes in Research Interdisciplinary Working Groups: The American Academy of Neurology affirms the value of this guideline as an educational tool for neurologists. *Circulation* **2007**, *115*, e478–e534. [CrossRef]
101. Shen, W.T.; Lee, J.; Kebebew, E.; Clark, O.H.; Duh, Q.Y. Selective use of steroid replacement after adrenalectomy: Lessons from 331 consecutive cases. *Arch. Surg.* **2006**, *141*, 771–774; discussion 774–776. [CrossRef]
102. de Graaf, J.S.; Lips, C.J.; Rutter, J.E.; van Vroonhoven, T.J. Subtotal adrenalectomy for phaeochromocytoma in multiple endocrine neoplasia type 2A. *Eur J. Surg.* **1999**, *165*, 535–538. [CrossRef] [PubMed]
103. van Heerden, J.A.; Sizemore, G.W.; Carney, J.A.; Grant, C.S.; ReMine, W.H.; Sheps, S.G. Surgical management of the adrenal glands in the multiple endocrine neoplasia type II syndrome. *World J. Surg.* **1984**, *8*, 612–621. [CrossRef] [PubMed]
104. Lamberts, S.W.; Bruining, H.A.; de Jong, F.H. Corticosteroid therapy in severe illness. *N. Engl. J. Med.* **1997**, *337*, 1285–1292. [CrossRef] [PubMed]
105. Liu, M.M.; Reidy, A.B.; Saatee, S.; Collard, C.D. Perioperative Steroid Management: Approaches Based on Current Evidence. *Anesthesiology* **2017**, *127*, 166–172. [CrossRef] [PubMed]
106. Bornstein, S.R.; Allolio, B.; Arlt, W.; Barthel, A.; Don-Wauchope, A.; Hammer, G.D.; Husebye, E.S.; Merke, D.P.; Murad, M.H.; Stratakis, C.A.; et al. Diagnosis and Treatment of Primary Adrenal Insufficiency: An Endocrine Society Clinical Practice Guideline. *J. Clin. Endocrinol. Metab.* **2016**, *101*, 364–389. [CrossRef] [PubMed]
107. Ortiz, D.I.; Findling, J.W.; Carroll, T.B.; Javorsky, B.R.; Carr, A.A.; Evans, D.B.; Yen, T.W.; Wang, T.S. Cosyntropin stimulation testing on postoperative day 1 allows for selective glucocorticoid replacement therapy after adrenalectomy for hypercortisolism: Results of a novel, multidisciplinary institutional protocol. *Surgery* **2016**, *159*, 259–265. [CrossRef]
108. Arlt, W. The approach to the adult with newly diagnosed adrenal insufficiency. *J. Clin. Endocrinol. Metab.* **2009**, *94*, 1059–1067. [CrossRef]
109. Grossman, A.B. Clinical Review#: The diagnosis and management of central hypoadrenalism. *J. Clin. Endocrinol. Metab.* **2010**, *95*, 4855–4863. [CrossRef] [PubMed]
110. Celik, H.; Celik, O.; Guldiken, S.; Inal, V.; Puyan, F.O.; Tugrul, A. Pheochromocytoma presenting with rhabdomyolysis and acute renal failure: A case report. *Ren. Fail.* **2014**, *36*, 104–107. [CrossRef]
111. Jin, Y.S.; Fan, M.X. Pheochromocytoma Characterizing Both Fever and Acute Renal Failure. *Chin. Med. J.* **2017**, *130*, 617–618. [CrossRef]
112. Pickard, J.L.; Ross, G., Jr.; Silver, D. Coexisting extraadrenal pheochromocytoma and renal artery stenosis: A case report and review of the pathophysiology. *J. Pediatr. Surg.* **1995**, *30*, 1613–1615. [CrossRef]
113. Kaufman, J.J. Pheochromocytoma and stenosis of the renal artery. *Surg. Gynecol. Obstet.* **1983**, *156*, 11–15. [PubMed]
114. Stanley, J.C.; Gewertz, B.L.; Bove, E.L.; Sottiurai, V.; Fry, W.J. Arterial fibrodysplasia. Histopathologic character and current etiologic concepts. *Arch. Surg.* **1975**, *110*, 561–566. [CrossRef] [PubMed]
115. Kota, S.K.; Kota, S.K.; Meher, L.K.; Jammula, S.; Panda, S.; Modi, K.D. Coexistence of pheochromocytoma with uncommon vascular lesions. *Indian J. Endocrinol. Metab.* **2012**, *16*, 962–971. [CrossRef] [PubMed]
116. Burns, A.P.; O'Connell, P.R.; Murnaghan, D.J.; Brady, M.P. Bilateral adrenal phaeochromocytomas associated with unilateral renal artery stenosis. *Postgrad. Med. J.* **1989**, *65*, 943–947. [CrossRef]
117. Gill, I.S.; Meraney, A.M.; Bravo, E.L.; Novick, A.C. Pheochromocytoma coexisting with renal artery lesions. *J. Urol.* **2000**, *164*, 296–301. [CrossRef]
118. Spergel, G.; Bleicher, S.J.; Ertel, N.H. Carbohydrate and fat metabolism in patients with pheochromocytoma. *N. Engl. J. Med.* **1968**, *278*, 803–809. [CrossRef]
119. Reynolds, C.; Wilkins, G.E.; Schmidt, N.; Doll, W.A.; Blix, P.M. Hyperinsulinism after removal of a pheochromocytoma. *Can. Med. Assoc. J.* **1983**, *129*, 349–353.
120. Auer, R.N. Hypoglycemic brain damage. *Metab. Brain Dis.* **2004**, *19*, 169–175. [CrossRef]
121. Levin, H.; Heifetz, M. Phaeochromocytoma and severe protracted postoperative hypoglycaemia. *Can. J. Anaesth.* **1990**, *37*, 477–478. [CrossRef]

122. Cryer, P.E.; Axelrod, L.; Grossman, A.B.; Heller, S.R.; Montori, V.M.; Seaquist, E.R.; Service, F.J.; Endocrine, S. Evaluation and management of adult hypoglycemic disorders: An Endocrine Society Clinical Practice Guideline. *J. Clin. Endocrinol. Metab.* **2009**, *94*, 709–728. [CrossRef] [PubMed]
123. Elliott, M.B.; Schafers, S.J.; McGill, J.B.; Tobin, G.S. Prediction and prevention of treatment-related inpatient hypoglycemia. *J. Diabetes Sci. Technol.* **2012**, *6*, 302–309. [CrossRef] [PubMed]
124. Brutsaert, E.; Carey, M.; Zonszein, J. The clinical impact of inpatient hypoglycemia. *J. Diabetes Complicat.* **2014**, *28*, 565–572. [CrossRef] [PubMed]
125. Fischer, K.F.; Lees, J.A.; Newman, J.H. Hypoglycemia in hospitalized patients. Causes and outcomes. *N. Engl. J. Med.* **1986**, *315*, 1245–1250. [CrossRef] [PubMed]
126. Meeke, R.I.; O'Keeffe, J.D.; Gaffney, J.D. Phaeochromocytoma removal and postoperative hypoglycaemia. *Anaesthesia* **1985**, *40*, 1093–1096. [CrossRef]
127. Eiland, L.; Goldner, W.; Drincic, A.; Desouza, C. Inpatient hypoglycemia: A challenge that must be addressed. *Curr. Diabetes Rep.* **2014**, *14*, 445. [CrossRef]
128. Hulkower, R.D.; Pollack, R.M.; Zonszein, J. Understanding hypoglycemia in hospitalized patients. *Diabetes Manag.* **2014**, *4*, 165–176. [CrossRef]
129. Araque, K.A.; Kadayakkara, D.K.; Gigauri, N.; Sheehan, D.; Majumdar, S.; Buller, G.; Flannery, C.A. Reducing severe hypoglycaemia in hospitalised patients with diabetes: Early outcomes of standardised reporting and management. *BMJ Open Qual.* **2018**, *7*, e000120. [CrossRef]
130. Kek, P.C.; Ho, E.T.; Loh, L.M. Phaeochromocytoma presenting with pseudo-intestinal obstruction and lactic acidosis. *Singap. Med. J.* **2015**, *56*, e131–e133. [CrossRef]
131. Osinga, T.E.; Kerstens, M.N.; van der Klauw, M.M.; Koornstra, J.J.; Wolffenbuttel, B.H.; Links, T.P.; van der Horst-Schrivers, A.N. Intestinal pseudo-obstruction as a complication of paragangliomas: Case report and literature review. *Neth. J. Med.* **2013**, *71*, 512–517.
132. Wu, H.W.; Liou, W.P.; Chou, C.C.; Chen, Y.H.; Loh, C.H.; Wang, H.P. Pheochromocytoma presented as intestinal pseudo-obstruction and hyperamylasemia. *Am. J. Emerg. Med.* **2008**, *26*, 971.e1–971.e4. [CrossRef] [PubMed]
133. Sohn, C.I.; Kim, J.J.; Lim, Y.H.; Rhee, P.L.; Koh, K.C.; Paik, S.W.; Rhee, J.C.; Chung, J.H.; Lee, M.S.; Yang, J.H. A case of ischemic colitis associated with pheochromocytoma. *Am. J. Gastroenterol.* **1998**, *93*, 124–126. [CrossRef] [PubMed]
134. Saunders, M.D. Acute colonic pseudo-obstruction. *Best Pract. Res. Clin. Gastroenterol.* **2007**, *21*, 671–687. [CrossRef] [PubMed]
135. Loftus, C.G.; Harewood, G.C.; Baron, T.H. Assessment of predictors of response to neostigmine for acute colonic pseudo-obstruction. *Am. J. Gastroenterol.* **2002**, *97*, 3118–3122. [CrossRef] [PubMed]
136. Eisen, G.M.; Baron, T.H.; Dominitz, J.A.; Faigel, D.O.; Goldstein, J.L.; Johanson, J.F.; Mallery, J.S.; Raddawi, H.M.; Vargo, J.J.; Waring, J.P.; et al. Acute colonic pseudo-obstruction. *Gastrointest. Endosc.* **2002**, *56*, 789–792. [CrossRef]
137. Yamaguchi, I.; Kopin, I.J. Differential inhibiton of alpha-1 and alpha-2 adrenoceptor-mediated pressor responses in pithed rats. *J. Pharmacol. Exp. Ther.* **1980**, *214*, 275–281. [PubMed]
138. Khafagi, F.A.; Lloyd, H.M.; Gough, I.R. Intestinal pseudo-obstruction in pheochromocytoma. *Aust. N. Z. J. Med.* **1987**, *17*, 246–248. [CrossRef]
139. Hashimoto, Y.; Motoyoshi, S.; Maruyama, H.; Sakakida, M.; Yano, T.; Yamaguchi, K.; Goto, K.; Sugihara, S.; Takano, S.; Kambara, T.; et al. The treatment of pheochromocytoma associated with pseudo-obstruction and perforation of the colon, hepatic failure, and DIC. *Jpn. J. Med.* **1990**, *29*, 341–346. [CrossRef]
140. Marik, P.E.; Rivera, R. Hypertensive emergencies: An update. *Curr. Opin. Crit. Care* **2011**, *17*, 569–580. [CrossRef]
141. Young, P.Y.; Khadaroo, R.G. Surgical site infections. *Surg. Clin. N. Am.* **2014**, *94*, 1245–1264. [CrossRef]
142. Darrah, D.M.; Griebling, T.L.; Silverstein, J.H. Postoperative urinary retention. *Anesthesiol. Clin.* **2009**, *27*, 465–484, table of contents. [CrossRef] [PubMed]

143. Pavlin, D.J.; Pavlin, E.G.; Gunn, H.C.; Taraday, J.K.; Koerschgen, M.E. Voiding in patients managed with or without ultrasound monitoring of bladder volume after outpatient surgery. *Anesth. Analg.* **1999**, *89*, 90–97. [PubMed]
144. Sarasin, S.M.; Walton, M.J.; Singh, H.P.; Clark, D.I. Can a urinary tract symptom score predict the development of postoperative urinary retention in patients undergoing lower limb arthroplasty under spinal anaesthesia? A prospective study. *Ann. R. Coll. Surg. Engl.* **2006**, *88*, 394–398. [CrossRef] [PubMed]

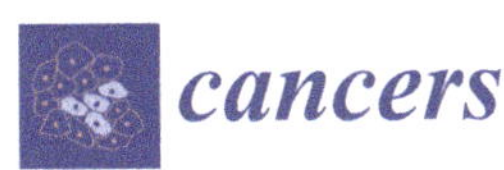

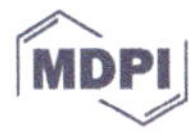

Article

FGF21 Levels in Pheochromocytoma/Functional Paraganglioma

Judita Klímová [1,*], Tomáš Zelinka [1], Ján Rosa [1], Branislav Štrauch [1], Denisa Haluzíková [2], Martin Haluzík [3,4], Robert Holaj [1], Zuzana Krátká [1], Jan Kvasnička [1], Viktorie Ďurovcová [1], Martin Matoulek [1], Květoslav Novák [5], David Michalský [6], Jiří Widimský Jr. [1] and Ondřej Petrák [1]

1. Third Department of Medicine, Department of Endocrinology and Metabolism of the First Faculty of Medicine, Charles University and General University Hospital in Prague, 128 00 Prague, Czech Republic; Tomas.Zelinka@vfn.cz (T.Z.); Jan.Rosa@vfn.cz (J.R.); Branislav.Strauch@vfn.cz (B.Š.); Robert.Holaj@vfn.cz (R.H.); Zuzana.Kratka@vfn.cz (Z.K.); Jan.Kvasnicka3@vfn.cz (J.K.); viktoria.durovcova@gmail.com (V.Ď.); martin.matoulek@vstj.cz (M.M.); Jiri.Widimsky@vfn.cz (J.W.J.); Ondrej.Petrak@vfn.cz (O.P.)
2. Institute of Sports Medicine, First Faculty of Medicine, Charles University and General University Hospital in Prague, 120 00 Prague, Czech Republic; Denisa.Haluzikova@vfn.cz
3. Centre for Experimental Medicine and Diabetes Centre, Institute for Clinical and Experimental Medicine, 140 21 Prague, Czech Republic; martin.haluzik@ikem.cz
4. Institute for Medical Biochemistry and Laboratory Diagnostics, Charles University and General University Hospital in Prague, 128 08 Prague, Czech Republic
5. Department of Urology of the First Faculty of Medicine, Charles University and General University Hospital in Prague, 128 00 Prague, Czech Republic; Kvetoslav.Novak@vfn.cz
6. First Department of Surgery of the First Faculty of Medicine, Charles University and General University Hospital in Prague, 128 00 Prague, Czech Republic; david.michalsky@vfn.cz

* Correspondence: Judita.Klimova@vfn.cz; Tel.: +420-224-962845

Received: 3 March 2019; Accepted: 2 April 2019; Published: 5 April 2019

Abstract: Fibroblast growth factor 21 (FGF21) is a hepatokine with beneficial effects on metabolism. Our aim was to evaluate the relationship between the serum FGF21, and energy and glucose metabolism in 40 patients with pheochromocytoma/functional paraganglioma (PPGL), in comparison with 21 obese patients and 26 lean healthy controls. 27 patients with PPGL were examined one year after tumor removal. Basic anthropometric and biochemical measurements were done. Energy metabolism was measured by indirect calorimetry (Vmax-Encore 29N). FGF21 was measured by ELISA. FGF21 was higher in PPGL than in controls (174.2 (283) pg/mL vs. 107.9 (116) pg/mL; $p < 0.001$) and comparable with obese (174.2 (283) pg/mL vs. 160.4 (180); p = NS). After tumor removal, FGF21 decreased (176.4 (284) pg/mL vs. 131.3 (225) pg/mL; $p < 0.001$). Higher levels of FGF21 were expressed, particularly in patients with diabetes. FGF21 positively correlated in PPGL with age ($p = 0.005$), BMI ($p = 0.028$), glycemia ($p = 0.002$), and glycated hemoglobin ($p = 0.014$). In conclusion, long-term catecholamine overproduction in PPGL leads to the elevation in serum FGF21, especially in patients with secondary diabetes. FGF21 levels were comparable between obese and PPGL patients, despite different anthropometric indices. We did not find a relationship between FGF21 and hypermetabolism in PPGL. Tumor removal led to the normalization of FGF21 and the other metabolic abnormalities.

Keywords: FGF21; pheochromocytoma; paraganglioma; diabetes mellitus; obesity; energy metabolism; calorimetry

---

1. Introduction

Fibroblast growth factor 21 (FGF21) is a metabolic regulator that has a systemic effect in promoting glucose uptake and oxidation [1,2]. The main site of FGF21 expression and production in humans is liver and, to a lesser degree, muscle and white adipose tissue (WAT) [3]. In rodents, FGF21 targets brown adipose tissue (BAT), where it induces mitochondrial uncoupling protein-1 (UCP1) gene expression and favors glucose oxidation and energy expenditure [4,5].

In humans, under conditions of enhanced adaptive energy expenditure, brown adipocyte-like cells appear at sites of WAT. This is called the "browning" of WAT, and cells resembling brown adipocytes arising in this process are called "beige" [6]. The promotion of WAT browning was documented in patients with pheochromocytoma and functional paragangliomas (PPGL) due to the tumor-mediated release of catecholamines [7,8]. Analysis of visceral adipose tissue from the perirenal and omental regions in small samples of pheochromocytoma confirmed the presence of beige adipose tissue with significant expression of FGF21 [9].

Furthermore, there is also an adipose-independent mechanism for FGF21 to be able to regulate metabolism [10,11]. FGF21 can cross the blood-brain barrier and is detectable in both human and rodent cerebrospinal fluid [12,13]. Continuous intracerebroventricular injection of FGF21 to obese rats increases energy expenditure and insulin sensitivity [14]. FGF21 has been shown to act on the central nervous system to increase systemic glucocorticoid levels, suppress physical activity, and alter circadian behavior [15,16].

PPGL represents a useful model for studying the influence of long-term catecholamine overproduction in metabolic disorders in humans. Catecholamine overproduction leads to a large variety of signs and symptoms, including sustained or paroxysmal arterial hypertension, hypermetabolic state with weight loss and disorders of glucose metabolism [17]. The aim of our study was to evaluate the changes of circulating levels of FGF21 and its relationship to energy and glucose metabolism in PPGL, before and one year after tumor removal. For comparison, at baseline, we used healthy lean controls and also obese patients with glucose metabolism disorder.

2. Results

2.1. Basic Characteristics of Groups

Biochemical, anthropometrical, and clinical characteristics of the studied groups are summarized in Table 1. Obese patients and controls contained significantly more females than PPGL ($p = 0.008$). As expected, obese patients had a higher body mass index (BMI) and body fat percentage in comparison with PPGL and controls ($p < 0.001$). Also their lipid profile differed in triglycerides (TAG) and high-density lipoprotein cholesterol (HDLc) ($p < 0.001$). Higher values of resting energy expenditure/basal energy expenditure (REE/BEE) were present in PPGL and obese in comparison with controls. Hypermetabolic state was detected in 49% of PPGL and 24% of obese. PPGL and obese also showed higher systolic blood pressure (sBP) than controls ($p = 0.002$). Fasting blood glucose (FBG) and glycated hemoglobin (HbA1c) levels in PPGL and obese were similar ($p =$ NS), but higher than in controls ($p < 0.001$). Insulin levels were lower in PPGL patients than in controls ($p = 0.037$) and expectedly higher in obese, together with HOMA-IR ($p < 0.001$). Adrenergic phenotype was seen in 61% of PPGL patients and noradrenergic phenotype in 39% of PPGL patients.

2.2. Effect of Tumor Removal in PPGL

A subgroup of 27 consecutive patients with PPGL was examined one year after tumor removal. The basic characteristics of patients before and after tumor removal are summarized in Table 2. The decrease in free plasma metanephrines and chromogranine reflects successful surgery ($p < 0.001$). Weight gain was significant in all parameters, including body fat percentage. No patient fulfilled the requirements for hypermetabolism after tumor removal. No significant decrease in office blood pressure measurements was present. Sustained hypertension remained in 22% of patients, but the total number of antihypertensives decreased. FBG and HbA1c decreased significantly. Unexpectedly, insulin levels did not normalize. On the contrary, normal glucose tolerance was present in the majority of patients (93%).

Table 1. Clinical and metabolic characteristics of study subjects.

Factors	Controls n = 26	Obese n = 21	PPGL n = 40	p
Female (n, %)	21 (81)	18 (86)	21 (53)	0.008
Age (years)	48.5 ± 10	54.6 ± 14	52.4 ± 14	0.262
Body mass index (kg/m^2)	23.9 ± 3	44.9 ± 9 *,†	25.1 ± 4	<0.001
Body fat percentage (%)	27.5 ± 11	51.4 ± 11 *,†	29.5 ± 8	<0.001
Resting energy expenditure (Kcal/day)	1467 ± 165	1943 ± 398 $^{+,*}$	1691 ± 327	<0.001
REE/BEE (%)	98.7 ± 8	101.9 ± 18 ‡	110.3 ± 12 $^{\bullet}$	0.007
Systolic blood pressure (mmHg)	114.7 ± 15	132.9 ± 17 ‡	131.7 ± 18 $^{\bullet}$	0.002
Diastolic blood pressure (mmHg)	71.3 ± 15	78.8 ± 10	75.9 ± 11	0.106
Mean arterial pressure (mmHg)	85.7 ± 12	96.8 ± 11 ‡	94.8 ± 13 $^{\bullet}$	0.013
Pulse pressure (mmHg)	50.1 ± 9	54.0 ± 10	55.7 ± 12	0.439
Fasting blood glucose (mmol/L)	4.2 (0.9)	6.0 (3) *	5.8 (2.1) $^{\circ}$	<0.001
HbA1c (mmol/mol)	34.0 (6)	44.0 (25) *	42.0 (16) $^{\bullet}$	<0.001
Insulin (mIU/L)	6.1 (4)	16.3 (9) ‡	3.7 (3) $^{\bullet,\dagger}$	<0.001
HOMA-IR	1.2 (1)	4.9 (7) †,*	0.95 (1)	<0.001
Total cholesterol (mmol/L)	5.1 ± 0.8	4.9 ± 1	4.6 ± 1	0.180
HDL cholesterol (mmol/L)	1.6 ± 0.4	1.1 ± 0.3 $^{+,*}$	1.5 ± 0,5	<0.001
LDL cholesterol (mmol/L)	3 ± 0.7	2.9 ± 0.9	2.6 ± 1	0.144
Triglycerides (mmol/L)	1.0 (0.4)	1.7 (0.4) *,†	0.9 (0.7)	<0.001
Fibroblast growth factor 21 (pg/mL)	107.9 (116)	160.4 (180) *	174.2 (283) $^{\circ}$	<0.001
Hypertension (n, %)	-	18 (86)	26 (65)	0.185
Diabetes Mellitus (n, %)	-	11 (52)	13 (33)	0.757
Obesity (n, %)	-	21 (100)	6 (15)	-
Dyslipidemia (n, %)	-	18 (86)	23 (58)	0.718
Metabolic syndrome (n, %)	-	19 (90)	20 (50)	0.118
Use of PAD (n, %)	-	10 (48)	10 (26)	0.025
Use of insulin (n, %)	-	4 (19)	3 (8)	-
Use of statins (n, %)	-	10 (48)	16 (40)	0.863
Number of antihypertensives (n)	-	2.38 ± 1.5	1.85 ± 1.1	0.038
Use of alpha blockers (n, %)	-	4 (19)	28 (70)	-
Use of beta blockers (n, %)	-	12 (57)	14 (35)	0.017

* <0.001 for Obese vs. Controls; † <0.001 for Obese vs. PPGL; $^{+}$ <0.05 for Obese vs. PPGL; ‡ <0.05 for Obese vs. Controls; $^{\bullet}$ <0.05 for PPGL vs. Controls; $^{\circ}$ <0.001 for PPGL vs. Controls. Abbreviations: PPGL, pheochromocytoma; REE, resting energy expenditure; BEE, basal energy expenditure; HbA1c, glycated hemoglobin; HOMA-IR, homeostasis model assessment of insulin resistance; HDL, high-density lipoprotein; LDL, low-density lipoprotein; PAD, peroral antidiabetics.

Table 2. PPGL patients before and after surgery.

Factors	Before n = 27	After n = 27	p
Female (n, %)	15 (56)	15 (56)	-
Age (years)	51.9 ± 13	53.0 ± 13	<0.001
Body mass index (kg/m^2)	24.7 ± 3	26.2 ± 4	<0.001
Body fat percentage (%)	29.3 ± 9	32.3 ± 9	0.034
BEE (Kcal/day)	1509 ± 252	1543 ± 266	0.001
REE (Kcal/day)	1655 ± 311	1477 ± 216	<0.001
REE/BEE (%)	110.8 ± 12	96.5 ± 7	<0.001
Systolic BP (mmHg)	131.8 ± 19	124.9 ± 17	0.084
Diastolic BP (mmHg)	75.7 ± 11	74.5 ± 11	0.598
MAP (mmHg)	94.4 ± 13	91.3 ± 12	0.253
Pulse pressure (mmHg)	56.11 ± 13	55.6 ± 19	0.888
FBG (mmol/L)	5.7 (1.7)	4.8 (0.8)	<0.001
HbA1c (mmol/mol)	42.0 (17)	40.0 (6)	0.018
Insulin (mIU/L)	3.3 ± 3	2.8 ± 3	<0.001

Table 2. *Cont.*

HOMA-IR	0.9 ± 0.9	0.6 ± 0.7	<0.001
Total cholesterol (mmol/L)	4.8 ± 1	4.6 ± 1.1	0.436
HDLc (mmol/L)	1.5 ± 0.5	1.4 ± 0.8	0.237
LDLc (mmol/L)	2.7 ± 1	2.7 ± 0.8	0.771
Triglycerides (mmol/L)	0.8 (0.6)	1.2 (0.7)	0.017
FGF21 (pg/mL)	176.4 (284)	131.3 (225)	<0.001
P-Metanephrine (nmol/L)	3.1 (9)	0.17 (0.2)	<0.001
P-Normetanephrine (nmol/L)	11.6 (14)	0.33 (0.4)	<0.001
Chromogranine (ng/mL)	334.8 (489)	39.6 (38)	<0.001
Hypertension (%)	19 (70)	6 (22)	0.071
Diabetes mellitus (%)	9 (33)	2 (7)	0.037
Obesity (*n*, %)	2 (7)	2 (7)	1.000
Dyslipidemia (*n*, %)	17 (63)	18 (67)	0.775
MS (*n*, %)	14 (52)	6 (22)	0.241
Use of PAD (*n*, %)	5 (19)	2 (7)	0.203
Use of insulin (*n*, %)	3 (11)	0 (0)	0.074
Use of statins (*n*, %)	11 (41)	13 (48)	0.583
Use of AHT (*n*)	1.93 ± 1	0.37 ± 0.7	<0.001

Abbreviations: PPGL, pheochromocytoma/paraganglioma; REE, resting energy expenditure; BEE, basal energy expenditure; BP, blood pressure; MAP, mean arterial pressure; FBG, fasting blood glucose; HbA1c; glycated hemoglobin; HOMA-IR, homeostasis model assessment of insulin resistance; HDLc, high-density lipoprotein cholesterol; LDLc, low-density lipoprotein cholesterol; FGF21, fibroblast growth factor 21; P-, plasma; MS; metabolic syndrome; PAD, peroral antidiabetics; AHT, antihypertensives.

2.3. FGF21 Levels and Correlation

FGF21 levels were broad in all groups. The correlation between FGF21 and other selected factors in patients with PPGL is shown in Table 3 and Figure 1. FGF21 was significantly higher in PPGL than in controls ($p < 0.001$) and comparable with obese (p = NS). PPGL patients with diabetes showed higher levels of FGF21 than those with normal glucose tolerance (NGT) (438.2 (337) pg/mL vs. 154.5 (97) pg/mL; $p = 0.007$) or those with prediabetes (438.2 (337) pg/mL vs. 154.5 (97) pg/mL; $p = 0.022$). Diabetic obese and obese with NGT showed similar results (314.1 (300) pg/mL vs. 140.5 (7) pg/mL; $p = 0.049$). Similar differences in FGF21 levels were present in diabetic and prediabetic obese (314.1 (300) pg/mL vs. 113.1 (54) pg/mL; $p = 0.024$). Those findings are summarized in Figure 2. PPGL with metabolic syndrome or dyslipidemia showed higher FGF21 than those without ($p < 0.001$). FGF21 levels differed in PPGL with adrenergic and noradrenergic phenotypes, but were slightly above the level of significance ($p = 0.062$]. A difference in FGF21 levels between hypermetabolic and normometabolic PPGL patients was not found (p = NS). FGF21 levels in all components of metabolic syndrome in PPGL are shown in Table 4.

Table 3. Selected factors associated with serum FGF21 levels in PPGL patients.

Factors	PPGL (*n* = 40)	
	r	*p*
Age	0.435	0.005
Weight	0.267	0.095
Body mass index	0.348	0.028
P-Metanephrine	0.212	0.194
P-Normetanephrine	0.086	0.602
Respiratory Quotient	−0.121	0.474
BEE (Kcal/day)	0.169	0.316
REE (Kcal/day)	0.163	0.336
REE/BEE (%)	0.018	0.915
Systolic blood pressure	0.194	0.231
Diastolic blood pressure	−0.047	0.755
Mean arterial pressure	0.058	0.721

Table 3. *Cont.*

Pulse pressure	0.338	0.032
Fasting blood glucose	0.459	0.002
HbA1c	0.426	0.014
Insulin	0.097	0.551
HOMA-IR	0.248	0.121
Total cholesterol	−0.045	0.785
HDL cholesterol	0.009	0.593
LDL cholesterol	−0.211	0.196
Triglycerides	0.255	0.113

Abbreviations: PPGL, pheochromocytoma/paraganglioma; P-, plasma; REE, resting energy expenditure; HbA1c, glycated hemoglobin; HOMA-IR, homeostasis model assessment of insulin resistance; HDL, high-density lipoprotein; LDL, low-density lipoprotein.

Table 4. FGF21 levels in PPGL patients with metabolic syndrome and its components.

Category	Occurrence	n	FGF21	p
Dyslipidemia	Yes	23	264.9 (343)	<0.001
	No	17	133.7 (102)	
Diabetes mellitus	Yes	13	438.2 (337)	0.001
	No	27	158.0 (170)	
Central Obesity	Yes	6	214.2 (326)	0.486
	No	34	167.1 (280)	
Metabolic syndrome	Yes	20	377.9 (333)	<0.001
	No	20	147.8 (94)	
Hypertension	Yes	26	214.2 (348)	0.085
	No	14	160.4 (131)	

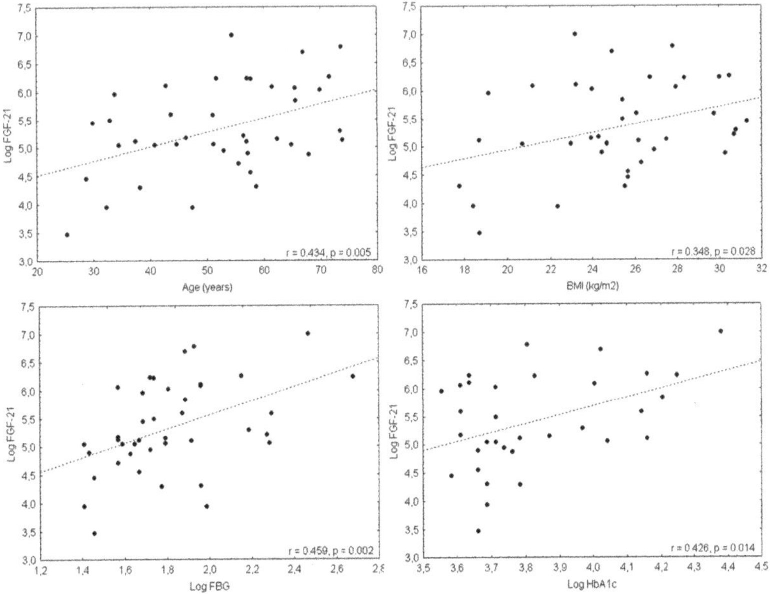

Figure 1. FGF21 levels and their correlation with selected factors in PPGL—age, BMI, FBG a HbA1c.

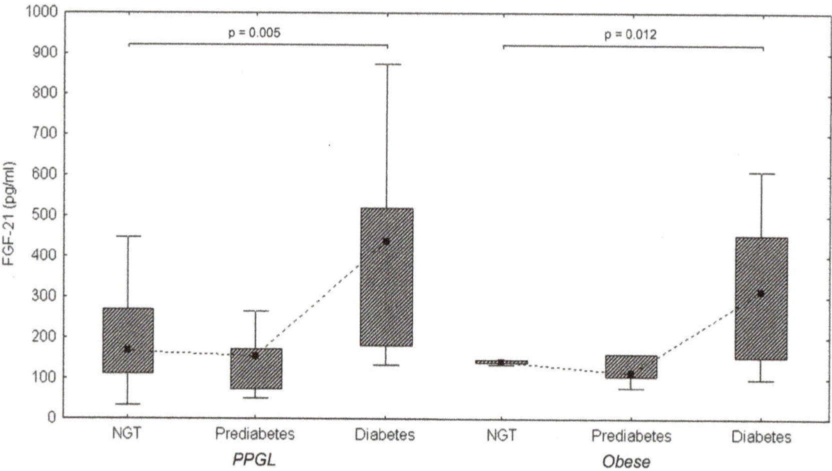

Figure 2. FGF21 levels in obese and PPGL with normal glucose tolerance (NGT), prediabetes, and diabetes mellitus.

3. Discussion

Our study shows that patients with PPGL have higher serum levels of FGF21 compared to healthy controls and these levels do not differ from obese patients. Furthermore, successful tumor removal significantly decreased FGF21 levels. Elevated FGF21 levels were more evident in patients with secondary diabetes mellitus and were related positively to fasting glucose levels and BMI in PPGL. We did not find a relationship between FGF21 and hypermetabolic state in PPGL.

We know from animal models that FGF21 stimulates whole-body energy expenditure and increases metabolic rate and physical activity [18]. In humans, conflicting results were published, depending on the studied population. In healthy lean volunteers, augmented FGF21 levels correlated positively with total energy expenditure during cold exposure [19]. In another study, fasting and postclamp FGF21 were positively related to REE, particularly in obese subjects [19]. On the other hand, no association between FGF21 and REE was reported in patients with hypercortisolism and a healthy population with low birth weight [20,21].

Catecholamine overproduction in PPGL leads to an increase in resting energy expenditure [22]. Although there are elevated levels of FGF21 in patients with PPGL, we have not found a link to hypermetabolic state. The causes of the hypermetabolic condition are likely to be much more complex and include the direct action of catecholamines on intermediate metabolism, fatty tissue, and inflammation [22–24]. In a fat biopsy study in PPGL, increased activity of brown adipose tissue in visceral fat, along with mRNA FGF21 was demonstrated, compared to patients undergoing elective cholecystectomy [9]. However, the study did not compare serum levels of FGF21. Thus we speculate that serum levels of FGF-12 may not reflect local paracrine production and activity in adipose tissue in PPGL. Another explanation can be found in the study by Douris and co-workers. They demonstrated that FGF21 also acts centrally in the brain through the activation of the sympathetic nervous system, which induces browning of WAT [11]. They also demonstrated that an intact beta-adrenergic receptor signaling pathway is necessary for the central actions of FGF21 [11]. It was shown that chronic overproduction of catecholamines could lead to desensitization of beta-adrenergic receptors in PPGL [25,26]. These findings and the existence of genetic polymorphisms of the beta-adrenergic receptor lead us back to actions (both, catecholamines and FGF21) on local levels.

Experimental studies have shown that it is noradrenaline which stimulates the production of FGF21 in brown adipose tissue, via beta-adrenoceptors [5]. In addition, this effect is not affected by the concomitant administration of an alpha-blocker [5]. Surprisingly, we did not find a link either between

FGF21 and both free plasmatic metanephrines or noradrenergic and adrenergic biochemical phenotype. In our study, we used free plasmatic metanephrines, which are the gold standard for the biochemical diagnosis of PPGL. They are produced continuously within PPGL tumor cells, and independently of catecholamine release, and they do not reflect the biochemical activity of tumors. We assume that this could explain the weak link between noradrenergic phenotype and serum FGF21 levels in our study.

Mraz and co-workers have demonstrated that FGF21 expression in the human liver was more than 100-fold higher relative to fat, suggesting that the liver remains the most important producer of this factor in humans [27]. Enhanced liver production of FGF21 has been linked to obesity, diabetes mellitus, and metabolic syndrome [27–29]. Our study reveals the same finding. Obese patients with metabolic syndrome had a higher level of FGF21, which correlates with blood glucose and BMI levels. In patients with PPGL, the findings were similar, despite significantly lower BMI. However, circulating levels of FGF21 were significantly higher in PPGL with secondary diabetes mellitus and signs of metabolic syndrome. The question remains whether it is the presence of hyperglycemia that stimulates the production of FGF21 in PPGL. According to available studies, human serum FGF21 levels are increased by oral boluses of fructose and glucose [30–32] and by 24-h hyperglycemia maintained via intravenous glucose infusion [33]. Furthermore, von Holstein-Rathlou et al. demonstrated in cell culture (HepG2) and mice models that glucose and fructose directly influence hepatocytes in the production of FGF21 [33]. On the other hand, Samms et al. showed that insulin rather than glucose "per se" increases total and bioactive FGF21 in the postprandial period in adult humans with and without type 2 DM according to oGTT and glucose clamp [34]. In our group with PPGL, basal insulin levels were significantly lower than in the obese and lean controls, and we did not find a relation to FGF21. It is possible that the mechanism of the insulin resistance state in PPGL is different. Insulin secretion is impaired, due to the inhibitory effect of catecholamines by the activation of α-adrenergic receptors in pancreatic β cells. In addition, catecholamines antagonize insulin action in target organs and thereby might trigger insulin resistance [35–37]. Komada et al. found impairment of insulin secretion particularly in the early phase of the insulin secretory response [38]. Our work shows that metabolic changes in PPGL are partially reversible. One year after adrenalectomy, we find an improvement in glucose metabolism and insulin resistance, followed by a decrease in FGF21, despite an increase in body weight due to the disappearance of the hypermetabolic effect of catecholamines.

The consequences of the elevation of FGF21 in PPGL are unclear. We cannot identify from our work whether the elevation of FGF21 is the result of a controversial "FGF21 resistance state", as is known in obese and diabetic patients [39–41], or whether FGF21 has some biological effect. However, in comparison to serum FGF21 levels in PPGL versus obese individuals, the levels in PPGL are most likely biologically significant. From the context mentioned above, we found that circulating FGF21 in PPGL reflects the metabolic abnormalities associated with diabetes mellitus and metabolic syndrome components, and we did not find a relation to hypermetabolism. Thus, it is possible that circulating levels of FGF21 originate predominantly from hepatic production, as demonstrated in the mice model [42]. Further investigation would be needed to assess the effect of FGF21 on metabolism and adipose tissue in PPGL.

Our study has several limitations. Firstly, the range of FGF21 serum concentration in human studies is very wide, making interpretation of clinical observations difficult. Secondly, our population was small and of a cross-sectional nature. Thirdly, we cannot exclude the influence of antihypertensive or antidiabetic therapy in both treated groups. Fourthly, we measured only total FGF21 and not the bioactive form of FGF21 and other important proteins such as fibroblast- activating protein. Finally, the lack of determination of urinary catecholamine levels to assess metabolic effects is another limitation of our study.

4. Patients and Methods

4.1. Recruitment and Background

87 subjects were included in the study (40 patients with PPGL, 26 healthy volunteers, and 21 obese individuals). Subjects with PPGL (38 pheochromocytoma and 2 abdominal paraganglioma) were examined during a short hospitalization in our department before and one year after tumor removal. Diagnosis of PPGL was based on free plasma metanephrines levels, visualization of the tumor by computer tomography or PET/CT with fluorodopa. The diagnosis was confirmed histopathologically. Five patients with familial, bilateral, or malignant PPGL were not examined after operation. Obese participants were investigated during hospitalization for weight reduction. All obese patients had hypercortisolism excluded. Healthy subjects had no history of chronic disease or medication. Written informed consent was obtained from all patients. The ethical committee of our institution approved the study (permission date: 21 May 2015, ethical code: 20/15). The study was done in accordance with the Declaration of Helsinki.

4.2. Anthropometric, Biochemical Measurements, and Indirect Calorimetry

Blood samples were withdrawn after overnight fasting between 6 and 7 a.m. Height (cm), weight (kg), and waist and hip circumference (cm) were measured. BMI was calculated as weight in kilograms divided by the square of height in meters. Obesity was defined by BMI >30 kg/m^2. Metabolic syndrome was classified according to the International Diabetes Federation by the presence of central obesity (BMI >30 kg/m^2 or waist circumference ≥94 cm in males or ≥80 cm in females), and any two of the following four factors: triglycerides ≥1.7 mmol/L or specific treatment for these lipid abnormalities; HDL cholesterol <1.03 mmol/L in males and <1.29 mmol/L in females or specific treatment for these lipid abnormalities; systolic blood pressure ≥130 or diastolic blood pressure ≥85 mmHg or treatment of previously diagnosed hypertension; fasting blood glucose ≥5.6 mmol/L or previously diagnosed type 2 diabetes.

Office arterial blood pressure was measured with an oscillometric sphygmomanometer according to the European Society of Hypertension guidelines. Arterial hypertension was defined in accordance with the European Society of Hypertension guidelines.

Basic laboratory tests, including serum glucose, lipid profile, glycated hemoglobin (HbA1c), were measured by standard methods in our institutional laboratory with international accreditation. Insulin was analyzed by the IRMA kit BI-INS-IRMA (Cis Bio International, Sark France). Homeostasis model assessment index-insulin resistance (HOMA-IR) was calculated as fasting glucose concentration multiplied by fasting insulin and divided by 22.5. Diabetes mellitus was defined by fasting plasma glucose levels ≥7.0 mmol/L or plasma glucose ≥11.1 mmol/L two hours after a 75 g oral glucose load or HbA1C ≥48 mmol/mol. Prediabetes was defined by fasting blood glucose levels from 5.6 to 6.9 mmol/L or plasma glucose ≥7.8 mmol/L, but not over 11.1 mmol/L, two hours after a 75 g oral glucose load according to the WHO 2006 definition.

Serum FGF21 levels were measured by a commercial ELISA kit (BioVendor, Modrice, Czech Republic), which is based on the polyclonal anti-human FGF21 antibody and biotin-labeled polyclonal anti-human FGF21 antibody. Plasma free metanephrines (normetanephrine and metanephrine) were quantified by liquid chromatography with electrochemical detection (HLPC-ED, Agilent 1100, Agilent Technologies, Inc., Wilmington, DE, USA). The noradrenergic biochemical phenotype was defined as: predominant increases of only normetanephrine, accompanied by either normal plasma concentrations of metanephrine or by increases of less than 5 % for metanephrine relative to the sum of increments for both hormones. The adrenergic biochemical phenotype was defined as: increases of plasma metanephrine above the upper reference limits and relative to the combined increments of both metabolites, of larger than 5 % for metanephrine [43].

Energy metabolism was quantified by indirect calorimetry with a ventilated canopy system (Vmax Encore 29 N system, VIASYS Healthcare Inc; SensorMedics, Yorba Linda, California).

Resting energy expenditure (REE) and respiratory quotient (RQ) were measured. The methodology was described in our previous article [22]. The Harris-Benedict formula was used for the calculation of predicted basal energy expenditure (BEE). REE was divided by BEE and multiplied by 100 to express the rate of metabolism (REE/BEE). Hypermetabolic state was classified as REE/BEE more than 110%. Free fat mass (FFM) was measured with a Bodystat 1500 device (Bodystat Ltd, Isle of Man, UK).

4.3. Statistical Analysis

Statistical analysis was performed by Statistica for Windows ver. 9.1 (StatSoft, Inc., Tulsa, OK, USA). Normally distributed data are shown as the mean ± SD (standard deviation). Data with abnormal distribution are expressed as median with interquartile range (IQR). Categorical variables are expressed as frequencies (%). All parameters were tested for normality by the Shapiro-Wilk test. Parameters without a normal distribution were logarithmically converted. Two independent groups were tested by the Student's *t*-test or Mann-Whitney test as appropriate. The dependent groups were tested by the Student's paired *t*-test or the Wilcoxon test as appropriate. For three and more groups, the Kruskal-Wallis test, or an ANOVA with Scheffe post-hoc test, was used. Correlations between variables were investigated by the Pearson correlation coefficient. Categorical variables were tested by chi-square or Fisher's exact test. p values of <0.05 were considered significant.

5. Conclusions

In conclusion, we found elevated levels of serum FGF21 levels in PPGL and their relation to secondary diabetes mellitus, but not to the hypermetabolic state. One year after tumor removal led to normalization of FGF21 and the other metabolic abnormalities.

Author Contributions: Conceptualization and methodology by T.Z. and O.P.; formal analysis by J.K. and O.P.; investigation by J.K. and O.P.; resources by D.M., K.N., and M.M.; data curation by all authors; writing—original draft preparation by J.K.; visualization by J.K.; project administration and supervision by J.W.J.; funding acquisition by O.P.

Funding: The study was supported by AZV 16-30345A grants from the Ministry of Health of the Czech Republic, RVO 64165 by General University Hospital and by Progres Q25 and Q28 research projects of Charles University.

Conflicts of Interest: The authors declare no conflict of interest.

References

1. Staiger, H.; Keuper, M.; Berti, L.; Hrabe de Angelis, M.; Haring, H.U. Fibroblast Growth Factor 21-Metabolic Role in Mice and Men. *Endocr. Rev.* **2017**, *38*, 468–488. [CrossRef]
2. BonDurant, L.D.; Potthoff, M.J. Fibroblast Growth Factor 21: A Versatile Regulator of Metabolic Homeostasis. *Annu. Rev. Nutr.* **2018**, *38*, 173–196. [CrossRef] [PubMed]
3. Domouzoglou, E.M.; Maratos-Flier, E. Fibroblast growth factor 21 is a metabolic regulator that plays a role in the adaptation to ketosis. *Am. J. Clin. Nutr.* **2011**, *93*, 901S–905S. [CrossRef]
4. Fisher, F.M.; Kleiner, S.; Douris, N.; Fox, E.C.; Mepani, R.J.; Verdeguer, F.; Wu, J.; Kharitonenkov, A.; Flier, J.S.; Maratos-Flier, E.; et al. FGF21 regulates PGC-1alpha and browning of white adipose tissues in adaptive thermogenesis. *Genes Dev.* **2012**, *26*, 271–281. [CrossRef]
5. Hondares, E.; Iglesias, R.; Giralt, A.; Gonzalez, F.J.; Giralt, M.; Mampel, T.; Villarroya, F. Thermogenic activation induces FGF21 expression and release in brown adipose tissue. *J. Biol. Chem.* **2011**, *286*, 12983–12990. [CrossRef] [PubMed]
6. Harms, M.; Seale, P. Brown and beige fat: Development, function and therapeutic potential. *Nat. Med.* **2013**, *19*, 1252–1263. [CrossRef] [PubMed]
7. Wang, Q.; Zhang, M.; Ning, G.; Gu, W.; Su, T.; Xu, M.; Li, B.; Wang, W. Brown adipose tissue in humans is activated by elevated plasma catecholamines levels and is inversely related to central obesity. *PLoS ONE* **2011**, *6*, e21006. [CrossRef]

8. Hadi, M.; Chen, C.C.; Whatley, M.; Pacak, K.; Carrasquillo, J.A. Brown fat imaging with (18)F-6-fluorodopamine PET/CT, (18)F-FDG PET/CT, and (123)I-MIBG SPECT: A study of patients being evaluated for pheochromocytoma. *J. Nucl. Med.* **2007**, *48*, 1077–1083. [CrossRef] [PubMed]
9. Hondares, E.; Gallego-Escuredo, J.M.; Flachs, P.; Frontini, A.; Cereijo, R.; Goday, A.; Perugini, J.; Kopecky, P.; Giralt, M.; Cinti, S.; et al. Fibroblast growth factor-21 is expressed in neonatal and pheochromocytoma-induced adult human brown adipose tissue. *Metabolism* **2014**, *63*, 312–317. [CrossRef] [PubMed]
10. BonDurant, L.D.; Ameka, M.; Naber, M.C.; Markan, K.R.; Idiga, S.O.; Acevedo, M.R.; Walsh, S.A.; Ornitz, D.M.; Potthoff, M.J. FGF21 Regulates Metabolism Through Adipose-Dependent and -Independent Mechanisms. *Cell Metab.* **2017**, *25*, 935–944. [CrossRef] [PubMed]
11. Douris, N.; Stevanovic, D.M.; Fisher, F.M.; Cisu, T.I.; Chee, M.J.; Nguyen, N.L.; Zarebidaki, E.; Adams, A.C.; Kharitonenkov, A.; Flier, J.S.; et al. Central Fibroblast Growth Factor 21 Browns White Fat via Sympathetic Action in Male Mice. *Endocrinology* **2015**, *156*, 2470–2481. [CrossRef] [PubMed]
12. Hsuchou, H.; Pan, W.; Kastin, A.J. The fasting polypeptide FGF21 can enter brain from blood. *Peptides* **2007**, *28*, 2382–2386. [CrossRef] [PubMed]
13. Tan, B.K.; Hallschmid, M.; Adya, R.; Kern, W.; Lehnert, H.; Randeva, H.S. Fibroblast growth factor 21 (FGF21) in human cerebrospinal fluid: Relationship with plasma FGF21 and body adiposity. *Diabetes* **2011**, *60*, 2758–2762. [CrossRef] [PubMed]
14. Sarruf, D.A.; Thaler, J.P.; Morton, G.J.; German, J.; Fischer, J.D.; Ogimoto, K.; Schwartz, M.W. Fibroblast growth factor 21 action in the brain increases energy expenditure and insulin sensitivity in obese rats. *Diabetes* **2010**, *59*, 1817–1824. [CrossRef] [PubMed]
15. Bookout, A.L.; de Groot, M.H.; Owen, B.M.; Lee, S.; Gautron, L.; Lawrence, H.L.; Ding, X.; Elmquist, J.K.; Takahashi, J.S.; Mangelsdorf, D.J.; et al. FGF21 regulates metabolism and circadian behavior by acting on the nervous system. *Nat. Med.* **2013**, *19*, 1147–1152. [CrossRef]
16. Liang, Q.; Zhong, L.; Zhang, J.; Wang, Y.; Bornstein, S.R.; Triggle, C.R.; Ding, H.; Lam, K.S.; Xu, A. FGF21 maintains glucose homeostasis by mediating the cross talk between liver and brain during prolonged fasting. *Diabetes* **2014**, *63*, 4064–4075. [CrossRef] [PubMed]
17. Martucci, V.L.; Pacak, K. Pheochromocytoma and paraganglioma: Diagnosis, genetics, management, and treatment. *Curr. Probl. Cancer* **2014**, *38*, 7–41. [CrossRef]
18. Xu, J.; Lloyd, D.J.; Hale, C.; Stanislaus, S.; Chen, M.; Sivits, G.; Vonderfecht, S.; Hecht, R.; Li, Y.S.; Lindberg, R.A.; et al. Fibroblast growth factor 21 reverses hepatic steatosis, increases energy expenditure, and improves insulin sensitivity in diet-induced obese mice. *Diabetes* **2009**, *58*, 250–259. [CrossRef] [PubMed]
19. Straczkowski, M.; Karczewska-Kupczewska, M.; Adamska, A.; Otziomek, E.; Kowalska, I.; Nikolajuk, A. Serum fibroblast growth factor 21 in human obesity: Regulation by insulin infusion and relationship with glucose and lipid oxidation. *Int. J. Obes. (Lond)* **2013**, *37*, 1386–1390. [CrossRef]
20. Vienberg, S.G.; Brons, C.; Nilsson, E.; Astrup, A.; Vaag, A.; Andersen, B. Impact of short-term high-fat feeding and insulin-stimulated FGF21 levels in subjects with low birth weight and controls. *Eur. J. Endocrinol.* **2012**, *167*, 49–57. [CrossRef]
21. Ďurovcová, V.; Marek, J.; Hána, V.; Matoulek, M.; Zikán, V.; Haluzíková, D.; Kaválková, P.; Lacinová, Z.; Kršek, M.; Haluzík, M. Plasma concentrations of fibroblast growth factors 21 and 19 in patients with Cushing's syndrome. *Physiol. Res.* **2010**, *59*, 415–422. [PubMed]
22. Petrák, O.; Haluzíkova, D.; Kaválková, P.; Štrauch, B.; Rosa, J.; Holaj, R.; Brabcová Vranková, A.; Michalský, D.; Haluzík, M.; Zelinka, T.; et al. Changes in energy metabolism in pheochromocytoma. *J. Clin. Endocrinol. Metab.* **2013**, *98*, 1651–1658. [CrossRef] [PubMed]
23. Zelinka, T.; Petrák, O.; Štrauch, B.; Holaj, R.; Kvasnička, J.; Mazoch, J.; Pacák, K.; Widimský, J., Jr. Elevated inflammation markers in pheochromocytoma compared to other forms of hypertension. *Neuroimmunomodulation* **2007**, *14*, 57–64. [CrossRef] [PubMed]
24. Bosanská, L.; Petrák, O.; Zelinka, T.; Mráz, M.; Widimský, J., Jr.; Haluzík, M. The effect of pheochromocytoma treatment on subclinical inflammation and endocrine function of adipose tissue. *Physiol. Res.* **2009**, *58*, 319–325. [CrossRef]
25. Tsujimoto, G.; Manger, W.M.; Hoffman, B.B. Desensitization of beta-adrenergic receptors by pheochromocytoma. *Endocrinology* **1984**, *114*, 1272–1278. [CrossRef] [PubMed]

26. Snavely, M.D.; Motulsky, H.J.; O'Connor, D.T.; Ziegler, M.G.; Insel, P.A. Adrenergic receptors in human and experimental pheochromocytoma. *Clin. Exp. Hypertens. A* **1982**, *4*, 829–848. [CrossRef]
27. Mráz, M.; Bartlová, M.; Lacinová, Z.; Michalský, D.; Kasalický, M.; Haluziková, D.; Matoulek, M.; Dostalová, I.; Humenanská, V.; Haluzík, M. Serum concentrations and tissue expression of a novel endocrine regulator fibroblast growth factor-21 in patients with type 2 diabetes and obesity. *Clin. Endocrinol.* **2009**, *71*, 369–375. [CrossRef] [PubMed]
28. Zhang, X.; Yeung, D.C.; Karpisek, M.; Stejskal, D.; Zhou, Z.G.; Liu, F.; Wong, R.L.; Chow, W.S.; Tso, A.W.; Lam, K.S.; et al. Serum FGF21 levels are increased in obesity and are independently associated with the metabolic syndrome in humans. *Diabetes* **2008**, *57*, 1246–1253. [CrossRef] [PubMed]
29. Semba, R.D.; Sun, K.; Egan, J.M.; Crasto, C.; Carlson, O.D.; Ferrucci, L. Relationship of serum fibroblast growth factor 21 with abnormal glucose metabolism and insulin resistance: The Baltimore Longitudinal Study of Aging. *J. Clin. Endocrinol. Metab.* **2012**, *97*, 1375–1382. [CrossRef] [PubMed]
30. Lin, Z.; Gong, Q.; Wu, C.; Yu, J.; Lu, T.; Pan, X.; Lin, S.; Li, X. Dynamic change of serum FGF21 levels in response to glucose challenge in human. *J. Clin. Endocrinol. Metab.* **2012**, *97*, E1224–E1228. [CrossRef] [PubMed]
31. Vienberg, S.G.; Jacobsen, S.H.; Worm, D.; Hvolris, L.E.; Naver, L.; Almdal, T.; Hansen, D.L.; Wulff, B.S.; Clausen, T.R.; Madsbad, S.; et al. Increased glucose-stimulated FGF21 response to oral glucose in obese nondiabetic subjects after Roux-en-Y gastric bypass. *Clin. Endocrinol.* **2017**, *86*, 156–159. [CrossRef] [PubMed]
32. Dushay, J.R.; Toschi, E.; Mitten, E.K.; Fisher, F.M.; Herman, M.A.; Maratos-Flier, E. Fructose ingestion acutely stimulates circulating FGF21 levels in humans. *Mol. Metab.* **2015**, *4*, 51–57. [CrossRef] [PubMed]
33. von Holstein-Rathlou, S.; BonDurant, L.D.; Peltekian, L.; Naber, M.C.; Yin, T.C.; Claflin, K.E.; Urizar, A.I.; Madsen, A.N.; Ratner, C.; Holst, B.; et al. FGF21 Mediates Endocrine Control of Simple Sugar Intake and Sweet Taste Preference by the Liver. *Cell Metab.* **2016**, *23*, 335–343. [CrossRef]
34. Samms, R.J.; Lewis, J.E.; Norton, L.; Stephens, F.B.; Gaffney, C.J.; Butterfield, T.; Smith, D.P.; Cheng, C.C.; Perfield, J.W., 2nd; Adams, A.C.; et al. FGF21 Is an Insulin-Dependent Postprandial Hormone in Adult Humans. *J. Clin. Endocrinol. Metab.* **2017**, *102*, 3806–3813. [CrossRef]
35. Colwell, J.A. Inhibition of insulin secretion by catecholamines in pheochromocytoma. *Ann. Intern. Med.* **1969**, *71*, 251–256. [CrossRef] [PubMed]
36. Isles, C.G.; Johnson, J.K. Phaeochromocytoma and diabetes mellitus: Further evidence that alpha 2 receptors inhibit insulin release in man. *Clin. Endocrinol.* **1983**, *18*, 37–41. [CrossRef]
37. Cryer, P.E. Adrenaline: A physiological metabolic regulatory hormone in humans? *Int. J. Obes Relat Metab Disord* **1993**, *17* (Suppl. 3), S43–S46; discussion S68. [PubMed]
38. Komada, H.; Hirota, Y.; So, A.; Nakamura, T.; Okuno, Y.; Fukuoka, H.; Iguchi, G.; Takahashi, Y.; Sakaguchi, K.; Ogawa, W. Insulin Secretion and Insulin Sensitivity Before and After Surgical Treatment of Pheochromocytoma or Paraganglioma. *J. Clin. Endocrinol. Metab.* **2017**, *102*, 3400–3405. [CrossRef] [PubMed]
39. Fisher, F.M.; Chui, P.C.; Antonellis, P.J.; Bina, H.A.; Kharitonenkov, A.; Flier, J.S.; Maratos-Flier, E. Obesity is a fibroblast growth factor 21 (FGF21)-resistant state. *Diabetes* **2010**, *59*, 2781–2789. [CrossRef]
40. Hale, C.; Chen, M.M.; Stanislaus, S.; Chinookoswong, N.; Hager, T.; Wang, M.; Veniant, M.M.; Xu, J. Lack of overt FGF21 resistance in two mouse models of obesity and insulin resistance. *Endocrinology* **2012**, *153*, 69–80. [CrossRef] [PubMed]
41. Markan, K.R. Defining "FGF21 Resistance" during obesity: Controversy, criteria and unresolved questions. *F1000Res* **2018**, *7*, 289. [CrossRef] [PubMed]
42. Markan, K.R.; Naber, M.C.; Ameka, M.K.; Anderegg, M.D.; Mangelsdorf, D.J.; Kliewer, S.A.; Mohammadi, M.; Potthoff, M.J. Circulating FGF21 is liver derived and enhances glucose uptake during refeeding and overfeeding. *Diabetes* **2014**, *63*, 4057–4063. [CrossRef] [PubMed]
43. Eisenhofer, G.; Lenders, J.W.; Goldstein, D.S.; Mannelli, M.; Csako, G.; Walther, M.M.; Brouwers, F.M.; Pacak, K. Pheochromocytoma catecholamine phenotypes and prediction of tumor size and location by use of plasma free metanephrines. *Clin. Chem.* **2005**, *51*, 735–744. [CrossRef] [PubMed]

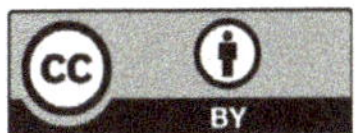

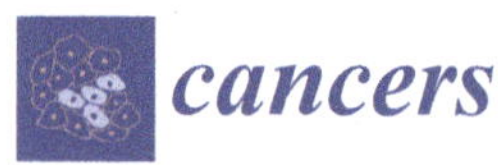 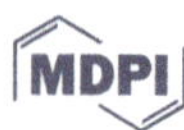

Article

Targeting Cyclooxygenase-2 in Pheochromocytoma and Paraganglioma: Focus on Genetic Background

Martin Ullrich [1,*], Susan Richter [2,3], Verena Seifert [1], Sandra Hauser [1], Bruna Calsina [4], Ángel M. Martínez-Montes [4], Marjolein ter Laak [5], Christian G. Ziegler [6], Henri Timmers [5], Graeme Eisenhofer [2,3], Mercedes Robledo [4,7] and Jens Pietzsch [1,8,*]

1 Department of Radiopharmaceutical and Chemical Biology, Helmholtz-Zentrum Dresden-Rossendorf, Institute of Radiopharmaceutical Cancer Research, 01328 Dresden, Germany; v.seifert@hzdr.de (V.S.); s.hauser@hzdr.de (S.H.)

2 Institute of Clinical Chemistry and Laboratory Medicine, University Hospital Carl Gustav Carus at the Technische Universität Dresden, 01307 Dresden, Germany; susan.richter@uniklinikum-dresden.de (S.R.); graeme.eisenhofer@uniklinikum-dresden.de (G.E.)

3 Faculty of Medicine Carl Gustav Carus, School of Medicine, Technische Universität Dresden, 01307 Dresden, Germany

4 Human Cancer Genetics Programme, Hereditary Endocrine Cancer Group, Spanish National Cancer Research Centre, 28029 Madrid, Spain; bcalsina@cnio.es (B.C.); ammontes@cnio.es (Á.M.M.-M.); mrobledo@cnio.es (M.R.)

5 Department of Internal Medicine; Sections of Endocrinology and Vascular Medicine, Radboud University Medical Centre, 6525 GA Nijmegen, The Netherlands; marjolein.terlaak@outlook.com (M.t.L.); henri.timmers@radboudumc.nl (H.T.)

6 Department of Medicine III, University Hospital Carl Gustav Carus at the TU Dresden, 01307 Dresden, Germany; christian.ziegler@uniklinikum-dresden.de

7 Centro de Investigación Biomédica en Red de Enfermedades Raras, 28029 Madrid, Spain

8 Faculty of Chemistry and Food Chemistry, School of Science, Technische Universität Dresden, 01069 Dresden, Germany

* Correspondence: m.ullrich@hzdr.de (M.U.); j.pietzsch@hzdr.de (J.P.); Tel.: +49-351-260-4046 (M.U.); +49-351-260-2622 (J.P.)

Received: 30 April 2019; Accepted: 24 May 2019; Published: 28 May 2019

Abstract: Cyclooxygenase 2 (COX-2) is a key enzyme of the tumorigenesis-inflammation interface and can be induced by hypoxia. A pseudohypoxic transcriptional signature characterizes pheochromocytomas and paragangliomas (PPGLs) of the cluster I, mainly represented by tumors with mutations in von Hippel–Lindau (*VHL*), endothelial PAS domain-containing protein 1 (*EPAS1*), or succinate dehydrogenase (*SDH*) subunit genes. The aim of this study was to investigate a possible association between underlying tumor driver mutations and COX-2 in PPGLs. *COX-2* gene expression and immunoreactivity were examined in clinical specimens with documented mutations, as well as in spheroids and allografts derived from mouse pheochromocytoma (MPC) cells. COX-2 in vivo imaging was performed in allograft mice. We observed significantly higher *COX-2* expression in cluster I, especially in *VHL*-mutant PPGLs, however, no specific association between *COX-2* mRNA levels and a hypoxia-related transcriptional signature was found. COX-2 immunoreactivity was present in about 60% of clinical specimens as well as in MPC spheroids and allografts. A selective COX-2 tracer specifically accumulated in MPC allografts. This study demonstrates that, although pseudohypoxia is not the major determinant for high COX-2 levels in PPGLs, COX-2 is a relevant molecular target. This potentially allows for employing selective COX-2 inhibitors as targeted chemotherapeutic agents and radiosensitizers. Moreover, available models are suitable for preclinical testing of these treatments.

Keywords: VHL; NF1; EPAS1; hypoxia-inducible factor; inflammation; radiosensitization; succinate dehydrogenase; mouse pheochromocytoma cells; immunohistochemistry; fluorescence imaging

1. Introduction

Over the past few decades, advances in genetic testing have substantially facilitated the identification of germline and somatic mutations in tumor susceptibility genes in about 60% of adrenal pheochromocytomas and their extra adrenal counterparts, paragangliomas (summarized as PPGLs) [1–4]. Gain-of-function mutations in proto-oncogenes such as rearranged during transfection (*RET*; germline or somatic), endothelial per-arnt-sim domain-containing protein 1 (*EPAS1*; somatic), and Harvey rat sarcoma viral oncogene homolog (*HRAS*; somatic); and loss-of-function mutations in tumor suppressor genes such as von Hippel–Lindau (*VHL*; germline or somatic), neurofibromin 1 (*NF1*; germline or somatic), transmembrane protein 127 (*TMEM127*; germline), and myc-associated factor X (*MAX*, germline or somatic), as well as mutations in all four succinate dehydrogenase subunits (*SDHD*, *SDHC*, *SDHB*, and *SDHA*; germline) and SDH assembly factor 2 (*SDHAF2*; germline) have been implicated in the tumorigenesis of PPGLs [2,5–11]. Beyond that, the number of PPGL susceptibility gene candidates is still increasing, e.g. [4,12–21], although most of them seem to play a minor role in PPGL according to the low proportion of patients related to these genes described so far.

Gene expression profiling provided the basis for classifying PPGLs according to their main transcriptional signatures underlying the aforementioned mutations: cluster I presents with activation of pseudohypoxic signaling pathways and includes mainly *VHL*-, *EPAS1*-, and *SDHx*-mutant cases; cluster II is enriched in kinase receptor signaling pathways and is comprised of *RET*-, *NF1*-, *TMEM127*-, *MAX*-, and *HRAS*-mutant cases [22,23]. Both pseudohypoxia and kinase receptor signaling are involved in regulating apoptosis, proliferation, invasion, and metastasis, and angiogenesis via different mechanisms, but can also contribute to inflammatory conditions in various tumor entities [24–27].

Cyclooxygenases (COX) 1 and 2, also referred to as prostaglandin-endoperoxide synthases (PTGS 1 and 2; EC 1.14.99.1), catalyze the conversion of arachidonic acid to prostaglandin H_2 (PGH_2). PGH_2 is then converted into a variety of other prostanoids, determined by certain downstream synthase and isomerase pathways. Prostanoids comprise other prostaglandins such as PGE_2 and $PGF_2\alpha$, prostacyclin (PGI_2) and thromboxanes (e.g., TXA_2). These compounds are ligands for G protein-coupled receptors and act as potent para- and endocrine mediators of metabolic processes in homeostasis, but also in inflammatory and neoplastic processes. In particular, the inducible isoenzyme COX-2 is a key enzyme of the tumorigenesis-inflammation interface. In this context, COX-2 overexpression has been shown in various tumor entities and is positively correlated with progression, malignancy and poor patient survival [28]. COX-2 overexpression also contributes to chemo- and radiation resistance [29–35]. Hypoxic and pseudo-hypoxic signaling additionally influences COX-2-mediated pathways [26,27,36]. Therefore, studies have been initiated on the use of selective COX-2 inhibitors (coxibs) as targeted chemotherapeutic agents and potential radiosensitizers [28,37].

Endoradiotherapy, e.g., with [^{177}Lu]Lu-DOTA-(Tyr^3)octreotate (^{177}Lu-DOTA-TATE) is currently investigated as a treatment option for inoperable or metastatic PPGLs, showing promising effects, but sometimes incomplete tumor remission in clinics as well as in preclinical PPGL models [38–40]. COX-2 is associated with chemo- and radiation resistance and poor patient outcome in a number of tumor entities [29–35] encouraging us to investigate whether COX-2 is a potential target in PPGLs.

The first report on COX-2 gene expression and immunohistochemistry in adrenal pheochromocytomas was published in 2001 suggesting that the enzyme might have a role in malignant transformation of these tumors [41]. Between 2007 and 2011, another four immunohistochemical studies were published supporting the value of COX-2 as surrogate marker that, in association with other factors, could potentially discriminate between benign and metastatic pheochromocytoma [42–45]. Due to literature showing that COX-2 is induced by hypoxia signaling [46,47], we hypothesized that cluster I PPGLs have a higher COX-2 expression than cluster II. Accordingly, COX-2 may be a promising molecular target for functional imaging and adjuvant treatment, in particular in cluster I PPGLs.

To address the above hypothesis, we evaluated COX-2 status of PPGLs with known mutational status for *VHL*, *SDHx*, *EPAS1*, *NF1*, *RET*, and *HRAS* on both mRNA and protein level. Furthermore, we characterized COX-2 immunoreactivity in tumor spheroids and allografts derived from mouse pheochromocytoma (MPC) cells with a heterozygous *Nf1* knockout [48,49] in order to assess the usefulness of these models for preclinical testing of COX-2-targeting adjuvant and, in particular, radiosensitizing treatments.

2. Results

2.1. COX-2 Gene Expression in Clinical PPGL Samples

COX-2 gene expression data were extracted from gene expression arrays [50,51] of 70 PPGL samples with documented mutations in tumor susceptibility genes (Table 1). This series reflects the expected age, location, and metastatic disease, according to the mutations involved. Most cases were adrenal pheochromocytomas (67%), followed by thoracic and abdominal paragangliomas (29%), and head and neck paragangliomas (7.1%). Germline mutations were documented in 60% of cases. At the time of investigation 8.6% of cases showed metastatic disease. Most of the tumors carried mutations in *SDHx* (23% comprising 5 *SDHD*, 2 *SDHC*, and 9 *SDHB*, cases) and *RET* (23%) followed by *VHL* (21%), *EPAS1* (16%), *HRAS* (11%), and *NF1* (5.7%). The *SDHx* subgroup showed the highest proportion of extra-adrenal paragangliomas (62% thoracic and abdominal, and 31% head and neck), followed by *EPAS1* (73% thoracic and abdominal). All other genetic subgroups included mostly adrenal pheochromocytomas (85–100%). All subgroups showed similar means in tumor diameters (4.4–5.9 cm). Metastatic disease was most frequently documented among *SDHx*-mutant cases (25%) compared to all other genetic subgroups (0–18%).

Table 1. Tumor characteristics and clinical features of 70 PPGL patients extracted from [50,51] for *COX-2* gene expression analysis; (A) adrenal; (TA) thoracic and abdominal; (HN) head and neck.

Mutant Gene	*VHL*	*SDHx* [1]	*EPAS1*	*NF1*	*RET*	*HRAS*	Total
Total cases (n)	15	16	11	4	16	8	70
Hereditary (n)	10	15	0	3	14	0	42
			Sex (n)				
Female	6	9	10	4	8	3	40
Male	9	7	1	0	8	2	27
Unknown	0	0	0	0	0	3	3
			Tumor location (n)				
A	13	1	5	4	16	8	47
A + TA	2	2	2	0	0	0	6
TA	0	8	4	0	0	0	14
HN	0	5	0	0	0	0	5
			Tumor diameter (n)				
<4 cm	1	6	3	0	4	0	14
≥ 4 and ≤ 8 cm	4	3	5	0	1	4	17
>8 cm	0	1	2	0	1	1	5
Unknown	10	6	1	4	10	3	34
Mean (cm)	4.4 ± 1.0	4.6±1.2	5.8 ± 1.2	n.a.	4.6 ± 1.2	5.9 ± 0.9	5.1 ± 0.5
			Age at diagnosis (years)				
Range	9–47	10–95	18–78	38–58	18–62	45–79	9–97
Unknown	1	0	0	1	0	2	4
Mean	24 ± 3.1 †	27 ± 7.9	42 ± 6.4	48 ± 5.8	38 ± 6.5	64 ± 4.6 ‡	36 ± 2.3
Metastatic (n)	0	4	2	0	0	0	6

[1] comprising 5 *SDHD*, 2 *SDHC*, and 9 *SDHB* cases; significance of differences tested with Mann–Whitney *U* test: † $p < 0.01$, ‡ $p < 0.001$; (n.a.) not available.

Statistical analysis taking into account the general clinico-morphologic features of the tumors showed that gender, tumor location, tumor diameter, age at diagnosis, or metastatic behavior had no relevant influences on *COX-2* gene expression (Table S1). On the other hand, *COX-2* expression was significantly higher in head and neck PPGLs ($p = 0.01$) compared to other locations. Of note, all head and neck PPGLs in this series were related to an *SDHD* germline mutation.

PPGLs carrying a *VHL* mutation showed the highest *COX-2* expression (0.30 ± 0.28), followed by cases with *SDHx* (−0.13 ± 0.22), *EPAS1* (−0.25 ± 0.13), *HRAS* (−0.55 ± 0.12), *RET* (−0.68 ± 0.14), and *NF1* (−0.96 ± 0.16) mutations (Figure 1). The mean *COX-2* expression among all cluster I tumors was higher (−0.01 ± 0.14) compared to cluster II (−0.68 ± 0.09). *COX-2* expression was similar in hereditary (−0.26 ± 0.15) and somatic cases (−0.31 ± 0.11). *COX-2* expression showed significant positive relationships with *VHL* mutations ($r = 0.371$, $p = 0.002$) and cluster I transcriptional signature ($r = 0.406$, $p < 0.001$), respectively.

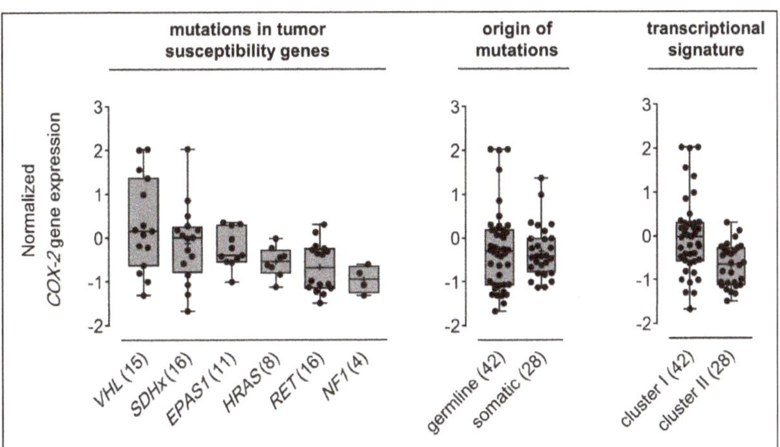

Figure 1. Normalized *COX-2* gene expression in PPGLs with regard to genetic background. gene expression array data were derived from Lopez-Jimenez et al. [50] and Qin et al. [51] mRNA expression series. Seventy samples with known genotype were included in this analysis and classified according to the specific gene mutated, origin of mutations, and transcriptional cluster; numbers in parentheses represent the number of samples investigated in each subgroup; see Table S1 for statistical analyses.

To further investigate a possible association between the pseudohypoxic signature and *COX-2* in cluster I PPGLs, unsupervised clustering for 97 hypoxia-related genes (see materials and methods for details) showed that *VHL*- and *SDHx*-mutant cases clustered together (Figure S1). Pearson correlation for *COX-2* expression and pseudohypoxic signature indicated significant relationships ($p < 0.05$) for 86 out of 171 probes, representing 65 out of 97 genes related to hypoxia in PPGLs (Table S2). Correlation coefficients ranged from 0.19 to 0.63 with 65 probes having only a weak correlation below 0.4. Exemplary, consistent with high *COX-2* expression, the analysis showed a significant positive relationship with mRNA levels of Ca^{2+}-dependent phospholipase A2 ($r = 0.564$, $p < 0.001$) since the enzyme is required for releasing arachidonic acid from phospholipid membranes as the specific substrate for cyclooxygenases.

2.2. COX-2 Immunoreactivity in Clinical PPGL Tissue Samples of a Second Cohort

COX-2 immunoreactivity was assessed in formalin-fixed paraffin-embedded tumor samples from a separate cohort sharing no case with the RNA sample cohort. This series included 96 PPGLs with a clinically documented mutation in tumor susceptibility genes (Table 2) and reflects the expected age, location, and metastatic disease, according to the mutations involved. Most cases were adrenal pheochromocytomas (52%), followed by thoracic and abdominal paragangliomas (26%), and head and neck paragangliomas (22%). Germline mutations were documented in 52% of cases. At the time of investigation, 13% of cases showed metastatic disease.

Table 2. Tumor characteristics and clinical features of 96 PPGL tissue samples available for COX-2 immunohistochemistry classified with regard to mutations in different tumor susceptibility genes; (A) adrenal; (TA) thoracic and abdominal; (HN) head and neck.

Mutant Gene	*VHL*	*SDHx* [1]	*EPAS1*	*NF1*	*RET*	*HRAS*	Total
Total cases (*n*)	14	39	7	21	9	6	96
Hereditary (*n*)	7	38	0	0	4	0	50
			Sex (*n*)				
Female	6	18	6	9	4	4	47
Male	8	21	1	12	5	2	49
			Tumor location (*n*)				
A	10	4	4	20	8	4	50
TA	3	15	3	1	1	2	25
HN	1	20	0	0	0	0	21
			Tumor diameter (*n*)				
<4 cm	3	22	2	6	2	2	35
≥4 and ≤8 cm	7	13	5	11	3	3	44
>8 cm	0	2	0	0	3	0	5
Unknown	4	2	0	4	1	0	12
Mean (cm)	4.6 ± 0.6	3.9 ± 0.4 *	4.5 ± 0.6	4.1 ± 0.3	7.2 ± 1.5 *	3.8 ± 0.5	4.4 ± 0.3
			Age at diagnosis (years)				
Range	9–49	14–71	17–75	20–74	33–72	28–81	9–81
Mean	25 ± 3.9 ‡	38 ± 2.7 †	42 ± 8.7	52 ± 2.8 †	49 ± 4.2	58 ± 7.2 *	42 ± 1.7
Metastatic (*n*)	1	8	0	1	1	1	12

[1] comprising 18 *SDHD*, 3 *SDHC*, 9 *SDHB*, 5 *SDHA*, and 4 *SDHAF2* cases; significance of differences tested with Mann–Whitney *U* test: * $p < 0.05$, † $p < 0.01$, ‡ $p < 0.001$.

Most of the cases carried a mutation in *SDHx* (41% comprising 18 *SDHD*, 3 *SDHC*, 9 *SDHB*, 5 *SDHA*, and 4 *SDHAF2* cases) followed by *NF1* (22%), *VHL* (15%), *RET* (9.4%), *EPAS1* (7.3%), and *HRAS* (6.3%). The *SDHx* subgroup showed the highest proportion of extra-adrenal paragangliomas (39% thoracic and abdominal, and 51% head and neck), whereas all other genetic subgroups included mostly adrenal pheochromocytomas (57–95%). Tumor diameters were significantly smaller in the *SDHx* subgroup (3.9 cm) and significantly higher in the *RET* subgroup (7.2 cm) compared to cases with other genetic backgrounds. Metastatic disease was most frequently documented among *SDHx* cases (21%) compared to all other genetic subgroups (0–17%).

COX-2 immunoreactivity was assessed by three observers using a three-mark score taking into account the percentage of positively stained tumor cells per tissue section (Figure 2). Sections with 'strong' (>50% of tumor cells stained) or 'moderate' score (20–50% of tumor cells stained) showed cytoplasmic COX-2 immunoreactivity in pheochromocytes and/or interconnected stromal cells. Tumors with 'negative or weak' score (<20% of tumor cells stained) showed COX-2 immunoreactivity predominantly in few stromal cells scatted over the tissue section. Interobserver variation statistics showed good agreement between the first two observers (weighted κ = 0.67). However, there were 14 cases of disagreement (15%) between 'negative or weak' and 'moderate' scores as well as 16 cases of disagreement (17%) between 'moderate' and 'strong' scores that where passed to a third observer for final decision.

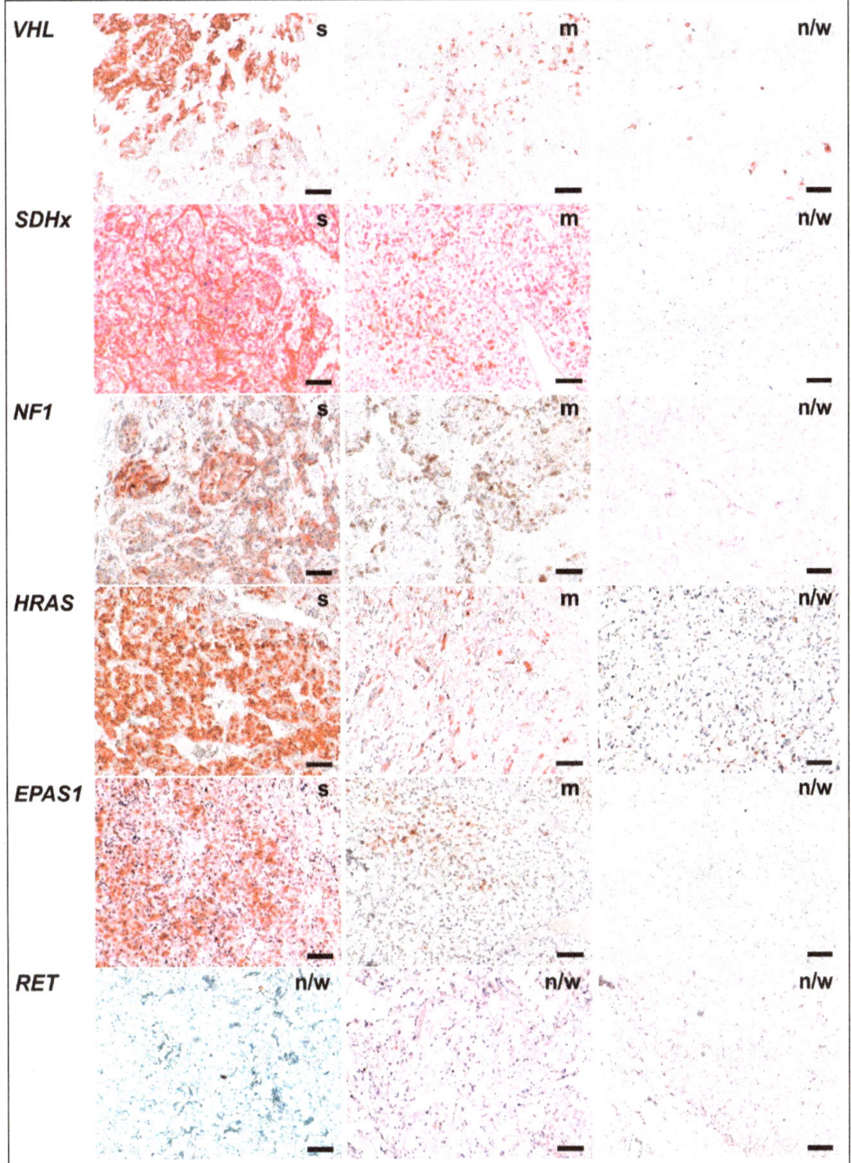

Figure 2. Scoring of COX-2 immunoreactivity in PPGL tissue samples; examples for cases carrying loss-of-function-mutations in *VHL*, *SDHx*, or *NF1*, or gain-of-function mutations in *HRAS*, *EPAS1*, or *RET*, (s) strong immunoreactivity, >50% of tumor cells were stained; (m) moderate immunoreactivity, 20–50% of tumor cells were stained; (n/w) negative or weak, <20% of tumor cells were stained; scale bars: 0.1 mm.

COX-2 immunoreactivity was strong in 23 samples (24%) and moderate in 35 samples (36%) whereas 38 samples (40%) showed negative or weak staining. Tumor location, tumor diameter, age at diagnosis, or metastatic behavior had no statistically relevant influences on COX-2 immunoreactivity

(Table S1). On the other hand, COX-2 immunoreactivity was significantly higher in samples from male patients compared to females and all genetic subgroups showed different sex ratios. However, multiple regression analyses, testing the relationships between COX-2 expression and the two independent variables 'genetic background' and 'sex' simultaneously, showed that trends in COX-2 immunoreactivity of the genetic subgroups were not artifacts of different sex ratios.

In tissue samples with different genetic backgrounds, a trend was observed with highest COX-2 immunoreactivity in PPGLs due to *VHL* mutations (36% strong, 43% moderate), followed by *NF1* (33% strong, 43% moderate), *SDHx* (23% strong, 41% moderate), *HRAS* (17% strong, 33% moderate), *EPAS1* (14% strong, 29% moderate), and RET (all samples negative or weak) (Figure 3). Of note, COX-2 immunoreactivity showed similar incidences in different *SDH* subtypes. However, due to higher numbers of *SDHD*-mutant cases compared to the other subtypes, multiple regression analyses (Table S2) taking also into account the sex of the patients showed a significant positive relationship between *SDHD* mutation and COX-2 immunoreactivity ($r = 0.867$, $p \leq 0.001$). A negative relationship was detected between *RET* mutation and COX-2 immunoreactivity ($r = -0.948$; $p < 0.001$). COX-2 immunoreactivity was similar in hereditary cases (24% strong, 37% moderate) compared to somatic cases (24% strong, 37% moderate). The trend for higher COX-2 immunoreactivity in cluster I (25% strong, 40% moderate) compared to cluster II (22% strong, 31% moderate) was related to different sex ratios in these groups ($r = 0.323$, $p = 0.043$).

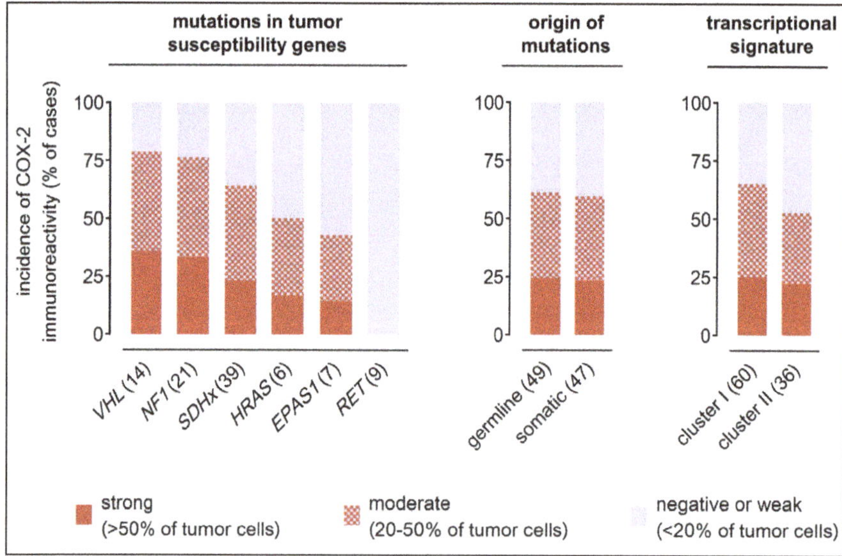

Figure 3. Comparison of COX-2 immunoreactivity in PPGLs in respect to genetic background; incidences of strong, moderate, and negative or weak COX-2 immunoreactivity observed among 96 tissue samples classified with regard to specific mutations in tumor susceptibility genes, origin of mutations, and transcriptional cluster; numbers in parentheses represent the number of samples investigated in each subgroup; see Table S1 for statistical analyses.

All 58 COX-2-positive PPGLs were further stratified in terms of their histologic staining pattern (Figure 4). Three different patterns of COX-2 immunoreactivity were observed: (pattern A) staining of pheochromocytes only, (pattern B) staining of both stromal cells and pheochromocytes, and (pattern C) staining of stromal cells only. Tumors with mutations in *SDHx* showed the highest proportion of COX-2 immunoreactivity with stromal cells involved (72%, pattern B+C), followed by *VHL* (45%, pattern B only), *NF1* (38%, pattern B+C), *HRAS* (33%, pattern B only), and *EPAS1* (0%). Pearson correlation showed a significant positive relationship between *SDHx* mutations and COX-2 immunoreactivity with stromal cells involved ($r = 0.266$, $p = 0.009$).

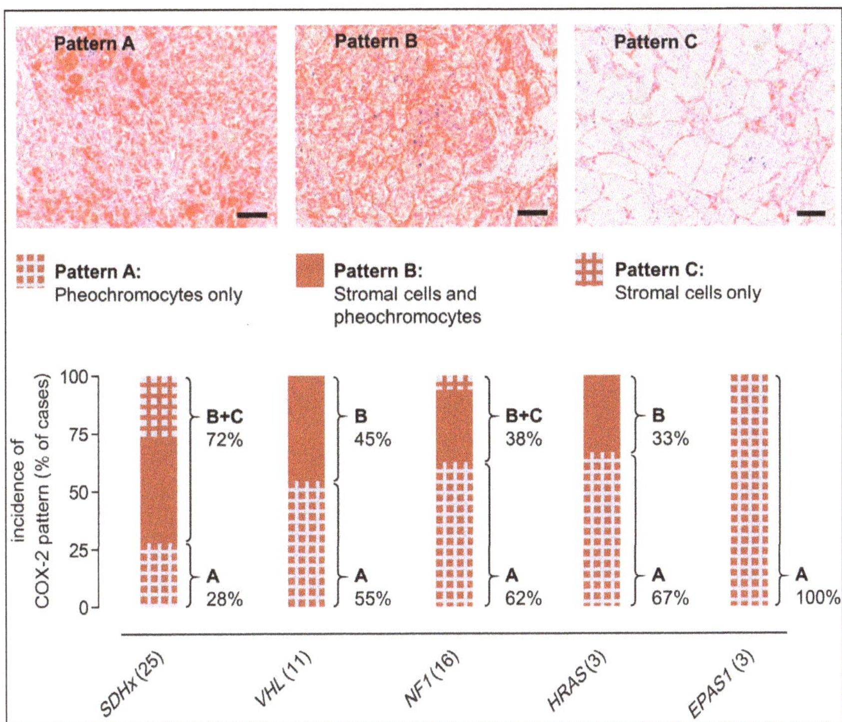

Figure 4. Immunoreactivity pattern in COX-2-positive PPGLs; COX-2 immunoreactivity with stromal cells involved was more frequently observed in tumors related to *SDHx* mutations (72%, pattern B+C) compared to other genetic background (0–45%); histologic examples: (pattern A) *HRAS* somatic mutation; (pattern B) *SDHD* germline mutation; (pattern C) *SDHD* germline mutation; see Table S1 for statistical analyses; scale bars: 0.1 mm.

2.3. COX-2 as Molecular Target in Preclinical PPGL Models

We further assessed the COX-2 status of a commonly used preclinical model of mouse pheochromocytoma (MPC) cells with heterozygous *Nf1* knockout. In vitro, MPC spheroids showed strong and homogeneous COX-2 immunoreactivity in pheochromocytes involving the most peripheral 8–10 cellular layers, whereas COX-2 immunoreactivity was absent in the necrotic core (Figure 5A). In vivo, MPC tumors in a subcutaneous allograft model showed strong tumor-specific uptake of a red-fluorescent COX-2 imaging probe (Figure 5B). Tissue sections from these allografts showed strong and homogenous COX-2 immunoreactivity predominantly involving pheochromocytes.

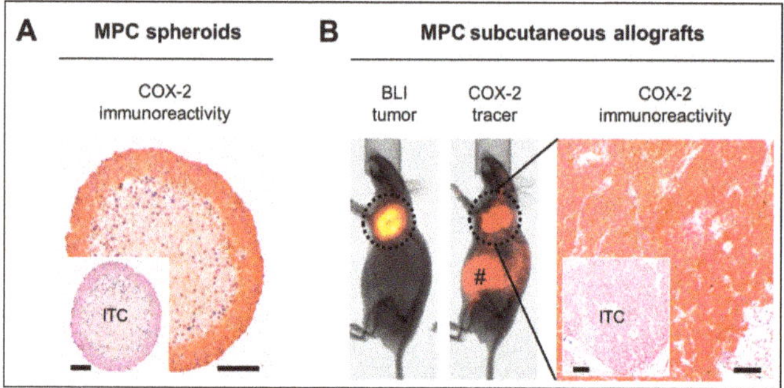

Figure 5. COX-2 as a molecular target in MPC spheroids and allografts harboring a heterozygous *Nf1* knockout; (**A**) COX-2 immunoreactivity in MPC spheroids; (**B**) COX-2 functional imaging and immunoreactivity in a luciferase-expressing subcutaneous MPC allograft model; (BLI) bioluminescence imaging of tumors; (COX-2 tracer) tumor uptake of a red-fluorescent COX-2 selective imaging probe; (#) residual non-specific accumulation of COX-2 tracer due to intraperitoneal injection; (ITC) IgG isotype control; scale bars: 0.1 mm

3. Discussion

Endoradiotherapy, e.g., with ^{177}Lu-DOTA-TATE is currently investigated as a treatment option for inoperable or metastatic PPGLs, showing promising effects, but sometimes incomplete tumor remission in clinics as well as in preclinical models [38–40]. COX-2 is associated with chemo- and radiation resistance and poor patient outcome in a number of tumor entities [29–35] encouraging us to investigate whether COX-2 is a potential target in PPGLs. Inhibition of COX-2 is considered a viable radiosensitization strategy [24,35]. In particular, selective COX-2 inhibitors (coxibs) have been suggested for combination radiotherapy of tumors, thereby enhancing radiosensitivity in various settings [28,35,37].

Expression of COX-2 was assessed on mRNA or protein level in two separate cohorts of PPGL patients with known tumor driver mutations. Both cohorts were comprised of tumors with a similar distribution of clinical features in respect to sex, tumor location, age at diagnosis, and metastatic behavior, reflecting previously described features of PPGLs [52].

Despite a significant increase in *COX-2* mRNA levels in cluster I compared to cluster II PPGLs, we did not find a significant relationship between the pseudohypoxic transcriptional signature of cluster I PPGLs and *COX-2* in clinical samples. COX-2 protein levels are consistent with these results showing also no significant difference between cluster I and cluster II PPGLs. This may be due to the fact that PPGLs are characterized by a high degree of intertumoral heterogeneity. Many different factors have been described to activate and interfere with COX-2 in cancer [28]. Amongst others, intratumoral differences in normoxic/hypoxic conditions, systemic chemotherapy, oxidative stress, or even tobacco smoking can interfere with COX-2 levels on gene expression and protein level, possibly masking a potential association with the pseudohypoxic signature of cluster I PPGLs. Nevertheless, trends were observed that may at least partially be explained by the underlying genetic background.

In cluster I PPGLs with loss-of-function mutations in *VHL* and *SDHx*, pseudohypoxic transcriptional phenotypes may contribute to COX-2 induction on gene expression and protein level. Functional defects of VHL, an E3 ubiquitin ligase, directly impair ubiquitin labeling of hypoxia-inducible factors (HIF-α) for regular proteasomal degradation. Functional defects of SDH indirectly impair ubiquitin-labeling of HIF-α caused by intracellular accumulation of succinate, an intrinsic inhibitor of prolyl hydroxylases. Therefore, both VHL and SDH defects are associated with enhanced HIF-α signaling even under normoxic conditions, a metabolic state referred to as pseudohypoxia [25]. From investigations on other tumor entities, in particular on colon cancer, it is known that both HIF-α isoforms (1 and 2) are capable of directly upregulating *COX-2* expression [26,27].

COX-2 mRNA levels as well as the percentage of moderate and high COX-2 immunoreactivity tended to be lower among cases carrying a gain-of function mutation in *EPAS1*, encoding the HIF-2α protein, compared to *VHL*- and *SDHx*-mutant cases. This observation suggests that activation of HIF-2α alone may not be sufficient for COX-2 upregulation in PPGLs.

In cluster II PPGLs with loss-of-function mutations in *NF1* gene, the trend for a relatively high COX-2 immunoreactivity is consistent with another report on elevated COX-2 and prostaglandin E2 (PGE_2) levels in *NF1* malignant peripheral nerve sheath tumors [53]. These observations raise the possibility that functional defects in NF1, a GTPase-activating protein, could indirectly contribute to the upregulation of *COX-2* expression. This may at least be partly explained by elevated levels of activated Ras-GTP leading to hyperactivation of mitogen-activated protein kinase (MAPK) pathways. Under normoxic conditions, *COX-2* expression can be induced through activation of oncogenic pathways such as Ras-MAPK and can even be further enhanced by HIF-1α during hypoxia [36]. The lack of high *COX-2* mRNA in the gene expression cohort might be due to the low number of *NF1*-mutant cases in this particular set of tumors. On the other hand, all *NF1* cases in the RNA sample cohort carried germline mutations, whereas all *NF1* cases in the tissue sample cohort carried somatic mutations. Whether there is a relationship between germ line or somatic *NF1* mutations and different COX-2 levels in PPGLs remains to be investigated.

In accordance with the observations in clinical PPGL samples, COX-2 immunoreactivity was also high in spheroids and subcutaneous allografts derived from mouse pheochromocytoma (MPC) cells with a heterozygous *Nf1* knockout. Therefore, these models are suitable for preclinical testing of COX-2-targeted treatments for the management of PPGLs. Since we did not find a significant relationship between tumor driver mutations and COX-2 in clinical PPGL samples, molecular imaging could be applied in a personalized approach to pre-estimate whether a tumor is susceptible to COX-2-targeted treatment. In our study, specific accumulation of a red-fluorescent COX-2 probe in subcutaneous MPC allografts demonstrates the potential value of COX-2 tracers for assessing the target status in PPGLs non-invasively. In order to translate this approach into clinical practice, studies have been initiated on the use of selective COX-2 inhibitors as PET radiotracers for cancer imaging [54–56].

In the case of HRAS and RET mutations, trends for lower *COX-2* mRNA levels in PPGLs are in agreement with COX-2 immunoreactivity. These findings suggest that both *HRAS* and *RET* have not major role in regulating *COX-2* expression in PPGLs. However, there have been reports on fibroblasts transformed with a mutant *HRAS* responding with a rapid induction of *COX-2* on gene expression and protein level [57]. It has also been reported that *HRAS* expression increases *COX-2* expression in intestinal epithelial cells [58]. In thyroid cancer, RET has been shown to activate Ras, and thus it could indirectly lead to *COX-2* activation, however, whether RET could activate *COX-2* in any other way is a matter of investigation [59].

The observation that tumor diameter and age at diagnosis had no statistically relevant impact on COX-2 levels is in accordance with previous studies [41–45]. In contrast to these reports, we did not detect a statistically relevant increase of *COX-2* mRNA and COX-2 immunoreactivity in primary tumors of metastatic PPGLs. This is most likely due to the relatively small number of metastatic cases in our cohorts. Significantly higher *COX-2* mRNA levels in head and neck PPGLs compared to other tumor locations is related to the fact that all head and neck PPGLs in this series carried an *SDHD* mutation. This raises the possibility that COX-2 expression may be regulated by *SDHD*-related metabolic alterations in particular in head & neck PPGLs. However, due to low sample numbers available in the *SDHD* subgroup, further studies focusing on COX-2 expression in specific *SDH* mutation subtypes are necessary to draw a conclusion from these initial observations. In our tissue series, head and neck PPGLs comprised of cases with different tumor driver mutations explaining why similar effects on COX-2 were not detected in this series. Significantly higher COX-2 protein in PPGLs from male patients compared to females is considered a specific characteristic of our tissue sample cohort since we did not detect a similar effect in the RNA samples.

Higher COX-2 immunoreactivity in stromal cells of PPGLs related to *SDHx* germline mutations compared to other tumor driver mutations indicates a systemic effect of partial *SDHx* loss on COX-2 levels. This pattern of COX-2 immunoreactivity may be related to structure-supporting sustentacular cells and/or a characteristic monocytic component in PPGLs that has recently been discovered [60]. Further histologic investigations are required to elucidate the specific cell populations of stromal COX-2 immunoreactivity in PPGLs. A report on COX-2 in cervical cancer showed that the ratio between COX-2 in tumor cells and COX-2 in stroma cells was very effective in distinguishing patients with low versus high risk of death from disease. A very strong relationship between both tumor *COX-2* expression and tumor-to-stromal COX-2 ratio has been shown to be highly correlated with response to chemotherapy while, high *COX-2* expression in the stroma was significantly associated with better survival, but failed to directly correlate with response to treatment [61]. Further studies are required to fully elucidate the role of COX-2 in PPGL tumorigenesis and therapy resistance.

4. Materials and Methods

4.1. Tumor Samples and Genetic Testing

For immunohistochemical analysis, a series of 96 tumors from patients with confirmed PPGL diagnosis were used for this study. The cohort was recruited in the four participating centers: Tumor and Normal Tissue Bank of the UCC/NCT at the Universal Hospital Carl Gustav Carus, Dresden, Germany, Spanish National Cancer Research Centre, Madrid, Spain, Radboud University Medical Centre, Nijmegen, The Netherlands, and University of Florence, Italy. All patients provided informed consent to collect clinical and genetic data, in accordance with institutional ethical-approved protocols for each center. Metastatic cases were defined based on clinical documentation of metastases or extensive local invasion. Genetic screening was performed in germline and tumor DNA using a next-generation sequencing panel (PheoSeq) as previously described [62].

4.2. Gene Expression Profiling and Data Processing

Gene expression array data were extracted from [50,51]. To investigate the association between a pseudohypoxic transcriptional signature and *COX-2* in cluster I PPGLs on RNA level, a published list of 782 genes significantly differentially expressed between *VHL*- and *SDHB*-mutant cases was taken into account [50]. These genes were compared with the hypoxia database including all genes theoretically related to hypoxia [63]. Unsupervised clustering was applied with 97 hypoxia-related genes overlapping from both lists (Figure S1). Pearson correlation coefficients® were calculated between *COX-2* expression and each of the 97 genes.

4.3. COX-2 Immunohistochemistry

Formalin-fixed and paraffin-embedded tumor and spheroid sections (3 μm) were dewaxed using Roticlear (Carl Roth, Karlsruhe, Germany) and rehydrated in a graded series of ethanol. Antigen retrieval was performed in 10 mmol/L citrate buffer pH 6 intermittently heated to 100 °C in 5 min intervals. Washing was performed using 0.05 mol/L Tris-buffered saline pH 8 containing 0.5% (v/v) Tween-20 (TBS-T). Endogenous peroxidase was quenched using 3% H_2O_2 in TBS-T. Endogenous avidin and biotin were blocked using a commercially available avidin/biotin quenching system (Agilent, Santa Clara, CA, USA). Non-specific binding sites were blocked using 10% fetal bovine serum (v/v) in TBS-T. COX-2 was detected using the primary antibody ab15191 (Abcam, Cambridge, UK). Isotype controls were incubated with non-specific rabbit IgG ab27478 (Abcam). Specific binding was detected using the biotinylated secondary antibody 111-065-003 (Dianova, Hamburg, Germany) and ExtrAvidin-peroxidase E2886 (Sigma-Aldrich, St. Louis, MO, USA) followed by staining with 3-amino-9-ethylcarbazole substrate (Sigma-Aldrich). Tumor sections were counterstained with Meyer's hematoxylin, mounted with Kaiser's glycerol gelatin (Carl Roth), and imaged using the AXIO Imager A1 microscope (Carl Zeiss, Oberkochen, Germany).

4.4. Scoring of COX-2 Immunoreactivity

For each case, COX-2 immunoreactivity was analyzed from a series of bright field images (magnification, ×100) contiguously captured along the diameter of one tumor section (images per section > 5). Perinuclear and cytoplasmic red-brown staining was considered positive. PPGLs form dense, reticular to glandular 'zellballen' or intermediate forms [64]. Typically, structure-supporting sustentacular cells are closely associated with tumor cells [65]. Taking into account these specific histologic features of PPGLs, our examination assessed COX-2 immunoreactivity in both inflammatory and sustentacular cells of the stromal compartment and/or pheochromocytes.

The percentage of COX-2-positive tumor cells was assessed using a three-mark score adapted from [41]: negative or weak (<20% of tumor cells); moderate (20–50% of tumor cells); strong (>50% of tumor cells). Samples were evaluated independently by two histologically experienced observers (Martin Ullrich and Verena Seifert) who were blinded to the genetic subtype of tumors. In cases of disagreement, samples were referred to a third observer for final decision (Sandra Hauser). Notably, our scoring system does not report on staining intensities that were observed to vary between samples from different centers most likely due to differences in tissue quality, preservation techniques, and storage time.

4.5. Spheroid Models

Mouse pheochromocytoma cells (MPC clone 4/30PRR [48]) were cultivated as previously described [49]. Spheroids were generated from MPC cells passage 34 as described elsewhere [66,67]. After 18 days of cultivation, spheroids (diameters between 500 and 600 µm) were fixed in paraformaldehyde and embedded in paraffin according to standard procedures ($n = 6$).

4.6. Tumor Allograft Models

Animal experiments were carried out at the Helmholtz-Zentrum Dresden-Rossendorf according to the guidelines of German Regulations for Animal Welfare and have been approved by the local Animal Ethics Committee for Animal Experiments (Landesdirektion Dresden, Germany). Subcutaneous tumor allografts were generated through injection of luciferase-expressing $MPC^{LUC/eGFP\text{-}ZEO}$ cells (abbreviated as $MPC^{LUC/GZ}$) passage 11 into female NMRI-nude mice (Rj:NMRI-*Foxn1*^{nu}, homozygous, T cell-deficient, hairless; Janvier Labs, Le Genest-Saint-Isle, France) as described previously. Five weeks after cell injection, optical in vivo imaging was performed (tumor diameters between 0.8 and 1.2 mm). After imaging, mice were sacrificed using CO_2 inhalation and cervical dislocation. Tumors were excised, fixed in paraformaldehyde, and embedded in paraffin according to standard procedures ($n = 6$).

4.7. Optical In Vivo Imaging

Optical tumor imaging in mice was performed on a preclinical In-Vivo Xtreme imaging system (Bruker, Billerica, MA, USA) under general anesthesia with inhalation of 10% (v/v) desflurane (Baxter, Unterschleißheim, Germany) in 30% (v/v) oxygen air. Location and morphology of luciferase-expressing $MPC^{LUC/GZ}$ allografts were assessed using bioluminescence imaging (BLI) as described previously [49]. Functional COX-2 imaging was performed using the RediJect COX-2 Fluorescent Imaging Probe (PerkinElmer, Waltham, MA, USA) injected intraperitoneally according to manufacturer's instructions. Fluorescence imaging (FLI) was performed three hours after injection. Specific fluorescence of the imaging probe was captured at $\lambda_{Ex/Em}$ = 570/600 nm and non-specific fluorescence was captured at $\lambda_{Ex/Em}$ = 480/535 nm. Tumor uptake was analyzed in processed images, showing specific fluorescence/non-specific fluorescence ratios.

4.8. Statistical Analysis

Graphs were drawn using Prism version 5.02 (GraphPad Software, San Diego, CA, USA). Incidences of COX-2 immunoreactivity within a defined subgroup are presented as percent of cases, n represents the number of cases. If not stated differently, data are presented as means ± standard error of the means. Significance of differences was tested for $n \geq 6$ using the Mann–Whitney U test. Multiple linear regression analysis was performed using OriginPro 2017G (OriginLab Corporation, Northhampton, MA, USA). Relationships were described with the regression coefficient r and considered significant at p-values < 0.05. Interobserver variation was calculated using online QuickCalcs κ statistics version 06/2014 (GraphPad Software, www.graphpad.com/quickcalcs/kappa1).

5. Conclusions

Moderate to high cyclooxygenase 2 (COX-2) gene expression and immunoreactivity in about 60% of PPGLs demonstrates that, for these patients, COX-2 is considered a clinically relevant molecular target for adjuvant, in particular radiosensitizing treatments using selective COX-2 inhibitors, e.g., in combination with ^{177}Lu-DOTA-TATE endoradiotherapy. However, taking into account the genetic background of the samples, is an indicator but not the major determinant for *COX-2* expression in PPGLs. High COX-2 immunoreactivity in tumor spheroids and subcutaneous tumor allografts derived from mouse pheochromocytoma (MPC) cells demonstrates that available PPGL models are suitable for preclinical in vitro and in vivo testing of COX-2-targeting treatments.

Supplementary Materials: The following are available online at http://www.mdpi.com/2072-6694/11/6/743/s1, Figure S1: Unsupervised clustering for 97 hypoxia-related genes in PPGLs applied to our mRNA expression series extracted from [50,51]; *VHL*- and *SDHx*-mutant cases clustered together whereas, other cases showed no homogeneous profile, Table S1: Statistical analyses of COX-2 status with regard to clinical characteristics and genetic background of tumors in two independent series of PPGL samples; data in parentheses were calculated from low sample numbers ($n < 7$); as Mann–Whitney U test showed significant sex-related differences in COX-2 immunoreactivity in tissue samples, multiple regression analyses was applied to distinguish whether the trends observed in the genetic subgroups were related to genetic background or different sex ratios only; levels of significance: * $p < 0.05$; † $p < 0.01$, ‡ $p < 0.001$, Table S2: Pearson correlation between expression of *COX-2* and 97 hypoxia-related genes in PPGLs in the mRNA expression series extracted from [50,51].

Author Contributions: Conceptualization, M.U., M.R., and J.P.; Methodology and validation, M.R.; Formal analysis, A.M.M.-M.; Investigation, M.U., V.S., S.H., B.C., A.M.M.-M., and M.T.L; Resources, H.T., G.E., M.R., and J.P.; Writing—original draft preparation, M.U. and S.R.; Writing—review and editing, C.G.Z, H.T, M.R., and J.P; Visualization, M.U. and A.M.M.-M.

Funding: This research was funded by Deutsche Forschungsgemeinschaft (DFG) grants BE-2607/1-2 (M.U. and J.P.), ZI-1362/2-2 (C.G.Z and G.E.), the Collaborative Research Center Transregio 205 "The Adrenal: Central Relay in Health and Disease" (CRC/TRR 205/1; M.U., S.R., V.S., G.E., C.G.Z., and J.P.) and the Paradifference Foundation (Consortium for Personalized Targeted Therapy for SDHB-mutated Metastatic PPGLs; M.U., S.R., V.S., B.C., M.T.L, H.T., G.E., M.R, and J.P). M.R. receives funding from Instituto de Salud Carlos III (ISCIII), through the "Acción Estratégica en Salud" (AES) (projects PI17/01796), cofounded by the European Regional Development Fund (ERDF). B.C. is supported by Becas de Excelencia 2017 from Rafael del Pino Foundation.

Acknowledgments: The authors greatly acknowledge the excellent technical assistance of Aline Morgenegg, Catharina Knöfel, and Johanna Wodtke (Department of Radiopharmaceutical and Chemical Biology, Institute of Radiopharmaceutical Cancer Research, Helmholtz-Zentrum Dresden-Rossendorf). The authors further thank Massimo Mannelli for providing PPGL samples from the University of Florence. MPC 4/30PRR cells were kindly provided by Arthur Tischler, James Powers, and Karel Pacak.

Conflicts of Interest: The authors declare no conflict of interest. The funders had no role in the design of the study; in the collection, analyses, or interpretation of data; in the writing of the manuscript, or in the decision to publish the results.

References

1. Gimenez-Roqueplo, A.P.; Dahia, P.L.; Robledo, M. An update on the genetics of paraganglioma, pheochromocytoma, and associated hereditary syndromes. *Horm. Metab. Res.* **2012**, *44*, 328–333. [CrossRef]
2. Crona, J.; Delgado Verdugo, A.; Maharjan, R.; Stalberg, P.; Granberg, D.; Hellman, P.; Bjorklund, P. Somatic mutations in h-ras in sporadic pheochromocytoma and paraganglioma identified by exome sequencing. *J. Clin. Endocrinol. Metab.* **2013**, *98*, E1266–E1271. [CrossRef]
3. Jochmanova, I.; Pacak, K. Genomic landscape of pheochromocytoma and paraganglioma. *Trends Cancer* **2018**, *4*, 6–9. [CrossRef] [PubMed]

4. Fishbein, L.; Leshchiner, I.; Walter, V.; Danilova, L.; Robertson, A.G.; Johnson, A.R.; Lichtenberg, T.M.; Murray, B.A.; Ghayee, H.K.; Else, T.; et al. Comprehensive molecular characterization of pheochromocytoma and paraganglioma. *Cancer Cell* **2017**, *31*, 181–193. [CrossRef] [PubMed]
5. Lorenzo, F.R.; Yang, C.; Ng Tang Fui, M.; Vankayalapati, H.; Zhuang, Z.; Huynh, T.; Grossmann, M.; Pacak, K.; Prchal, J.T. A novel EPAS1/hif2a germline mutation in a congenital polycythemia with paraganglioma. *J. Mol. Med. (Berl.)* **2013**, *91*, 507–512. [CrossRef] [PubMed]
6. Comino-Mendez, I.; de Cubas, A.A.; Bernal, C.; Alvarez-Escola, C.; Sanchez-Malo, C.; Ramirez-Tortosa, C.L.; Pedrinaci, S.; Rapizzi, E.; Ercolino, T.; Bernini, G.; et al. Tumoral EPAS1 (hif2a) mutations explain sporadic pheochromocytoma and paraganglioma in the absence of erythrocytosis. *Hum. Mol. Genet.* **2013**, *22*, 2169–2176. [CrossRef]
7. Dahia, P.L. The genetic landscape of pheochromocytomas and paragangliomas: Somatic mutations take center stage. *J. Clin. Endocrinol. Metab.* **2013**, *98*, 2679–2681. [CrossRef] [PubMed]
8. Qin, Y.; Yao, L.; King, E.E.; Buddavarapu, K.; Lenci, R.E.; Chocron, E.S.; Lechleiter, J.D.; Sass, M.; Aronin, N.; Schiavi, F.; et al. Germline mutations in TMEM127 confer susceptibility to pheochromocytoma. *Nat. Genet.* **2010**, *42*, 229–233. [CrossRef]
9. Burnichon, N.; Briere, J.J.; Libe, R.; Vescovo, L.; Riviere, J.; Tissier, F.; Jouanno, E.; Jeunemaitre, X.; Benit, P.; Tzagoloff, A.; et al. SDHA is a tumor suppressor gene causing paraganglioma. *Hum. Mol. Genet.* **2010**, *19*, 3011–3020. [CrossRef]
10. Burnichon, N.; Vescovo, L.; Amar, L.; Libe, R.; de Reynies, A.; Venisse, A.; Jouanno, E.; Laurendeau, I.; Parfait, B.; Bertherat, J.; et al. Integrative genomic analysis reveals somatic mutations in pheochromocytoma and paraganglioma. *Hum. Mol. Genet.* **2011**, *20*, 3974–3985. [CrossRef]
11. Comino-Mendez, I.; Gracia-Aznarez, F.J.; Schiavi, F.; Landa, I.; Leandro-Garcia, L.J.; Leton, R.; Honrado, E.; Ramos-Medina, R.; Caronia, D.; Pita, G.; et al. Exome sequencing identifies max mutations as a cause of hereditary pheochromocytoma. *Nat. Genet.* **2011**, *43*, 663–667. [CrossRef] [PubMed]
12. Yang, C.; Zhuang, Z.; Fliedner, S.M.; Shankavaram, U.; Sun, M.G.; Bullova, P.; Zhu, R.; Elkahloun, A.G.; Kourlas, P.J.; Merino, M.; et al. Germ-line PHD1 and PHD2 mutations detected in patients with pheochromocytoma/paraganglioma-polycythemia. *J. Mol. Med. (Berl.)* **2015**, *93*, 93–104. [CrossRef] [PubMed]
13. Pang, Y.; Gupta, G.; Yang, C.; Wang, H.; Huynh, T.T.; Abdullaev, Z.; Pack, S.D.; Percy, M.J.; Lappin, T.R.J.; Zhuang, Z.; et al. A novel splicing site IRP1 somatic mutation in a patient with pheochromocytoma and JAK2(V617F) positive polycythemia vera: A case report. *BMC Cancer* **2018**, *18*, 286. [CrossRef] [PubMed]
14. Richter, S.; Gieldon, L.; Pang, Y.; Peitzsch, M.; Huynh, T.; Leton, R.; Viana, B.; Ercolino, T.; Mangelis, A.; Rapizzi, E.; et al. Metabolome-guided genomics to identify pathogenic variants in isocitrate dehydrogenase, fumarate hydratase, and succinate dehydrogenase genes in pheochromocytoma and paraganglioma. *Genet. Med.* **2019**, *21*, 705–717. [CrossRef]
15. Cascon, A.; Comino-Mendez, I.; Curras-Freixes, M.; de Cubas, A.A.; Contreras, L.; Richter, S.; Peitzsch, M.; Mancikova, V.; Inglada-Perez, L.; Perez-Barrios, A.; et al. Whole-exome sequencing identifies MDH2 as a new familial paraganglioma gene. *J. Natl. Cancer Inst.* **2015**, *107*, 1–5. [CrossRef] [PubMed]
16. Remacha, L.; Comino-Mendez, I.; Richter, S.; Contreras, L.; Curras-Freixes, M.; Pita, G.; Leton, R.; Galarreta, A.; Torres-Perez, R.; Honrado, E.; et al. Targeted exome sequencing of krebs cycle genes reveals candidate cancer-predisposing mutations in pheochromocytomas and paragangliomas. *Clin. Cancer Res.* **2017**, *23*, 6315–6324. [CrossRef]
17. Remacha, L.; Pirman, D.; Mahoney, C.E.; Coloma, J.; Calsina, B.; Curras-Freixes, M.; Leton, R.; Torres-Perez, R.; Richter, S.; Pita, G.; et al. Recurrent germline dlst mutations in individuals with multiple pheochromocytomas and paragangliomas. *Am. J. Hum. Genet.* **2019**, *104*, 651–664. [CrossRef]
18. Remacha, L.; Curras-Freixes, M.; Torres-Ruiz, R.; Schiavi, F.; Torres-Perez, R.; Calsina, B.; Leton, R.; Comino-Mendez, I.; Roldan-Romero, J.M.; Montero-Conde, C.; et al. Gain-of-function mutations in dnmt3a in patients with paraganglioma. *Genet. Med.* **2018**, *20*, 1644–1651. [CrossRef] [PubMed]
19. Buffet, A.; Morin, A.; Castro-Vega, L.J.; Habarou, F.; Lussey-Lepoutre, C.; Letouze, E.; Lefebvre, H.; Guilhem, I.; Haissaguerre, M.; Raingeard, I.; et al. Germline mutations in the mitochondrial 2-oxoglutarate/malate carrier slc25a11 gene confer a predisposition to metastatic paragangliomas. *Cancer Res.* **2018**, *78*, 1914–1922. [CrossRef] [PubMed]

20. Letouze, E.; Martinelli, C.; Loriot, C.; Burnichon, N.; Abermil, N.; Ottolenghi, C.; Janin, M.; Menara, M.; Nguyen, A.T.; Benit, P.; et al. Sdh mutations establish a hypermethylator phenotype in paraganglioma. *Cancer Cell* **2013**, *23*, 739–752. [CrossRef]
21. Calsina, B.; Curras-Freixes, M.; Buffet, A.; Pons, T.; Contreras, L.; Leton, R.; Comino-Mendez, I.; Remacha, L.; Calatayud, M.; Obispo, B.; et al. Role of MDH2 pathogenic variant in pheochromocytoma and paraganglioma patients. *Genet. Med.* **2018**, *20*, 1652–1662. [CrossRef]
22. Dahia, P.L.; Ross, K.N.; Wright, M.E.; Hayashida, C.Y.; Santagata, S.; Barontini, M.; Kung, A.L.; Sanso, G.; Powers, J.F.; Tischler, A.S.; et al. A HIF1alpha regulatory loop links hypoxia and mitochondrial signals in pheochromocytomas. *PLoS Genet.* **2005**, *1*, 72–80. [CrossRef]
23. Dahia, P.L. Pheochromocytoma and paraganglioma pathogenesis: Learning from genetic heterogeneity. *Nat. Rev. Cancer* **2014**, *14*, 108–119. [CrossRef]
24. Deorukhkar, A.; Krishnan, S. Targeting inflammatory pathways for tumor radiosensitization. *Biochem. Pharmacol.* **2010**, *80*, 1904–1914. [CrossRef]
25. Jochmanova, I.; Yang, C.; Zhuang, Z.; Pacak, K. Hypoxia-inducible factor signaling in pheochromocytoma: Turning the rudder in the right direction. *J. Natl. Cancer Inst.* **2013**, *105*, 1270–1283. [CrossRef]
26. Xue, X.; Shah, Y.M. Hypoxia-inducible factor-2alpha is essential in activating the COX2/mpges-1/PGE2 signaling axis in colon cancer. *Carcinogenesis* **2013**, *34*, 163–169. [CrossRef]
27. Kaidi, A.; Qualtrough, D.; Williams, A.C.; Paraskeva, C. Direct transcriptional upregulation of cyclooxygenase-2 by hypoxia-inducible factor (HIF)-1 promotes colorectal tumor cell survival and enhances HIF-1 transcriptional activity during hypoxia. *Cancer Res.* **2006**, *66*, 6683–6691. [CrossRef]
28. Hashemi Goradel, N.; Najafi, M.; Salehi, E.; Farhood, B.; Mortezaee, K. Cyclooxygenase-2 in cancer: A review. *J. Cell. Physiol.* **2019**, *234*, 5683–5699. [CrossRef]
29. Nix, P.; Lind, M.; Greenman, J.; Stafford, N.; Cawkwell, L. Expression of cox-2 protein in radioresistant laryngeal cancer. *Ann. Oncol.* **2004**, *15*, 797–801. [CrossRef]
30. Lin, F.; Luo, J.; Gao, W.; Wu, J.; Shao, Z.; Wang, Z.; Meng, J.; Ou, Z.; Yang, G. COX-2 promotes breast cancer cell radioresistance via p38/mapk-mediated cellular anti-apoptosis and invasiveness. *Tumor Biol.* **2013**, *34*, 2817–2826. [CrossRef]
31. Suzuki, K.; Gerelchuluun, A.; Hong, Z.; Sun, L.; Zenkoh, J.; Moritake, T.; Tsuboi, K. Celecoxib enhances radiosensitivity of hypoxic glioblastoma cells through endoplasmic reticulum stress. *Neuro-Oncology* **2013**, *15*, 1186–1199. [CrossRef]
32. Terakado, N.; Shintani, S.; Yano, J.; Chunnan, L.; Mihara, M.; Nakashiro, K.; Hamakawa, H. Overexpression of cyclooxygenase-2 is associated with radioresistance in oral squamous cell carcinoma. *Oral Oncol.* **2004**, *40*, 383–389. [CrossRef]
33. Choy, H.; Milas, L. Enhancing radiotherapy with cyclooxygenase-2 enzyme inhibitors: A rational advance? *J. Natl. Cancer Inst.* **2003**, *95*, 1440–1452. [CrossRef]
34. Tessner, T.G.; Muhale, F.; Riehl, T.E.; Anant, S.; Stenson, W.F. Prostaglandin E2 reduces radiation-induced epithelial apoptosis through a mechanism involving akt activation and bax translocation. *J. Clin. Investig.* **2004**, *114*, 1676–1685. [CrossRef]
35. Laube, M.; Kniess, T.; Pietzsch, J. Development of antioxidant COX-2 inhibitors as radioprotective agents for radiation therapy-a hypothesis-driven review. *Antioxidants (Basel)* **2016**, *5*, 14. [CrossRef]
36. Greenhough, A.; Smartt, H.J.; Moore, A.E.; Roberts, H.R.; Williams, A.C.; Paraskeva, C.; Kaidi, A. The COX-2/PGE2 pathway: Key roles in the hallmarks of cancer and adaptation to the tumour microenvironment. *Carcinogenesis* **2009**, *30*, 377–386. [CrossRef]
37. Bechmann, N.; Hauser, S.; Hofheinz, F.; Kniess, T.; Pietzsch, J. Nitric oxide-releasing selective cyclooxygenase-2 inhibitors as promising radiosensitizers in melanoma cells in vitro. *Ann. Radiat. Ther. Oncol.* **2017**, *1*, 1010.
38. van Essen, M.; Krenning, E.P.; Kam, B.L.; de Herder, W.W.; van Aken, M.O.; Kwekkeboom, D.J. Report on short-term side effects of treatments with ^{177}Lu-octreotate in combination with capecitabine in seven patients with gastroenteropancreatic neuroendocrine tumours. *Eur. J. Nucl. Med. Mol. Imaging* **2008**, *35*, 743–748. [CrossRef]
39. Castinetti, F.; Kroiss, A.; Kumar, R.; Pacak, K.; Taieb, D. 15 years of paraganglioma: Imaging and imaging-based treatment of pheochromocytoma and paraganglioma. *Endocr. Relat. Cancer* **2015**, *22*, T135–T145. [CrossRef]

40. Ullrich, M.; Bergmann, R.; Peitzsch, M.; Zenker, E.F.; Cartellieri, M.; Bachmann, M.; Ehrhart-Bornstein, M.; Block, N.L.; Schally, A.V.; Eisenhofer, G.; et al. Multimodal somatostatin receptor theranostics using [^{64}Cu]Cu-/[^{177}Lu]Lu-DOTA-(Tyr^{3})octreotate and AN-238 in a mouse pheochromocytoma model. *Theranostics* **2016**, *6*, 650–665. [CrossRef]
41. Salmenkivi, K.; Haglund, C.; Ristimaki, A.; Arola, J.; Heikkila, P. Increased expression of cyclooxygenase-2 in malignant pheochromocytomas. *J. Clin. Endocrinol. Metab.* **2001**, *86*, 5615–5619. [CrossRef]
42. Cadden, I.S.; Atkinson, A.B.; Johnston, B.T.; Pogue, K.; Connolly, R.; McCance, D.; Ardill, J.E.; Russell, C.F.; McGinty, A. Cyclooxygenase-2 expression correlates with phaeochromocytoma malignancy: Evidence for a bcl-2-dependent mechanism. *Histopathology* **2007**, *51*, 743–751. [CrossRef]
43. Zhu, Y.; He, H.C.; Yuan, F.; Zhang, J.; Rui, W.B.; Zhao, J.P.; Shen, Z.J.; Ning, G. Heparanase-1 and cyclooxygenase-2: Prognostic indicators of malignancy in pheochromocytomas. *Endocrine* **2010**, *38*, 93–99. [CrossRef] [PubMed]
44. Feng, F.; Zhu, Y.; Wang, X.; Wu, Y.; Zhou, W.; Jin, X.; Zhang, R.; Sun, F.; Kasoma, Z.; Shen, Z. Predictive factors for malignant pheochromocytoma: Analysis of 136 patients. *J. Urol.* **2011**, *185*, 1583–1590. [CrossRef] [PubMed]
45. Saffar, H.; Sanii, S.; Heshmat, R.; Haghpanah, V.; Larijani, B.; Rajabiani, A.; Azimi, S.; Tavangar, S.M. Expression of galectin-3, nm-23, and cyclooxygenase-2 could potentially discriminate between benign and malignant pheochromocytoma. *Am. J. Clin. Pathol.* **2011**, *135*, 454–460. [CrossRef]
46. Xing, Y.; Wang, R.; Chen, D.; Mao, J.; Shi, R.; Wu, Z.; Kang, J.; Tian, W.; Zhang, C. COX2 is involved in hypoxia-induced TNF-alpha expression in osteoblast. *Sci. Rep.* **2015**, *5*, 10020. [CrossRef] [PubMed]
47. Campillo, N.; Torres, M.; Vilaseca, A.; Nonaka, P.N.; Gozal, D.; Roca-Ferrer, J.; Picado, C.; Montserrat, J.M.; Farre, R.; Navajas, D.; et al. Role of cyclooxygenase-2 on intermittent hypoxia-induced lung tumor malignancy in a mouse model of sleep apnea. *Sci. Rep.* **2017**, *7*, 44693. [CrossRef]
48. Powers, J.F.; Evinger, M.J.; Tsokas, P.; Bedri, S.; Alroy, J.; Shahsavari, M.; Tischler, A.S. Pheochromocytoma cell lines from heterozygous neurofibromatosis knockout mice. *Cell Tissue Res.* **2000**, *302*, 309–320. [CrossRef]
49. Ullrich, M.; Liers, J.; Peitzsch, M.; Feldmann, A.; Bergmann, R.; Sommer, U.; Richter, S.; Bornstein, S.R.; Bachmann, M.; Eisenhofer, G.; et al. Strain-specific metastatic phenotypes in pheochromocytoma allograft mice. *Endocr. Relat. Cancer* **2018**, *25*, 993–1004. [CrossRef] [PubMed]
50. Lopez-Jimenez, E.; Gomez-Lopez, G.; Leandro-Garcia, L.J.; Munoz, I.; Schiavi, F.; Montero-Conde, C.; de Cubas, A.A.; Ramires, R.; Landa, I.; Leskela, S.; et al. Research resource: Transcriptional profiling reveals different pseudohypoxic signatures in SDHB and VHL-related pheochromocytomas. *Mol. Endocrinol.* **2010**, *24*, 2382–2391. [CrossRef]
51. Qin, N.; de Cubas, A.A.; Garcia-Martin, R.; Richter, S.; Peitzsch, M.; Menschikowski, M.; Lenders, J.W.; Timmers, H.J.; Mannelli, M.; Opocher, G.; et al. Opposing effects of HIF1α and HIF2α on chromaffin cell phenotypic features and tumor cell proliferation: Insights from myc-associated factor x. *Int. J. Cancer* **2014**, *135*, 2054–2064. [CrossRef]
52. Pamporaki, C.; Hamplova, B.; Peitzsch, M.; Prejbisz, A.; Beuschlein, F.; Timmers, H.; Fassnacht, M.; Klink, B.; Lodish, M.; Stratakis, C.A.; et al. Characteristics of pediatric vs adult pheochromocytomas and paragangliomas. *J. Clin. Endocrinol. Metab.* **2017**, *102*, 1122–1132. [CrossRef]
53. Deadwyler, G.D.; Dang, I.; Nelson, J.; Srikanth, M.; De Vries, G.H. Prostaglandin E_2 metabolism is activated in schwann cell lines derived from human NF1 malignant peripheral nerve sheath tumors. *Neuron Glia Biol.* **2004**, *1*, 149–155. [CrossRef]
54. Kniess, T.; Laube, M.; Bergmann, R.; Sehn, F.; Graf, F.; Steinbach, J.; Wuest, F.; Pietzsch, J. Radiosynthesis of a ^{18}F-labeled 2,3-diarylsubstituted indole via McMurry coupling for functional characterization of cyclooxygenase-2 (COX-2) in vitro and in vivo. *Bioorg. Med. Chem.* **2012**, *20*, 3410–3421. [CrossRef]
55. Laube, M.; Gassner, C.; Sharma, S.K.; Gunther, R.; Pigorsch, A.; Konig, J.; Kockerling, M.; Wuest, F.; Pietzsch, J.; Kniess, T. Diaryl-substituted (dihydro)pyrrolo[3,2,1-hi]indoles, a class of potent COX-2 inhibitors with tricyclic core structure. *J. Org. Chem.* **2015**, *80*, 5611–5624. [CrossRef]
56. Laube, M.; Kniess, T.; Pietzsch, J. Radiolabeled COX-2 inhibitors for non-invasive visualization of COX-2 expression and activity—A critical update. *Molecules* **2013**, *18*, 6311–6355. [CrossRef]
57. Sheng, H.; Williams, C.S.; Shao, J.; Liang, P.; DuBois, R.N.; Beauchamp, R.D. Induction of cyclooxygenase-2 by activated ha-ras oncogene in rat-1 fibroblasts and the role of mitogen-activated protein kinase pathway. *J. Biol. Chem.* **1998**, *273*, 22120–22127. [CrossRef]

58. Sheng, H.; Shao, J.; Dixon, D.A.; Williams, C.S.; Prescott, S.M.; DuBois, R.N.; Beauchamp, R.D. Transforming growth factor-beta1 enhances ha-Ras-induced expression of cyclooxygenase-2 in intestinal epithelial cells via stabilization of mrna. *J. Biol. Chem.* **2000**, *275*, 6628–6635. [CrossRef]
59. Lam, A.K.; Montone, K.T.; Nolan, K.A.; Livolsi, V.A. Ret oncogene activation in papillary thyroid carcinoma: Prevalence and implication on the histological parameters. *Hum. Pathol.* **1998**, *29*, 565–568. [CrossRef]
60. Farhat, N.A.; Powers, J.F.; Shepard-Barry, A.; Dahia, P.; Pacak, K.; Tischler, A.S. A previously unrecognized monocytic component of pheochromocytoma and paraganglioma. *Endocr. Pathol.* **2019**, 1–6. [CrossRef]
61. Ferrandina, G.; Lauriola, L.; Zannoni, G.F.; Distefano, M.G.; Legge, F.; Salutari, V.; Gessi, M.; Maggiano, N.; Scambia, G.; Ranelletti, F.O. Expression of cyclooxygenase-2 (COX-2) in tumour and stroma compartments in cervical cancer: Clinical implications. *Br. J. Cancer* **2002**, *87*, 1145–1152. [CrossRef]
62. Curras-Freixes, M.; Pineiro-Yanez, E.; Montero-Conde, C.; Apellaniz-Ruiz, M.; Calsina, B.; Mancikova, V.; Remacha, L.; Richter, S.; Ercolino, T.; Rogowski-Lehmann, N.; et al. Pheoseq: A targeted next-generation sequencing assay for pheochromocytoma and paraganglioma diagnostics. *J. Mol. Diagn.* **2017**, *19*, 575–588. [CrossRef] [PubMed]
63. Khurana, P.; Sugadev, R.; Jain, J.; Singh, S.B. Hypoxiadb: A database of hypoxia-regulated proteins. *Database (Oxf.)* **2013**, *2013*, bat074. [CrossRef]
64. Salmenkivi, K.; Heikkila, P.; Haglund, C.; Arola, J. Malignancy in pheochromocytomas. *APMIS* **2004**, *112*, 551–559. [CrossRef]
65. Unger, P.; Hoffman, K.; Pertsemlidis, D.; Thung, S.; Wolfe, D.; Kaneko, M. S100 protein-positive sustentacular cells in malignant and locally aggressive adrenal pheochromocytomas. *Arch. Pathol. Lab. Med.* **1991**, *115*, 484–487.
66. Seifert, V.; Liers, J.; Kniess, T.; Richter, S.; Bechmann, N.; Feldmann, A.; Bachmann, M.; Eisenhofer, G.; Pietzsch, J.; Ullrich, M. Fluorescent mouse pheochromocytoma spheroids expressing hypoxia-inducible factor 2 alpha: Morphologic and radiopharmacologic characterization. *J. Cell. Biotechnol.* **2019**, in press.
67. Bechmann, N.; Poser, I.; Seifert, V.; Greunke, C.; Ullrich, M.; Qin, N.; Walch, A.; Peitzsch, M.; Robledo, M.; Pacak, K.; et al. Impact of extrinsic and intrinsic hypoxia on catecholamine biosynthesis in absence or presence of HIF2α in pheochromocytoma cells. *Cancers* **2019**, *11*, 594. [CrossRef]

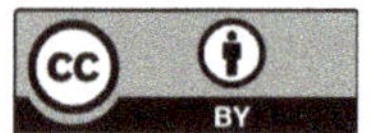

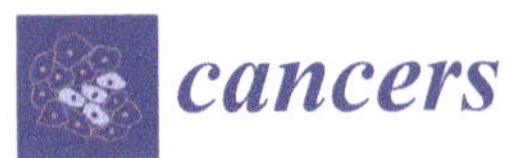

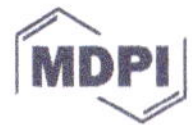

Review

A Developmental Perspective on Paragangliar Tumorigenesis

Lavinia Vittoria Lotti [1], Simone Vespa [2,3], Mattia Russel Pantalone [4], Silvia Perconti [2,3], Diana Liberata Esposito [2,3], Rosa Visone [2,3], Angelo Veronese [5], Carlo Terenzio Paties [6], Mario Sanna [7], Fabio Verginelli [8], Cecilia Soderberg Nauclér [4] and Renato Mariani-Costantini [2,3,*]

1 Department of Experimental Medicine, "La Sapienza" University, Viale Regina Elena 324, 00161 Rome, Italy; laviniavittoria.lotti@uniroma1.it
2 Center of Sciences on Aging and Translational Medicine (CeSI-MeT), "G. d'Annunzio" University, Via Luigi Polacchi 11, 66100 Chieti, Italy; sv85@libero.it (S.V.); percontisilvia@gmail.com (S.P.); d.esposito@unich.it (D.L.E); r.visone@unich.it (R.V.)
3 Department of Medical, Oral and Biotechnological Sciences, "G. d'Annunzio" University, Via dei Vestini 31, 66100 Chieti, Italy
4 Department of Medicine (Solna), Division of Microbial Pathogenesis, BioClinicum, Karolinska Institutet, 17164 Stockholm, Sweden; mattia.pantalone@ki.se (M.R.P.); cecilia.naucler@ki.se (C.S.N.)
5 Department of Medicine and Aging Sciences, "G. d'Annunzio" University, Via Luigi Polacchi 11, 66100 Chieti, Italy; a.veronese@unich.it
6 Department of Oncology-Hematology, Service of Anatomic Pathology, "Guglielmo da Saliceto" Hospital, Via Taverna 49, 29100 Piacenza, Italy; carlopaties@yahoo.it
7 Skull Base Unit, "Gruppo Otologico" Piacenza-Roma, Via Antonio Emmanueli, 42, 29121 Piacenza, Italy; mario.sanna@gruppootologico.it
8 Department of Pharmacy, "G. d'Annunzio" University, Via dei Vestini 31, 66100 Chieti, Italy; verginelli@unich.it
* Correspondence: rmc@unich.it

Received: 30 January 2019; Accepted: 21 February 2019; Published: 26 February 2019

Abstract: In this review, we propose that paraganglioma is a fundamentally organized, albeit aberrant, tissue composed of neoplastic vascular and neural cell types that share a common origin from a multipotent mesenchymal-like stem/progenitor cell. This view is consistent with the pseudohypoxic footprint implicated in the molecular pathogenesis of the disease, is in harmony with the neural crest origin of the paraganglia, and is strongly supported by the physiological model of carotid body hyperplasia. Our immunomorphological and molecular studies of head and neck paragangliomas demonstrate in all cases relationships between the vascular and the neural tumor compartments, that share mesenchymal and immature vasculo-neural markers, conserved in derived cell cultures. This immature, multipotent phenotype is supported by constitutive amplification of NOTCH signaling genes and by loss of the microRNA-200s and -34s, which control *NOTCH1*, *ZEB1*, and *PDGFRA* in head and neck paraganglioma cells. Importantly, the neuroepithelial component is distinguished by extreme mitochondrial alterations, associated with collapse of the $\Delta\Psi$m. Finally, our xenograft models of head and neck paraganglioma demonstrate that mesenchymal-like cells first give rise to a vasculo-angiogenic network, and then self-organize into neuroepithelial-like clusters, a process inhibited by treatment with imatinib.

Keywords: carotid body; angiogenesis; mitochondria; neural crest; neurogenesis; paraganglioma; stem-like tumor cells; vasculogenesis; xenograft

1. Introduction

1.1. Intersections between Tumorigenesis, Histogenesis, and Tissue Regeneration

Tumors are capable of autonomous and aberrant growth, but, as normal tissues, can grow only after achieving a structural organization, which requires the coordinated contribution of different cell types, the establishment of appropriate cell–cell and cell–matrix interactions and the development of specific scaffolds and vascular networks [1]. However, much of the basic information about the structural and functional organization of neoplastic tissues is still lacking. For instance, the key question of whether tumors contain cells able to transdifferentiate into both vascular and parenchymal cell types is still debated [2]. We do not know to what extent tumors follow the histogenetic blueprint of their normal tissue counterparts, and we do not fully understand which of the several tumor-resident cell types can regenerate neoplastic tissue after damage inflicted by therapy [3–6]. Nonetheless, it is clear that evolutionarily conserved developmental programs and signaling pathways intersect tumorigenesis, histo/organogenesis, and tissue repair/regeneration [1,6]. In particular, invasive and/or metastatic tumors essentially imitate the organogenetic program of the neural crest, a transient embryonic structure that characterizes the evolution of procraniates and craniates (*Cristozoa*) [7]. The temporary neural crest milieu defines a highly plastic population of migratory and multipotent cells that, in response to complex signals—including morphogen gradients, cell–cell interactions, availability of oxygen and nutrients, and topography—dedifferentiate via the epithelial–mesenchymal transition (EMT) program, migrate, proliferate, and again re-differentiate via the reverse mesenchymal–epithelial transition (MET) program, giving rise to an amazing variety of cell types and tissues throughout the axial body region [4,8]. While the embryonic population of neural crest cells is ephemeral, it appears that in postnatal tissues and organs the perivascular niche preserves multipotent stem/progenitor-like cells that retain tissue-specific histogenetic instructions that are reactivated during regeneration and repair [4,9–12]. Such cells might link development, tissue regeneration, and neoplasia.

1.2. Paragangliomas and Pheochromocytomas

Paragangliomas (PGLs) are rare, generally sluggish but invasive and potentially lethal tumors arising from the neural crest-derived paraxial autonomic ganglia (paraganglia) of parasympathetic (mainly head and neck) or sympathoadrenal (mainly truncal) lineage [13]. Pheochromocytomas are in essence catecholamine-producing tumors that arise mainly from the chromaffin cells of the adrenal medulla, also of neural crest origin, and present with a constellation of symptoms secondary to catecholamine overload, eventually leading to severe cardiovascular disorders and death [14]. It is estimated that 10–20% of all pheochromocytomas and PGLs (collectively termed PPGLs) manifest a malignant behavior, in terms of synchronous or metachronous metastatic spread, generally associated with poor prognosis [15]. Metastatic progression seems less common in head and neck PGLs (HNPGL, $\approx$5%) and pheochromocytomas ($\approx$10%) than in thoraco-abdominal PGLs (15% to 35%) [15–17]. However, despite intensive research, no clinicopathological, molecular, or genetic criteria that unequivocally distinguish PPGLs with metastatic potential have been identified [15–18]. Therefore, to overcome diagnostic problems, the WHO Endocrine Tumor Classification recently acknowledged metastatic potential to all PPGLs [19,20]. This implies life-long follow-up after surgery for all cases and additional risk stratification according to pathological, clinical, biochemical, and genetic evidence [17,21].

Collectively, PPGLs may provide important insights into the intersection(s) between organogenesis and tumorigenesis, as it is plainly evident that their basically conserved histostructure mimics that shared by their normal tissue counterparts, the extramedullary paraganglia and the adrenal medulla. In fact, as exemplified in Figure 1, PPGL tissue quite invariably consists in nests or ribbons of more or less dysplastic neurosecretory cells, fairly circumscribed and "nursed" by glial cells, with the whole resting on a highly vascular framework composed of dysplastic endothelia and pericytes that may assume frankly angiomatous features [22]. Thus, PPGLs provide a model for "organoid" tumors, i.e., tumors consisting of a tridimensional assemblage of cells of more than one type, arranged to form predictable tissue-like structures mimicking those of the organ of origin.

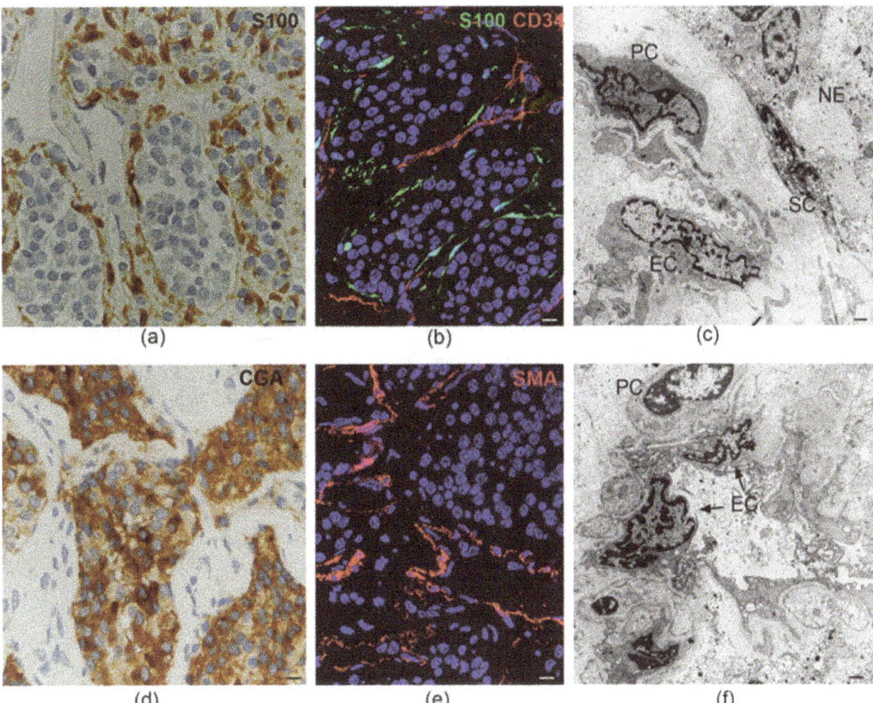

Figure 1. Tissue-like organization in paraganglioma. (**a**) Dark brown immunohistochemical staining for S100, a glial marker, highlights the sustentacular cell component surrounding the alveolar nests ("zellballen") of neuroepithelial ("chief") cells (avidin-biotin immunoperoxidase counterstained with hematoxylin and eosin, bar = 10 µm). (**b**) Immunofluorescence highlights thin sustentacular cells at the edges of neuroepithelial "zellballen," identified by labeling with antibody to S100 (green). The endothelial lining of the capillaries in the surrounding stroma is labeled in red with CD34 (double immunofluorescence on semithin frozen section, bar = 10 µm). (**c**) Transmission electron micrograph showing the cytological features and topological relationships of the four main cell types that organize the paraganglioma microenvironment (endothelial cells, EC; pericytes, PC; sustentacular cells, SC; neuroepithelial cells, NE). Note the nuclear pleomorphism and similarities between chromatin patterns (bar = 2 µm). (**d**) Dark brown cytoplasmic staining for chromogranin A (CGA), a marker for neuroendocrine neoplasia, highlights neuroepithelial cell nests ("zellballen") (avidin-biotin immunoperoxidase counterstained with hematoxylin and eosin, bar = 10 µm). (**e**) Immunofluorescence highlights the pericytic/mural cell component of the paraganglioma vasculature, identified by red labeling with antibody to smooth muscle actin (SMA, immunofluorescence on semithin frozen section, bar = 10 µm). (**f**) Ultrastructural cross section of a paraganglioma capillary showing the atypical cytological features of endothelial cells (EC) and pericytes (PC), two cell types whose roles in paragangliar tumorigenesis have been thus far scarcely considered (bar = 2 µm).

Intriguingly, PPGLs are among the tumors most frequently associated with autosomal dominant genetic predisposition, found in up to ≈40% of the cases [23–25]. The genes most commonly involved are those encoding the four subunits of the succinate dehydrogenase (SDH) enzyme, namely *SDHA*, *SDHB*, *SDHC*, and *SDHD*, and the SDH assembly co-factor, i.e., *SDHAF2*. Furthermore, PPGLs have been associated with germline mutations in other genes, including *RET*, *NF1*, *VHL*, *EPAS1*, *FH*, *MDH2*, *EGLN1/2*, *TMEM127*, and *MAX*, some of which are linked to hereditary neoplastic syndromes including other neural crest tumors, such as multiple endocrine neoplasia (*RET*), von-Hippel-Lindau syndrome (*VHL*), neurofibromatosis type 1 (*NF1*), and Carney–Stratakis syndrome (*SDH* genes) [23–25]. Notably, a maternal parent-of-origin effect, interpreted as evidence for "imprinting," is implicated in the transmission of *SDHD*, *SDHAF2*, and *MAX* mutations [26]. Regardless of this effect, which may result in generation skipping, the penetrance of the mutations in the *SDH* genes that are most commonly associated with PPGL is surprisingly low; in fact, it has been reliably estimated at only 1.7% for *SDHA*, 22.0% for *SDHB*, and 8.3% for *SDHC* [27]. Furthermore, mice mutated in *sdhb*, the human *SDHB* homolog, do not develop any type of cancer [28]. All this suggests that germline *SDH* mutations predispose to PPGL, but are not sufficient for tumorigenesis. The environmental and/or constitutional factors that might modulate hereditary PPGL risk and contribute to PPGL, even in the absence of genetic predisposition, are currently unknown, with the exception, for carotid body PGL, of exposure to chronic hypoxia, such as in people living at high altitudes or in patients affected with chronic obstructive pulmonary disease or cyanotic heart defects [29–32].

Importantly, the most relevant genes implicated in PPGL predisposition, namely the *SDH* genes and *VHL*, as well as *EPAS1*, *FH*, *MDH2*, and *EGLN1/2*, link PPGL tumorigenesis to pseudohypoxia, a cellular phenotype characterized by the constitutive expression of proteins involved in the adaptive responses to low partial pressures of oxygen [23–25]. Among other pleiotropic effects on metabolism, the EMT, vasculoangiogenesis, etc., pseudohypoxia deregulates growth factor signaling and attenuates cell death, promoting the expansion of immature cell populations [33]. The same processes, induced to various extents by chronic environmental hypoxia, are implicated in the adaptive growth of the carotid body, the paraganglion at the basis of the homeostatic oxygen-sensing system. Notably, the carotid body is the most frequent site of origin of head and neck PGL (HNPGL) [34].

2. The Physiological Model of Carotid Body Hyperplasia Under Chronic Hypoxia May Illuminate Paraganglioma Development

Carotid body development has been recently delineated in a notable series of elegant studies from Ricardo Pardal's group [35–37]. The carotid body is implicated in the organismal adaptation to chronic hypoxia, as in people living at high altitudes or in patients with cardiorespiratory diseases, in which cases, this organelle sustains marked hyperplasia and hypertrophy, reflecting the combined expansion of the neural and vascular tissue components, as in PGL. Pardal's lab has clearly shown that this adaptive process is made possible via hypoxia inducible factor (HIF)-dependent reactivation of neural crest-derived resident stem-like cells retaining mesectodermal differentiation potential [36,37]. Such cells, overlooked because of lack of distinctive markers, remain quiescent under normoxia, but, under low partial pressure of oxygen, acquire a nestin+/GFAP- stem/progenitor cell phenotype and convert not only into new sustentacular and neuroepithelial cells, but also into endothelial and pericytic/mural cells, thus contributing to the impressive vasculoangiogenesis that sustains the hyperplastic carotid body. This capability of vasculo/neural transdifferentiation is consistent with the fact that both the neural ganglia of the autonomic nervous system and the cardiovascular structures of the upper trunk originate from the cephalic neural crest during embryogenesis [36]. Furthermore, it has been shown that stem-like neural cells can convert into vascular cells in vitro, and that neoplastic stem-like cells from neural tumors, such as glioblastoma, can give rise to tumor-derived endothelia in immunodeficient mice. This process, defined as vasculogenic mimicry, rather than being aberrant, might reflect the conservation of a physiological developmental potential, which is probably useful for tissue repair/regeneration [2,37–39].

Despite functional differences and the fact that they originate from distinct axial levels of the neural crest, the carotid body and the adrenal medulla are very much alike in tissue structure and cell types, and this similarity is maintained in the derived tumors. Furthermore, as demonstrated in several mammals, including humans, the adrenal medulla is also hypoxia-sensitive, particularly in the neonatal period of life [40]. All this suggests that the developmental and genetic pathways responsible for the growth and homeostasis of the carotid body and of the adrenal medulla could be very similar. In support of this hypothesis, studies based on genetic cell fate tracing and on genetic ablation of Schwann cell precursors in avian and mammalian models revealed that the adrenal medulla originates from neural crest-derived multipotent precursors with a glial phenotype ("Schwann cell precursors"), that migrate along the developing sympathetic nerve to the adrenal area to differentiate into postsynaptic neuroendocrine chromaffin cells [41,42]. Surprisingly, the conclusions of these publications, highly relevant to our understanding of PGL and pheochromocytoma, have yet to be incorporated into the mainstream pathological and molecular interpretation of PPGL tumorigenesis.

In fact, it is currently assumed that the phenotypic plasticity of PPGL cells is circumscribed within the neuroepithelial lineage, a theory backed by the neuroepithelial-specific loss of SDHB protein in the *SDH*-related PPGLs, which conforms to the widely accepted two-hit hypothesis of tumor suppressor genes [43–46]. This would imply that a uniquely neoplastic neuroepithelial cell population drives PPGL growth stimulating angiogenesis and gliogenesis from adjacent normal blood vessels and nerves. Thus, the vascular (endothelial and pericytic) and the glial (sustentacular) PPGL components are relegated to ancillary roles. Such a view is incongruent with the hypothesis that PPGL tumorigenesis could aberrantly recapitulate the histogenesis of the carotid body and of the adrenal medulla [47,48]. Thus, the origin(s) and the nature of PPGL remain undefined and controversial.

3. Molecular Heterogeneities Do Not Exclude a Developmental Model of Paragangliar Tumorigenesis

PPGLs have been linked to germline and/or somatic mutations in more than 20 genes considered tumor-initiators and/or -drivers [23–25]. PPGL tissues bear the distinguishable molecular signatures of these gene mutations, and, on such a basis, can be subdivided into at least three major molecular clusters [49]. The first and largest cluster, identified by pseudohypoxic signaling, is related to loss-of-function mutations that stabilize HIFA, either indirectly, via metabolic inhibition of the α-ketoglutarate-dependent dioxygenases, as in the case of mutations in the Krebs cycle genes encoding the SDH enzyme subunits (*SDHA/B/C/D*), the SDH assembly factor (*SDHAF2*), fumarate hydratase (*FH*) and malate dehydrogenase 2 (*MDH2*); or directly, via disruption of HIFA proteasomal targeting, as in the case of *VHL* and of the genes encoding the prolyl hydroxylases 1 and 2 (*EGLN1/2*). Additionally, gain-of-function mutations in *EPAS1*, encoding HIF2A, contribute to this cluster. Functionally, the pseudohypoxic cluster is characterized by steady HIFA signaling, even under normoxia, and by a cascade of downstream effects, including a metabolic shift towards glycolysis, impaired oxidative phosphorylation, production of reactive oxygen species, DNA and histone hypermethylation, inhibition of collagen maturation and activation of the EMT, which is the widely recognized driver of the migratory mesenchymal-like cell phenotype and of vasculoangiogenesis [50].

With the exception of the *VHL*-related PPGLs, frequently located in the adrenals, the pseudohypoxic cluster encompasses mainly noradrenergic extra-adrenal PGLs and is clinically important because it includes the *SDHB/FH*-related PGLs associated with higher metastatic potential and higher risk of disease multiplicity/recurrence [51]. The second cluster, designated the kinase signaling cluster, bears the molecular signature of aberrant PI3K/AKT and RAS/MAPK activation. Tumors in this cluster are mainly pheochromocytomas and have mutations in various genes involved in protein kinase signaling networks, including *NF1*, *KIF1B*, *MAX*, *RET*, *TMEM127*, *H-RAS*, *ATRX*, and, more rarely, *K-RAS* and *FGFR* [52]. PPGL-associated fusion genes involving *NGFR*, *BRAF*, or *NF1* also contribute to this group. Although lacking the central pseudohypoxic footprint, the kinase signaling cluster relies on a glycolytic and glutaminolytic switch, necessary for cell proliferation and survival, as well as for chromatin remodeling. Clinically, the PPGLs in this cluster do not display a particularly aggressive behavior, except those associated with *ATRX* mutations [52]. Finally, the third cluster, also mainly adrenal, designated the Wnt signaling cluster, is associated with mutations in the cold shock domain containing E1 (*CSDE1*) gene and with fusion genes involving the mastermind-like transcriptional coactivator 3 (*MAML3*). The PPGLs in this cluster tend to be hypomethylated and overexpress genes of the Wnt and Hedgehog pathways, known to play key roles in development [25]. Thus, the genomic landscape of PPGLs demonstrates clinically-relevant heterogeneity, but it is not granted that the distinctive molecular phenotypes entail substantial divergence in fundamental processes responsible for PPGL tissue development and growth. In fact, the molecular pathways defining the three major PPGL clusters are interrelated and participate in developmental processes [53–55]. Indeed, the relative uniformity of the organoid tissue organization of PPGLs suggests that different mutational backgrounds and molecular phenotypes converge on encouraging the aberrant activation of a single, pre-determined morphogenetic program that most likely retraces the developmental footsteps of paragangliar hyperplasia, as in the physiological model of the carotid body [37,56]. Furthermore, molecular phenotypes reflect microenvironmental interactions, which in complex tissues that contain cells of more than one type, like PPGLs, are likely modulated by the composition of the resident cell populations [57,58]. In this regard, PPGLs remain essentially faithful to their characteristic vasculo-neural architecture, but the extent to which the various vascular and neural cell types are represented in individual tumors, and their levels of differentiation, are variable [22,56]. Thus, the PPGL molecular clusters might reflect microenvironmental footprints, rather than differences in fundamental biological programs.

4. Ultrastructural and Immunomorphological Relationships Between the Vascular and Neural Compartments of Head and Neck Paragangliomas

In the past decade, we have tried to understand the relationships between the diverse PPGL cell types and to devise ways to capture the processes underlying PPGL development. Based on the characteristics of our patients, recruited at a skull base surgery center, we focused on HNPGLs, which mostly arise at the carotid bifurcation, in or around the jugular bulb, in the cervical tract of the vagus, or within the temporal bone. HNPGLs cause important morbidity and, when inoperable, are inevitably lethal [59].

We proceeded through sequential steps including: (1) analysis of the ultrastructural and immunomorphological relationships between the various resident HNPGL cell types; (2) identification of genes and molecular pathways common to HNPGLs; (3) localization of relevant protein products at the cellular and subcellular levels; (4) development and characterization of in vitro and in vivo models of HNPGL; and (5) use of such models, in conjunction with information derived from the preceding steps, to investigate HNPGL tissue development and evaluate the potential of specifically-targeted therapy [22,56]. None of the HNPGL cases recruited in our studies revealed evidence of metastasis, therefore our focus is on the reconstruction of the fundamental natural history of the disease, and not on factors linked to metastatic potential.

Using standard immunohistochemistry, classical electron microscopy (EM), and frozen section immunofluorescence (Figure 1), we confirmed that the endothelial, pericytic, glial, and neuroepithelial PGL cell types were clearly discriminated by specific markers (e.g., CD34, CD31, β2-microglobulin for endothelial cells; smooth muscle actin, S100, and GFAP for sustentacular cells; and chromogranin A and β3-tubulin for neuroepithelial cells). However, we also found that these allegedly distinct HNPGL cells coexpressed, to variable extents, markers associated with pluripotent mesenchymal stem-like state, vasculo/neurogenesis, and hypoxia (e.g., vimentin, nestin, CD44/HCAM, KIT/CD117, HIF2A, GLUT4, ZEB1, NOTCH1, DLK1, PDGFRA, VEGFR1/2) [22,56]. This was in agreement with flow cytometry, which highlighted within freshly-dissociated HNPGLs cell populations positive for stem-like mesenchymal cell markers (e.g., CD44/HCAM, CD73, CD90, CD105, and CD133). Further, the cells sorted for CD34 included subsets positive for stem (CD133, CD44/HCAM), neural (NCAM), or glial (GFAP) cell markers, suggesting pluripotency. A pluripotent potential was also consistent with the strong positivity of the endothelia for CD34, a sialomucin also expressed in mesenchymal progenitors and in gastrointestinal stromal tumors (GISTs), which co-occur with PGL in some *SDH*-related PGL syndromes [46,60], and for β2-microglobulin, a major histocompatibility complex

(MHC) class I component associated with infection, the EMT, and cancer [61]. Furthermore, EM, that we extensively utilized, revealed aberrant features in the contiguous vascular (endothelial/pericytic) and neural (glial/neuroepithelial) HNPGL compartments [56], and highlighted widespread contacts between the pervasive dendritic processes of the sustentacular cells and the plasma membranes of the neuroepithelial cells, suggesting contact-mediated sustentacular nurturing [22]. Most notably, at the ultrastructural level, the HNPGL cell types demonstrated a gradient in mitochondrial alterations, limited to occasional swelling of the cristae in the endothelial, pericytic, and sustentacular cells, but striking in the neuroepithelial cells, where the mitochondria were massively increased in number, extremely swollen, and presented convoluted or disrupted cristae [56]. Additionally, the mitochondria tended to form tight perinuclear clustering, a subcellular redistribution connected to an oxidant-rich nuclear microenvironment that promotes hypoxia-induced transcription [62]. These aberrant mitochondria appeared to be incompatible with normal respiration. In fact, the mitochondrial membrane potential ($\Delta\Psi m$) collapsed in the neuroepithelial PGL component relative to autologous normal adipose tissue, while the $\Delta\Psi m$ was only slightly decreased in the vascular component. This lineage-related pattern of mitochondrial alterations was found in all the HNPGLs analyzed, both mutated and unmutated in the *SDH* genes. However, larger mitochondria were significantly associated with the HNPGLs from *SDHB/C/D* gene mutation carriers [56].

5. Our Approach to the Study of Genes and Pathways Shared Among Head and Neck Paragangliomas

Back in 2013, we used high-density genome-wide copy number variation (CNV) analysis to identify HNPGL-related genes and pathways [22]. This analysis, then conducted on a pilot series of 24 tumors, including *SDH*-related and unrelated cases, versus matched blood, revealed in all cases a high level of chromosomal instability. A group of 104 genes, then mostly new to PPGL, was significantly over-represented among those affected by CNVs. We confirmed with orthogonal assays some of the most frequently amplified hits, including *IDUA* (4p16.3), *NOTCH1* (9q34.3), *JAG2* (14q32), *HES5* (1p36.32), *DVL1* (1p36), and *CTBP1* (4p16) [22]. Interestingly, *IDUA*, whose loss-of-function mutations are linked to type 1 mucopolysaccharidosis, a lysosomal storage disease (LSD) [63], showed the highest concordance for CN gains ($p = 0.000002$ by Fisher's exact test). Notably, the HNPGL-derived *IDUA* gene sequences did not show mutations. By frozen section immunofluorescence, alpha-L-iduronidase, the *IDUA*-encoded enzyme, was strongly expressed in the neuroepithelial component of all tested PGLs, including cases not amplified at the *IDUA* locus (Figure 2) [22]. Alpha-L-iduronidase is necessary for the lysosomal hydrolysis of iduronic acid-containing glycosaminoglycans, such as dermatan sulfate and heparan sulfate, important microenvironmental cofactors of cell behavior in development and cancer, that act as receptors for viruses, exosomes, lipoproteins, and growth factors and control Fibroblast Growth Factor (FGF) and Sonic Hedgehog signaling [64–66]. While the above reported functions may be relevant to tumorigenesis, the link between *IDUA* and PGL can be better understood considering that mucopolysaccharidosis type 1 is associated with the accumulation of morpho-functionally altered mitochondria in neural cells, an alteration ascribed to impaired mitophagy due to alpha-L-iduronidase deficiency [67]. In fact, in carriers of loss-of-function *IDUA* mutations, mitochondrial clearance is compromised, leading to the intraneuronal accumulation of pathological mitochondria, characterized by low $\Delta\Psi m$ and swelling, loss of cristae, and vacuolation [67]. Contrariwise, in HNPGLs, alpha-L-iduronidase expression is high and the IDUA gene is unmutated [22], which suggests that the accumulation of dysfunctional mitochondria is due to primary factors and not to deficient clearance [56]. Indeed, high alpha-L-iduronidase expression might reflect upregulation of the mitophagic machinery, in response to the large and dysfunctional mitochondrial pool [68], a hypothesis supported by the frequent ultrastructural evidence of mitophagy in HNPGL neuroepithelial cells and by positivity of the mitochondria for LC3 and sequestosome (Figure 2).

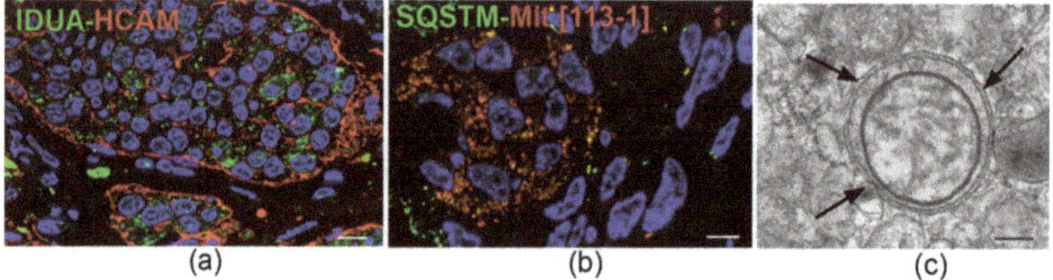

Figure 2. IDUA protein immunostaining and mitophagy in head and neck paraganglioma. (**a**) Immunofluorescence detects cytoplasmic IDUA protein labeling (green) in the neuroepithelial zellballen of paraganglioma. The zellballen are outlined in red by mainly peripheral labeling with antibody to HCAM/CD44, a surface stem cell marker that functions as a receptor for hyaluronan, a glycosaminoglycan degraded by the IDUA product (double immunofluorescence on semithin frozen section, bar = 10 μm). (**b**) Immunofluorescence highlights spots of colocalization (yellow) between anti-p62 antibody (Sequestosome-1, SQSTM, green) and anti-mitochondrial antibody 113-1 (ABCAM, red) (double immunofluorescence on semithin frozen section, bar = 10 μm). (**c**) Ultrastructural cross section of an autophagosome (indicated by arrows) containing a swollen mitochondrion, detected in the cytoplasm of a neuroepithelial paraganglioma cell (transmission electron micrograph, bar = 1 μm).

6. Constitutive Notch Signaling in Head and Neck Paraganglioma

Bioinformatics analyses of tumor-derived gene databases are inherently biased toward better known pathways, which may divert attention from novelty. Nonetheless, it was notable that in our 2013 genome-wide CNV analysis of HNPGLs, "Notch signaling" stood out as the pathway with the highest statistical significance [22]. This pathway controls stem cell maintenance and binary cell fate specification in the vascular and parenchymal compartments, and directly affects nuclear and mitochondrial functions [69–71].

The statistical emergence of Notch signaling rested on five Notch signaling-related genes targeted by recurrent amplifications [22]. These included *NOTCH1*, prototype of the NOTCH receptor family, *JAG2*, a NOTCH ligand linked to vasculogenesis and the EMT, *HES5*, a NOTCH1-activated transcriptional repressor involved in neural stem cells induction [72,73], *DVL1*, hub of the interactions between Notch and Wnt signaling [74], and *CTBP1*, a transcription regulator sensitive to the reduced form of nicotinamide-adenine dinucleotide (NADH), that in melanoma cells links NOTCH signaling to the drop of the intracellular NAD+:NADH ratio caused by aerobic glycolysis [75,76]. NOTCH1 signaling is mediated by the NOTCH1 intracellular domain (NICD1), released by proteolysis of transmembrane NOTCH1 after ligand-induced activation, which relocates to the mitochondria and to the nucleus. In the mitochondria NICD1 inhibits BAX and deregulates complex I, an effect that could contribute to explain the deregulation of complex I activity reported in the *SDH*-mutated PGLs [77,78]. In the nucleus, NICD1 forms a transcriptional regulatory complex with Suppressor of Hairless and Mastermind, which prevents the expression of cell differentiation factors and mediates the HIFA-induced metabolic changes resulting in the Warburg effect [79,80]. Importantly, NOTCH and HIFA signaling are linked in a positive loop: hypoxia promotes NOTCH activation, and NOTCH signaling upregulates HIF2A, the driver of the pseudo-hypoxic phenotype [81]. As investigated using immunohistochemistry, immunofluorescence, and cryo-immuno-EM (Figure 3), the protein products of the top-amplified NOTCH1-related genes were highly expressed in all the PGLs analyzed, independently of CNV status at the respective loci and of presence or absence of germline *SDHx* mutations [22]. However, for some of these proteins, the levels and the subcellular localizations of the immunostaining varied with cell type. JAG2 was mainly expressed in the sustentacular cells, including their dendritic processes, which establish multiple contacts with the neuroepithelial cells [22]. Membrane NOTCH1 was strongest in the endothelial and sustentacular cells, while mitochondrial and nuclear NOTCH1 was more conspicuous in the neuroepithelial component, where the mitochondria are severely altered and contiguous to the nuclear envelope (Figure 3), suggesting a mitochondrial role in the nuclear delivery of NICD1 [22,56].

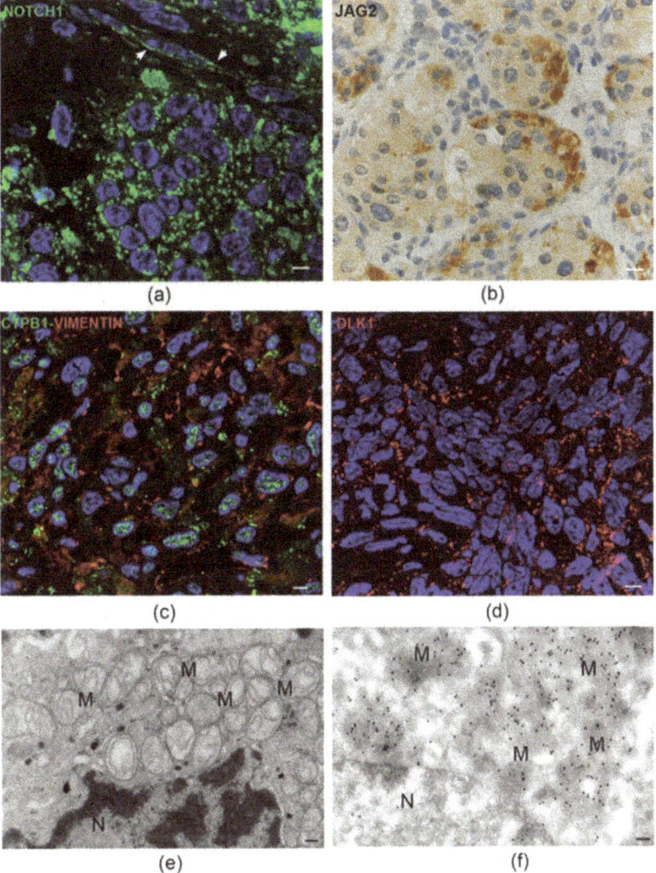

Figure 3. Notch pathway proteins in head and neck paraganglioma. (**a**) Semithin paraganglioma frozen section stained using immunofluorescence with an antibody that recognizes both membrane NOTCH1 and its active intracellular domain, NICD1 (green). In neuroepithelial cells, labeling is mainly concentrated in discrete cytoplasmic spots, suggesting mitochondrial localizations of NICD1. The adjacent endothelia (arrowheads) mainly reveal cell membrane NOTCH1 labeling (bar = 10 μm). (**b**) Immunohistochemical staining for the NOTCH ligand JAG2 is intense at the periphery of the neuroepithelial cell clusters, a typical location of the sustentacular cells (standard avidin-biotin immunoperoxidase counterstained with hematoxylin and eosin, bar = 10 μm). (**c**) Double immunofluorescence on semithin paraganglioma frozen section highlights punctate CTBP1 nuclear labeling in most cells. Red labeling identifies cells staining positive for vimentin, a mesenchymal marker (double immunofluorescence on semithin frozen section, bar = 10 μm). (**d**) Punctate membrane staining pattern (red) of the atypical NOTCH ligand DLK1 in paraganglioma cells (immunofluorescence on semithin frozen section, bar = 10 μm). (**e**) Electron micrograph of a neuroepithelial ("chief") paraganglioma cell showing the accumulation of swollen mitochondria with disrupted cristae (M) next to the envelope of the nucleus (N) (bar = 1 μm). (**f**) Immunoelectron microscopic view of a similar ultrastructural field, showing dense NICD1 labeling of the perinuclear mitochondria with gold particles (ultrathin frozen section immunoelectronmicroscopy, bar = 1 μm).

The strong association of the NOTCH signaling pathway with HNPGLs may not simply reflect a pathological condition. In fact, we recently performed a limited immunohistochemical study on scarce paraffin-embedded sections of a warm autopsy-derived normal human carotid body, which revealed NOTCH1 immunostaining of the vascular and neural tissue components, less intense but similar to that observed in the HNPGLs (Figure 4), hinting to a physiological role of NOTCH1 signaling in paraganglia. In this respect, it is intriguing that complex I deregulation is necessary for normal carotid body function [82]. All this may exemplify the repurposing of developmental and morphogenetic pathways in HNPGL tumorigenesis.

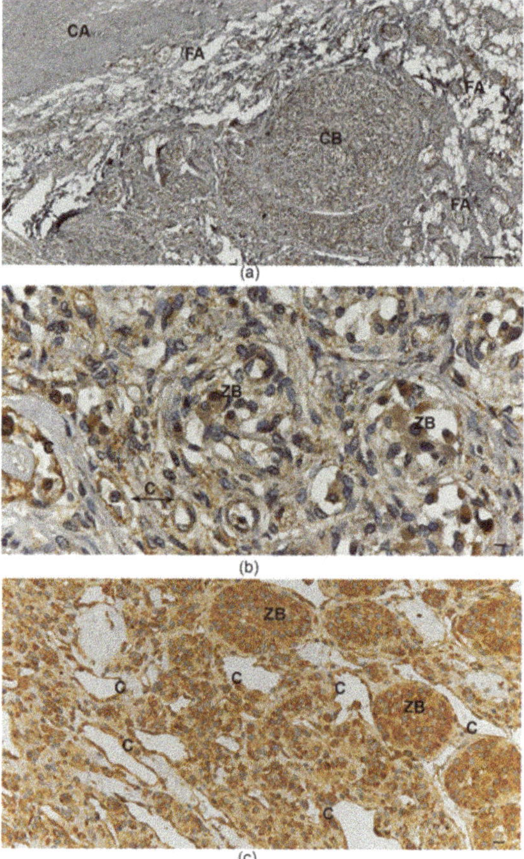

Figure 4. NOTCH1 protein immunostaining in normal carotid body and in carotid body paraganglioma. (**a**) Low-power view of the fibroadipose tissue located at the carotid bifurcation, which contains paragangliar tissue immunostained (brown) with NOTCH1 antibody (avidin-biotin immunoperoxidase counterstained with hematoxylin and eosin, CA: carotid artery; FA: fibroadipose tissue; CB: carotid body; bar = 100 µm). (**b**) High-power view of the carotid body tissue immunostained (brown) with NOTCH1 antibody. Both capillary endothelia and neuroepithelial cells within "zellballen" are immunostained (avidin-biotin immunoperoxidase counterstained with hematoxylin and eosin, C: capillaries; ZB: "zellballen"; bar = 20 µm). (**c**) Paraganglioma tissue immunostained (brown) with NOTCH1 antibody. Ectatic capillaries and "zellballen" are immunostained (avidin-biotin immunoperoxidase counterstained with hematoxylin and eosin, C: capillaries; ZB: "zellballen"; bar = 25 µm).

7. Patient-Derived Head and Neck Paraganglioma Cultures Exhibit a Multipotent Mesenchymal-Like Phenotype

The lack of human PPGL-derived cell lines may reflect the difficulty of maintaining neuroepithelial PPGL cells under culture conditions. In fact, these cells are thought to be the unique neoplastic component of the tumor tissue [44–46]. However, a developmental origin of PPGL would rather be consistent with a multipotent stem/progenitor phenotype of PPGL cells in culture. We generated several primary and at least four lentivirus-immortalized HNPGL cell cultures [56]. Both the primary and the immortalized cultures demonstrated quite homogeneous flow cytometric profiles, positive for classic mesenchymal markers (CD73, CD90, CD105), for embryonic and neural stem cell markers (SOX2 and nestin), and for GFAP and PDGFRA. Such characteristics were common to cultures from PGLs with and without constitutional *SDH* gene mutations. Immunofluorescence confirmed expression of the immature mesenchymal, hypoxic, and vascular/neural markers shared by the diverse tissue components of the PGLs of origin (e.g., vimentin, nestin, CD44/HCAM, KIT/CD117, HIF2A, GLUT4, ZEB1, NOTCH1, DLK1, PDGFRA, and VEGFR1/2). In tridimensional foci, randomly formed under standard culture conditions, and in neurospheres, formed under non-adhesive conditions, the outer shell of cells exposed to the medium was vimentin-positive and nestin-negative, while the reverse occurred in the putatively hypoxic inner cell core. In matrigel, which allows tridimensional growth, the cells readily generated pseudovascular networks expressing CD34 together with DLK1 and PDGFRA, known components of the molecular mechanisms involved in vasculogenesis [56]. Notably, both the primary and the immortalized HNPGL cells had normal tubular mitochondria with high $\Delta\Psi m$, implying normal respiratory functions. However, mitochondrial alterations similar to those found in the HNPGLs of origin where observed in cell-derived xenografts (CDXs) formed after subcutaneous transplantation into nude mice [56]. This indicates that the dysfunctional mitochondria observed in the neuroepithelial HNPGL component are not exclusively determined by genetic alterations, but develop under the influence of microenviromental and differentiation-related factors.

8. The microRNA-200s and -34s Modulate NOTCH1, ZEB1, and PDGFRA Levels in Paraganglioma

We addressed the hypothesis that microRNAs (miRNAs) could contribute to the establishment of an immature mesenchymal phenotype in HNPGL. We therefore compared the miRNA profiles of HNPGLs (13 independent tumors) to those of pools of normal Jacobson's nerves (JN), a parasympathetic nerve that is a frequent site of origin of tympanic HNPGL [22]. JN has the unique advantage of being recoverable, as it must be removed during petrosectomy, and has never been used as a reference tissue for HNPGL by other authors. Genome-wide miRNA expression profiling on the Illumina platform, validated using reverse transcription quantitative PCR (RT-qPCR), revealed that 16 miRNAs were significantly downregulated in the HNPGLs, and only three were significantly upregulated [22]. Notably, the miRNAs most significantly downregulated included the miR-200a,b,c, which inhibit the EMT and promote cell differentiation and senescence by targeting the E-cadherin transcriptional repressors *ZEB1* and *ZEB2* [83,84], and the miR-34b, a mediator of TP53 function [85]. Enforcing Mir expression via transfection in the SH-SY5Y neuroblastoma cell model, or via lentiviral infection in our primary or immortalized HNPGL cells, we proved that the miR-200b,c and the miR-34b directly target NOTCH1 and that miR-200a indirectly influences the NOTCH pathway [22]. We also confirmed in the same models that the miR-200a,b/429 cluster strongly reduces both PDGFRA and ZEB1 RNA and protein levels, while the miR-34b,c cluster strongly downregulates PDGFRA, but not ZEB1 [56]. Reintroduction of these miRs in PGL cells was followed by cell death accompanied by upregulation of BAX protein expression, indicating activation of an apoptotic response [22,56]. In conclusion, the loss of miR-200 and miR-34 family members influences the molecular and cellular HNPGL microenvironment by promoting the upregulation of key EMT- and mesenchymal-related genes. This may be of translational relevance: in fact, PDGFRA, together with KIT/CD117, also expressed in HNPGLs [56], are key targets of imatinib, a drug highly effective in the prevention and treatment of GISTs [86,87]. Furthermore, the NOTCH pathway and ZEB1 are major inducers of chemo- and radio-resistance [88].

9. The Lesson of the Xenograft Models

The formation of patient-derived tumor xenografts (PDXs) in immunosuppressed mice is predicted to depend on cells that survive ischemic necrosis during the prolonged avascular phase that follows surgery and lasts until a new vascular network links the PDX to the murine circulation [56]. To investigate the cells that survive in PGL tissue after devascularization, we analyzed ex vivo-cultured PGL samples corresponding in size to those xenografted in mice. Light microscopy and EM showed extensive coagulative necrosis by day 10 post-surgery, but also revealed areas recolonized and remodeled by endogenous smooth muscle actin/vimentin-positive, collagen-producing mesenchymal-like cells showing phagocytic capability, plausibly useful for the recovery of nutrients from necrotic tissue. These cells were similar to those found at an early phase of subcutaneous PDX formation in immunodeficient mice (3 weeks) [56]. We further analyzed the ultrastructural and light microscopic morphology of 90 PDX samples from different HNPGL patients, all implanted subcutaneously into the flanks or neck. The overall take-rate at 4.5–10 months was high (89%) and unrelated to *SDH* mutation carrier status. The PDX tissues, including the vasculature, proved to be of human origin, as demonstrated by mitochondrial DNA analysis and immunoreactivity with antibodies recognizing human, but not mouse, antigens [56]. Permeation with intracardiacally-injected India ink solution demonstrated connections to the murine circulation. Typically, given the transplantation sites, the PDXs infiltrated the cutaneous branches of the dorsal spinal nerves, imitating the perineural growth typical of HNPGL. However, despite the locally aggressive behavior, the PDXs never exceeded ≈6 mm in maximum diameter, a size consistent with the slow growth of HNPGLs in patients [56]. EM and thin section immunofluorescence revealed that PDX tissue organization initiated with a vasculogenic process, schematized in Figure 5, which led to the formation of endothelial tubes [56]. Such tubes originated from the self-assembly of individual endothelial precursors, that first developed intracytoplasmic lumina through cytoplasmic vacuolization (cell hollowing), as in HUVECs and in drosophila and zebrafish embryos [89,90]. The lumenized tubes were positive for human β2-microglobulin, CD31, and CD34, as HNPGL endothelium, and defined a perivascular niche that attracted mesenchymal-like, smooth muscle actin-positive cells [56,91]. The adherence of these cells to the abluminal endothelial cell membranes was associated with dichotomic branching of the endothelial tube, a morphology pointing to intussusceptive angiogenesis, a form of nonsprouting angiogenesis that allows the rapid bifurcation of neoformed vasculature via endothelial invaginations [56,92]. Notably, in this process, membrane NOTCH1 was uniquely present on the abluminal endothelial membrane, in contact with adhering perivascular cells strongly positive for DLK1, a HIF-induced non-canonical NOTCH antagonist known as a cancer pericyte antigen [56,93]. These DLK1-positive cells also coexpressed smooth muscle actin and PDGFRA, assuming the ultrastructural and immunophenotypic characteristics of mural cells or pericytes [56]. The initial vasculo-angiogenic network was supported by autonomously synthesized collagen I, an EMT-related collagen [56,94]. With the formation of structured vessels, supported by mural cells or pericytes, the perivascular matrix was enriched with collagen IV, a key component of basement membranes [56,95]. Such microenvironmental modification was associated with the development of neuroepithelial-like cell clusters, often encircled by glia-like spindle cells (Figure 5).

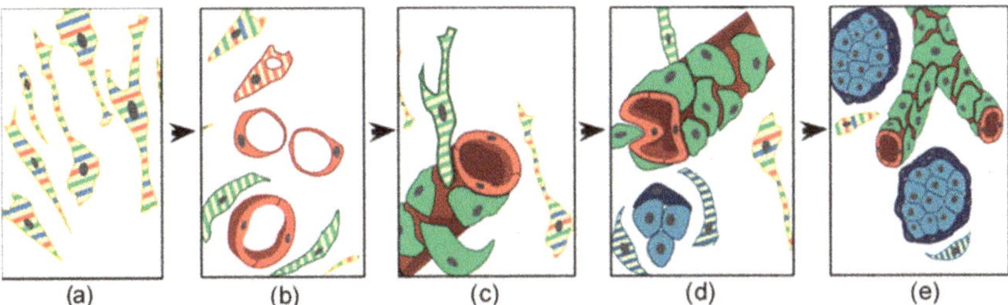

Figure 5. Schematic representation of the histogenesis of head and neck paraganglioma, based on patient- and cell-derived xenograft models. The thin elongated stem-like cells (**a**), stabilized and expanded in paraganglioma cell cultures, co-express (stripes) multipotent stem/progenitor cell markers. In vivo, (**b**) these cells grow on autonomously synthesized extracellular matrix, develop intracytoplasmic vacuoles of increasing size (cells with red stripes only), and coalesce (uniformly red cells), giving rise to endothelial tubes (vasculogenesis via cytoplasmic hollowing). The endothelium then recruits adjacent stem-like cells (cells with green stripes only), which, after contact with the abluminal endothelial membranes (**c**), differentiate into mural cells (uniformly green). (**d**) The panel outlines two remarkable consequences of mural stabilization. First, mural impingement results in intraluminal endothelial intussusceptions, which divide the flow, giving rise to Y-shaped vascular ramifications (intussusceptive angiogenesis, a process detectable only with whole-mount confocal microscopy and/or transmission electron microscopy, as used in our study [56]). Secondly, vascular stabilization results in perivascular deposition of collagen IV [56], which supports the development of cell clusters with neural phenotype (cells with blue stripes only, then uniformly blue). As shown in (**e**), these clusters develop into "zellballen"-like neuroepithelial nests (uniform light blue), bound by spindle-shaped glia-like cells (uniform dark blue). Notably, while mesenchymal paraganglioma stem-like cells have normal mitochondria, paraganglioma tissue organization is associated with increasing mitochondrial dysfunction (swelling and loss of membrane potential), culminating in the neuroepithelial component. Original art by Giulio Pandolfelli, adapted and modified from Verginelli et al., 2018 [56].

These cell nests revealed positivity for the immature mesenchymal, hypoxic, and vasculoneurogenic markers found in the neuropithelial component of PGLs (e.g., vimentin, nestin, CD44/HCAM, KIT/CD117, HIF2A, GLUT4, ZEB1, NOTCH1, DLK1, PDGFRA, and VEGFR1/2), but lacked advanced neuroendocrine markers, such as chromogranin A and synaptophysin. Ultrastructurally, most PDX cells, and particularly those of the neuroepithelial-like nests, exhibited hyperplastic and swollen mitochondria with vesicular or disrupted cristae, as in the neuroepithelial cells of the HNPGLs of origin [56]. Cell-derived xenografts (CDXs) were similarly obtained after subcutaneous injection of an immortalized HNPGL cell line (PTJ64i) into immunodeficient mice. At 45 days from transplantation the cells formed flat red-brown patches of 4–6 mm in diameter that, as the PDXs, comprised a vasculo-angiogenic network supporting nests of neuroepithelial-like cells (Figure 6) [56]. As noted before, the CDX cells developed hyperplastic and swollen mitochondria, resembling those of the neuroepithelial HNPGL component.

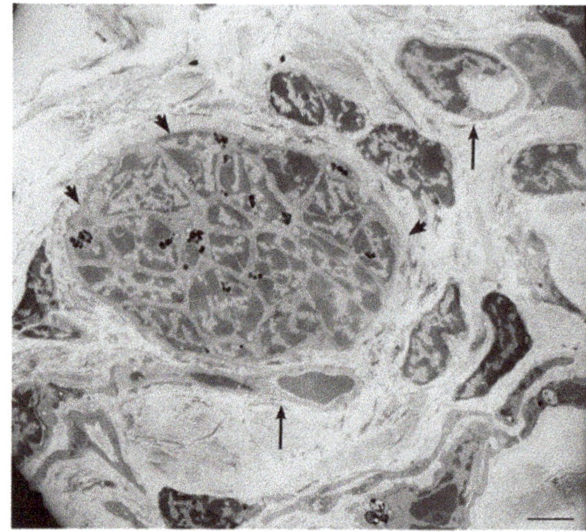

Figure 6. Ultrastructural view of paraganglioma xenograft tissue. The electron micrograph, derived from a xenograft obtained by subcutaneous injection of an immortalized tympano-jugular paraganglioma cell line (PTJ64i), shows a tight neuroepithelial-like cell cluster (arrowheads, dark spots are lipofuscins) in the context of a vasculogenic tissue revealing endothelial-like cells with cytoplasmic hollowing and capillary-like structures (arrows) (bar = 5 μm).

Overall, despite their slow development and small size, our HNPGL xenograft models support the view that HNPGL histogenesis does not depend on neurogenesis and ancillary sprouting angiogenesis, but on primary vasculogenesis of the embryonic type, followed by neurogenesis [56]. This is in agreement with the physiological model of the hyperplastic carotid body [36] and emphasizes the link between HNPGL development and embryogenesis, where vasculogenesis precedes and guides histo/organogenesis, a sequence recapitulated in postnatal tissue regeneration [96,97].

10. Imatinib Blocks HNPGL Cell Growth and Inhibits Xenograft Formation

The evidence that HNPGLs express PDGFRA and KIT/CD117, the receptor tyrosine kinases targeted by imatinib, brought us to test the effects of this drug on our HNPGL models [56]. At low dose (10 μM), imatinib inhibited the growth of four HNPGL cell cultures tested, three primary and one immortalized, that are representative of *SDH*-related and unrelated HNPGLs. Imatinib treatment was followed by global protein dephosphorylation, downregulation of the ZEB1, PDGFRA, and PDGFRB proteins, upregulation of Beclin 1, core component of the autophagy machinery, activation of the caspases 3/7 and induction of BAX. Treatment was also followed by mainly upward variation in the levels of miR-200a/b/c and miR-34b/c, consistent with the observed downregulation of the ZEB1 and PDGFRA proteins. Imatinib also significantly prevented CDX formation in immunodeficient mice. In this case imatinib (50 mg/kg for 20 days, then 16.6 mg/kg for 20 additional days) was given by intra-peritoneal injection, starting at 72 hours from the subcutaneous inoculation of the immortalized HNPGL cell line PTJ64i. Only 2 CDXs were detected at 10 heterotransplant sites in the imatinib-treated group versus 11 at 12 sites in the control group ($p = 0.0015$). Furthermore, the 2 CDXs found in the treated mice contained only disorganized or apoptotic cells with diffuse evidence of autophagic vacuoles [56], suggesting that imbalanced autophagic flux contributed to imatinib-induced growth arrest and apoptosis, as previously demonstrated by other authors in several mammalian cell types [98].

11. Conclusions

This perspective review challenges the prevalent view postulating that PPGLs are exclusively neuroendocrine tumors [44–46]. In fact, we propose that HNPGL arises from mesenchymal stem-like cells with vasculo-neural differentiation potential, in keeping with the neural crest derivation of paraganglia [8,41,42] and with the hyperplastic carotid body model, where the vascular and the neural components arise from resident stem-like cells retaining mesectodermal differentiation potential, reactivated by chronic hypoxia [36]. In support of this, retention of mesenchymal markers is evident in all the distinct HNPGL tissue components. Furthermore, mesenchymal stem-like cells persist in HNPGL tissue, and after damage, might be regenerated via EMT from more differentiated vascular and/or neural cells [56].

HNPGL xenografts can be viewed as attempts to HNPGL regeneration after devascularization. In patients, tumor regeneration after embolization, radiotherapy or chemotherapy could follow in the same footsteps. In essence, our xenograft models, based on tumors related and unrelated to *SDH* gene mutations, show that the vascular and neural HNPGL tissue components sequentially emerge following an endogenous developmental program [56]. Primordial endothelial tubulogenesis seems to be the earliest histogenetic event, as in embryonic development. This process is complemented by angiogenesis, which does not follow the well-known sprouting model, but exploits endothelial intussusception [56], a stochastic intravascular process of dichotomic branching, mediated by largely unexplored paracrine and contact-mediated signals [99,100]. Interestingly, during the development of the early vasculo-angiogenic network, the interaction between endothelial and pericytic/mural cells involves compartmentalized expression of the NOTCH1, PDGFRA, and DLK1 proteins [56,101]. NOTCH1 is localized on the abluminal endothelial membrane, i.e., the original plasma membrane of the mesenchymal-like cell that, by vacuolization, differentiates towards the endothelial lineage (Figure 5), whereas PDGFRA and the atypical NOTCH ligand DLK1 are expressed by the smooth muscle actin-positive periendothelial cells engaged in pericytic/mural differentiation, which physically interact with the NOTCH1-labeled endothelial membranes [56].

The dependence of HNPGL histogenesis on a primordial vasculo-angiogenic phase provides a rationale for targeted preventive and therapeutic interventions, which, however, would require a better understanding of the molecular mechanisms underlying endothelial tubulogenesis and intussusceptive angiogenesis. Nonetheless, imatinib, which targets the recruitment of PDGFRA-positive mural/pericytic cells necessary for the stabilization of endothelial tubes [87,91], strongly prevented CDX formation in our murine model. Given that tumor maintenance and tumor development are distinct phenomena [102], this may not be translated into the conclusion that imatinib could effectively target structured HNPGL tissue in patients, but raises the intriguing possibility of whether this drug could be given in a preventive setting after surgery, embolization, or radiotherapy in order to reduce the risk of HNPGL regeneration. This important question remains to be addressed with appropriate study designs. Interestingly, vasculo-angiogenesis, as well as the EMT, are predicted to be negatively controlled by the miR-200a,b,c and by the miR-34b [103,104], which were significantly downregulated in our HNPGLs relative to our normal parasympathetic neural control, JN [22]. *ZEB1*, *NOTCH1*, and *PDGFRA* are coordinately targeted by these miRs, thus the high levels of the relative protein products in our HNPGLs can be at least partly explained by the loss of miRNA-mediated regulation [22,56]. Additionally, the significant amplification of NOTCH pathway genes, demonstrated by us for *NOTCH1*, *JAG2*, *HES5*, *DVL1*, and *CTBP1*, must concur with the constitutive upregulation of NOTCH1 signaling in HNPGLs. This might contribute to link cell fate decisions to metabolism via the coordinated transcriptional effects exerted by NICD1, at the mitochondrial and nuclear levels, and by nuclear CTBP1, a sensor of the NAD+/NADH ratio. NOTCH1 signaling is likely fundamental not only for the development, but also for the homeostasis of HNPGL. In fact, neuroepithelial dependence on NOTCH1 signaling via JAG2, delivered by sustentacular cells, may account for the extensive interactions between dendritic sustentacular processes and neuroepithelial cells, where BAX inhibition and complex I deregulation, contributed by NICD1, might help to sustain dysfunctional mitochondria.

Furthermore, in connection with the upregulation of ZEB1 and the EMT, NOTCH signaling is predicted to promote resistance to chemo/radiotherapy and to antiangiogenic agents, which are major problems in PPGL therapy [105–109].

Widespread mitochondrial alterations, that correlate with neuroepithelial differentiation and loss of ΔΨm, implying glycolytic dependence, are a key ultrastructural feature basically common to HNPGLs, again independently of their genetic backgrounds [56]. Such alterations, not present in our cultured mesenchymal-like HNPGL cells, are acquired after in vivo transplantation, which links these mitochondrial changes to microenvironment-related factors. In this regard, the role of complex I deregulation is probably central, but is still debated. In fact, several studies reported loss of complex I activity in PPGLs and in *SDHB*-mutated cell models [77,110,111], whereas Pang and coworkers recently found an upregulation of complex I, accompanied by a strengthened NAD+ metabolism, in *SDHB*-mutated PPGLs [78]. The latter finding suggests that complex I could compensate for the primary loss of complex II activity characteristic of *SDH*-mutated PPGLs, an effect of potential relevance in the clinical setting, as it could account for differential sensitivities to chemotherapeutic agents [78]. The question is clearly open, and in our opinion, could be addressed taking into account the microenvironmental contexts. In fact, viewing each neuroepithelial PPGL cell and each PPGL tissue as an ecosystem, it could be hypothesized that complex I activity is balanced in the mitochondrial populations to meet specific metabolic needs that contribute to the homeostasis of stressed neuroepithelial cells in the variable tumor microenvironment. This is an area that is currently addressed in our laboratories in Chieti and Stockholm.

To sum up, we challenge the view of PGL as the prototype of "Warburg tumors" [43]. In this perspective, PGL cells would be constrained into a pre-defined role conforming to "classic" two-hit or multiple-hit, gene-centered paradigms, where random genetic and epigenetic changes, driven by "selective pressures," result in the emergence of heterogeneous and uncoordinated clonal tumor subpopulations. Instead, we believe that, regardless of genetic heterogeneities, HNPGL tumorigenesis essentially adheres to a finalized and pre-defined histogenetic program, most likely retracing the footsteps of carotid body histogenesis [10,35,36]. Our findings likely bear on the development of PPGLs in general and could open up to a new understanding of the disease.

Author Contributions: S.V., M.R.P., S.P., D.L.E., F.V., R.V., A.V. and C.T.P. generated and critically interpreted the original articles upon which this review is based; L.V.L. and S.V. prepared the original figures; M.S. and C.S.N. contributed with their ideas to the drafting and revision of the article; L.V.L. and R.M.-C. wrote the manuscript.

Funding: This research was funded by the Associazione Italiana per la Ricerca sul Cancro (AIRC), grant number IG16932 (2015–2019).

Acknowledgments: We acknowledge the services provided by the Mario Sanna Foundation Onlus, Piacenza, Italy (http://www.gruppootologico.com/en/institutional/mario-sanna-foundation), dedicated to the prevention and treatment of skull base tumors. We thank Ms. Anna Nassani, Dipartimento di Oncologia-Ematologia, Servizio di Anatomia Patologica, Ospedale Guglielmo da Saliceto, Piacenza, Italy, and the staff of the Unità di Chirurgia della Base Cranica, Gruppo Otologico Piacenza-Roma, Italy, for their continuous expert and kind assistance.

Conflicts of Interest: The authors declare no conflict of interest.

References

1. Kho, A.T.; Zhao, Q.; Cai, Z.; Butte, A.J.; Kim, J.Y.; Pomeroy, S.L.; Rowitch, D.H.; Kohane, I.S. Conserved mechanisms across development and tumorigenesis revealed by a mouse development perspective of human cancers. *Genes Dev.* **2004**, *18*, 629–640. [CrossRef] [PubMed]
2. Krishna Priya, S.; Nagare, R.P.; Sneha, V.S.; Sidhanth, C.; Bindhya, S.; Manasa, P.; Ganesan, T.S. Tumour angiogenesis-Origin of blood vessels. *Int. J. Cancer* **2016**, *139*, 729–735. [CrossRef] [PubMed]
3. Beachy, P.A.; Karhadkar, S.S.; Berman, D.M. Tissue repair and stem cell renewal in carcinogenesis. *Nature* **2004**, *432*, 324–331. [CrossRef] [PubMed]
4. Levin, M. Morphogenetic fields in embryogenesis, regeneration, and cancer: Non-local control of complex patterning. *Biosystems* **2012**, *109*, 243–261. [CrossRef] [PubMed]

5. Simon, M.C.; Keith, B. The role of oxygen availability in embryonic development and stem cell function. *Nat. Rev. Mol. Cell Biol.* **2008**, *9*, 285–296. [CrossRef] [PubMed]
6. Egeblad, M.; Nakasone, E.S.; Werb, Z. Tumors as organs: Complex tissues that interface with the entire organism. *Dev. Cell* **2010**, *18*, 884–901. [CrossRef] [PubMed]
7. Maguire, L.H.; Thomas, A.R.; Goldstein, A.M. Tumors of the neural crest: Common themes in development and cancer. *Dev. Dyn.* **2015**, *244*, 311–322. [CrossRef] [PubMed]
8. Dupin, E.; Sommer, L. Neural crest progenitors and stem cells: From early development to adulthood. *Dev. Biol.* **2010**, *366*, 83–95. [CrossRef] [PubMed]
9. Wolsky, A. Regeneration and cancer. *Growth* **1978**, *42*, 425–426. [PubMed]
10. Dvorak, H.F. Tumors: Wounds that do not heal. Similarities between tumor stroma generation and wound healing. *N. Engl. J. Med.* **1986**, *315*, 1650–1659. [PubMed]
11. Bianco, P. "Mesenchymal" stem cells. *Annu. Rev. Cell Dev. Biol.* **2014**, *30*, 677–704. [CrossRef] [PubMed]
12. Sacchetti, B.; Funari, A.; Remoli, C.; Giannicola, G.; Kogler, G.; Liedtke, S.; Cossu, G.; Serafini, M.; Sampaolesi, M.; Tagliafico, E.; et al. No Identical "Mesenchymal Stem Cells" at Different Times and Sites: Human Committed Progenitors of Distinct Origin and Differentiation Potential Are Incorporated as Adventitial Cells in Microvessels. *Stem Cell Rep.* **2016**, *14*, 897–913. [CrossRef] [PubMed]
13. Martucci, V.L.; Pacak, K. Pheochromocytoma and paraganglioma: Diagnosis, genetics, management, and treatment. *Curr. Probl. Cancer* **2014**, *38*, 7–41. [CrossRef] [PubMed]
14. Kantorovich, V.; Eisenhofer, G.; Pacak, K. Pheochromocytoma: An endocrine stress mimicking disorder. *Ann. N. Y. Acad. Sci.* **2008**, *1148*, 462–468. [CrossRef] [PubMed]
15. Harari, A.; Inabnet, W.B., 3rd. Malignant pheochromocytoma: A review. *Am. J. Surg.* **2011**, *201*, 700–708. [CrossRef] [PubMed]
16. Kim, K.Y.; Kim, J.H.; Hong, A.R.; Seong, M.W.; Lee, K.E.; Kim, S.J.; Kim, S.W.; Shin, C.S.; Kim, S.Y. Disentangling of Malignancy from Benign Pheochromocytomas/Paragangliomas. *PLoS ONE* **2016**, *11*, e0168413. [CrossRef] [PubMed]
17. Kimura, N.; Takekoshi, K.; Naruse, M. Risk Stratification on Pheochromocytoma and Paraganglioma from Laboratory and Clinical Medicine. *J. Clin. Med.* **2018**, *7*, 242. [CrossRef] [PubMed]
18. Thompson, L.D.; Young, W.F.; Kawashima, A.; Komminoth, P. Malignant adrenal phaeochromocytoma. In *World Health Organization Classification of Tumours Pathology & Genetics, Tumours of Endocrine Organs*, 3rd ed.; DeLellis, R.A., Lloyd, R.V., Eds.; IARC: Lyon, France, 2004; pp. 147–150.
19. Kimura, N.; Capella, C. Extraadrenal paraganglioma. In *WHO Classification of Tumors of Endocrine Organs*, 4th ed.; Lloyd, R.V., Osamura, R.Y., Kloppel, G., Eds.; IARC Press: Lyons, France, 2017; pp. 190–195.
20. Tischler, A.S.; de Krijger, R.R. Phaeochromocytoma. In *WHO Classification of Tumors of Endocrine Organs*, 4th ed.; Lloyd, R.V., Osamura, R.Y., Kloppel, G., Eds.; IARC Press: Lyons, France, 2017; pp. 183–189.
21. Lenders, J.W.M.; Duh, Q.-Y.; Eisenhofer, G.; Gimenez-Roqueplo, A.-P.; Grebe, S.K.G.; Murad, M.H.; Naruse, M.; Pacak, K.; Young, W.F., Jr. Pheochromocytoma and paraganglioma: An endocrine society clinical practice guideline. *J. Clin. Endocrinol. Metab.* **2014**, *99*, 1915–1942. [CrossRef] [PubMed]
22. Cama, A.; Verginelli, F.; Lotti, L.V.; Napolitano, F.; Morgano, A.; D'Orazio, A.; Vacca, M.; Perconti, S.; Pepe, F.; Romani, F.; et al. Integrative genetic, epigenetic and pathological analysis of paraganglioma reveals complex dysregulation of NOTCH signaling. *Acta Neuropathol.* **2013**, *126*, 575–594. [CrossRef] [PubMed]
23. Favier, J.; Amar, L.; Gimenez-Roqueplo, A.P. Paraganglioma and phaeochromocytoma: From genetics to personalized medicine. *Nat. Rev. Endocrinol.* **2015**, *11*, 101–111. [CrossRef] [PubMed]
24. Zhikrivetskaya, S.O.; Snezhkina, A.V.; Zaretsky, A.R.; Alekseev, B.Y.; Pokrovsky, A.V.; Golovyuk, A.L.; Melnikova, N.V.; Stepanov, O.A.; Kalinin, D.V.; Moskalev, A.A.; et al. Molecular markers of paragangliomas/pheochromocytomas. *Oncotarget* **2017**, *8*, 25756–25782. [CrossRef] [PubMed]
25. Jochmanova, I.; Pacak, K. Genomic Landscape of Pheochromocytoma and Paraganglioma. *Trends Cancer* **2018**, *4*, 6–9. [CrossRef] [PubMed]
26. Bayley, J.-P.; Oldenburg, R.A.; Nuk, J.; Hoekstra, A.S.; van der Meer, C.A.; Korpershoek, E.; McGillivray, B.; Corssmit, E.P.M.; Dinjens, W.N.M.; de Krijger, R.R.; et al. Paraganglioma and pheochromocytoma upon maternal transmission of SDHD mutations. *BMC Med. Genet.* **2014**, *15*, 111. [CrossRef] [PubMed]
27. Benn, D.E.; Zhu, Y.; Andrews, K.A.; Wilding, M.; Duncan, E.L.; Dwight, T.; Tothill, R.W.; Burgess, J.; Crook, A.; Gill, A.J.; et al. Bayesian approach to determining penetrance of pathogenic SDH variants. *J. Med. Genet.* **2018**, *55*, 729–734. [CrossRef] [PubMed]

28. Piruat, J.I.; Millán-Uclés, Á. Genetically Modeled Mice with Mutations in Mitochondrial Metabolic Enzymes for the Study of Cancer. *Front. Oncol.* **2014**, *4*, 200. [CrossRef] [PubMed]
29. Saldana, M.J.; Salem, L.E.; Travezan, R. High altitude hypoxia and chemodectomas. *Hum. Pathol.* **1973**, *4*, 251–263. [CrossRef]
30. Chedid, A.; Jao, W. Hereditary tumors of the carotid bodies and chronic obstructive pulmonary disease. *Cancer* **1974**, *33*, 1635–1641. [CrossRef]
31. Hirsch, J.H.; Killien, F.C.; Troupin, R.H. Bilateral carotid body tumors and cyanotic heart disease. *AJR Am. J. Roentgenol.* **1980**, *134*, 1073–1075. [CrossRef] [PubMed]
32. Cerecer-Gil, N.Y.; Figuera, L.E.; Llamas, F.J.; Lara, M.; Escamilla, J.G.; Ramos, R.; Estrada, G.; Hussain, A.K.; Gaal, J.; Korpershoek, E.; et al. Mutation of SDHB is a Cause of Hypoxia-Related High-Altitude Paraganglioma. *Clin. Cancer Res.* **2010**, *16*, 4148–4154. [CrossRef] [PubMed]
33. Lee, S.; Nakamura, E.; Yang, H.; Wei, W.; Linggi, M.S.; Sajan, M.P.; Farese, R.V.; Freeman, R.S.; Carter, B.D.; Kaelin, W.G., Jr.; et al. Neuronal apoptosis linked to EglN3 prolyl hydroxylase and familial pheochromocytoma genes: Developmental culling and cancer. *Cancer Cell* **2005**, *8*, 155–167. [CrossRef] [PubMed]
34. Wieneke, J.A.; Smith, A. Paraganglioma: Carotid body tumor. *Head Neck Pathol.* **2009**, *3*, 303–306. [CrossRef] [PubMed]
35. Pardal, R.; Ortega-Sáenz, P.; Durán, R.; López-Barneo, J. Glia-like stem cells sustain physiologic neurogenesis in the adult mammalian carotid body. *Cell* **2007**, *131*, 364–377. [CrossRef] [PubMed]
36. Annese, V.; Navarro-Guerrero, E.; Rodríguez-Prieto, I.; Pardal, R. Physiological Plasticity of Neural-Crest-Derived Stem Cells in the Adult Mammalian Carotid Body. *Cell Rep.* **2017**, *19*, 471–478. [CrossRef] [PubMed]
37. Sobrino, V.; Annese, V.; Navarro-Guerrero, E.; Platero-Luengo, A.; Pardal, R. The carotid body: A physiologically relevant germinal niche in the adult peripheral nervous system. *Cell. Mol. Life Sci.* **2018**, 1–13. [CrossRef] [PubMed]
38. Nakagomi, T.; Kubo, S.; Nakano-Doi, A.; Sakuma, R.; Lu, S.; Narita, A.; Kawahara, M.; Taguchi, A.; Matsuyama, T. Brain vascular pericytes following ischemia have multipotential stem cell activity to differentiate into neural and vascular lineage cells. *Stem Cells* **2015**, *33*, 1962–1974. [CrossRef] [PubMed]
39. Farahani, R.M.; Rezaei-Lotfi, S.; Simonian, M.; Xaymardan, M.; Hunter, N. Neural microvascular pericytes contribute to human adult neurogenesis. *J. Comp. Neurol.* **2019**, *527*, 780–796. [CrossRef] [PubMed]
40. Salman, S.; Buttigieg, J.; Nurse, C.A. Ontogeny of O_2 and CO_2//H+ chemosensitivity in adrenal chromaffin cells: Role of innervation. *J. Exp. Biol.* **2014**, *217 Pt 5*, 673–681. [CrossRef]
41. Furlan, A.; Dyachuk, V.; Kastriti, M.E.; Calvo-Enrique, L.; Abdo, H.; Hadjab, S.; Chontorotzea, T.; Akkuratova, N.; Usoskin, D.; Kamenev, D.; et al. Multipotent peripheral glial cells generate neuroendocrine cells of the adrenal medulla. *Science* **2017**, *357*, eaal3753. [CrossRef] [PubMed]
42. Hockman, D.; Adameyko, I.; Kaucka, M.; Barraud, P.; Otani, T.; Hunt, A.; Hartwig, A.C.; Sock, E.; Waithe, D.; Franck, M.C.M.; et al. Striking parallels between carotid body glomus cell and adrenal chromaffin cell development. *Dev. Biol.* **2018**, pii: S0012-1606(17)30905-3. [CrossRef] [PubMed]
43. Bayley, J.P.; Devilee, P. Warburg tumours and the mechanisms of mitochondrial tumour suppressor genes. Barking up the right tree? *Curr. Opin. Genet. Dev.* **2010**, *20*, 324–329. [CrossRef] [PubMed]
44. van Schothorst, E.M.; Beekman, M.; Torremans, P.; Kuipers-Dijkshoorn, N.J.; Wessels, H.W.; Bardoel, A.F.; van der Mey, A.G.; van der Vijver, M.J.; van Ommen, G.J.; Devilee, P.; et al. Paragangliomas of the head and neck region show complete loss of heterozygosity at 11q22-q23 in chief cells and the flowsorted DNA aneuploid fraction. *Hum. Pathol.* **1998**, *29*, 1045–1049. [CrossRef]
45. Douwes Dekker, P.B.; Corver, W.E.; Hogendoorn, P.C.; van der Mey, A.G.; Cornelisse, C.J. Multiparameter DNA flow-sorting demonstrates diploidy and SDHD wild-type gene retention in the sustentacular cell compartment of head and neck paragangliomas: Chief cells are the only neoplastic component. *J. Pathol.* **2004**, *202*, 456–462. [CrossRef] [PubMed]
46. Gill, A.J. Succinate dehydrogenase (SDH)-deficient neoplasia. *Histopathology* **2018**, *72*, 106–116. [CrossRef] [PubMed]
47. Hendrix, M.J.C.; Seftor, E.A.; Hess, A.R.; Seftor, R.E.B. Vasculogenic mimicry and tumour-cell plasticity: Lessons from melanoma. *Nat. Rev. Cancer* **2003**, *3*, 411–421. [CrossRef] [PubMed]

48. Kuratani, S.; Kusakabe, R.; Hirasawa, T. The neural crest and evolution of the head/trunk interface in vertebrates. *Dev. Biol.* **2018**, in press. [CrossRef] [PubMed]
49. Fishbein, L.; Leshchiner, I.; Walter, V.; Danilova, L.; Robertson, A.G.; Johnson, A.R.; Lichtenberg, T.M.; Murray, B.A.; Ghayee, H.K.; Else, T.; et al. Comprehensive Molecular Characterization of Pheochromocytoma and Paraganglioma. *Cancer Cell* **2017**, *31*, 181–193. [CrossRef] [PubMed]
50. Sun, B.; Zhang, D.; Zhao, N.; Zhao, X. Epithelial-to-endothelial transition and cancer stem cells: Two cornerstones of vasculogenic mimicry in malignant tumors. *Oncotarget* **2016**, *8*, 30502–30510. [CrossRef] [PubMed]
51. Turkova, H.; Prodanov, T.; Maly, M.; Martucci, V.; Adams, K.; Widimsky, J., Jr.; Chen, C.C.; Ling, A.; Kebebew, E.; Stratakis, C.A.; et al. Characteristics and outcomes of metastatic SDHB and sporadic pheochromcytoma/paraganglioma: An National Institutes of Halth Study. *Endocr. Pract.* **2016**, *22*, 302–314. [CrossRef] [PubMed]
52. Comino-Méndez, I.; Tejera, Á.M.; Currás-Freixes, M.; Remacha, L.; Gonzalvo, P.; Tonda, R.; Letón, R.; Blasco, M.A.; Robledo, M.; Cascón, A. ATRX driver mutation in a composite malignant pheochromocytoma. *Cancer Genet.* **2016**, *209*, 272–277. [CrossRef] [PubMed]
53. Folmes, C.D.L.; Terzic, A. Metabolic determinants of embryonic development and stem cell fate. *Reprod. Fertil. Dev.* **2014**, *27*, 82–88. [CrossRef] [PubMed]
54. Chisolm, D.A.; Weinmann, A.S. Connections Between Metabolism and Epigenetics in Programming Cellular Differentiation. *Annu. Rev. Immunol.* **2018**, *36*, 221–246. [CrossRef] [PubMed]
55. Janke, R.; Dodson, A.E.; Rine, J. Metabolism and Epigenetics. *Annu. Rev. Cell Dev. Biol.* **2015**, *31*, 473–496. [CrossRef] [PubMed]
56. Verginelli, F.; Perconti, S.; Vespa, S.; Schiavi, F.; Prasad, S.C.; Lanuti, P.; Cama, A.; Tramontana, L.; Esposito, D.L.; Guarnieri, S.; et al. Paragangliomas arise through an autonomous vasculo-angio-neurogenic program inhibited by imatinib. *Acta Neuropathol.* **2018**, *135*, 779–798. [CrossRef] [PubMed]
57. Lyssiotis, C.A.; Kimmelman, A.C. Metabolic Interactions in the Tumor Microenvironment. *Trends Cell Biol.* **2017**, *27*, 863–875. [CrossRef] [PubMed]
58. Lopes-Coelho, F.; Gouveia-Fernandes, S.; Serpa, J. Metabolic cooperation between cancer and non-cancerous stromal cells is pivotal in cancer progression. *Tumour Biol.* **2018**, *40*. [CrossRef] [PubMed]
59. Taïeb, D.; Kaliski, A.; Boedeker, C.C.; Martucci, V.; Fojo, T.; Adler, J.R.; Pacak, K. Current Approaches and Recent Developments in the Management of Head and Neck Paragangliomas. *Endocr. Rev.* **2014**, *35*, 795–819. [CrossRef] [PubMed]
60. Sidney, L.E.; Branch, M.J.; Dunphy, S.E.; Dua, H.S.; Hopkinson, A. Concise review: Evidence for CD34 as a common marker for diverse progenitors. *Stem Cells* **2014**, *32*, 1380–1389. [CrossRef] [PubMed]
61. Li, L.; Dong, M.; Wang, X.G. The Implication and Significance of Beta 2 Microglobulin: A Conservative Multifunctional Regulator. *Chin. Med. J.* **2016**, *129*, 448–455. [CrossRef] [PubMed]
62. Al-Mehdi, A.B.; Pastukh, V.M.; Swiger, B.M.; Reed, D.J.; Patel, M.R.; Bardwell, G.C.; Pastukh, V.V.; Alexeyev, M.F.; Gillespie, M.N. Perinuclear mitochondrial clustering creates an oxidant-rich nuclear domain required for hypoxia-induced transcription. *Sci. Signal.* **2012**, *5*, ra47. [CrossRef] [PubMed]
63. Clarke, L.A. Mucopolysaccharidosis Type I. Available online: https://www.ncbi.nlm.nih.gov/books/NBK1162/ (accessed on 12 December 2018).
64. Afratis, N.; Gialeli, C.; Nikitovic, D.; Tsegenidis, T.; Karousou, E.; Theocharis, A.D.; Pavao, M.; Tzanakakis, G.M.; Karamanos, N.K. Glycosaminoglycans: Key players in cancer cell biology and treatment. *FEBS J.* **2012**, *279*, 1177–1197. [CrossRef] [PubMed]
65. Christianson, H.C.; Belting, M. Heparan sulfate proteoglycan as a cell-surface endocytosis receptor. *Matrix Biol.* **2014**, *35*, 51–55. [CrossRef] [PubMed]
66. He, H.; Huang, M.; Sun, S.; Wu, Y.; Lin, X. Epithelial heparan sulfate regulates Sonic Hedgehog signaling in lung development. *PLoS Genet.* **2017**, *13*, e1006992. [CrossRef] [PubMed]
67. de la Mata, M.; Cotán, D.; Villanueva-Paz, M.; de Lavera, I.; Álvarez-Córdoba, M.; Luzón-Hidalgo, R.; Suárez-Rivero, J.M.; Tiscornia, G.; Oropesa-Ávila, M. Mitochondrial Dysfunction in Lysosomal Storage Disorders. *Diseases* **2016**, *4*, 31. [CrossRef] [PubMed]
68. Kotiadis, V.N.; Duchen, M.R.; Osellame, L.D. Mitochondrial quality control and communications with the nucleus are important in maintaining mitochondrial function and cell health. *Biochim. Biophys. Acta* **2014**, *1840*, 1254–1265. [CrossRef] [PubMed]

69. Caolo, V.; Molin, D.G.; Post, M.J. Notch regulation of hematopoiesis, endothelial precursor cells, and blood vessel formation: Orchestrating the vasculature. *Stem Cells Int.* **2012**, *2012*, 805602. [CrossRef] [PubMed]
70. Kofler, N.M.; Shawber, C.J.; Kangsamaksin, T.; Reed, H.O.; Galatioto, J.; Kitajewski, J. Notch signaling in developmental and tumor angiogenesis. *Genes Cancer* **2011**, *2*, 1106–1116. [CrossRef] [PubMed]
71. Imayoshi, I.; Kageyama, R. The role of Notch signaling in adult neurogenesis. *Mol. Neurobiol.* **2011**, *44*, 7–12. [CrossRef] [PubMed]
72. Pietras, A.; von Stedingk, K.; Lindgren, D.; Påhlman, S.; Axelson, H. JAG2 induction in hypoxic tumor cells alters Notch signaling and enhances endothelial cell tube formation. *Mol. Cancer Res.* **2011**, *9*, 626–636. [CrossRef] [PubMed]
73. Hitoshi, S.; Ishino, Y.; Kumar, A.; Jasmine, S.; Tanaka, K.F.; Kondo, T.; Kato, S.; Hosoya, T.; Hotta, Y.; Ikenaka, K. Mammalian Gcm genes induce Hes5 expression by active DNA demethylation and induce neural stem cells. *Nat. Neurosci.* **2011**, *14*, 957–964. [CrossRef] [PubMed]
74. Gao, C.; Chen, Y.G. Dishevelled: The hub of Wnt signaling. *Cell. Signal.* **2010**, *22*, 717–727. [CrossRef] [PubMed]
75. Blevins, M.A.; Huang, M.; Zhaoa, R. The role of CtBP1 in oncogenic processes and its potential as a therapeutic target. *Mol. Cancer Ther.* **2017**, *16*, 981–990. [CrossRef] [PubMed]
76. Deng, Y.; Li, H.; Yin, X.; Liu, H.; Liu, J.; Guo, D.; Shi, Z. C-Terminal Binding Protein 1 Modulates Cellular Redox via Feedback Regulation of MPC1 and MPC2 in Melanoma Cells. *Med. Sci. Monit.* **2018**, *24*, 7614–7624. [CrossRef] [PubMed]
77. Lorendeau, D.; Rinaldi, G.; Boon, R.; Spincemaille, P.; Metzger, K.; Jäger, C.; Christen, S.; Dong, X.; Kuenen, S.; Voordeckers, K.; et al. Dual loss of succinate dehydrogenase (SDH) and complex I activity is necessary to recapitulate the metabolic phenotype of SDH mutant tumors. *Metab. Eng.* **2017**, *43*, 187–197. [CrossRef] [PubMed]
78. Pang, Y.; Lu, Y.; Caisova, V.; Liu, Y.; Bullova, P.; Huynh, T.T.; Zhou, Y.; Yu, D.; Frysak, Z.; Hartmann, I.; et al. Targeting NAD+/PARP DNA Repair Pathway as a Novel Therapeutic Approach to SDHB-Mutated Cluster I Pheochromocytoma and Paraganglioma. *Clin. Cancer Res.* **2018**, *24*, 3423–3432. [CrossRef] [PubMed]
79. Perumalsamy, L.R.; Nagala, M.; Sarin, A. Notch-activated signaling cascade interacts with mitochondrial remodeling proteins to regulate cell survival. *Proc. Natl. Acad. Sci. USA* **2010**, *107*, 6882–6887. [CrossRef] [PubMed]
80. Basak, N.P.; Roy, A.; Banerjee, S. Alteration of mitochondrial proteome due to activation of Notch1 signaling pathway. *J. Biol. Chem.* **2014**, *289*, 7320–7334. [CrossRef] [PubMed]
81. Mutvei, A.P.; Landor, S.K.-J.; Fox, R.; Braune, E.-B.; Tsoi, Y.L.; Phoon, Y.P.; Sahlgren, C.; Hartman, J.; Bergh, J.; Jin, S.; et al. Notch signaling promotes a HIF2α-driven hypoxic response in multiple tumor cell types. *Oncogene* **2018**, *37*, 6083–6095. [CrossRef] [PubMed]
82. Fernández-Agüera, M.C.; Gao, L.; González-Rodríguez, P.; Pintado, C.O.; Arias-Mayenco, I.; García-Flores, P.; García-Pergañeda, A.; Pascual, A.; Ortega-Sáenz, P.; López-Barneo, J. Oxygen Sensing by Arterial Chemoreceptors Depends on Mitochondrial Complex I Signaling. *Cell Metab.* **2015**, *22*, 825–837. [CrossRef] [PubMed]
83. Park, S.M.; Gaur, A.B.; Lengyel, E.; Peter, M.E. The miR-200 family determines the epithelial phenotype of cancer cells by targeting the E-cadherin repressors ZEB1 and ZEB2. *Genes Dev.* **2008**, *22*, 894–907. [CrossRef] [PubMed]
84. Grego-Bessa, J.; Díez, J.; Timmerman, L.; de la Pompa, J.L. Notch and epithelial-mesenchyme transition in development and tumor progression: Another turn of the screw. *Cell Cycle* **2004**, *3*, 718–721. [CrossRef] [PubMed]
85. Rokavec, M.; Li, H.; Jiang, L.; Hermeking, H. The p53/miR-34 axis in development and disease. *J. Mol. Biol.* **2014**, *6*, 214–230. [CrossRef] [PubMed]
86. Farahani, R.M.; Xaymardan, M. Platelet-Derived Growth Factor Receptor Alpha as a Marker of Mesenchymal Stem Cells in Development and Stem Cell Biology. *Stem Cells Int.* **2015**, *2015*, 362753. [CrossRef] [PubMed]
87. Mei, L.; Smith, S.C.; Faber, A.C.; Trent, J.; Grossman, S.R.; Stratakis, C.A.; Boikos, S.A. Gastrointestinal Stromal Tumors: The GIST of Precision Medicine. *Trends Cancer* **2018**, *4*, 74–91. [CrossRef] [PubMed]
88. Wang, J.; Wakeman, T.P.; Lathia, J.D.; Hjelmeland, A.B.; Wang, X.F.; White, R.R.; Rich, J.N.; Sullenger, B.A. Notch promotes radioresistance of glioma stem cells. *Stem Cells* **2010**, *28*, 17–28. [CrossRef] [PubMed]
89. Kamei, M.; Saunders, W.B.; Bayless, K.J.; Dye, L.; Davis, G.E.; Weinstein, B.M. Endothelial tubes assemble from intracellular vacuoles in vivo. *Nature* **2006**, *442*, 453–456. [CrossRef] [PubMed]
90. Iruela-Arispe, M.L.; Beitel, G.J. Tubulogenesis. *Development* **2013**, *140*, 2851–2855. [CrossRef] [PubMed]

91. Klein, D.; Meissner, N.; Kleff, V.; Jastrow, H.; Yamaguchi, M.; Ergün, S.; Jendrossek, V. Nestin(+) tissue-resident multipotent stem cells contribute to tumor progression by differentiating into pericytes and smooth muscle cells resulting in blood vessel remodeling. *Front. Oncol.* **2014**, *4*, 169. [CrossRef] [PubMed]
92. Mentzer, S.J.; Konerding, M.A. Intussusceptive angiogenesis: Expansion and remodeling of microvascular networks. *Angiogenesis* **2014**, *17*, 499–509. [CrossRef] [PubMed]
93. Kim, Y.; Lin, Q.; Zelterman, D.; Yun, Z. Hypoxia-regulated delta-like 1 homologue enhances cancer cell stemness and tumorigenicity. *Cancer Res.* **2009**, *69*, 9271–9280. [CrossRef] [PubMed]
94. Payne, L.S.; Huang, P.H. The pathobiology of collagens in glioma. *Mol. Cancer Res.* **2013**, *11*, 1129–1140. [CrossRef] [PubMed]
95. Kruegel, J.; Miosge, N. Basement membrane components are key players in specialized extracellular matrices. *Cell. Mol. Life Sci.* **2010**, *67*, 2879–2895. [CrossRef] [PubMed]
96. Hawkins, K.E.; Joy, S.; Delhove, J.M.K.M.; Kotiadis, V.N.; Fernandez, E.; Fitzpatrick, L.M.; Whiteford, J.R.; King, P.J.; Bolanos, J.P.; Duchen, M.R.; et al. NRF2 Orchestrates the Metabolic Shift during Induced Pluripotent Stem Cell Reprogramming. *Cell Rep.* **2016**, *14*, 1883–1891. [CrossRef] [PubMed]
97. Ramasamy, S.K.; Kusumbe, A.P.; Adams, R.H. Regulation of tissue morphogenesis by endothelial cell-derived signals. *Trends Cell Biol.* **2015**, *25*, 148–157. [CrossRef] [PubMed]
98. Ertmer, A.; Huber, V.; Gilch, S.; Yoshimori, T.; Erfle, V.; Duyster, J.; Elsässer, H.P.; Schätzl, H.M. The anticancer drug imatinib induces cellular autophagy. *Leukemia* **2007**, *21*, 936–942. [CrossRef] [PubMed]
99. Pozzi, A.; Zent, R. Extracellular matrix receptors in branched organs. *Curr. Opin. Cell Biol.* **2011**, *23*, 547–553. [CrossRef] [PubMed]
100. Hannezo, E.; Scheele, C.L.G.J.; Moad, M.; Drogo, N.; Heer, R.; Sampogna, R.V.; van Rheenen, J.; Simons, B.D. A Unifying Theory of Branching Morphogenesis. *Cell* **2017**, *171*, 242–255. [CrossRef] [PubMed]
101. Casaletto, J.B.; McClatchey, A.I. Spatial regulation of receptor tyrosine kinases in development and cancer. *Nat. Rev. Cancer* **2012**, *12*, 387–400. [CrossRef] [PubMed]
102. Sonnenschein, C.; Soto, A.M.; Rangarajan, A.; Kulkarni, P. Competing views on cancer. *J. Biosci.* **2014**, *39*, 281–302. [CrossRef] [PubMed]
103. Pecot, C.V.; Rupaimoole, R.; Yang, D.; Akbani, R.; Ivan, C.; Lu, C.; Wu, S.; Han, H.D.; Shah, M.Y.; Rodriguez-Aguayo, C.; et al. Tumour angiogenesis regulation by the miR-200 family. *Nat. Commun.* **2013**, *4*, 2427. [CrossRef] [PubMed]
104. Zhao, T.; Li, J.; Chen, A.F. MicroRNA-34a induces endothelial progenitor cell senescence and impedes its angiogenesis via suppressing silent information regulator 1. *Am. J. Physiol. Endocrinol. Metab.* **2010**, *299*, E110–E116. [CrossRef] [PubMed]
105. Zhang, P.; Sun, Y.; Ma, L. ZEB1: At the crossroads of epithelial-mesenchymal transition, metastasis and therapy resistance. *Cell Cycle* **2015**, *14*, 481–487. [CrossRef] [PubMed]
106. Barker, H.E.; Paget, J.T.; Khan, A.A.; Harrington, K.J. The tumour microenvironment after radiotherapy: Mechanisms of resistance and recurrence. *Nat. Rev. Cancer* **2015**, *15*, 409–425. [CrossRef] [PubMed]
107. van Beijnum, J.R.; Nowak-Sliwinska, P.; Huijbers, E.J.; Thijssen, V.L.; Griffioen, A.W. The great escape; the hallmarks of resistance to antiangiogenic therapy. *Pharmacol. Rev.* **2015**, *67*, 441–461. [CrossRef] [PubMed]
108. Jimenez, C. Treatment for Patients with Malignant Pheochromocytomas and Paragangliomas: A Perspective from the Hallmarks of Cancer. *Front. Endocrinol.* **2018**, *9*, 277. [CrossRef] [PubMed]
109. Prasad, S.C.; Mimoune, H.A.; D'Orazio, F.; Medina, M.; Bacciu, A.; Mariani-Costantini, R.; Piazza, P.; Sanna, M. The role of wait-and-scan and the efficacy of radiotherapy in the treatment of temporal bone paragangliomas. *Otol. Neurotol.* **2014**, *35*, 922–931. [CrossRef] [PubMed]
110. Favier, J.; Briere, J.J.; Burnichon, N.; Riviere, J.; Vescovo, L.; Benit, P.; Giscos-Douriez, I.; De Reynies, A.; Bertherat, J.; Badoual, C.; et al. The Warburg effect is genetically determined in inherited pheochromocytomas. *PLoS ONE* **2009**, *4*, e7094. [CrossRef] [PubMed]
111. Cardaci, S.; Zheng, L.; MacKay, G.; van den Broek, N.J.; MacKenzie, E.D.; Nixon, C.; Stevenson, D.; Tumanov, S.; Bulusu, V.; Kamphorst, J.J.; et al. Pyruvate carboxylation enables growth of SDH-deficient cells by supporting aspartate biosynthesis. *Nat. Cell Biol.* **2015**, *17*, 1317–1326. [CrossRef] [PubMed]

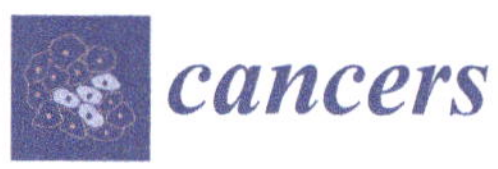

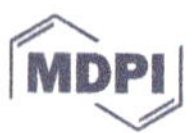

Article

Chromogranin A in the Laboratory Diagnosis of Pheochromocytoma and Paraganglioma

Radovan Bílek [1,*], Petr Vlček [2], Libor Šafařík [3], David Michalský [4], Květoslav Novák [5], Jaroslava Dušková [6], Eliška Václavíková [1], Jiří Widimský Jr. [7] and Tomáš Zelinka [7]

1 Institute of Endocrinology, Národní 8, 116 94 Prague, Czech Republic; evaclavikova@endo.cz
2 Department of Nuclear Medicine and Endocrinology, Motol Teaching Hospital and Second Faculty of Medicine, Charles University, V Úvalu 84, 15006 Prague 5, Czech Republic; petr.vlcek@fnmotol.cz
3 Urology Clinic, V Pražské bráně 74, 26601 Beroun, Czech Republic; lsafarik@centrum.cz
4 1st Department of Surgery-Department of Abdominal, Thoracic Surgery and Traumatology, First Faculty of Medicine, Charles University and General University Hospital, U Nemocnice 2, 12808 Prague 2, Czech Republic; david.michalsky@lf1.cuni.cz
5 Department of Urology, First Faculty of Medicine, Charles University and General University Hospital, Ke Karlovu 4, 12808 Prague 2, Czech Republic; kvetoslav.novak@vfn.cz
6 Institute of Pathology, First Faculty of Medicine, Charles University in Prague and General University Hospital, Studničkova 2, 12800 Prague 2, Czech Republic; jaroslava.duskova@lf1.cuni.cz
7 Center for Hypertension, 3rd Medical Department-Department of Endocrinology and Metabolism, First Faculty of Medicine, Charles University and General University Hospital, U Nemocnice 1, 12808 Prague 2, Czech Republic; jwidi@lf1.cuni.cz (J.W.J.); Tomas.Zelinka@lf1.cuni.cz (T.Z.)
* Correspondence: rbilek@endo.cz; Tel.: +420-224-905-251

Received: 17 March 2019; Accepted: 17 April 2019; Published: 25 April 2019

Abstract: This work discusses the clinical performance of chromogranin A (CGA), a commonly measured marker in neuroendocrine neoplasms, for the diagnosis of pheochromocytoma/ paraganglioma (PPGL). Plasma CGA (cut-off value 150 μg/L) was determined by an immunoradiometric assay. Free metanephrine (cut-off value 100 ng/L) and normetanephrine (cut-off value 170 ng/L) were determined by radioimmunoassay. Blood samples were collected from PPGL patients preoperatively, one week, six months, one year and two years after adrenal gland surgery. The control patients not diagnosed with PPGL suffered from adrenal problems or from MEN2 and thyroid carcinoma. The clinical sensitivity in the PPGL group of patients (n = 71) based on CGA is 90% and is below the clinical sensitivity determined by metanephrines (97%). The clinical specificity based on all plasma CGA values after surgery (n = 98) is 99% and is the same for metanephrines assays. The clinical specificity of CGA in the control group (n = 85) was 92% or 99% using metanephrines tests. We can conclude that plasma CGA can serve as an appropriate complement to metanephrines assays in laboratory diagnosis of PPGL patients. CGA is elevated in PPGLs, as well as in other neuroendocrine or non-neuroendocrine neoplasia and under clinical conditions increasing adrenergic activity.

Keywords: chromogranin A; metanephrines; pheochromocytoma; paraganglioma

1. Introduction

In this work we present our experiences with radioimmunoassay of plasma chromogranin A (CGA) in the laboratory diagnosis of neuroendocrine tumors classified as pheochromocytoma (PCC) and paraganglioma (PGL). Radioimmunoassay of plasma methanephrines were also performed.

Neuroendocrine cells are widely dispersed cells with dense core granules similar to those dense core granules present in serotonergic neurons (neuro properties), which store bioactive amines and peptide hormones (endocrine properties) [1,2]. These cells do not contain synapses [1,3]. Neuroendocrine neoplasms are a heterogeneous group of tumors, including malignancies from several anatomic areas that also include pheochromocytomas and paragangliomas, commonly denoted PPGLs. Neuroendocrine neoplasms are classified into well-differentiated neuroendocrine tumors, poorly differentiated neuroendocrine carcinomas, and mixed adenoneuroendocrine carcinomas showing more than 30% of neuroendocrine cells and additional components [4,5]. Neuroendocrine neoplasms can be divided into functional and non-functional tumors; the former ones are usually diagnosed at an earlier stage due to endocrine symptoms related to hormonal production, whereas the non-functional tumors remain silent and are frequently diagnosed when metastasis has already occurred [2,5]. Neuroendocrine neoplastic cells have been described in the central nervous system, respiratory tract, the larynx, gastrointestinal tract, thyroid, skin, urogenital system, breast and lung [2]. Well differentiated neuroendocrine tumor cells synthesize, store and secrete chromogranin A (CGA) and amines; metastatic neuroendocrine carcinomas have fewer cytoplasmic secretory granules [1]. Serum CGA is a commonly measured marker in neuroendocrine neoplasms [3].

PPGLs are rare neuroendocrine tumors of a chromaffin cell origin usually found in the adrenal medulla and other ganglia of the nervous system [6]. PCC is a tumor arising from adrenomedullary chromaffin cells that commonly produces catecholamines. PGL is a tumor derived from extra-adrenal chromaffin cells of the sympathetic paravertebral ganglia (thorax, abdomen, pelvis) producing catecholamines or parasympathetic ganglia located in the neck and at the base of the skull, which is often non-secretory [7–9]. PGLs were identified in the head and neck, being most frequent in the carotid body, followed by jugulotympanic paraganglia, vagal nerve and ganglion nodosum, as well as laryngeal paraganglia. Abdominal sites include urinary bladder tumors; other unusual sites are peri-adrenal, para-aortic, inter-aortocaval, and paracaval retroperitoneal sites, as well as tumors in the thyroid, parathyroid, pituitary, gut, pancreas, liver, mesentery, lung, heart and mediastinum [10]. The adrenal tumor localization is usually found in 80–85% of patients, and extra-adrenal sympathetic and parasympathetic PGL are observed in 10–20% of patients [11,12]. While most PPGLs are benign, approximately 10% of the PCCs and 20–25% of the PGLs are malignant [8,13,14].

PPGLs have considerable genetic heterogeneity [15] associated with various clusters based to different patient outcomes and underlying genetics. The *pseudohypoxia group* is characterized by somatic or germline mutations and silent or dopaminergic and/or noradrenergic secretory profiles in the tricarboxylic acid cycle related to succinate dehydrogenase subunits *SDHA*, *SDHB*, *SDHC*, *SDHD*, *SDHAF1*, *SDHAF2* (together *SDHx*) or in fumarate hydratase (*FH*), a second enzyme in the tricarboxylic acid cycle, in von Hippel-Lindau disease (*VHL*), endothelial PAS domain 1 (*EPAS10*, also known as hypoxia–inducible factor 2α (*HIF2A*)), and prolylhydroxylases *PHD1* and *PHD2*. The *wnt signaling group* includes somatic mutations in cold shock domain containing E1 (*CSDE1*), α thalassemia/mental retardation syndrome X-linked (*ATRX*) and mastermind-like transcriptional coactivator (3*MAML3*) with mixed noradrenergic and adrenergic secretory phenotype. The *kinase signaling group* consists of germline or somatic mutations in *RET* proto-oncogene (syndrome MEN 2A, 2B), neurofibromin 1 (*NF1*), transmembrane protein 127 (*TMEM127*), MYC-associated factor X (*MAX*), kinesin-like protein (*KIF1BB*), receptor tyrosine kinase (*MET*) and GTPase, Harvey rat sarcoma viral oncogene homolog (*HRAS*) with adrenergic or mixed noradrenergic and adrenergic secretory profiles [10,15]. Mutations in the mitochondrial succinate dehydrogenase enzyme complex subunit B (*SDHB*) and the tumor suppressor gene Von Hippel-Lindau (*VHL*) are mainly associated with malignancy [13].

Elevated levels of circulating CGA have been associated with almost all types of neuroendocrine neoplasms including PPGLs [5]. CGA belongs to the family of secretory chromogranin and secretogranin proteins (CGA, chromogranin B, chromogranin C or secretogranin II, secretogranins III, IV, V, VI, VII and VIII). These proteins are the driving force for the biogenesis of secretory chromaffin granules present in the diffuse neuroendocrine system [16]. CGA is an acidic hydrophilic glycoprotein abundantly expressed in large dense core vesicles of neuroendocrine cells [17]. CGA comprises at least 40% of the soluble proteins of the adrenal chromaffin granules [18]. Human CGA is encoded by the *CHGA* gene, located in chromosome 14q32.12 with eight exons and seven introns. It is transcribed and translated into a 439 amino acids protein with a molecular weight of 48 kDa which is co-stored and co-released with catecholamines [5,16]. The N-terminal domain of CGA is responsible for directing CGA into the secretory granules [19], and for binding to secretogranin III, the receptor for CGA requiring the presence of Ca^{2+} [4]. The CGA structure is described in Uniprot/SWISS-PROT database under the accession number P10645 and it consists of 18 amino acids (aa) long signal peptide (CGA 1–18) and 439 aa long CGA (together 457 aa). It includes multiple dibasic cleavage sites [5]. CGA is processed to a lesser extent within the secretory granules to yield bioactive peptides [20]. These peptide hormones such as vasostatin-1 (CGA 19–94), vasostatin-2 (CGA 19–131), pancreastatin (CGA 272–319), catestatin (CGA 370–390), parastatin (CGA 347–419), serpinin (CGA 429–454), chromofugin (CGA 47–66), chromostatin (CGA 124–143), chromactin I (CGA 173–194), chromactin II (CGA 195–221) or WE14 (CGA 316–329) have different biological functions. Generally the peptide hormones negatively modulate the neuroendocrine function [4,5] and are involved in regulation of the cardiovascular system, metabolism, innate immunity, angiogenesis and tissue repair [21].

The main biological role of CGA is to regulate calcium-mediated exocytosis [22]. The granin family has the capacity to bind calcium ions and the ability to form aggregates [5]. They are involved in vesicle sorting, in the generation of bioactive peptides and in the accumulation of soluble species such as catecholamines and Ca^{2+} at low pH to large dense core vesicles. CGA is synthesized in the rough endoplasmic reticulum, transported to the Golgi complex and packaged together with other secretory proteins/peptides and amines into immature granules, where it may be cleaved into the various derived peptides by specific processing enzymes. Upon acidification, secretory granules mature, and are ready for stimulation–induced release. Intact CGA controls the dense core granule biogenesis as well as the sorting and secretion of other bioactive molecules, and participates in the regulation of cytosolic calcium stores and granule exocytosis [5,23]. The pH gradient across the membrane of large dense core vesicles is responsible for maintaining the high concentrations of amines, Ca^{2+} and ATP inside the vesicles. The pH gradient depends on the activity of a vesicular H^+-proton pump ATPase, which is continuously pumping H^+ to acidify the vesicles [24]. Treatment of patients with proton pump inhibitors (PPIs) can increase the concentrations of CGA in circulation.

CGA is an essential protein for PPGLs [25]. High levels of CGA, co-stored and co-secreted with catecholamines, may indicate tumor mass and malignancy in PPGL patients and can be used to monitor response and relapse [13]. Although non-specific for PPGL, CGA may facilitate diagnostic evaluation of e.g., SDHB-related PPGL, especially where the measurement of plasma metanephrines could otherwise be delayed by decreased availability or cost restriction [26]. High levels of CGA at the time of PPGL diagnosis were associated with the presence of metastases according to the histological evaluation of primary PPGL tumors with a PASS scoring scale, which is based on the histological evaluation of large nest or diffuse growth (>10% of tumor volume) (2 points), central or confluent necrosis (2 points), high cellularity (2 points), cellular monotony (2 points), tumor cell spindling (2 points), mitoses >3/10 HPF (2 points), atyp. mitoses (2 points), periadrenal fat infiltration (2 points), angioinvasion (1 point), transcapsular invasion (1 point), extreme pleomorphism (1 point) and nuclear hyperchromasia (1 point) [27]. The PASS score of PPGL patients usually exceeds 4 points [28]. A value of less than four out of 20 points indicates the benign character of a tumor [27]. The PASS score shows the possibility of malignancy, and its value higher than four indicates uncertain biological behavior. Increasing the score increases the likelihood of malignancy. However, the real evidence of malignancy is only the presence of metastasis in PPGL patients [7]. CGA is physiologically released via exocytosis by both functioning and non-functioning tumors [29]. A significant positive relationship was demonstrated between tumor mass and serum CGA levels [30–32]. Abnormally high circulating CGA levels are a typical feature of patients with neuroendocrine tumors and the detection of circulating CGA has a high sensitivity and specificity for the diagnosis of these tumors [29]. Plenty of misdiagnoses or delayed diagnoses still occur due to silent or weak clinical manifestation, especially for non-functioning neuroendocrine tumors [33]. CGA is a widely used biomarker for the assessment of neuroendocrine neoplasms, mainly of a gastroenteropancreatic origin [4]. It is elevated in approximately 90% of gut neuroendocrine tumors; the highest values are noted in ileal and gastrointestinal neuroendocrine tumors associated with MEN1.

Pancreatic neuroendocrine tumors also have elevated values [1]. CGA was significantly higher in patients affected by hepatocellular carcinoma [34], gastroenteropancreatic neuroendocrine tumors [35], and in primary and metastatic small intestinal neuroendocrine tumors [36]. Gastric type I, pituitary and parathyroid tumors had lower values [1]. CGA is more frequently elevated in well-differentiated tumors compared to poorly differentiated neuroendocrine tumors [1].

Falsely elevated CGA levels are observed in patients treated with proton pump inhibitors (PPIs) or other acid-blocking medications [1,4,5,37]. This effect of the PPIs is fully eliminated after discontinuation of the PPI for 2 weeks [38]. Chronic renal insufficiency (CRI) can also substantially increase the concentration of circulated CGA [39] and may led to concentrations of CGA as high as those detected in patients with neuroendocrine neoplasm [40]. Other diseases of the alimentary tract affecting CGA concentration are chronic gastritis [41], chronic hepatitis, liver cirrhosis [42], pancreatitis, irritable bowel, and inflammatory bowel diseases [43]. Its concentration in circulation is also increased after myocardial infarction, acute coronary syndrome and heart failure [21,44,45]. The cardiovascular complications were observed in nearly 20% of patients with PPGLs due to an increased level of catecholamines [46].

We have presented in this study our experiences with the radioimmunoanalytical determination of plasma CGA in groups of patients who suffered from PPGLs. These data were partly published in the literature [47], and commentary on the data is given in the Discussion section. Patients with various endocrine disorders other than PPGLs were used as the control group.

2. Results

In all PPGL patients, CGA and methanephrines were determined by radioimmunoassay in EDTA plasma. The nature of the PPGL was differentiated by colored solid symbols as given in the legend of Figure 1. Plasma CGA results were not statistically dependent on either age or gender.

As seen in Figure 1, clinical specificity and sensitivity was considerably influenced by administering proton pump inhibitors and in patients by chronic renal insufficiency. Recurrence of the disease (REC) was observed in two patients one week or two years after surgery. These results concerning PPI, CRI or REC were not included in the clinical specificity and sensitivity calculations listed in Tables 1 and 2 since such increased values can be normalized by not administering PPI to patients, or long-term kidney failure or the recurrence of PPGL must be taken into consideration when interpreting the results as the case may be. Figure 1 describes CGA concentration in EDTA plasma of all samples of 78 PPGL patients and 86 controls in a given time period. Metanephrine (MN) and normetanephrine (NMN) using radioimmunoassay in EDTA plasma were also determined in these patients. Data from 71 PPGL patients were used for determination of sensitivity, the remaining seven patients were excluded from the study due to PPI, CRI, or REC (Table 1). One patient out of 86 control samples was also excluded from the same cause (CRI), so the calculation of specificity was done from a group of 85 patients.

Table 1. The clinical sensitivity and specificity of PPGL patients based on the plasma chromogranin A (CGA) determinations before and after the adrenal surgery. The meaning of abbreviations is pheochromocytoma (PCC); paraganglioma (PGL); together denoted as PPGL; mutations in genes *RET*; *VHL*; *NF1*; *MAX*; *MET*; *SDHB* and *SDHD*; number (n); standard deviation (SD).

			PPGL—Patients with Pheochromocytoma (PCC) or Paraganglioma (PGL)																					
			2 ± 3 Weeks before Surgery						1 ± 0.5 Week after Surgery				6 Months (30 ± 10 Weeks) after Surgery				1 Year (54 ± 6 Weeks) after Surgery				2 Years (96 ± 22 Weeks) after Surgery			
Disease	Genetics	Gender	n	AGE (Years)		CGA (µg/L)		Clinical Sensitivity	n	CGA (µg/L)		Clinical Specificity	n	CGA (µg/L)		Clinical Specificity	n	CGA (µg/L)		Clinical Specificity	n	CGA (µg/L)		Clinical Specificity
				Mean	SD	Mean	SD			Mean	SD			Mean	SD			mean	SD			Mean	SD	
PPGL	total	total	71	49	17	618.9	479.7	90	27	76	24.4	100	31	75.9	33.8	97	29	73.1	28.6	100	11	59.2	16.7	100
		males	38	47	16	638.7	512	92	15	69.1	21.5	100	17	71.6	28.6	100	16	73.1	31	100	6	64.1	16.6	100
		females	33	50	18	596.1	446.5	88	12	84.6	26	100	14	81.2	39.7	93	13	73.2	26.6	100	5	53.4	16.7	100
PCC	total	total	62	48	17	657.1	492.7	90	25	76	24	100	30	76.2	34.3	97	27	74.9	28.6	100	9	57.0	17.9	100
		males	35	48	16	667.4	522.8	91	14	70.7	21.3	100	16	71.8	29.5	100	15	73.7	32	100	4	61.5	20.8	100
		females	27	48	18	643.7	460.4	89	11	82.8	26.5	100	14	81.2	39.7	93	12	76.4	25	100	5	53.4	16.7	100
	not specified	total	45	52	16	718.9	506	96	20	77.1	26.4	100	20	71.2	27.3	100	20	74.8	27.5	100	6	55.0	13.6	100
		males	25	52	15	758.4	543.4	100	10	70.6	24.6	100	11	70.7	24.8	100	10	70	30	100	3	54.3	18.2	100
		females	20	52	16	669.6	464.2	90	10	83.7	27.8	100	9	71.8	31.5	100	10	79.6	25.5	100	3	55.7	11.4	100
	RET	total	7	34	9	614.8	482.6	86	-	-	-	-	2	129	82.8	50	2	60.5	20	100	1	83.3	-	100
		males	3	42	6	693.7	603	67	-	-	-	-	-	-	-	-	-	-	-	-	1	83.3	-	100
		females	4	28	5	555.6	460.9	100	-	-	-	-	2	129	82.8	50	2	60.5	20	100	-	-	-	-
	VHL	total	5	32	21	427.9	482.5	60	2	70.9	14.9	100	3	85	52.2	100	2	99.1	62.6	100	2	49.9	28.5	100
		males	3	22	2	244.2	127.4	67	2	70.9	14.9	100	2	82.3	73.5	100	2	99.1	62.6	100	-	-	-	-
		females	2	46	34	703.6	803.5	50	-	-	-	100	1	90.3	-	100	-	-	-	-	2	49.9	28.5	100
	NF1	total	3	54	10	220.2	128.8	67	2	71.4	15.4	100	2	56.2	16.9	100	2	57.8	7.5	100	-	-	-	-
		males	3	54	10	220.2	128.8	67	2	71.4	15.4	100	2	56.2	16.9	100	2	57.8	7.5	100	-	-	-	-
		females	-	-	-	-	-	-	-	-	-	-	-	-	-	-	-	-	-	-	-	-	-	-
	MAX	total	1	60	-	357.9	-	100	1	74.2	-	100	2	71.5	2.1	100	-	-	-	-	-	-	-	-
		males	-	-	-	-	-	-	-	-	-	-	-	-	-	-	-	-	-	-	-	-	-	-
		females	1	60	-	357.9	-	100	1	74.2	-	100	2	71.5	2.1	100	-	-	-	-	-	-	-	-
	MET	total	1	47	-	925	-	100	-	-	-	-	1	94.4	-	100	1	92	-	100	-	-	-	-
		males	1	47	-	925	-	100	-	-	-	-	1	94.4	-	100	1	92	-	100	-	-	-	-
		females	-	-	-	-	-	-	-	-	-	-	-	-	-	-	-	-	-	-	-	-	-	-
PGL	total	total	9	52	20	355.9	270.8	89	2	74.9	40.4	100	1	67.3	-	100	2	49.3	20.7	100	2	69.1	2.8	100
		males	3	36	12	303.7	145.1	100	1	46.4	-	100	1	67.3	-	100	1	64	-	100	2	69.1	2.8	100
		females	6	61	18	382	326.3	83	1	103.5	-	100	-	-	-	-	1	34.6	-	100	-	-	-	-
	not specified	total	6	56	22	258.2	181.1	83	1	103.5	-	100	-	-	-	-	1	34.6	-	100	1	71.1	-	100
		males	1	32	-	197.1	-	100	-	-	-	-	-	-	-	-	-	-	-	-	1	71.1	-	100
		females	5	61	20	270.5	199.7	80	1	103.5	-	100	-	-	-	-	1	34.6	-	100	-	-	-	-
	SDHB	total	2	55	7	592.2	190.9	100	-	-	-	-	-	-	-	-	-	-	-	-	1	67.1	-	100
		males	1	50	-	245.1	-	100	-	-	-	-	-	-	-	-	-	-	-	-	1	67.1	-	100
		females	1	60	-	939.4	-	100	-	-	-	-	-	-	-	-	-	-	-	-	-	-	-	-
	SDHD	total	1	26	-	469	-	100	1	46.4	-	100	1	67.3	-	100	1	64	-	100	-	-	-	-
		males	1	26	-	469	-	100	1	46.4	-	100	1	67.3	-	100	1	64	-	100	-	-	-	-
		females	-	-	-	-	-	-	-	-	-	-	-	-	-	-	-	-	-	-	-	-	-	-

Table 2. The clinical specificity determined from the control group of patients with various adrenal disorders; but not afflicted by pheochromocytoma or paraganglioma. The meaning of abbreviations is plasma chromogranin A (CGA); multiple endocrine neoplasia (MEN) type 2A (MEN2A) or 2B (MEN2B); medullary (MTC); papillary (PTC) or follicular (FTC) thyroid carcinoma; number (n); standard deviation (SD).

Controls							
Syndrome	**Gender**	**n**	**AGE (years)**		**CGA μg/L)**		**Clinical Specificity**
			Mean	**SD**	**Mean**	**SD**	
total	total	85	53	19	125.3	259.3	92
	males	29	53	21	102.6	128.9	93
	females	56	54	18	134	306.3	91
adrenocortical adenoma	total	44	63	11	178.5	352.7	84
	males	15	65	6	135.2	173.3	87
	females	29	62	13	200.9	417.7	83
adrenocortical adenoma + MTC, FTC	total	1	71	-	31.8	-	100
	males	-	-	-	-	-	-
	females	1	71	-	31.8	-	100
adrenocortical adenoma + PTC	total	1	75	-	108.4	-	100
	males	-	-	-	-	-	-
	females	1	75	-	108.4	-	100
hypertension	total	8	45	16	43.2	11	100
	males	4	41	22	50.2	9.1	100
	females	4	48	8	36.3	8.3	100
MEN 2A	total	2	10	4	70.6	15.2	100
	males	1	13	-	81.3	-	100
	females	1	7	-	59.8	-	100
MEN 2A + MTC	total	7	26	14	69.5	35.5	100
	males	3	20	12	71.8	24.9	100
	females	4	30	16	67.7	45.7	100
MEN 2B + MTC	total	3	30	16	90.7	53.9	100
	males	1	17	-	146.2	-	100
	females	2	37	16	62.9	34.4	100
MTC	total	9	56	13	76.9	36.2	100
	males	2	51	17	51.3	10.9	100
	females	7	57	13	84.2	38.1	100
MTC + PTC	total	1	70	-	42.3	-	100
	males	1	70	-	42.3	-	100
	females	-	-	-	-	-	-
PTC	total	4	58	22	81.1	40.4	100
	males	1	80	-	102.6	-	100
	females	3	50	20	73.9	46.2	100
thyroid disorders	total	5	36	18	70.2	12.2	100
	males	1	51	-	54.6	-	100
	females	4	32	18	74.1	9.9	100

PPGL patients are divided into PCC and PGL groups (total, males, females) with specified or not specified mutations in Table 1. Six of the PCC patients (none of the PGL patients) were metastatic (1 case of *RET* mutation, other mutations were not specified), two of these patients died prior to surgery. Nine PGL patients with preoperative CGA concentrations 355.9 ± 270.8 μg/L (Table 1) showed only noradrenergic phenotype with increased NMN and normal MN with one exception in which both MN and NMN were normal. Preoperative CGA concentrations 657.1 ± 492.7 μg/L (Table 1) were found in

62 PCC patients. According to Eisenhofer et al. [48], there was an adrenergic phenotype with elevated MN and variable NMN levels in 36 patients with a CGA concentration equal to 767.7 ± 513.7 µg/L. A noradrenergic phenotype with elevated NMN and normal or slightly increased MN to 120 µg/L was found in 25 patients with a CGA concentration of 516.9 ± 428.8 µg/L. Both MN and NMN were in normal reference ranges in one PCC patient. In general, the adrenergic phenotype of PPGL patients did not have a statistically significantly higher concentration of CGA than the noradrenergic phenotype. The CGA concentration of the adrenergic and noradrenegic phenotype is shown in Figure 2 as the notched box plot.

The clinical sensitivity of 71 PPGL patients based on plasma CGA values greater than 150 µg/L before surgery is equal to 90%. A total of seven patients (three not specified, one *RET*, two *VHL*, one *NF1*) had pre-surgery CGA values below 150 µg/L (Figure 1). Five of these patients had a tumor volume less than 20 mm^3, and in one PCC patient diagnosed in 2002 with VHL gene mutation, recurrence was observed in 2003, 2005 and 2014. A kidney tumor was removed from him in 2014. The last patient was treated with vasodilating and antithrombotic drugs. Clinical sensitivity based on the concentrations of plasma MN and NMN was 97%.

Clinical specificity of PPGL patients based on all plasma CGA values during one week, six months, one year and two years after surgery less than 150 µg/L is equal to 99% (n = 98, CGA 73.2 ± 28.4 [29.7–187.6] µg/L). One result concerning the specificity of CGA 188 µg/L six months after surgery was a false positive. There was also a clinical specificity of 99% for PPGL patients determined by the concentration of metanephrines.

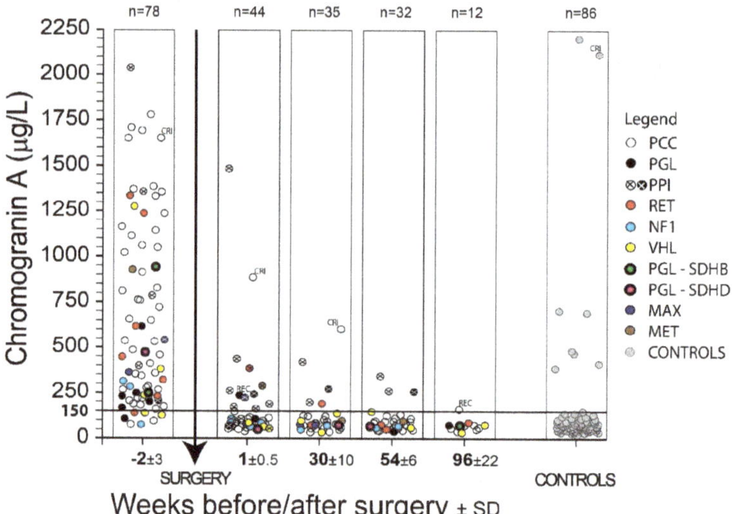

Figure 1. The results of chromogranin A (CGA) determination in PPGL patients before and after surgery. Symbols indicate the type of PPGL and found mutations in genes *RET*; *NF1*; *VHL*; *SDHB*; *SDHD*; *MAX*; *MET*. The meaning of abbreviations is pheochromocytoma (PCC); paraganglioma (PGL); patients treated with proton pump inhibitors (PPI); patients with chronic renal insufficiency (CRI); patients with a recurrence of the disease (REC).

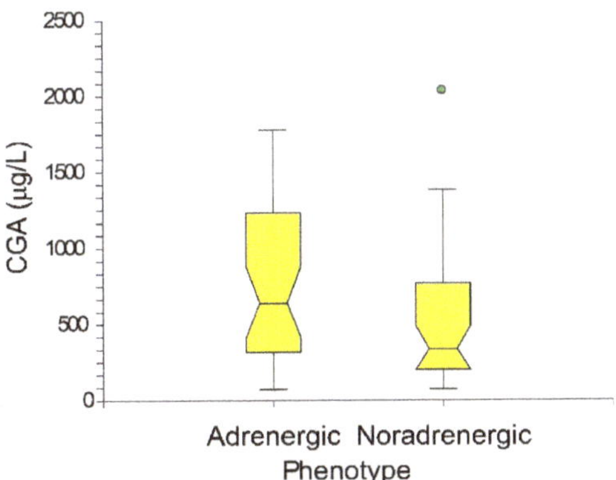

Figure 2. The notched box plot of CGA concentrations in adrenergic and noradrenergic phenotype of PPGL patients.

Results concerning the clinical specificity of CGA in the group of control patients without PCC or PGL are shown in Table 2. Some of these control patients had a diagnosis closely related to PPGL. This concerned 44 patients with adrenocortical adenoma or one patient with adrenocortical adenoma together with medullary thyroid carcinoma (MTC), follicular thyroid carcinoma (FTC) or papillary thyroid carcinoma (PTC), two patients with MEN2A syndrome or seven patients with MEN2A and MTC, three patients with MEN2B and MTC, or nine patients with merely somatic MTC. There was one patient with MTC and PTC and four patients with PTC, nine patients with hypertension, and five cases in which patients suffered from thyroid diseases (one goiter, one thyroiditis, three thyroid nodules). This concerned a total of 86 cases. One of these patients with hypertension labeled CRI in Figure 1 was not included in the control group because he suffered from chronic renal insufficiency (4th degree hypertensive nephrosclerosis), so Table 2 shows a total of 85 patients. The CGA clinical specificity of the control group is 92%; seven out of 85 had a CGA higher than 150 μg/L. All of these patients were diagnosed with adenoma of the adrenal gland, which was accompanied by two serious cases of cardiovascular disease and two cases of hypertension. MN and NMN values of these patients were inside the reference range. The clinical specificity of the control patients, based on the concentration of metanephrines, was 99%.

The mass of the operated PPGL tumors was determined in 59 of a total of 78 PPGL patients. Of these 59 patients, five patients who received PPI and one patient with CRI were excluded. The correlation between mass of PPGL tumors and corresponding CGA was calculated in 53 patients according to the following equation:

$$\text{Mass (g)} = 16.2481 + 0.2073 \times \text{CGA}(\mu\text{g/L});\ n = 53,\ \text{correlation } r = 0.4490,\ \text{significance level } p = 0.0007.$$

The volume of the operated PPGL tumors was determined in 47 of a total of 78 PPGL patients. Of these 47 patients, six patients who received PPI and one patient with CRI were excluded. The correlation between volume of PPGL tumors and corresponding CGA was calculated in 40 patients according to the equation:

$$\text{Volume (mm}^3) = -23.6810 + 0.3131 \times \text{CGA } (\mu\text{g/L});\ n = 40,\ \text{correlation } r = 0.7300,\ \text{significance level } p = 0.0000.$$

The PASS score [29] was determined in 65 of a total of 78 PPGL patients (PASS score mean ± SD = 5 ± 3, range 1–11 points). Of these 65 patients, six patients who received PPI and one patient with CRI were excluded. The correlation between PASS scores and the corresponding CGA was calculated in 58 patients according to the equation:

$$\text{PASS} = 3.7643 + 0.0023 \times \text{CGA } (\mu\text{g/L});\ n = 58, \text{ correlation } r = 0.4322, \text{ significance level } p = 0.0007.$$

3. Discussion

In a pilot study of 25 PPGL patients in 2008, we examined the utility of the CGA radioimmunoassay for the diagnosis of PPGL [30]. The results were so hopeful that by 2017 radioimmunoassays with CGA and plasma free metanephrines were determined in our institute in another 55 PPGL patients and results were published in 2017 [47]. This article includes all data on CGA and free plasma metanephrines concerning 78 PPGL patients measured by radioimmunoassays in our institute. Data were revised according to clinical diagnosis, consistently purified from all results of PPI-mediated analyses, chronic renal insufficiency or recurrence of the disease. Based on the revised results, we had to reduce clinical sensitivity for CGA from 93% [47] to 90%, and for metanephrines we increased the clinical sensitivity from 96% [47] to 97%. The combined clinical specificity calculated from the results of PPGL patients four months and more after surgery and from the control group (151 analyses) was 96% for CGA and 100% for metanephrines [47] and it was decreased in this set (156 analyses) to 95% for CGA and 99% for metanephrines. In this study the clinical specificity of PPGL patients after surgery (98 analyses over one week to two years after the operation of PPGL; analyses influenced by PPI, CRI or REC were excluded—see Figure 1) was 99% for CGA and 99% for metanephrines. The clinical specificity of the control group (85 analyses, one patient with CRI was excluded) was 92% for CGA, 99% for metanephrines. In all cases the combination of metanephrines and CGA gave 100% results of clinical sensitivity.

The clinical sensitivity of CGA in the PPGL group of patients is 90% and is therefore below the clinical sensitivity determined by MN and NMN (97%). But the sensitivity of metanephrines is not equal to 100%. In our PPGL patient population, metanephrines were falsely negative in one case of PGL and in one case of PCC (the kind of genetic mutation is unknown), while CGA levels were increased. In the PGL case the preoperative concentrations of CGA and NMN were increased, while MN was normal. The patient was designated for resection of sympathetic paraganglioma due to identical results of imaging procedures using MIBG and FDG PET, respectively. The PGL located on the abdominal aorta was removed during the first operation and one week after surgery the CGA concentration was increased, NMN and MN were within the normal reference range. Further measurements after 6 months have shown that the CGA level is still elevated, but MN and NMN are normal. By the imaging procedure (PET/CT with FDOPA) another deposit was found and PGL was surgically removed in the area of the right adrenal gland after 10 months. One week after surgery the concentrations of CGA, MN and NMN were within the normal reference range. Table 1 does not state that one PGL patient with recurrence of the disease had MN and NMN within the reference range in the first week after surgery, while the CGA was greater than the CGA cut-off value. Zuber et al. [26] showed that CGA is a valuable complementary biomarker in the workup of SDHB-related PCC/PGL. Combined with plasma NMN, CGA further enhance tumor detection by 22% with minimal loss in specificity. Unlike the previous quote, other literature [49] states that plasma CGA levels are increased in only a small portion (16%) of patients with biochemically silent hereditary head and neck paragangliomas, but the finding that nine out of 62 PGL patients with a biochemically silent tumor had an elevated CGA level possesses diagnostic significance. The CGA can be increased in a number of neuroendocrine neoplasias, so it cannot be used alone to diagnose PPGL. Metanephrines also have an advantage over CGA that they are unaffected by PPI use, and renal insufficiency should not affect their value. However, the combination of CGA and plasma metanephrines increases the predictive value in terms of clinical sensitivity and specificity and it is evident that CGA determination can be an appropriate addition to MN and NMN assays in laboratory diagnostics of PPGL patients.

The clinical specificity of PPGL patients after surgery based on all plasma CGA values (n = 98) purified from results with PPI, CRI or REC (Figure 1) is 99% and is the same as the 99% specificity based on the MN and NMN assays. CGA determination was also in this case an appropriate addition to the MN and NMN tests, and vice versa.

The clinical specificity of CGA in the control group was 92%, while the clinical specificity based on the MN and NMN tests was 99%. In 1 case of a patient with adrenocortical adenoma and MTC without diagnosis of PPGL, the NMN was falsely positive increased (197 ng/L), while the CGA 115 μg/L was below the 150 μg/L cut-off value.

A PASS score was absent in the nine patients without surgery and it was not determined in four patients. Of the 58 PPGL patients who had determined the PASS score, 46 patients (79%) had the PASS score equal to or greater than 4. In four metastatic PCC patients, PASS score was also equal to or greater than 4 (mean PASS ± SD = 7 ± 3). A PASS score equal or higher than 4 indicates uncertain biological behavior and increases the likelihood of malignancy. From this perspective, the PASS score was clinically relevant in malignant PPGL patients. We found in the literature [50] that the overall sensitivity for the PASS algorithm to correctly identify a malignant PCC (n = 105) was 97%, whereas the specificity of benign PCC (n = 704) was 68%. The sensitivity of the PASS score in malignant PGL (n = 13) was 100%, the specificity of benign PGL (n = 29) was 72%.

In the monitored PPGL and control group, increased values of CGA were found in connection with the PPGL diagnosis, while for patients with MEN syndrome and MTC or with differentiated cancer of thyroid gland (PTC, FTC) without the presence of PCC or PGL, CGA values were within the reference range.

Although PPGLs are rare tumors of chromaffin cells, it has serious consequences to the health of afflicted patients. Its familiar occurrence in individuals with a genetic predisposition is common in young people and often consists of bilateral tumors with aggressive biological behavior [7]. Unlike the determination of MN or NMN, the determination of CGA is not influenced by hypertensive drugs, substances and activities affecting biosynthesis and the secretion of catecholamines [7,12], but the value of CGA determination in patient taking proton pump inhibitors and in patients with severe renal insufficiency is limited [4,5] (see Figure 1).

The Endocrine Society [7] recommends that initial screening for PPGLs should include measurement of plasma-free metanephrines or urine-fractionated metanephrines using liquid chromatography with mass spectrometric or electrochemical detection methods. The CGA in circulation seems to be in general a biomarker of neuroendocrine tumors which can improve diagnosis, serve to estimate prognosis and monitor the course of treatment [5]. CGA is an essential protein for PPGLs and if immunohistochemistry for CGA is negative, PPGLs should be ruled out [25]. According to the European Society of Endocrinology [51], CGA should be preoperatively measured in patients with normal preoperative plasma or urinary levels of MN, NMN and 3-methoxytyramine (3MT), and also 2–6 weeks and every year after surgery. Elevated preoperative CGA levels can be used to screen for local or metastatic recurrences or new tumors. The postoperative determination of CGA is recommended in cases with preoperative elevated CGA and normal metanephrines. Our experience corresponds to the recommendations of the European Endocrinology Society. We think that if there is any doubt about metanephrines in the laboratory diagnosis of PPGL, CGA should also be determined.

A problem in the immunoanalytical determination of CGA lies in the fact that immunoassays are not standardized, and the results of various kit producers are different. This is due to the different specificity and sensitivity of the antibodies used, as well as to the different format of the given immunoassays [5]. CGA is highly acidic, it binds Ca^{2+} ions and aggregates rapidly. If the Ca^{2+} concentration is limited in EDTA plasma samples, there CGA does not form aggregates and concentrations of free CGA are immunoanalytically detected in comparison with serum samples [52]. The principal limitation of CGA evaluation is its low clinical specificity and sensitivity. The CGA is elevated in PPGLs, however, as well as in other neuroendocrine or non-neuroendocrine neoplasia and in clinical conditions with increased adrenergic activity [4]. The advantage of the immunoassay approach is that these methods are common in a clinical-biochemical laboratory and do not require additional expensive instrumentation. Limitations are given by the immunoassay principle in which, owing to interference, the immunological quantity does not have to correspond to the biological activity.

4. Materials and Methods

4.1. The Group of Patients

Included in the study were the group of PPGL patients and the control group without PPGL diagnosis. Patients with PCC or PGL consisted of 78 patients aged 49 ± 17 (18–78) years, 36 females aged 52 ± 18 (18–78) years, 42 males aged 48 ± 15 (20–76) years. PCC occurred in 68 patients, PGL in 10 patients. In the PCC group, mutations in the *RET* gene were found in seven patients, three were diagnosed with MEN2A and MTC, four had MEN2B and MTC. Mutations in the *VHL* gene were observed in five patients, in three patients were mutations in the *NF1* gene, two patients had mutations in the *MAX* gene, one patient in the *MET* gene, and in 50 patients the mutations were not determined. In the PGL group, mutations in the *SDHB* gene were found in two patients, while mutation in the *SDHD* gene was observed in one patient. Mutations were not determined in seven patients.

A sampling of biological materials was performed preoperatively (2 ± 3 weeks before surgery) and about one week (1 ± 0.5 weeks), six months (30 ± 10 weeks), one year (54 ± 6 weeks) and two years (96 ± 22 weeks) after surgery. A blood basal sampling was performed 20 min after the introduction of cannula in supine position. Four collections (before surgery, one week, six months, one year after surgery) were conducted in 27 patients (25 PCC, 2 PGL); 19 blood samplings were from patients treated with proton pump inhibitors. Three collections (before surgery, one week, six months after surgery) were from seven PCC patients, in which four samplings were from patients treated with PPI and one patient suffered from chronic renal insufficiency (CRI). Three collections (before surgery, one week, one year after surgery) were from one PCC and one PGL patient, one sampling of PGL patient was treated with PPI. Two collections (before surgery, one week after surgery) were from six PCC patients and two PGL patients, three samplings were from patients treated with PPI, one PGL patient had a recurrence of the disease (REC). Two collections were in one patient (before surgery, six months after surgery), two collections (before surgery, one year after surgery) were from three PCC patients. Two collections were in 10 PCC patients and two PGL patients (before surgery, two years after surgery), two PCC patients had REC of the disease. One collection was in 15 PCC patients and three PGL patients before surgery.

The control group consisted of 86 patients aged 53 ± 19 (7–84) years, 57 females and 29 males without diagnosis of PCC or PGL. These patients, however, had adrenal problems, or were diagnosed with MEN syndrome and with medullary, papillary or follicular thyroid carcinoma. The rest of the control group suffered from thyroid diseases (goiter, thyroiditis, thyroid nodules). Forty six patients had adrenocortical adenoma, two of whom suffered from hypertension; two patients had serious cardiovascular problems, one adenoma was accompanied by MTC and FTC, one adenoma was accompanied by PTC. Nine patients suffered from hypertension, one of these patients had severe chronic renal insufficiency. Nine patients had MEN2A syndrome, which was associated with MTC in seven patients. MTC was detected in addition to MEN2B in three patients. Ten patients suffered from MTC, one of whom was also diagnosed with PTC. Four other patients were found to have PTC. Five patients had thyroid disease (one goiter, one thyroiditis, and three thyroid nodules). The study was approved by the Internal Grant Agency, Ministry of Health of the Czech Republic, grant No. NT/12336-4 and local Ethical Committee, which also examined and adopted the informed consent of the patient.

4.2. Laboratory Examination

CGA was determined in the EDTA-plasma using a commercially available a solid-phase two-site immunoradiometric assay with primary immobilized monoclonal antibodies and secondary radioiodinated monoclonal antibodies, both directed against sterically remote sites on the CGA molecule (manufacturer Cisbio Bioassays, Codolet, France; code CGA-RIACT). The cut-off value of

CGA in the EDTA plasma 150 μg/L was determined on the basis of our results and information from the Cisbio company that 97% of healthy persons (n = 60) had CGA below 97 μg/L with a maximum concentration of 146 μg/L.

Free MN and NMN were determined in human EDTA plasma by competitive radioimmunoassay using a MetCombi Plasma RIA kit (IBL International GmbH, Hamburg, Germany, code RE29111). The cut-off values were 100 ng/L for metanephrine and 170 ng/L for normetanephrine.

4.3. Statistics

All statistical calculations were made using the computer program NCSS 2004 (Number Cruncher Statistical Systems, Kaysville, UT, USA).

5. Conclusions

We can conclude that plasma CGA determined by immunoassay, which is simple without the necessity of special laboratory equipment, is an effective marker of PPGLs and can serve as an appropriate complement to MN and NMN assays in laboratory diagnosis of PPGL patients. Based on 90% clinical sensitivity, CGA can provide additional information to metanephrines, but absence of elevated CGA should not be relied on to rule out PPGL. In all cases of PPGL patients under investigation the combination of metanephrines and CGA gave 100% results of clinical sensitivity. Plasma CGA also exerts an association to PASS score, tumor mass and tumor volume.

Author Contributions: Conceptualization, R.B., L.Š. and T.Z.; Methodology, R.B., L.Š., D.M., K.N., J.D. and E.V.; Software, R.B., Validation, R.B., L.Š., J.D., E.V., J.W.J. and T.Z.; Resources, R.B., P.V., L.Š. and T.Z.; Data Curation, R.B., P.V., L.Š. and T.Z.; Writing—Original Draft Preparation, R.B.; Writing—Review and Editing, R.B. and T.Z.; Supervision, J.W.J.; Project Administration, R.B.; Funding Acquisition, R.B.

Funding: This research was funded by grants IGA MZ CR NT/12336-4, MH CZ-DRO (Institute of Endocrinology-EÚ, 00023761); MZ CR 16-30345 and PROGRES Q28/LF1 (research program of Charles University).

Conflicts of Interest: The authors declare no conflict of interest.

References

1. Modlin, I.M.; Gustafsson, B.I.; Moss, S.F.; Pavel, M.; Tsolakis, A.V.; Kidd, M. Chromogranin A-biological function and clinical utility in neuro endocrine tumor disease. *Ann. Surg. Oncol.* **2010**, *17*, 2427–2443. [CrossRef]
2. Modlin, I.M.; Oberg, K.; Chung, D.C.; Jensen, R.T.; de Herder, W.W.; Thakker, R.V.; Caplin, M.; Delle Fave, G.; Kaltsas, G.A.; Krenning, E.P.; et al. Gastroenteropancreatic neuroendocrine tumours. *Lancet Oncol.* **2008**, *9*, 61–72. [CrossRef]
3. Oronsky, B.; Ma, P.C.; Morgensztern, D.; Carter, C.A. Nothing but NET: A Review of Neuroendocrine Tumors and Carcinomas. *Neoplasia* **2017**, *19*, 991–1002. [CrossRef] [PubMed]
4. Di Giacinto, P.; Rota, F.; Rizza, L.; Campana, D.; Isidori, A.; Lania, A.; Lenzi, A.; Zuppi, P.; Baldelli, R. Chromogranin A: From Laboratory to Clinical Aspects of Patients with Neuroendocrine Tumors. *Int. J. Endocrinol.* **2018**, *2018*, 8126087. [CrossRef]
5. Marotta, V.; Zatelli, M.C.; Sciammarella, C.; Ambrosio, M.R.; Bondanelli, M.; Colao, A.; Faggiano, A. Chromogranin A as circulating marker for diagnosis and management of neuroendocrine neoplasms: More flaws than fame. *Endocr. Relat. Cancer* **2018**, *25*, R11–R29. [CrossRef] [PubMed]
6. Tischler, A.S. Molecular and cellular biology of pheochromocytomas and extra-adrenal paragangliomas. *Endocr. Pathol.* **2006**, *17*, 321–328. [CrossRef]
7. Lenders, J.W.; Duh, Q.Y.; Eisenhofer, G.; Gimenez-Roqueplo, A.P.; Grebe, S.K.; Murad, M.H.; Naruse, M.; Pacak, K.; Young, W.F., Jr. Endocrine Society. Pheochromocytoma and paraganglioma: An endocrine society clinical practice guideline. *J. Clin. Endocrinol. Metab.* **2014**, *99*, 1915–1942. [CrossRef]
8. Pacak, K.; Tella, S.H. Pheochromocytoma and Paraganglioma. Available online: https://www.ncbi.nlm.nih.gov/books/NBK481899/ (accessed on 5 November 2018).

9. Eisenhofer, G.; Lenders, J.W.; Pacak, K. Biochemical diagnosis of pheochromocytoma. *Front. Horm. Res.* **2004**, *31*, 76–106.
10. Asa, S.L.; Ezzat, S.; Mete, O. The Diagnosis and Clinical Significance of Paragangliomas in Unusual Locations. *J. Clin. Med.* **2018**, *7*, 280. [CrossRef] [PubMed]
11. Chen, H.; Sippel, R.S.; O'Dorisio, M.S.; Vinik, A.I.; Lloyd, R.V.; Pacak, K. North American Neuroendocrine Tumor Society (NANETS): The North American Neuroendocrine Tumor Society consensus guideline for the diagnosis and management of neuroendocrine tumors: Pheochromocytoma; paraganglioma; and medullary thyroid cancer. *Pancreas* **2010**, *39*, 775–783. [CrossRef]
12. Van Berkel, A.; Lenders, J.W.; Timmers, H.J. Diagnosis of endocrine disease: Biochemical diagnosis of phaeochromocytoma and paraganglioma. *Eur. J. Endocrinol.* **2014**, *170*, R109–R119. [CrossRef]
13. Andersen, K.F.; Altaf, R.; Krarup-Hansen, A.; Kromann-Andersen, B.; Horn, T.; Christensen, N.J.; Hendel, H.W. Malignant pheochromocytomas and paragangliomas—The importance of a multidisciplinary approach. *Cancer Treat. Rev.* **2011**, *37*, 111–119. [CrossRef] [PubMed]
14. Lenders, J.W.; Eisenhofer, G.; Mannelli, M.; Pacak, K. Phaeochromocytoma. *Lancet* **2005**, *366*, 665–675. [CrossRef]
15. Crona, J.; Taieb, D.; Pacak, K. New Perspectives on Pheochromocytoma and Paraganglioma: Toward a Molecular Classification. *Endocr. Rev.* **2017**, *38*, 489–515. [CrossRef] [PubMed]
16. D'amico, M.A.; Ghinassi, B.; Izzicupo, P.; Manzoli, L.; Di Baldassarre, A. Biological function and clinical relevance of chromogranin A and derived peptides. *Endocr. Connect.* **2014**, *3*, R45–R54. [CrossRef] [PubMed]
17. D'Herbomez, M.; Do Cao, C.; Vezzosi, D.; Borzon-Chasot, F.; Baudin, E.; Groupe des tumeurs endocrines (GTE France). Chromogranin A assay in clinical practice. *Ann. Endocrinol.* **2010**, *71*, 274–280. [CrossRef]
18. Helman, L.J.; Ahn, T.G.; Levine, M.A.; Allison, A.; Cohen, P.S.; Cooper, M.J.; Cohn, D.V.; Israel, M.A. Molecular cloning and primary structure of human chromogranin A (secretory protein I) cDNA. *J. Biol. Chem.* **1988**, *263*, 11559–11563. [PubMed]
19. Courel, M.; Rodemer, C.; Nguyen, S.T.; Pance, A.; Jackson, A.P.; O'Connor, D.T.; Taupenot, L. Secretory granule biogenesis in sympathoadrenal cells: Identification of a granulogenic determinant in the secretory prohormone chromogranin A. *J. Biol. Chem.* **2006**, *281*, 38038–38051. [CrossRef] [PubMed]
20. Koshimizu, H.; Kim, T.; Cawley, N.X.; Loh, Y.P. Reprint of: Chromogranin A: A new proposal for trafficking; processing and induction of granule biogenesis. *Regul. Pept.* **2010**, *165*, 95–101. [CrossRef] [PubMed]
21. Corti, A.; Marcucci, F.; Bachetti, T. Circulating chromogranin A and its fragments as diagnostic and prognostic disease markers. *Pflugers Arch.* **2018**, *470*, 199–210. [CrossRef]
22. Borges, R.; Díaz-Vera, J.; Domínguez, N.; Arnau, M.R.; Machado, J.D. Chromogranins as regulators of exocytosis. *J. Neurochem.* **2010**, *114*, 335–343. [CrossRef] [PubMed]
23. Yoo, S.H. Secretory granules in inositol 1;4;5-trisphosphate-dependent Ca^{2+} signaling in the cytoplasm of neuroendocrine cells. *FASEB J.* **2010**, *24*, 653–664. [CrossRef]
24. Nelson, N.; Harvey, W.R. Vacuolar and plasma membrane proton-adenosinetriphosphatases. *Physiol. Rev.* **1999**, *79*, 361–385. [CrossRef]
25. Kimura, N.; Takekoshi, K.; Naruse, M. Risk Stratification on Pheochromocytoma and Paraganglioma from Laboratory and Clinical Medicine. *J. Clin. Med.* **2018**, *7*, 242. [CrossRef]
26. Zuber, S.; Wesley, R.; Prodanov, T.; Eisenhofer, G.; Pacak, K.; Kantorovich, V. Clinical utility of chromogranin A in SDHx-related paragangliomas. *Eur. J. Clin. Investig.* **2014**, *44*, 365–371. [CrossRef] [PubMed]
27. Thompson, L.D. Phaeochromocytoma of the adrenal gland scoring scale (PASS) to separate benign from malignant neoplasms. A clinicopathologic and immunophenotypic study of 100 cases. *Am. J. Surg. Pathol.* **2002**, *26*, 551–566. [CrossRef] [PubMed]
28. Szalat, A.; Fraenkel, M.; Doviner, V.; Salmon, A.; Gross, D.J. Malignant pheochromocytoma: Predictive factors of malignancy and clinical course in 16 patients at a single tertiary medical center. *Endocrine* **2011**, *39*, 160–166. [CrossRef] [PubMed]
29. Yang, X.; Yang, Y.; Li, Z.; Cheng, C.; Yang, T.; Wang, C.; Liu, L.; Liu, S. Diagnostic value of circulating chromogranin a for neuroendocrine tumors: A systematic review and meta-analysis. *PLoS ONE* **2015**, *10*, e0124884. [CrossRef]
30. Bilek, R.; Safarik, L.; Ciprova, V.; Vlcek, P.; Lisa, L. Chromogranin A; a member of neuroendocrine secretory proteins as a selective marker for laboratory diagnosis of pheochromocytoma. *Physiol. Res.* **2008**, *57*, S171–S179.

31. D'Herbomez, M.; Gouze, V.; Huglo, D.; Nocaudie, M.; Pattou, F.; Proye, C.; Wemeau, J.L.; Marchandise, X. Chromogranin A assay and (131)I-MIBG scintigraphy for diagnosis and follow-up of pheochromocytoma. *J. Nucl. Med.* **2001**, *42*, 993–997. [PubMed]
32. Giovanella, L.; Squin, N.; Ghelfo, A.; Ceriani, L. Chromogranin A immunoradiometric assay in diagnosis of pheochromocytoma: Comparison with plasma metanephrines and 123I-MIBG scan. *Q. J. Nucl. Med. Mol. Imaging* **2006**, *50*, 344–347. [PubMed]
33. Vinik, A.I.; Woltering, E.A.; Warner, R.R.; Caplin, M.; O'Dorisio, T.M.; Wiseman, G.A.; Coppola, D.; Go, V.L.; North American Neuroendocrine Tumor Society (NANETS). North American Neuroendocrine Tumor Society (NANETS). NANETS consensus guidelines for the diagnosis of neuroendocrine tumor. *Pancreas* **2010**, *39*, 13–34. [CrossRef] [PubMed]
34. Malaguarnera, M.; Vacante, M.; Fichera, R.; Cappellani, A.; Cristaldi, E.; Motta, M. Chromogranin A (CgA) serum level as a marker of progression in hepatocellular carcinoma (HCC) of elderly patients. *Arch. Gerontol. Geriatr.* **2010**, *51*, 81–85. [CrossRef] [PubMed]
35. Lawrence, B.; Gustafsson, B.I.; Kidd, M.; Pavel, M.; Svejda, B.; Modlin, I.M. The clinical relevance of chromogranin A as a biomarker for gastroenteropancreatic neuroendocrine tumors. *Endocrinol. Metab. Clin. N. Am.* **2011**, *40*, 111–134. [CrossRef]
36. Giovinazzo, F.; Schimmack, S.; Svejda, B.; Alaimo, D.; Pfragner, R.; Modlin, I.; Kidd, M. Chromogranin A and its fragments as regulators of small intestinal neuroendocrine neoplasm proliferation. *PLoS ONE* **2013**, *8*, e81111. [CrossRef]
37. Korse, C.M.; Muller, M.; Taal, B.G. Discontinuation of proton pump inhibitors during assessment of chromogranin A levels in patients with neuroendocrine tumours. *Br. J. Cancer* **2011**, *105*, 1173–1175. [CrossRef]
38. Mosli, H.H.; Dennis, A.; Kocha, W.; Asher, L.J.; Van Uum, S.H. Effect of short-term proton pump inhibitor treatment and its discontinuation on chromogranin A in healthy subjects. *J. Clin. Endocrinol. Metab.* **2012**, *97*, E1731–E1735. [CrossRef]
39. O'Connor, D.T.; Pandlan, M.R.; Carlton, E.; Cervenka, J.H.; Hslao, R.J. Rapid radioimmunoassay of circulating chromogranin A: In vitro stability; exploration of the neuroendocrine character of neoplasia; and assessment of the effects of organ failure. *Clin. Chem.* **1989**, *35*, 1631–1637.
40. Mikkelsen, G.; Asberg, A.; Hultström, M.E.; Aasarod, K.; Hov, G.G. Reference limits for chromogranin A; CYFRA 21-1; CA 125; CA 19-9 and carcinoembryonic antigen in patients with chronic kidney disease. *Int. J. Biol. Markers* **2017**, *32*, e461–e466. [CrossRef]
41. Peracchi, M.; Gebbia, C.; Basilisco, G.; Quatrini, M.; Tarantino, C.; Vescarelli, C.; Massironi, S.; Conte, D. Plasma chromogranin A in patients with autoimmune chronic atrophic gastritis; enterochromaffin-like cell lesions and gastric carcinoids. *Eur. J. Endocrinol.* **2005**, *152*, 443–448. [CrossRef]
42. Massironi, S.; Fraquelli, M.; Paggi, S.; Sangiovanni, A.; Conte, D.; Sciola, V.; Ciafardini, C.; Colombo, M.; Peracchi, M. Chromogranin A levels in chronic liver disease and hepatocellular carcinoma. *Dig. Liver. Dis.* **2009**, *41*, 31–35. [CrossRef] [PubMed]
43. Sidhu, R.; McAlindon, M.E.; Leeds, J.S.; Skilling, J.; Sanders, D.S. The role of serum chromogranin A in diarrhoea predominant irritable bowel syndrome. *J. Gastrointestin. Liver. Dis.* **2009**, *18*, 23–26.
44. Estensen, M.E.; Hognestad, A.; Syversen, U.; Squire, I.; Ng, L.; Kjekshus, J.; Dickstein, K.; Omland, T. Prognostic value of plasma chromogranin A levels in patients with complicated myocardial infarction. *Am. Heart J.* **2006**, *152*, e1–e6. [CrossRef]
45. Jansson, A.M.; Rosjo, H.; Omland, T.; Karlsson, T.; Hartford, M.; Flyvbjerg, A.; Caidahl, K. Prognostic value of circulating chromogranin A levels in acute coronary syndromes. *Eur. Heart J.* **2009**, *30*, 25–32. [CrossRef]
46. Zelinka, T.; Petrak, O.; Turkova, H.; Holaj, R.; Strauch, B.; Krsek, M.; Vrankova, A.B.; Musil, Z.; Dusková, J.; Kubinyi, J.; et al. High incidence of cardiovascular complications in pheochromocytoma. *Horm. Metab. Res.* **2012**, *44*, 379–384. [CrossRef]
47. Bilek, R.; Zelinka, T.; Vlcek, P.; Duskova, J.; Michalsky, D.; Novak, K.; Vaclavikova, E.; Widimsky, J., Jr. Radioimmunoassay of chromogranin A and free metanephrines in diagnosis of pheochromocytoma. *Physiol. Res.* **2017**, *66*, S397–S408.
48. Eisenhofer, G.; Lenders, J.W.; Goldstein, D.S.; Mannelli, M.; Csako, G.; Walther, M.M.; Brouwers, F.M.; Pacak, K. Pheochromocytoma catecholamine phenotypes and prediction of tumor size and location by use of plasma free metanephrines. *Clin. Chem.* **2005**, *51*, 735–744. [CrossRef]

49. Van Duinen, N.; Kema, I.P.; Romijn, J.A.; Corssmit, E.P. Plasma chromogranin A levels are increased in a small portion of patients with hereditary head and neck paragangliomas. *Clin. Endocrinol.* **2011**, *74*, 160–165. [CrossRef] [PubMed]
50. Stenman, A.; Zedenius, J.; Juhlin, C.C. The Value of Histological Algorithms to Predict the Malignancy Potential of Pheochromocytomas and Abdominal Paragangliomas. A Meta-Analysis and Systematic Review of the Literature. *Cancers* **2019**, *11*, 225. [CrossRef]
51. Plouin, P.F.; Amar, L.; Dekkers, O.M.; Fassnacht, M.; Gimenez-Roqueplo, A.P.; Lenders, J.W.; Lussey-Lepoutre, C.; Steichen, O.; Guideline Working Group. European Society of Endocrinology Clinical Practice Guideline for long-term follow-up of patients operated on for a phaeochromocytoma or a paraganglioma. *Eur. J. Endocrinol.* **2016**, *174*, G1–G10. [CrossRef]
52. Yoo, S.H.; Albanesi, J.P. Ca2(+)-induced conformational change and aggregation of chromogranin A. *J. Biol. Chem.* **1990**, *265*, 14414–14421. [PubMed]

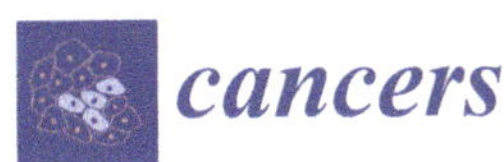 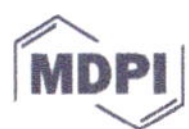

Article

Impact of Extrinsic and Intrinsic Hypoxia on Catecholamine Biosynthesis in Absence or Presence of Hif2α in Pheochromocytoma Cells

Nicole Bechmann [1,*], Isabel Poser [1], Verena Seifert [2], Christian Greunke [3], Martin Ullrich [2], Nan Qin [4,5,6,7], Axel Walch [3], Mirko Peitzsch [1], Mercedes Robledo [8], Karel Pacak [9], Jens Pietzsch [2,10], Susan Richter [1] and Graeme Eisenhofer [1,11]

1 Institute of Clinical Chemistry and Laboratory Medicine, University Hospital Carl Gustav Carus, Technische Universität Dresden, Fetscherstrasse 74, 01307 Dresden, Germany; Isabel.poser@uniklinikum-dresden.de (I.P.); Mirko.peitzsch@uniklinikum-dresden.de (M.P.); susan.richter@uniklinikum-dresden.de (S.R.); Graeme.eisenhofer@uniklinikum-dresden.de (G.E.)
2 Department of Radiopharmaceutical and Chemical Biology, Helmholtz-Zentrum Dresden-Rossendorf, Institute of Radiopharmaceutical Cancer Research, Bautzner Landstrasse 400, 01328 Dresden, Germany; v.seifert@hzdr.de (V.S.); m.ullrich@hzdr.de (M.U.); j.pietzsch@hzdr.de (J.P.)
3 Research Unit Analytical Pathology, Helmholtz Zentrum München, German Research Center for Environmental Health (GmbH), Neuherberg, Germany; Ingolstädter Landstraße 1, 85764 Neuherberg, Germany; christian.greunke@gmx.de (C.G.); axel.walch@helmholtz-muenchen.de (A.W.)
4 Division of Pediatric Neuro-Oncogenomics, German Cancer Research Center (DKFZ), 69120 Heidelberg, Germany; nan.qin@med.uni-duesseldorf.de
5 German Consortium for Translational Cancer Research (DKTK), partner site Essen/Düsseldorf, 45147 Düsseldorf, Germany
6 Department of Pediatric Oncology, Hematology, and Clinical Immunology, Medical Faculty, University Hospital Düsseldorf, 40225 Düsseldorf, Germany
7 Department of Neuropathology, Medical Faculty, Heinrich-Heine University Düsseldorf, 40225 Düsseldorf, Germany
8 Hereditary Endocrine Cancer Group, CNIO, Madrid, Spain and Centro de Investigación Biomédica en Red de Enfermedades Raras (CIBERER), 28029 Madrid, Spain; mrobledo@cnio.es
9 Section on Medical Neuroendocrinology, Eunice Kennedy Shriver National Institute of Child Health and Human Development, National Institutes of Health, Bethesda, MD 20892, USA; karel@mail.nih.gov
10 Department of Chemistry and Food Chemistry, School of Science, Technische Universität Dresden, Mommsenstrasse 9, 01062 Dresden, Germany
11 Department of Medicine III, University Hospital Carl Gustav Carus, Technische Universität Dresden, Fetscherstrasse 74, 01307 Dresden, Germany
* Correspondence: Nicole.bechmann@uniklinikum-dresden.de; Tel.: +49-351-45819687

Received: 26 March 2019; Accepted: 25 April 2019; Published: 28 April 2019

Abstract: Pheochromocytomas and paragangliomas (PPGLs) with activated pseudohypoxic pathways are associated with an immature catecholamine phenotype and carry a higher risk for metastasis. For improved understanding of the underlying mechanisms we investigated the impact of hypoxia and pseudohypoxia on catecholamine biosynthesis in pheochromocytoma cells naturally lacking *Hif2α* (MPC and MTT) or expressing both *Hif1α* and *Hif2α* (PC12). Cultivation under extrinsic hypoxia or in spheroid culture (intrinsic hypoxia) increased cellular dopamine and norepinephrine contents in all cell lines. To distinguish further between *Hif1α*- and *Hif2α*-driven effects we expressed *Hif2α* in MTT and MPC-mCherry cells (naturally lacking *Hif2α*). Presence of *Hif2α* resulted in similarly increased cellular dopamine and norepinephrine under hypoxia as in the control cells. Furthermore, hypoxia resulted in enhanced phosphorylation of tyrosine hydroxylase (TH). A specific knockdown of *Hif1α* in PC12 diminished these effects. Pseudohypoxic conditions, simulated by expression of *Hif2α* under normoxia resulted in increased TH phosphorylation, further stimulated by extrinsic hypoxia. Correlations with PPGL tissue data led us to conclude that catecholamine biosynthesis under hypoxia is mainly mediated through increased phosphorylation of TH, regulated as a short-term response (24–48 h) by HIF1α. Continuous activation of hypoxia-related genes under pseudohypoxia leads to a HIF2α-mediated phosphorylation of TH (permanent status).

Keywords: hypoxia; pseudohypoxia; spheroids; HIF; EPAS1; catecholamine; pheochromocytoma and paraganglioma; phosphorylation tyrosine hydroxylase

---

1. Introduction

Pheochromocytomas and extra-adrenal paragangliomas (PPGLs) are rare catecholamine-producing neuroendocrine tumors with variable aggressiveness. PPGLs with activated pseudohypoxic pathways (cluster 1), including those with mutations in genes encoding hypoxia-inducible factor (*HIF*) *2α* (also known as *EPAS1*), von Hippel-Lindau tumor suppressor (*VHL*), prolyl hydroxylase domain (*PHD*), fumarate hydratase, and succinate dehydrogenase subunits (*SDHx*) are characterized by an immature catecholamine phenotype and higher risk of metastasis particularly prevalent in SDHx-mutated tumors [1–3]. In contrast, PPGLs with genetic alterations associated with activated kinase signaling pathways (cluster 2) are mostly benign and show a mature catecholamine phenotype with strong expression of phenylethanolamine *N*-methyltransferase (PNMT), the enzyme that converts norepinephrine (NEpi) to epinephrine (Epi) [3,4]. Increased stabilization of HIFs and resulting activation of hypoxia-related pathways seem to play a central role in the development and progression of PPGLs [5]. Under normoxic conditions, the oxygen-sensitive HIFα subunit of the HIFα/HIFβ complex is degraded by PHD- and VHL-mediated mechanisms. Insufficient oxygen (≤1% oxygen), also known as hypoxia, leads to stabilization of the HIFα subunit resulting in the regulation of numerous HIF-target genes, either by interaction with HIF1β followed by the transactivation of the hypoxia responsive element (HRE) or by interactions with NOTCH, WNT, and MYC pathways [6].

There are two main HIFα isoforms, HIF1α and HIF2α, with partly overlapping functions, regulating numerous processes including angiogenesis, cell survival, stem cell self-renewal and pro-metastatic features of tumor cells. Gene expression profiling and immunohistochemical studies have established enhanced expression of HIF2α, but no differences in expression of HIF1α, in cluster 1 compared to cluster 2 PPGLs [4,7–9]. In chromaffin cells, HIF2α seems to be responsible for maintaining the balance between differentiation and stemness of the sympathoadrenal lineage, with both HIFα subunits regulating biosynthesis, storage and secretion of catecholamines [10]. Expression of tyrosine hydroxylase (TH), the rate-limiting enzyme in catecholamine biosynthesis and responsible for conversion of tyrosine to L-dihydroxyphenylalanine (L-DOPA), is inducible by hypoxia. Both HIFα subunits are able to bind at the HRE of the *TH* promoter, thereby increasing TH expression [11]. Besides altered expression, TH enzyme activity further depends on posttranslational phosphorylation at serine 8, 19, 31, and 40 [12,13]. A specific knockdown of *Hif2α* by RNA interference had no effect on *Th* mRNA expression in a rat adrenomedullary chromaffin cell line; in contrast, an influence on DOPA decarboxylase (*Ddc*), the enzyme responsible for conversion of L-DOPA to dopamine (DA), was established by changes in mRNA expression [14]. Park and coworkers investigated impacts of HIF1α protein stabilization on catecholamine-induced expression of vascular endothelial growth factor (VEGF) and showed that treatment with NEpi stimulated HIF1α protein stabilization associated with increased angiogenesis [15]. Furthermore, PNMT expression seemed to be predominantly regulated by HIF1α [16,17]. These findings suggest that HIF1α is the major player for the stress-induced fight-or-flight response (short-term response) by regulating the biosynthesis of Epi. In contrast, HIF2α seems to be more important for the regulation of developmental processes (long-term response), such as those associated with immature chromaffin cell features including absence of PNMT expression with missing production of Epi in cluster 1 PPGLs [18,19] and promotes an aggressive phenotype [20].

Three-dimensional tumor cell spheroids provide an excellent in vitro model to study the influence of hypoxia (intrinsic hypoxia) under conditions close to the in vivo situation within tumors. This is because in contrast to monolayer culture, tumor cell spheroids mimic the tumor microenvironment and the structure of the spheroid encourages the formation of an oxygen and nutrient gradient (Figure 1A).

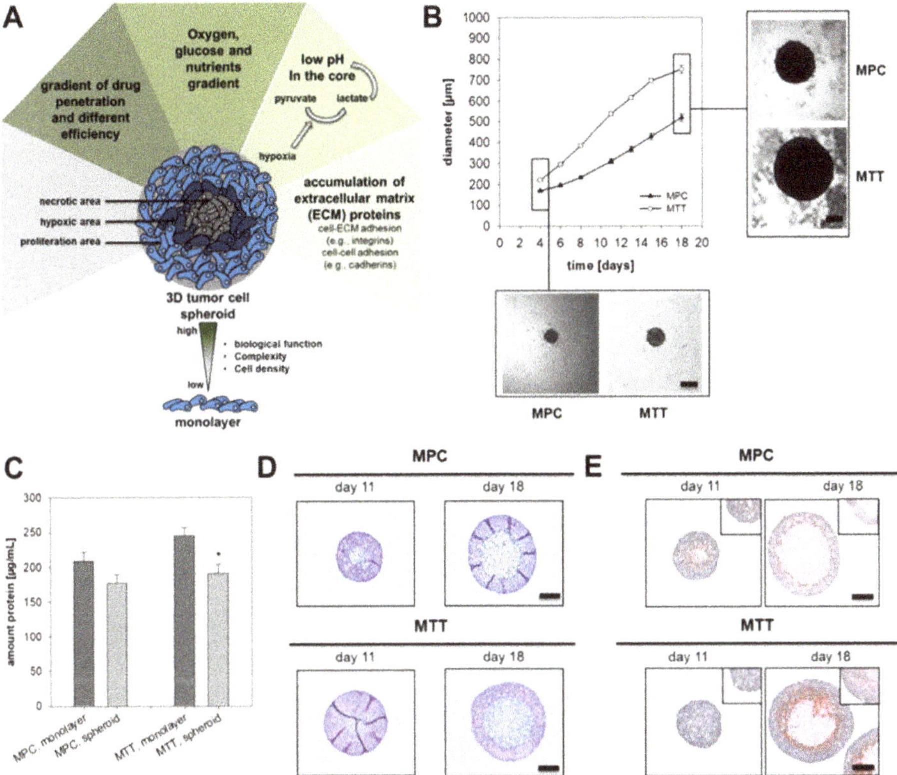

Figure 1. Characterization of pheochromocytoma cell spheroids. (**A**) Tumor cell spheroids are characterized by a necrotic core surrounded by hypoxic cell layers and an external zone of proliferating cells. This structure encourages the formation of an oxygen, pH and nutrient gradient and leads to accumulation of extracellular matrix proteins. Complexity and comparability with the structure of a metastasis offers an important tool for drug screening. (**B**) Growth pattern of MPC and MTT cell spheroids generated by using methylcellulose method. Four independent experiments (n = 15–20). Mean ± SEM. (**C**) Impact of spheroid cultivation on the amount of protein produced by 500 cells over a time-period of eight days in comparison to monolayer conditions. Four independent experiments (n = 16). Mean ± SEM. ANOVA and Bonferroni post hoc test comparison vs. monolayer, * $p < 0.05$. (**D**) Representative section of pheochromocytoma cell spheroids stained with Hematoxylin and Eosin (nuclei: blue, cytosol: violet). (**E**) Covalent binding of pimonidazole confirmed the development of a hypoxic region (red) surrounding the necrotic core of the spheroids (nuclei: blue). Scale bar: 200 µm.

Several studies have shown the excellent suitability of this model for drug screenings [21,22] and investigations of the microenvironment [23] also on pheochromocytoma cell lines. The present study investigates the hypothesis, that pheochromocytoma cell spheroids provide a suitable model to examine chromaffin cell features such as catecholamine biosynthesis in vitro. Therefore, mouse pheochromocytoma cells (MPC) generated from a neurofibromin 1 knockout mouse model [24] and its more aggressive derivate, the MTT cell line [25], were used as models and cultivated under intrinsic or extrinsic (monolayer culture with 1% oxygen) hypoxia. Cellular catecholamine contents were analyzed as a reflection of catecholamine biosynthesis, storage and turnover. We further addressed the question, about whether HIF1α or HIF2α is the key regulator of TH biosynthesis under hypoxic and pseudohypoxic conditions. Specific knockin or knockdown models were utilized to answer this question and in vitro data were compared to gene expression in PPGL tumor tissue.

2. Results

2.1. Spheroid Growth Pattern and Characteristics

In accordance with growth in monolayer culture, MTT cells showed an enhanced growth pattern in spheroid culture compared to MPC cells (Figure 1B). MPC cell spheroids reached a diameter of approximately 550 μm after 18 days in culture, whereas the MTT cell spheroids already achieved a diameter of 600 μm after 14 days. For both cell lines an optimized cell number (Figure S3) of 500 cells per well were used for spheroid generation to reach an exponential growth pattern over 18 days. Cultivation under spheroid conditions diminished protein contents, an expected finding due to reduced nutrient supply within spheroids (Figure 1C). In comparison to other methods (Figure S3–S5) the use of methyl cellulose leads to uniform spheroids without verifiable outgrowth. Pheochromocytoma spheroids were characterized by a necrotic core surrounded by a narrow hypoxic zone and an external zone of proliferating cells as confirmed by the covalent binding of pimonidazole (Figure 1D,E). MALDI mass spectrometry imaging (MALDI-MSI) was used to analyze the distribution of phosphatidylinositol (PIP) within the spheroids. Higher contents in the proliferating cell layers indicated that the membrane of the cells remained intact, while PIP contents in the necrotic core were reduced (Figure S7). Higher levels of hexose monophosphate in the outer cell layers of the spheroid indicated an enhanced metabolic activity in the hexose monophosphate shunt (Figure S7).

2.2. Impact of Extrinsic and Intrinsic Hypoxia on Catecholamine Biosynthesis

Hypoxia is an important contributor to intra- and inter-tumor cell diversity and is associated with reduced differentiation, as shown in neuroblastoma and breast cancer cells [26,27]. Furthermore, alterations in hypoxia-associated genes in pseudohypoxic cluster 1 PPGLs are associated with an immature catecholamine phenotype [3,18]. The establishment of pheochromocytoma cell spheroids allowed us for the first time to distinguish between short-term effects (extrinsic) and long-term effects (intrinsic) of hypoxia on chromaffin cell characteristics. Long-term exposure to extrinsic hypoxia is not suitable for the currently available pheochromocytoma cell lines, because of the complete loss of cell growth characteristics [28]. We investigated the impact of extrinsic ($O_2 \leq 1\%$) and intrinsic hypoxia on catecholamine biosynthesis in several pheochromocytoma cell lines (Figure S6). In MTT cells cultivated under extrinsic hypoxia or spheroid conditions TH protein levels (Figure 2A) were not affected but instead showed increased phosphorylation at Ser40, an indicator of enhanced catalytic activity (Figure 2B). Immunohistochemical staining showed increased expression of TH in the necrotic core and the surrounding hypoxic area of the spheroid (Figure 2C). MPC cells contained lower amounts of basal catecholamines compared to MTT cells. Extrinsic as well as intrinsic hypoxia led to a significant increase of cellular DA in both cell lines (Figure 2D,E). Cultivation under spheroid conditions further increased cellular NEpi. The hypoxic regions and necrotic core of the spheroid enlarged with increasing cultivation time; this was also reflected by enhanced DA and NEpi contents comparing 11- and 18-days old spheroids. Especially in MPC cell spheroids, DA and NEpi were much higher compared to the monolayer culture under extrinsic hypoxia. This indicates an additional impact of necrosis on catecholamine biosynthesis in spheroids.

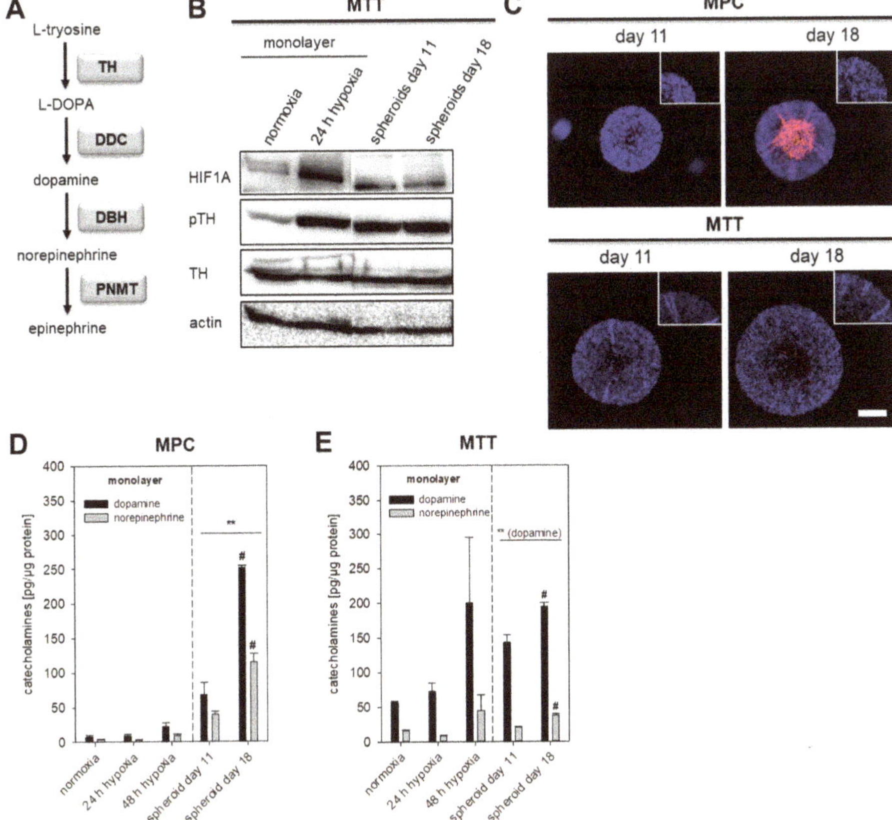

Figure 2. Impact of extrinsic and intrinsic hypoxia on catecholamine biosynthesis. (**A**) Section of biosynthetic pathways of catecholamines. Squares highlighted the underlying enzymes (TH: tyrosine hydroxylase; DDC: DOPA decarboxylase; DBH: dopamine β-hydroxylase; PNMT: phenylethanolamine *N*-methyltransferase). (**B**) Effect of extrinsic and intrinsic hypoxia on the protein expression and phosphorylation of TH at Ser40 in MTT cells. (**C**) Immunohistochemical staining showed an increased expression of TH (red) in the necrotic and hypoxic core of the spheroid (DAPI, blue). Scale bar: 200 µm. Catecholamine content of (**D**) MPC and (**E**) MTT cell spheroids in comparison to monolayer cultivation under normoxic or hypoxic conditions. Three independent experiments (n = 3–6). Mean ± SEM. ANOVA and Bonferroni post hoc test comparison vs. normoxia, ** $p < 0.01$, or vs. spheroid day 11, # $p < 0.05$ or, ## $p < 0.01$.

2.3. *HIF1α- and HIF2α-Mediated Effects on Catecholamine Biosynthesis*

MPC and MTT cells naturally lack *Hif2α*. To clarify whether *Hif1α* or *Hif2α* drives the induction of catecholamine biosynthesis under extrinsic hypoxia, we analyzed cellular catecholamines of the rat PC12 cell line expressing both *Hif1α* and *Hif2α*. PC12 cells were unable to form spheroids using different methods for spheroid generation (described in Supplementary Materials). Quantitative real-time polymerase chain reaction (qRT-PCR) showed enhanced expression of *Th* under extrinsic hypoxic conditions, whereas the expression of *Ddc* and *Dbh* remained unchanged (Figure 3B). Cultivation under extrinsic hypoxia led to an increased phosphorylation of TH at Ser40 (Figure 3C) and accumulation of DA in PC12 cells (Figure 3A). Presence of *Hif2α* in PC12 cells seemed not to have any effect on hypoxia-induced catecholamine biosynthesis.

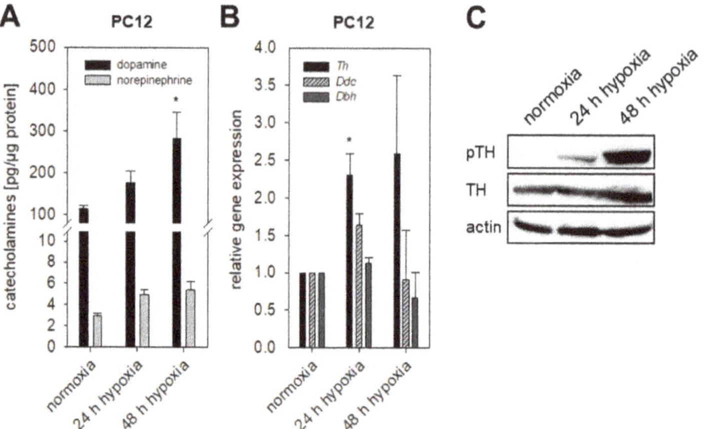

Figure 3. Impact of extrinsic hypoxia in presence of *Hif1α* and *Hif2α*. (**A**) Cellular catecholamines in PC12 cells in dependence of hypoxia. Presence of *Hif1α* and *Hif2α* led to an increase of dopamine within the cells. Three independent experiments (n = 6–9). Mean ± SEM. ANOVA and Bonferroni post hoc test comparison vs. normoxia, * $p < 0.05$. (**B**) Hypoxia resulted in a significant up-regulation of *Th* expression in PC12 cells under extrinsic hypoxia, whereas expression of *Ddc* and *Dbh* remained unaffected. Four independent experiments (n = 4). Mean ± SEM. ANOVA and Bonferroni post hoc test comparison vs. normoxia, * $p < 0.05$. (**C**) Hypoxia further enhanced phosphorylation of TH at Ser40 investigated by Western blot analysis. Shown is a representative section out of three independent experiments.

To mimic pseudohypoxic conditions, we expressed codon optimized *Hif2α* in MTT cells (MTT H2A) naturally lacking *Hif2α*. The counterpart cell line, transfected with an empty vector (MTT control), was used as a control (Table S1). The relative *Th* expression (Figure 4A) was not affected by the expression of *Hif2α* (pseudohypoxia). No differences in cellular DA and NEpi content between MTT H2A cells and MTT control cells were observed. Cultivation under extrinsic and intrinsic hypoxia increased cellular DA contents in both cell lines (Figure 4B). Spheroid culture conditions furthermore increased NEpi significantly. The relative expression of *Ddc* and *Dbh* was not affected by the incubation under extrinsic hypoxic conditions (Figure 4C). *Hif2α* expression led to increased phosphorylation of TH while the total amount of TH protein remained unaffected (Figure 4D). In the presence of *Hif2α* (pseudohypoxia), the exposure to extrinsic hypoxia only had a negligible effect on the TH phosphorylation. To confirm the previous results, we used MPC-mCherry cells (no *Hif2α* expression) with expression of *Hif2α* (MPC-mCherry H2A) and their counterpart cell line (MPC-mCherry control) [22]. Similar to the MTT H2A cells, expression of *Hif2α* in MPC-mCherry cells had no effect on *Th* gene expression and basal DA and NEpi contents under normoxic conditions (Figure 4E,F). Independent of *Hif2α* expression, cultivation under hypoxia resulted in increased DA and NEpi contents in both cell lines, indicating a predominantly *Hif1α*-mediated effect under extrinsic hypoxia (Figure 4F). Under extrinsic hypoxia, no effect on *Th* and *Dbh* expression was observed, but the expression of *Ddc* was significantly increased in MPC-mCherry H2A cells (Figure 4G). The expression of *Hif2α* (pseudohypoxia) was accompanied by an enhanced phosphorylation of TH that further increased in both cell lines under extrinsic hypoxia (Figure 4H). The generation of a pseudohypoxic environment by expression of *Hif2α* in MPC and MTT cells permitted comparison of catecholamine biosynthesis, gene expression and TH activation under both extrinsic and intrinsic hypoxia in presence or absence of a pseudohypoxic cellular environment.

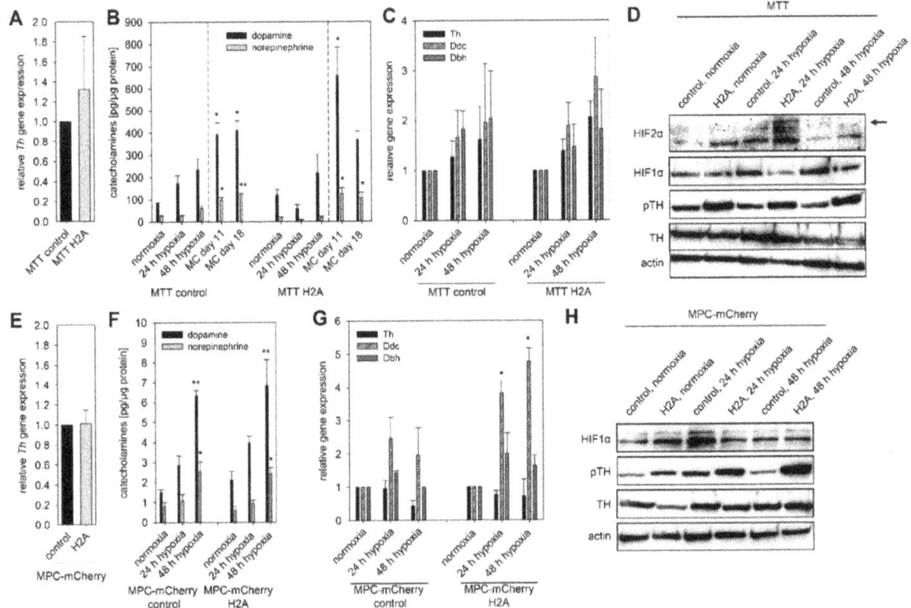

Figure 4. Expression of *Hif2α* in mouse pheochromocytoma cells (pseudohypoxic conditions) enhanced the basal phosphorylation (pseudohypoxic conditions) of TH, which was further increased by the exposure to hypoxia. (**A**) Expression of *Hif2α* in MTT cells had no effect on the relative *Th* expression determined by qRT-PCR. Three independent experiments ($n = 3$). Mean ± SEM. (**B**) In both cell lines with different *Hif2α* expression, exposure to extrinsic or intrinsic hypoxia led to elevated DA and NEpi, especially in spheroids generated with the methyl cellulose (MC) method. Three independent experiments ($n = 9$). Mean ± SEM. ANOVA and Bonferroni post hoc test comparison vs. normoxia, * $p < 0.05$, or ** $p < 0.01$. (**C**) In MTT cells, expression of *Th*, *Ddc* and *Dbh* increased by the exposure to hypoxia independent of their *Hif2α* expression. Three independent experiments ($n = 3$). Mean ± SEM. (**D**) Pseudohypoxia, simulated by the expression of *Hif2α* as well as extrinsic hypoxia led to an enhance phosphorylation of TH at Ser40 in MTT cells. Representative sections of three independent Western blot analysis were shown. To confirm these results MPC-mCherry cells expressing *Hif2α* and their counterpart cell line were used. (**E**) Expression of *Hif2α* in MPC-mCherry cells had no impact on the relative *Th* expression. Six independent experiments ($n = 6$). Mean ± SEM. (**F**) Similar to MTT cells the exposure to hypoxia resulted in enhanced DA and NEpi in both MPC-mCherry cell lines. Three independent experiments ($n = 9$). Mean ± SEM. ANOVA and Bonferroni post hoc test comparison vs. normoxia, * $p < 0.05$, or ** $p < 0.01$. (**G**) Expression of *Hif2α* was associated with increased expression of *Ddc* under extrinsic hypoxia. Four independent experiments ($n = 4$). Mean ± SEM. ANOVA and Bonferroni post hoc test comparison vs. normoxia, * $p < 0.05$. (**H**) Western blot analysis confirmed the enhanced phosphorylation of TH at Ser40 under pseudohypoxic conditions in MPC-mCherry cells. Extrinsic hypoxia further increased this effect. Three independent experiments.

Exposure to extrinsic hypoxia led to a time-dependent upregulation of *Hif1α* and *Hif2α* in PC12 (Figure 5A). In the next step, we reduced the expression of *Hif1α* in PC12 cells using RNA interference. A stable knockdown efficiency of 42.1 ± 5.7% was achieved over at least 72 h, also under extrinsic hypoxia (Figure 5B,C). The knockdown of *Hif1α* had no effect on expression of *Hif2α* (Figure 5B). Specific knockdown of *Hif1α* reduced hypoxia-induced DA content of PC12 cells significantly (Figure 5C). Moreover, specific knockdown of *Hif1α* led to reduced phosphorylation of TH at Ser40, while the total TH protein amount remained unaffected (Figure 5D).

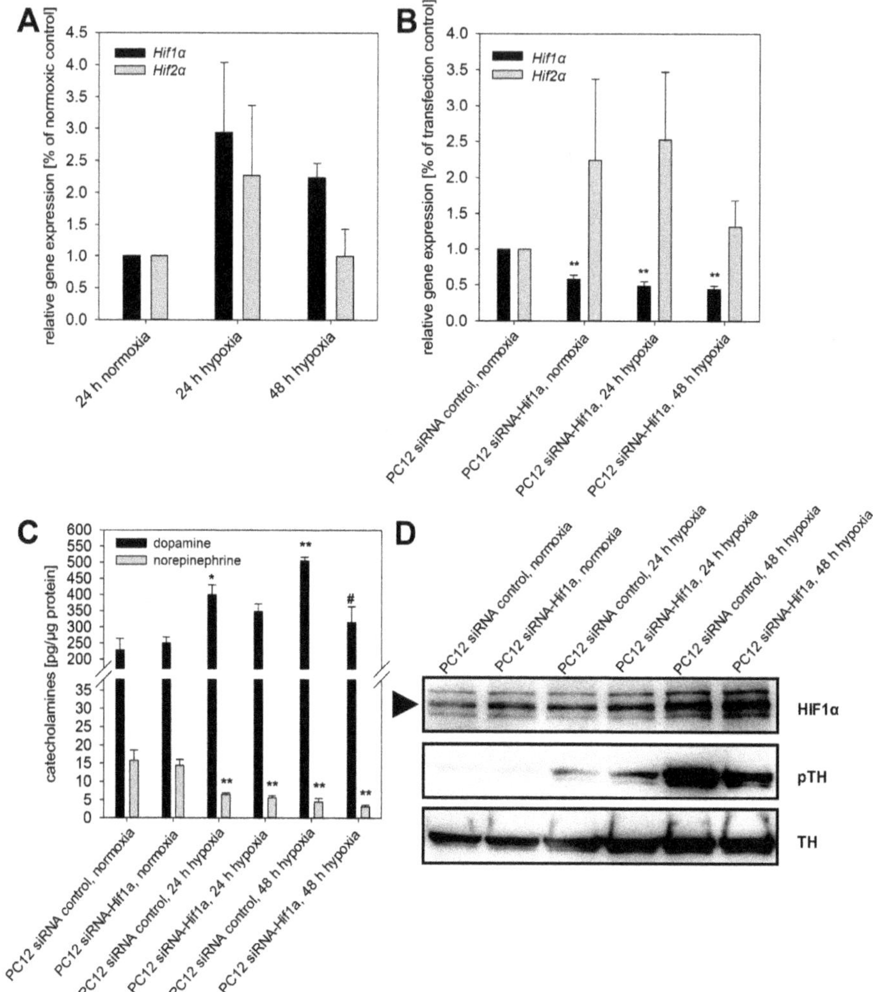

Figure 5. Specific knockdown of *Hif1α* diminished phosphorylation of tyrosine hydroxylase and thereby reduced cellular dopamine content in PC12 cells. (**A**) Extrinsic hypoxia led to a time-dependent upregulation of *Hif1α* and *Hif2α* in PC12. (**B**) RNA interference using siRNA against *Hif1α* repressed the expression of *Hif1α* also under extrinsic hypoxia while *Hif2α* remains unaffected. (**C**) Extrinsic hypoxia increased cellular dopamine content in PC12 control cells (transfection without siRNA). This effect was diminished by knockdown of *Hif1α*. (**D**) Furthermore, phosphorylation of TH was decreased by knockdown of *Hif1α*. Three independent experiments (n = 3–6). Mean ± SEM. ANOVA and Bonferroni post hoc test comparison vs. normoxia, * $p < 0.05$ or, ** $p < 0.01$, or vs. PC12 siRNA control 24 or 48 h hypoxia, # $p < 0.05$.

2.4. TH Expression under Pseudohypoxic Conditions In Vitro and In Vivo

In contrast to extrinsic and intrinsic hypoxia, pseudohypoxic conditions are characterized by the presence of oxygen with simultaneous activation of hypoxia-related pathways. We simulated pseudohypoxic conditions in vitro by the expression of *Hif2α* in MPC-mCherry and MTT cells under normoxic conditions (Figure 4). Expression of *Hif2α* had no effect on the expression of *Th* and cellular DA and NEpi contents. To correlate these findings with the in vivo situation, the *TH*, *HIF1α* and *HIF2α* expression in tumors from PPGL patients with known genetic mutation (Figure 6A) were analyzed using qRT-PCR (Figure 6C–E). Similar to other pseudohypoxic cluster 1 (5 *VHL*, 4 *SDHB*, 3 *SDHD*) PPGLs, tumors with a somatic gain-of-function mutation in *EPAS1/HIF2α* (n = 3) showed an increased expression of *HIF2α* compared to cluster 2 tumors (4 *NF1*, 6 *MEN2*), confirming previous results [4] in the present cohort (Figure 6A,C). All three groups (*EPAS1/HIF2α* vs. cluster 1 vs. cluster 2) showed a similar *TH* expression independent of *HIF2α* expression (Figure 6C), which is in accordance with our in vitro findings using mouse pheochromocytoma cells expressing *Hif2α* (Figure 4A,E). The three patients with *EPAS1/HIF2α* mutation consistently showed a doubling of NEpi in comparison to other cluster 1 tumors (Figure 6B). In mature cluster 2 PPGLs Epi was significantly elevated in comparison to immature cluster 1 tumors. Regression analysis demonstrated a significant correlation between the expression of *TH* and both *HIFα* subunits (Figure 6D,E).

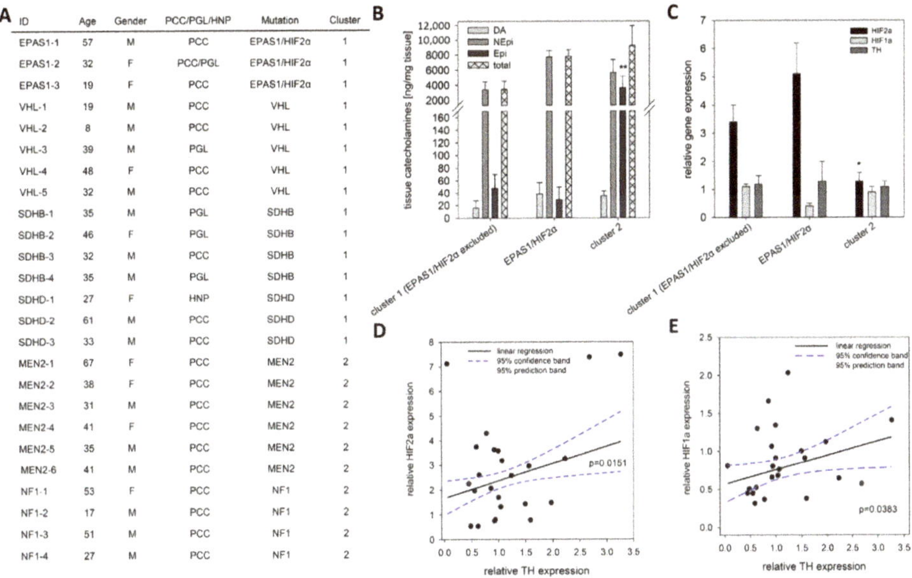

ID	Age	Gender	PCC/PGL/HNP	Mutation	Cluster
EPAS1-1	57	M	PCC	EPAS1/HIF2α	1
EPAS1-2	32	F	PCC/PGL	EPAS1/HIF2α	1
EPAS1-3	19	F	PCC	EPAS1/HIF2α	1
VHL-1	19	M	PCC	VHL	1
VHL-2	8	M	PCC	VHL	1
VHL-3	39	M	PGL	VHL	1
VHL-4	48	F	PCC	VHL	1
VHL-5	32	M	PCC	VHL	1
SDHB-1	35	M	PGL	SDHB	1
SDHB-2	46	F	PGL	SDHB	1
SDHB-3	32	M	PCC	SDHB	1
SDHB-4	35	M	PGL	SDHB	1
SDHD-1	27	F	HNP	SDHD	1
SDHD-2	61	M	PCC	SDHD	1
SDHD-3	33	M	PCC	SDHD	1
MEN2-1	67	F	PCC	MEN2	2
MEN2-2	38	F	PCC	MEN2	2
MEN2-3	31	M	PCC	MEN2	2
MEN2-4	41	F	PCC	MEN2	2
MEN2-5	35	M	PCC	MEN2	2
MEN2-6	41	M	PCC	MEN2	2
NF1-1	53	F	PCC	NF1	2
NF1-2	17	M	PCC	NF1	2
NF1-3	51	M	PCC	NF1	2
NF1-4	27	M	PCC	NF1	2

Figure 6. Expression pattern of *EPAS1/HIF2α*, *HIF1α* and *TH* in human tumor tissue. (**A**) Clinical characteristics of the included patients with confirmed mutation in well-described cluster 1 or cluster 2 related genes. (**B**) Tumor tissue from patients carrying a somatic gain-of-function mutation in *EPAS1/HIF2α* (n = 3) showed twice as much NEpi than other cluster 1 tumors that is also reflected by the total amount of catecholamines (sum of DA, NEpi and Epi). An elevated content of Epi was observed for mature cluster 2 tumors in comparison to the immature cluster 1 tumors. Mean ± SEM. ANOVA and Bonferroni post hoc test comparison vs. cluster 1 and EPAS1/HIF2α, ** $p < 0.01$. (**C**) qRT-PCR analysis showed an elevated *EPAS1/HIF2α* expression in cluster 1 PPGLs; whereas the *TH* expression remains unaffected by the underlying mutations in the different cluster. Mean ± SEM. ANOVA and Bonferroni post hoc test comparison vs. cluster 1 and EPAS1/HIF2α, * $p < 0.05$. (**D**) A significant linear correlation between the expression of *EPAS1/HIF2α* and *TH* could be detected (f = 1.667 + 0.681x, r = 0.490, $R^2 = 0.2399$). (**E**) A similar correlation was also observed for the expression of *HIF1α* and *TH* (f = 0.566 + 0.190x, r = 0.4252, $R^2 = 0.1808$).

3. Discussion

Hypoxia and the associated activation of hypoxia-related pathways contribute to tumor aggressiveness and therapy resistance [29,30]. As an alternative to extrinsic hypoxia, tumor cell spheroids provide a useful model to investigate the impact of hypoxia in vitro. Our study shows for the first time that the chromaffin cell features of pheochromocytoma cell lines remain unchanged during cultivation under spheroid conditions. This confirms the suitability of the model for investigations related to chromaffin cell features such as catecholamine biosynthesis, storage and secretion. For the tested cell lines, induction of spheroid formation via cultivation in the presence of methyl cellulose provided the most reproducible spheroids (Figures S1 and S2). Beside the described methods (Supplementary Materials), we also tested the agar-based liquid overlay technique [31–33] for all three pheochromocytoma cell lines. This method, however, resulted in multiple, small spheroids that were not useful for our purposes. The utilized methyl cellulose method is also suitable for the generation of endothelial cell spheroids [34]. This provides an opportunity for a future generation of multicellular spheroids consisting of pheochromocytoma cells, endothelial cells and/or fibroblasts providing a closer model to the in vivo situation within the tumor microenvironment.

Extrinsic as well as intrinsic hypoxia led to an up-regulation of total catecholamine contents of different pheochromocytoma cell lines with a cluster 2-like phenotype presumably reflecting increased phosphorylation of TH (Figure 7).

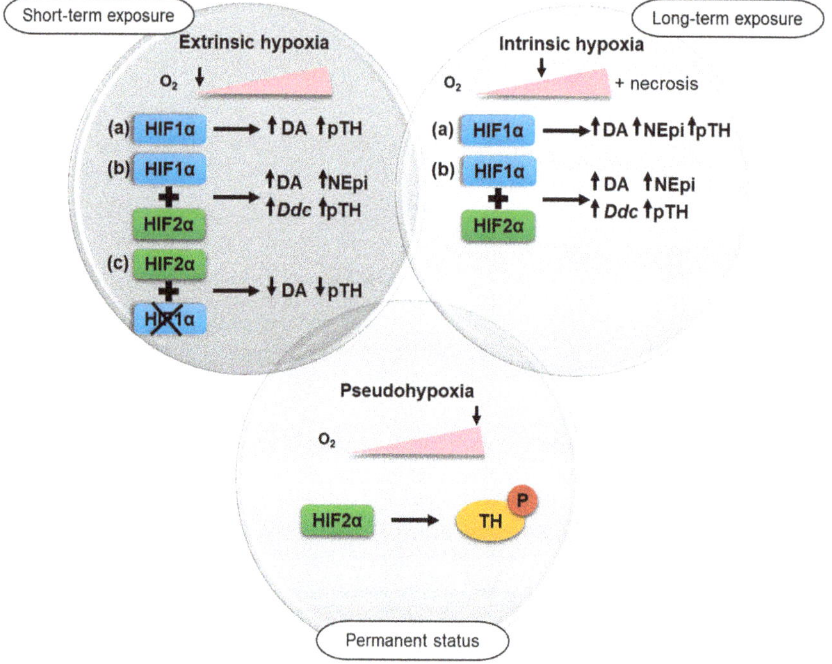

Figure 7. In the present study, the impact of three different types of hypoxia on the catecholamine biosynthesis of pheochromocytoma cells was investigated. Short-term exposure (24–48 h) to ≤ 1% oxygen under extrinsic hypoxia in *Hif2α*-deficient cells (**a**) led to an up-regulation of tyrosine phosphorylase (TH) phosphorylation and dopamine (DA). This effect was increased by long-term exposure to intrinsic hypoxia along with elevated norepinephrine (NEpi). Under both conditions similar effects could be observed after expression of *Hif2α* (**b**) in these cells. Expression of *Hif2α* further resulted in enhanced *Ddc* expression after hypoxic stimulation. The impact of extrinsic hypoxia could be reduced by a specific knockdown of *Hif1α* (**c**). Pseudohypoxia, characterized by permanent activation of hypoxia-related pathways in presence of oxygen, also led to an enhanced phosphorylation of TH.

It is also possible that a reduced turnover of catecholamines due to influences on secretion or intracellular metabolism could also contribute to the increased catecholamine content under hypoxic conditions. Under spheroid conditions, an additional impact of necrosis on catecholamine turnover is conceivable. Different protein kinases and protein phosphatases mediate the phosphorylation of TH at serine residues Ser8, Ser19, Ser31 and Ser40. TH activity is nevertheless predominantly dependent on the phosphorylation at Ser40; phosphorylation at Ser31 also enhances TH activity but to a much lesser extent than for Ser40, and phosphorylation at Ser19 or Ser8 has no effect on the enzyme activity [13]. Protein kinase (PK) A, PKG, and PKC are primarily responsible for the phosphorylation of Ser40, whereas dephosphorylation is regulated by protein phosphatase 2A and 2C. Goldberg and coworkers showed that exposure to hypoxia led to an increased activation of different PKC isoforms [35]. A reactive oxygen species (ROS)-mediated activation of PKC was postulated as a mechanism for the increased secretory capacity of mouse adrenal chromaffin cells under chronic intermittent hypoxia [36]. Lee et al. documented a PKA-dependent effect on TH phosphorylation at Ser40, which seems to be responsible for elevated dopamine in PC12 cells under intermittent hypoxia [37]. In human cervical adenocarcinoma cells, hypoxia activated PKC-δ led to both increased HIF1α transcription and stability [38]. On the other hand, expression of PKA-α repressed the activity of HIF1α in PC12 cells [39]. The data of the present study further indicate an impact of Hif2α on TH phosphorylation. Expression of *Hif2α* in MTT and MPC-mCherry cells naturally lacking *Hif2α* led to an increased phosphorylation of TH under normoxic conditions. In further studies, it should be addressed if Hif2α-mediated phosphorylation of TH is directly or indirectly regulated by PKs independence on various hypoxic conditions (extrinsic, intrinsic and pseudohypoxic). The three tumors bearing a mutation in *EPAS1/HIF2α* consistently showed a doubling of NEpi in comparison to other cluster 1 PPGLs. For a final characterization of these tumors, the sample number needs to be increased. Differences in *TH* expression could not be observed. This suggests an increased phosphorylation of TH (Figure 6B) or reduced catecholamine turnover in vivo. Furthermore, expression of *Hif2α* in MPC-mCherry cells enhanced hypoxia-stimulated expression of *Ddc* (Figure 4). Brown and coworkers described two putative hypoxia response elements for HIF2α binding in the promoter region of *Ddc* [14]. This could be responsible for the enhanced *Ddc* expression in presence of *Hif1α* and *Hif2α*.

The present study allows for the first time a differentiation between HIF1α- and HIF2α-driven effects on the catecholamine biosynthesis under hypoxic conditions (Figure 7). The regulation of the catecholamine biosynthesis in pheochromocytoma cells seems to be primarily regulated by HIF1α under extrinsic hypoxia. A specific knockdown of *Hif1α* reduced hypoxia-induced dopamine synthesis and diminished TH phosphorylation significantly (Figure 5), while the expression of *Hif2α* had no additional effect (Figure 4). This is in line with findings of other groups showing that HIF2α is dispensable for the response to hypoxia [40,41]. Extrinsic hypoxia as performed in our study reflects only the effect of a short-term exposure (24–48 h) to reduced oxygen mainly leading in a stabilization of HIF1α. Tumor cell spheroids provide an excellent model to study long-term effects of hypoxia in vitro, but with considerations that results reflect a mixture of (a) proliferating cells under normoxia, (b) hypoxic cells, and (c) necrotic cells (Figure 1). In all cell lines cultivation under spheroid conditions increased cellular DA and NEpi contents compared to monolayer culture (Figures 2 and 4), indicating an additional impact of necrosis. Immunohistochemical staining for TH showed an elevated expression in the necrotic core of the MTT and MPC spheroids (Figure 2). Little is known about the impact of necrosis on catecholamine biosynthesis, storage and turnover. Our data provide the first indication that necrosis enhances the biosynthesis of catecholamines in vitro.

The cellular catecholamine contents of pheochromocytoma cells in response to hypoxia seem to be primarily regulated through an increased phosphorylation of TH at Ser40. In short-term response (24–48 h), HIF1α regulates catecholamine biosynthesis, while HIF2α is dispensable for the direct response to hypoxia. A permanent activation of HIF2α, as shown in pseudohypoxic cluster 1 PPGLs for example, led to HIF2α-mediated phosphorylation of TH seen in MPC and MTT cells. Targeted inhibition of HIF2α possibly provides an excellent therapeutic approach for advanced PPGLs [42] and is moreover able to modulate catecholamine biosynthesis within the tumor cells.

4. Materials and Methods

If not indicated otherwise, all solutions and reagents were of the highest purity available from Sigma Aldrich GmbH (St. Louis, MO, USA). Cell culture medium and additives were obtained from Gibco (Thermo Fisher Scientific, Waltham, MA, USA) with the exception of fetal calf serum (Biowest, Riverside, MO, USA).

4.1. Cell Culture

Mouse pheochromocytoma cells (MPC 4/30/PRR) generated from heterozygous neurofibromatosis knockout mice and its more aggressive derivate termed MTT were used as models [24,25]. MPC cells were cultivated with RPMI-1640 containing 10% horse serum (HS), 5% fetal calf serum (FCS) and 2 mM Glutamax. For MTT cells Dulbecco's Modified Eagle Medium (DMEM) + Glutamax supplemented with 10% HS, 5% FCS and 1 mM sodium pyruvate were used. For the cultivation of the PC12 rat pheochromocytoma cell line RPMI-1640 containing 10% horse serum (HS) and 5% fetal calf serum (FCS) were used [43]. All media were named complete medium in the following sections. All cell lines were acquired from Arthur Tischler (Department of Pathology and Laboratory Medicine, Tufts University School of Medicine, Boston, MA, USA and Karel Pacak. In general, cells were cultured at 37 °C, 5% CO_2 and 95% humidity. MycoAlert Mycoplasma Detection Kit (Lonza, Basel, Switzerland) was used for testing cells to be mycoplasma free. After trypsinization (trypsin/EDTA; 0.05%/0.02%) cells were diluted with complete medium and counted by using C-CHIPs (Neubauer improved). Cultivation and all experiments were performed in absence of antibiotics. Cultivation and experiments in monolayer culture were performed using collagen A coated cell culture dishes. To generate extrinsic hypoxia, cells were cultivated under reduced oxygen partial pressure (≤1% oxygen) in an incubator furnished with an oxygen sensor (Sanyo InCuSafe O_2/CO_2 Incubator, Model MCO-5M, Osaka, Japan).

4.2. *Hif2a* Gene Knockin in MPC-mCherry and MTT Cells

MPC-mCherry H2A, expressing *Hif2α*, and their counterpart cell line MPC-mCherry control, transfected with an empty vector, were cultivated in collagen coated flask with antibiotic selection as previously described [22,44,45]. For the generation of *Hif2α* expressing MTT cells we used cells with stable expression of a non-targeting shRNA construct (SHC002V) [46]. These cells were transfected with pcDNA3.1+ carrying a codon-optimized version of the murine *Epas1* gene (MTT H2A; Genescript, Piscataway, NJ, USA) via nucleofection (4D-Nucleofector™ System, Lonza). At the same time, an empty-vector control cell line was generated (MTT control). Both cell lines were maintained after geneticin (250 µg/mL; Thermo Fisher Scientific) selection (Table S1). All experiments were performed in absence of antibiotics.

4.3. HIF1α Gene Knockdown in PC12 Cells

To achieve a specific HIF1α gene knockdown in PC12 cells rat HIF1α siRNA (sc-45919, Santa Cruz Biotechnology, Dallas, TX, USA) was used. A transfection efficiency of 57.9 ± 5.7% was achieved by using 12.5 nM siRNA per well in presence of lipofectamine RNAiMAX (Thermo Fisher Scientific). As control, aqua was utilized for transfection instead of siRNA.

4.4. Spheroid Generation

Cells were trypsinized from monolayer culture and an optimized cell number of 500 cells per spheroid were used for spheroid generation using the methyl cellulose (MC) method as previously described by us [28]. Additionally, two other methods for the generation of the spheroids were tested. A comparison of all three methods, (A) methyl cellulose method, (B) medium method, and (C) NunClon method, is shown in the Supplementary Materials. In general, spheroids were grown under standard culture conditions (5% CO_2, 37 °C). Spheroid formation was considered as completed four days after seeding (Figure S1); thereafter medium was replaced by fresh complete medium with or without addition of 0.24% methyl cellulose after three to four days of cultivation. Spheroids were harvested 11 or 18 days after generation.

4.5. Protein Measurement

For measurements of protein, 500 cells were seeded in a 24-well plate (monolayer) or spheroids were generated as previously described. Spheroids and cells in monolayer culture were cultivated for eight days without changing medium for comparable conditions. After cultivation, two spheroids were combined in an Eppendorf tube. Spheroids and cells in monolayer culture were washed with PBS. Cell lysis was performed by using CellLytic^{TM} M with protease inhibitor. Protein amounts per spheroid or per well of 24-well plates were analyzed using the Bradford assay (Bio-Rad Laboratories, Hercules, CA, USA) according to manufacturer specifications.

4.6. Catecholamine Measurements

For measurements of catecholamines 12–24 spheroids were combined in an Eppendorf tube, washed in PBS and homogenized with at least five volumes of 0.4 M perchloric acid containing 0.5 mM ethylenediaminetetraacetic acid (50 µL) on ice. For cells in monolayer culture, 1×10^5 cells were plated in a 24-well plate. After three days of cultivation, cells were washed and homogenized with 100 µL perchloric acid as described. All samples were centrifuged (1500× *g*, 15 min, 4 °C), supernatants were collected and catecholamines were analyzed by liquid chromatography with electrochemical detection as described previously [47]. Concentrations of catecholamines calculated relative to total protein. Therefore, a separate well of the 24-well plate or a separate Eppendorf tube containing the same number of spheroids was lysed and analyzed using the Bradford assay outlined above.

4.7. Hematoxylin and Eosin Staining

Spheroids were transferred in a Eppendorf tube, washed twice with ice-cold PBS and fixed with phosphate-buffered paraformaldehyde (4%) for 2 h. Fixed spheroids were stored in PBS containing 0.1% sodium azide (pH 7.2) at 4 °C. Spheroids were dehydrated with a series of processed alcohol ending with isopropanol and embedded in paraffin. For immunohistochemical or Hematoxylin and Eosin (H&E) staining 4-µm-thick sections were fixed on SuperFrost Plus slides and air-dried. Sections were deparaffinizedusing Neo-Clear and hydrated via descending ethanol series ending with 70% ethanol. For the H&E staining, sections were dyed with hematoxylin (Gill III), rinsed with 0.1% hydrochloric acid, differentiated with flowing water and stained with 0.5% aqueous eosin G solution. After rinsing in water, sections were rehydrated with processed alcohol series ending with 100% ethanol. Sections were mounted with Neo-Mount.

4.8. Immunohistochemistry

Paraffin sections were deparaffinized and hydrated as described above ending with distilled water. Spheroid sections were demarcated, washed with PBS and blocked for 1 h at room temperature with 1% bovine serum albumin in PBS containing 5% goat serum (blocking solution 1) followed by an overnight incubation at 4 °C with polyclonal rabbit anti-tyrosine hydroxylase (NB300-109, Novus Biologicals, Centennial, CO, USA, 1:100 in blocking solution 1). After incubation, sections were washed three times with PBS and incubated for 1 h with the secondary antibody Cy^{TM}3 AffiniPure goat anti-rabbit IgG (111-165-144, Jackson Immunoresearch, Cambridgeshire, UK, 1:500 in PBS). After three washing steps with PBS, sections were counterstained with 4′,6-diamidino-2-phenylindole (DAPI; Sigma-Aldrich, 1:1000 in PBS) for 1.5 min, washed again with PBS and mounted with fluorescence mounting medium.

4.9. Pimonidazole Staining

Hypoxic areas within the spheroids were stained using the Hypoxyprobe-Kit (Hypoxyprobe, Burlington, MA, USA). Spheroids cultivated for 11 or 18 days were incubated with pimonidazole

(20 µg/mL in phosphate-buffered saline, 30 min), fixed with formaldehyde, and embedded in paraffin. After dewaxing with RotiClear (Carl Roth GmbH & Co. KG, Karlsruhe, Germany) and rehydration in a graded series of ethanol solutions (100, 80, 70, 60, 50%, H_2O) spheroids were de-masked via incubation in citric acid buffer (10 mmol/L, pH 6, 100 °C, 20 min). Thereafter endogenous peroxidase was blocked using hydrogen peroxide (3% in Tris-buffered saline, 10 min). Nonspecific binding sites were blocked for 1 h using blocking solution (10% fetal bovine serum (*v*/*v*) in Tris-buffered saline). Spheroid sections were incubated for 1 h with primary anti-pimonidazole antibody (PAb2627, Hypoxyprobe, 1:200 in blocking solution) and secondary biotinylated donkey anti-rabbit antibody (RPN1004V1, Amersham Biosciences, Little Chalfont, UK, 1:200 in blocking solution), respectively. For isotype control, spheroids were incubated with IgG rabbit (ab37415, Abcam, Cambridge, UK) instead of primary antibody. Specific binding was detected using extra-avidin-peroxidase (E2886, Sigma Aldrich, 1:50 in Tris-buffered saline, 30 min) followed by incubation with 3-Amino-9-ethylcarbazole (Thermo Fisher Scientific) and counterstaining with hematoxylin.

4.10. SDS-PAGE and Western Blot Analysis

HIF-1α, HIF-2α, PNMT, TH, pTH, and actin were analyzed by Western blot. After incubation under normoxic or hypoxic (≤1% O_2) conditions, cells were washed with PBS, detached (typsin/EDTA) and resuspended in cold medium. After centrifugation at 4 °C, pellets were washed twice with PBS and stored at −80 °C. Sixty spheroids were transferred to each Eppendorf tube, washed three times with PBS and stored at −80 °C. Lysates were prepared on ice using CellLytic^{TM} M (Sigma-Aldrich, C2978) with protease inhibitors (1:100, Sigma-Aldrich; P8340). After 30 min incubation on ice and thoroughly mixing, cell lysates were centrifuged to remove cell debris. Protein concentration of all lysates were quantified using the Bradford assay. Fifty µg protein were mixed with LDS sample buffer (C.B.S. Scientific, San Diego, CA, USA; FB31010) and 5% mercaptoethanol. After denaturation at 99 °C for 5 min, proteins were separated on a 10% SDS-polyacrylamide gel and transferred to a polyvinylidine difluoride membrane (0.45 µm; Whatman, Buckinghamshire, UK) by semi-dry electroblotting. Non-specific binding sites on the membrane were blocked (5% skimmed milk powder plus 2% bovine serum albumin in TBS-T, blocking solution) at room temperature. Membranes were incubated with primary antibodies anti-PNMT (1:500; ab90862; abcam plc., Cambridge, UK), anti-tyrosine hydroxylase (1:1000, NB300-109, Novus Biologicals), anti-tyrosine hydroxylase phospho S40 (1:500, ab51206; abcam plc.), anti-HIF-1 alpha (1:200; NB10-479; Novus Biologicals), anti-HIF-2 alpha (1:200; NB10-479; Novus Biologicals), and anti-actin (1:1000; MAB1501R, Millipore, Massachusetts, USA) for 2 h at room temperature followed by an overnight incubation at 4 °C. After three washing steps in TBS-T, membranes were incubated for 1 h at room temperature with peroxidase-conjugated secondary antibody goat anti-rabbit IgG (1:5000; sc-2004; Santa Cruz Biotechnology) or goat anti-mouse IgG (1:5000; sc-2005; Santa Cruz Biotechnology). All antibodies were diluted in blocking solution. Protein visualization was performed as previously described [28].

4.11. Tumor Procurement and Genetic Testing

Snap frozen tumor tissue was collected directly after surgery from 25 patients with PPGL. Patients were enrolled in two different studies (Dresden/Germany, NIH/Bethesda/USA). All patients from Dresden are part of the PMT study (https://pmt-study.pressor.org/), ethic code EK 189062010; all patients from NIH were enrolled under the IRB Protocol 00-CH-0093. All patients have signed informed consent. Patients or tumor tissue were tested for germline and/or somatic mutations in established susceptibility by the CNIO institute in Madrid through a collaborative multi-center study (prospective monoamine-producing tumor study, https://pmt-study.pressor.org/) as previously described [48].

4.12. RNA Isolation and qRT-PCR

RNA from cells, spheroid pellets, or human PPGL tissue was isolated using RNeasy Plus Mini kit (Qiagen, Hilden, Germany) in accordance with manufacturer's instructions. Reverse transcription of

RNA and qRT-PCR was performed as described previously by us [28]. Sequence of each primer pair is summarized in detail in the supporting material (Table S2).

4.13. Statistical Analysis

Descriptive data are expressed as means ± SEM with statistical analyses taking into considerations numbers (n) of technical and biological replicates within independent experiments. Statistical analyses were carried out by one-way analysis of variance with post hoc Bonferroni tests using SigmaPlot 12.5 (Systat Software GmbH, Erkrath, Germany).

5. Conclusions

Our present study showed for the first time the suitability of pheochromocytoma spheroids to analyze the impact of hypoxia and necrosis on chromaffin cell features. Using either this model or extrinsic hypoxia in presence or absence of *Hif1α* or *Hif2α*, we demonstrated that Hif1α predominantly regulates catecholamines during short-term responses (24–48 h) to hypoxia, while Hif2α is dispensable for the direct response. Continuous activation of hypoxia-related genes under pseudohypoxic conditions leads to Hif2α-mediated activation of the catecholamine biosynthesis (permanent status).

Supplementary Materials: The following are available online at http://www.mdpi.com/2072-6694/11/5/594/s1, Figure S1: MPC cell spheroid formation, Figure S2: MTT cell spheroid formation, Figure S3: Determining the optimal cell number to generate MTT cell spheroids, Figure S4: Growth curves and protein amount of MPC and MTT cell spheroids generated by three different methods, Figure S5: Pheochromocytoma cell spheroids stained with pimonidazole to visualize hypoxic regions, Figure S6: Impact of extrinsic and intrinsic hypoxia on catecholamine biosynthesis, Figure S7: Distribution of hexose-monophosphate (HMP) and phosphatidylinositol (PIP) in MTT cell spheroids, Table S1: Gene expression of MTT H2A cells compared to the MTT control cells was analyzed by reverse transcriptase polymerase chain reaction, Table S2: Primer sequences and targeted genes.

Author Contributions: Conceptualization, N.B. and G.E.; methodology, N.B., I.P., V.S., C.G., M.U. and M.R.; validation, N.B., I.P., V.S., C.G., M.U. and M.R.; formal analysis, N.B. and C.G.; investigation, N.B, I.P., V.S. and C.G.; resources, N.Q., K.P., S.R. and G.E.; writing—original draft preparation, N.B., I.P., V.S., C.G., M.U., N.Q., A.W., M.P., M.R., K.P., J.P., S.R. and G.E.; writing—review and editing, N.B., I.P., V.S., C.G., M.U., N.Q., A.W., M.P., M.R., K.P., J.P., S.R. and G.E.; visualization, N.B.; supervision, A.W., J.P. and G.E.; project administration, M.P., A.W., J.P., S.R. and G.E.; funding acquisition, A.W., M.P., J.P., S.R. and G.E.

Funding: This research was funded by the Deutsche Forschungsgemeinschaft (DFG) within the CRC/Transregio 205/1 (project number: 314061271-TRR 205), Project No. B12 (N.B. and G.E.), Project No. B10 (S.R., J.P. and M.U.) and Project No. S01 (A.W., C.G. and M.P.) "The Adrenal: Central Relay in Health and Disease", and by the Paradifference Foundation (N.B., I.P., S.R. and G.E.).

Acknowledgments: The authors thank Arthur Tischler for providing the MPC and PC12 cell lines. The excellent technical assistance of Tina Fleischer, Linda Friedrich, Daniela Stanke, Mareike Barth, Johanna Pufe, Claudia-Mareike Pflüger and Cristina Huebner Freitas is greatly acknowledged. The authors thank the University of Technology Dresden (TU Dresden) for covering the publication fee.

Conflicts of Interest: The authors declare no conflict of interest. The funding sponsors had no role in the design of the study; in the collection, analyses, or interpretation of data; in the writing of the manuscript, and in the decision to publish the results.

References

1. Fishbein, L.; Leshchiner, I.; Walter, V.; Danilova, L.; Robertson, A.G.; Johnson, A.R.; Lichtenberg, T.M.; Murray, B.A.; Ghayee, H.K.; Else, T. Comprehensive molecular characterization of pheochromocytoma and paraganglioma. *Cancer Cell* **2017**, *31*, 181–193. [CrossRef] [PubMed]
2. Matro, J.; Giubellino, A.; Pacak, K. Current and future therapeutic approaches for metastatic pheochromocytoma and paraganglioma: Focus on sdhb tumors. *Horm. Metab. Res.* **2013**, *45*, 147–153. [CrossRef]
3. Eisenhofer, G.; Pacak, K.; Huynh, T.-T.; Qin, N.; Bratslavsky, G.; Linehan, W.M.; Mannelli, M.; Friberg, P.; Grebe, S.K.; Timmers, H.J. Catecholamine metabolomic and secretory phenotypes in phaeochromocytoma. *Endocr. Relat. Cancer* **2011**, *18*, 97–111. [CrossRef] [PubMed]
4. Eisenhofer, G.; Huynh, T.; Pacak, K.; Brouwers, F.; Walther, M.; Linehan, W.; Munson, P.; Mannelli, M.; Goldstein, D.; Elkahloun, A. Distinct gene expression profiles in norepinephrine-and epinephrine-producing

hereditary and sporadic pheochromocytomas: Activation of hypoxia-driven angiogenic pathways in von hippel–lindau syndrome. *Endocr. Relat. Cancer* **2004**, *11*, 897–911. [CrossRef]

5. Jochmanová, I.; Yang, C.; Zhuang, Z.; Pacak, K. Hypoxia-inducible factor signaling in pheochromocytoma: Turning the rudder in the right direction. *J. Natl. Cancer Inst.* **2013**, *105*, 1270–1283. [CrossRef] [PubMed]
6. Kaelin Jr, W.G.; Ratcliffe, P.J. Oxygen sensing by metazoans: The central role of the hif hydroxylase pathway. *Mol. Cell* **2008**, *30*, 393–402. [CrossRef]
7. Burnichon, N.; Vescovo, L.; Amar, L.; Libé, R.; de Reynies, A.; Venisse, A.; Jouanno, E.; Laurendeau, I.; Parfait, B.; Bertherat, J. Integrative genomic analysis reveals somatic mutations in pheochromocytoma and paraganglioma. *Hum. Mol. Genet.* **2011**, *20*, 3974–3985. [CrossRef] [PubMed]
8. López-Jiménez, E.; Gómez-López, G.; Leandro-García, L.J.; Muñoz, I.; Schiavi, F.; Montero-Conde, C.; De Cubas, A.A.; Ramires, R.; Landa, I.; Leskelä, S. Research resource: Transcriptional profiling reveals different pseudohypoxic signatures in sdhb and vhl-related pheochromocytomas. *Mol. Endocrinol.* **2010**, *24*, 2382–2391. [CrossRef]
9. Favier, J.; Brière, J.-J.; Burnichon, N.; Rivière, J.; Vescovo, L.; Benit, P.; Giscos-Douriez, I.; De Reyniès, A.; Bertherat, J.; Badoual, C. The warburg effect is genetically determined in inherited pheochromocytomas. *PloS ONE* **2009**, *4*, e7094. [CrossRef] [PubMed]
10. Richter, S.; Qin, N.; Pacak, K.; Eisenhofer, G. Role of hypoxia and hif2α in development of the sympathoadrenal cell lineage and chromaffin cell tumours with distinct catecholamine phenotypic features. *Adv. Pharmacol.* **2013**, *68*, 285–317. [CrossRef] [PubMed]
11. Schnell, P.O.; Ignacak, M.L.; Bauer, A.L.; Striet, J.B.; Paulding, W.R.; Czyzyk-Krzeska, M.F. Regulation of tyrosine hydroxylase promoter activity by the von hippel–lindau tumor suppressor protein and hypoxia-inducible transcription factors. *J. Neurochem.* **2003**, *85*, 483–491. [CrossRef] [PubMed]
12. Fukuda, T.; Ishii, K.; Nanmoku, T.; Isobe, K.; Kawakami, Y.; Takekoshi, K. 5-aminoimidazole-4-carboxamide-1-β-4-ribofuranoside stimulates tyrosine hydroxylase activity and catecholamine secretion by activation of amp-activated protein kinase in pc12 cells. *J. Neuroendocrinol.* **2007**, *19*, 621–631. [CrossRef] [PubMed]
13. Dunkley, P.R.; Bobrovskaya, L.; Graham, M.E.; Von Nagy-Felsobuki, E.I.; Dickson, P.W. Tyrosine hydroxylase phosphorylation: Regulation and consequences. *J Neurochem* **2004**, *91*, 1025–1043. [CrossRef]
14. Brown, S.T.; Kelly, K.F.; Daniel, J.M.; Nurse, C.A. Hypoxia inducible factor (hif)-2α is required for the development of the catecholaminergic phenotype of sympathoadrenal cells. *J. Neurochem.* **2009**, *110*, 622–630. [CrossRef] [PubMed]
15. Park, S.Y.; Kang, J.H.; Jeong, K.J.; Lee, J.; Han, J.W.; Choi, W.S.; Kim, Y.K.; Kang, J.; Park, C.G.; Lee, H.Y. Norepinephrine induces vegf expression and angiogenesis by a hypoxia-inducible factor-1α protein-dependent mechanism. *Int. J. Cancer* **2011**, *128*, 2306–2316. [CrossRef] [PubMed]
16. Evinger, M.J.; Cikos, S.; NWAFOR-ANENE, V.; Powers, J.F.; Tischler, A.S. Hypoxia activates multiple transcriptional pathways in mouse pheochromocytoma cells. *Ann. N. Y. Acad. Sci.* **2002**, *971*, 61–65. [CrossRef] [PubMed]
17. Wong, D.L.; Tai, T.; Wong-Faull, D.C.; Claycomb, R.; Siddall, B.J.; Bell, R.A.; Kvetnansky, R. Stress and adrenergic function: Hif1α, a potential regulatory switch. *Cell. Mol. Neurobiol.* **2010**, *30*, 1451–1457. [CrossRef]
18. Qin, N.; De Cubas, A.A.; Garcia-Martin, R.; Richter, S.; Peitzsch, M.; Menschikowski, M.; Lenders, J.W.; Timmers, H.J.; Mannelli, M.; Opocher, G. Opposing effects of hif1α and hif2α on chromaffin cell phenotypic features and tumor cell proliferation: Insights from myc-associated factor x. *Int. J. Cancer* **2014**, *135*, 2054–2064. [CrossRef] [PubMed]
19. Pietras, A.; Johnsson, A.S.; Påhlman, S. The hif-2α-driven pseudo-hypoxic phenotype in tumor aggressiveness, differentiation, and vascularization. *Curr. Top. Microbiol. Immunol.* **2010**, *345*, 1–20. [CrossRef] [PubMed]
20. Holmquist-Mengelbier, L.; Fredlund, E.; Löfstedt, T.; Noguera, R.; Navarro, S.; Nilsson, H.; Pietras, A.; Vallon-Christersson, J.; Borg, Å.; Gradin, K.; et al. Recruitment of hif-1α and hif-2α to common target genes is differentially regulated in neuroblastoma: Hif-2α promotes an aggressive phenotype. *Cancer Cell* **2006**, *10*, 413–423. [CrossRef]
21. Chatzinikolaidou, M. Cell spheroids: The new frontiers in in vitro models for cancer drug validation. *Drug Discov. Today* **2016**, *21*, 1553–1560. [CrossRef] [PubMed]
22. Seifert, V.; Liers, J.; Kniess, T.; Richter, S.; Bechmann, N.; Feldmann, A.; Bachmann, M.; Eisenhofer, G.; Pietzsch, J.; Ullrich, M. Fluorescent mouse pheochromocytoma spheroids expressing hypoxia-inducible factor 2 alpha: Morphologic and radiopharmacologic characterization. *J. Cell. Biotechnol.* **2019**, in press.

23. D'Antongiovanni, V.; Martinelli, S.; Richter, S.; Canu, L.; Guasti, D.; Mello, T.; Romagnoli, P.; Pacak, K.; Eisenhofer, G.; Mannelli, M. The microenvironment induces collective migration in sdhb-silenced mouse pheochromocytoma spheroids. *Endocr. Relat. Cancer* **2017**, *24*, 555–564. [CrossRef] [PubMed]
24. Powers, J.; Evinger, M.; Tsokas, P.; Bedri, S.; Alroy, J.; Shahsavari, M.; Tischler, A. Pheochromocytoma cell lines from heterozygous neurofibromatosis knockout mice. *Cell Tissue Res.* **2000**, *302*, 309–320. [CrossRef]
25. Martiniova, L.; Lai, E.W.; Elkahloun, A.G.; Abu-Asab, M.; Wickremasinghe, A.; Solis, D.C.; Perera, S.M.; Huynh, T.-T.; Lubensky, I.A.; Tischler, A.S. Characterization of an animal model of aggressive metastatic pheochromocytoma linked to a specific gene signature. *Clin. Exp. Metastasis* **2009**, *26*, 239–250. [CrossRef]
26. Axelson, H.; Fredlund, E.; Ovenberger, M.; Landberg, G.; Påhlman, S. Hypoxia-induced dedifferentiation of tumor cells–a mechanism behind heterogeneity and aggressiveness of solid tumors. *Semin. Cell Dev. Biol.* **2005**, *16*, 554–563. [CrossRef] [PubMed]
27. Edsjö, A.; Holmquist, L.; Påhlman, S. Neuroblastoma as an experimental model for neuronal differentiation and hypoxia-induced tumor cell dedifferentiation. *Semin. Cancer Biol.* **2007**, *17*, 248–256. [CrossRef] [PubMed]
28. Bechmann, N.; Ehrlich, H.; Eisenhofer, G.; Ehrlich, A.; Meschke, S.; Ziegler, C.G.; Bornstein, S.R. Anti-tumorigenic and anti-metastatic activity of the sponge-derived marine drugs aeroplysinin-1 and isofistularin-3 against pheochromocytoma in vitro. *Mar. Drugs* **2018**, *16*, 172. [CrossRef]
29. Verduzco, D.; Lloyd, M.; Xu, L.; Ibrahim-Hashim, A.; Balagurunathan, Y.; Gatenby, R.A.; Gillies, R.J. Intermittent hypoxia selects for genotypes and phenotypes that increase survival, invasion, and therapy resistance. *PloS ONE* **2015**, *10*, e0120958. [CrossRef]
30. Muz, B.; de la Puente, P.; Azab, F.; Azab, A.K. The role of hypoxia in cancer progression, angiogenesis, metastasis, and resistance to therapy. *Hypoxia* **2015**, *3*, 83. [CrossRef]
31. Carlsson, J.; Yuhas, J. Liquid-overlay culture of cellular spheroids. *Recent Results Cancer Res.* **1984**, *95*, 1–23. [PubMed]
32. Friedrich, J.; Seidel, C.; Ebner, R.; Kunz-Schughart, L.A. Spheroid-based drug screen: Considerations and practical approach. *Nat Protoc* **2009**, *4*, 309. [CrossRef] [PubMed]
33. Kunz-Schughart, L.A.; Freyer, J.P.; Hofstaedter, F.; Ebner, R. The use of 3-d cultures for high-throughput screening: The multicellular spheroid model. *J. Biomol. Screen.* **2004**, *9*, 273–285. [CrossRef] [PubMed]
34. Augustin, H.G. Methods in Endothelial Cell Biology. Springer Science & Business Media. 2004. Available online: https://www.springer.com/gb/book/9783540213970 (accessed on 12 January 2019).
35. Goldberg, M.; Zhang, H.L.; Steinberg, S.F. Hypoxia alters the subcellular distribution of protein kinase c isoforms in neonatal rat ventricular myocytes. *J. Clin. Invest.* **1997**, *99*, 55–61. [CrossRef] [PubMed]
36. Kuri, B.A.; Khan, S.A.; Chan, S.A.; Prabhakar, N.R.; Smith, C.B. Increased secretory capacity of mouse adrenal chromaffin cells by chronic intermittent hypoxia: Involvement of protein kinase c. *J. Physiol.* **2007**, *584*, 313–319. [CrossRef]
37. Kumar, G.K.; Kim, D.-K.; Lee, M.-S.; Ramachandran, R.; Prabhakar, N.R. Activation of tyrosine hydroxylase by intermittent hypoxia: Involvement of serine phosphorylation. *J. Appl. Physiol.* **2003**. [CrossRef]
38. Lee, J.W.; Park, J.A.; Kim, S.H.; Seo, J.H.; Lim, K.J.; Jeong, J.W.; Jeong, C.H.; Chun, K.H.; Lee, S.K.; Kwon, Y.G. Protein kinase c-δ regulates the stability of hypoxia-inducible factor-1α under hypoxia. *Cancer Sci.* **2007**, *98*, 1476–1481. [CrossRef] [PubMed]
39. Torii, S.; Okamura, N.; Suzuki, Y.; Ishizawa, T.; Yasumoto, K.-i.; Sogawa, K. Cyclic amp represses the hypoxic induction of hypoxia-inducible factors in pc12 cells. *J. Biochem.* **2009**, *146*, 839–844. [CrossRef]
40. Compernolle, V.; Brusselmans, K.; Franco, D.; Moorman, A.; Dewerchin, M.; Collen, D.; Carmeliet, P. Cardia bifida, defective heart development and abnormal neural crest migration in embryos lacking hypoxia-inducible factor-1α. *Cardiovasc. Res.* **2003**, *60*, 569–579. [CrossRef]
41. Hu, C.-J.; Wang, L.-Y.; Chodosh, L.A.; Keith, B.; Simon, M.C. Differential roles of hypoxia-inducible factor 1α (hif-1α) and hif-2α in hypoxic gene regulation. *Mol. Cell. Biol.* **2003**, *23*, 9361–9374. [CrossRef]
42. Toledo, R.A. New hif2α inhibitors: Potential implications as therapeutics for advanced pheochromocytomas and paragangliomas. *Endoc. Relat. Cancer* **2017**, *24*, C9–C19. [CrossRef] [PubMed]
43. Tischler, A.S.; Greene, L.A.; Kwan, P.W.; Slayton, V.W. Ultrastructural effects of nerve growth factor on pc 12 pheochromocytoma cells in spinner culture. *Cell Tissue Res.* **1983**, *228*, 641–648. [CrossRef] [PubMed]
44. Ullrich, M.; Bergmann, R.; Peitzsch, M.; Zenker, E.F.; Cartellieri, M.; Bachmann, M.; Ehrhart-Bornstein, M.; Block, N.L.; Schally, A.V.; Eisenhofer, G.; et al. Multimodal somatostatin receptor theranostics using

[(64)cu]cu-/[(177)lu]lu-dota-(tyr(3))octreotate and an-238 in a mouse pheochromocytoma model. *Theranostics* **2016**, *6*, 650–665. [CrossRef] [PubMed]

45. Ullrich, M.; Bergmann, R.; Pietzsch, J.; Ehrhart-Bornstein, M.; Bornstein, S.R.; Ziegler, C.G.; Eisenhofer, G.; Qin, N.; Peitzsch, M.; Cartellieri, M.; et al. In vivo fluorescence imaging and urinary monoamines as surrogate biomarkers of disease progression in a mouse model of pheochromocytoma. *Endocrinology* **2014**, *155*, 4149–4156. [CrossRef] [PubMed]
46. Richter, S.; D'Antongiovanni, V.; Martinelli, S.; Bechmann, N.; Riverso, M.; Poitz, D.M.; Pacak, K.; Eisenhofer, G.; Mannelli, M.; Rapizzi, E. Primary fibroblast co-culture stimulates growth and metabolism in sdhb-impaired mouse pheochromocytoma mtt cells. *Cell Tissue Res.* **2018**, *374*, 473–485. [CrossRef] [PubMed]
47. Eisenhofer, G.; Goldstein, D.S.; Stull, R.; Keiser, H.R.; Sunderland, T.; Murphy, D.L.; Kopin, I.J. Simultaneous liquid-chromatographic determination of 3,4-dihydroxyphenylglycol, catecholamines, and 3,4-dihydroxyphenylalanine in plasma, and their responses to inhibition of monoamine oxidase. *Clin. Chem.* **1986**, *32*, 2030–2033. [PubMed]
48. Richter, S.; Gieldon, L.; Pang, Y.; Peitzsch, M.; Huynh, T.; Leton, R.; Viana, B.; Ercolino, T.; Mangelis, A.; Rapizzi, E.; et al. Metabolome-guided genomics to identify pathogenic variants in isocitrate dehydrogenase, fumarate hydratase, and succinate dehydrogenase genes in pheochromocytoma and paraganglioma. *Genet. Med.* **2019**, *21*, 705–717. [CrossRef] [PubMed]

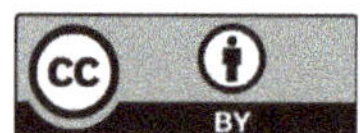

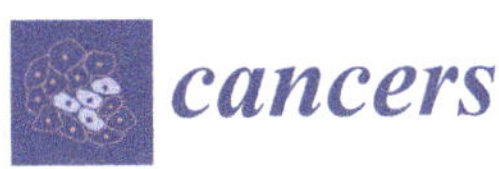 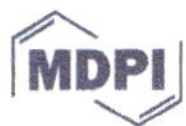

Article

Molecular Alterations in Dog Pheochromocytomas and Paragangliomas

Esther Korpershoek [1,*], Daphne A. E. R. Dieduksman [1], Guy C. M. Grinwis [2], Michael J. Day [3], Claudia E. Reusch [4], Monika Hilbe [5], Federico Fracassi [6], Niels M. G. Krol [1], André G. Uitterlinden [7], Annelies de Klein [8], Bert Eussen [8], Hans Stoop [1], Ronald R. de Krijger [9], Sara Galac [10] and Winand N. M. Dinjens [1]

1 Department of Pathology, Erasmus MC Cancer Institute, University Medical Center, 3015 GD Rotterdam, The Netherlands; daphne93@live.nl (D.A.E.R.D.); a.krol@erasmusmc.nl (N.M.G.K.); j.stoop@erasmusmc.nl (H.S.); w.dinjens@erasmusmc.nl (W.N.M.D.)
2 Department of Pathobiology, Faculty of Veterinary Medicine, Utrecht University, 3584 CL Utrecht, The Netherlands; G.C.M.Grinwis@uu.nl
3 School of Veterinary and Life Sciences, Murdoch University, Murdoch 6150, WA, Australia; profmjday@gmail.com
4 Clinic for Small Animal Internal Medicine, University of Zurich, 8057 Zurich, Switzerland; creusch@vetclinics.uzh.ch
5 Institute of Veterinary Pathology, University of Zurich, 8057 Zurich, Switzerland; hilbe@vetpath.uzh.ch
6 Department of Veterinary Medical Science, University of Bologna, 40064 Ozzano dell'Emilia, Italy; federico.fracassi@unibo.it
7 Genetic Laboratory, Erasmus MC University Medical Center, 3015 GD Rotterdam, The Netherlands; a.g.uitterlinden@erasmusmc.nl
8 Department of Clinical Genetics, Erasmus MC University Medical Center, 3015 GD Rotterdam, The Netherlands; a.deklein@erasmusmc.nl (A.d.K.); h.eussen@erasmusmc.nl (B.E.)
9 Department of Pathology University Medical Center/Princess Maxima Center for Pediatric Oncology, 3584 CS Utrecht, The Netherlands; R.R.deKrijger@umcutrecht.nl
10 Department of Clinical Sciences of Companion Animals, Faculty of Veterinary Medicine, Utrecht University, 3584 CL Utrecht, The Netherlands; S.Galac@uu.nl
* Correspondence: e.korpershoek.1@erasmusmc.nl; Tel.: +31-10-7043496

Received: 21 February 2019; Accepted: 18 April 2019; Published: 30 April 2019

Abstract: Recently, genetic alterations in the genes encoding succinate dehydrogenase subunit B and D (*SDHB* and *SDHD*) were identified in pet dogs that presented with spontaneously arising pheochromocytomas (PCC) and paragangliomas (PGL; together PPGL), suggesting dogs might be an interesting comparative model for the study of human PPGL. To study whether canine PPGL resembled human PPGL, we investigated a series of 50 canine PPGLs by immunohistochemistry to determine the expression of synaptophysin (SYP), tyrosine hydroxylase (TH) and succinate dehydrogenase subunit A (SDHA) and B (SDHB). In parallel, 25 canine PPGLs were screened for mutations in *SDHB* and *SDHD* by Sanger sequencing. To detect large chromosomal alterations, single nucleotide polymorphism (SNP) arrays were performed for 11 PPGLs, including cases for which fresh frozen tissue was available. The immunohistochemical markers stained positive in the majority of canine PPGLs. Genetic screening of the canine tumors revealed the previously described variants in four cases; *SDHB* p.Arg38Gln ($n = 1$) and *SDHD* p.Lys122Arg ($n = 3$). Furthermore, the SNP arrays revealed large chromosomal alterations of which the loss of chromosome 5, partly homologous to human chromosome 1p and chromosome 11, was the most frequent finding (100% of the six cases with chromosomal alterations). In conclusion, canine and human PPGLs show similar genomic alterations, suggestive of common interspecies PPGL-related pathways.

Keywords: dog; pheochromocytoma; paraganglioma; *SDHB*; *SDHD*; mutation; chromosomal alteration; comparative genomics

1. Introduction

Pheochromocytomas (PCCs) and paragangliomas (PGLs; together PPGLs) are tumors arising from chromaffin tissue inside (PCC) and outside the adrenal glands (PGL). These tumors occur in the context of several hereditary syndromes, such as Von Hippel Lindau (VHL), Multiple Endocrine Neoplasia type 2, Neurofibromatosis type 1, and the PCC-PGL syndrome, with underlying germline mutations in the *VHL*, rearranged during transfection (*RET*), neurofibromin 1 (*NF1*), and the *SDH*-genes, respectively [1]. Both germline and somatic mutations can be found in more than 20 genes [2,3]. Although approximately 10% of PPGL patients, in general, will present with (distant) metastases, this frequency is much higher in patients with succinate dehydrogenase subunit B (*SDHB*) germline mutations. During follow-up, more than 35% of *SDHB* patients will present with PPGL metastases [4,5].

In an effort to unravel the mechanisms behind malignant behavior of PPGLs, and more specifically the metastatic behavior of *SDHB*-related tumors, several attempts have been made to generate knock-out mouse models. These models either proved lethal during embryogenesis or the mice did not develop PPGL or other *SDH*-related tumors [6]. The only mouse models that presented with high frequencies of PCCs were based on conditional homozygous inactivation of *Pten* and heterozygous conventional inactivation of *Nf1* [7]. However, human PPGLs have never been associated with phosphatase and tensin homolog (*PTEN*) mutations [8]. In addition, *NF1*-related PPGLs are relatively benign with metastatic behavior seen in fewer than 10% of cases [9]. So, although these PPGL mouse models are interesting, there remains a need for an appropriate animal model to study *SDH*-related PPGL.

Recently, Holt et al. reported genetic screening of eight canine PPGLs and identified four genetic variants that might be potentially pathogenic; one in *SDHB* (p.Arg38Gln) and three in succinate dehydrogenase subunit D (*SDHD*; p.Lys122Arg), of which one was somatic [10]. Because these alterations occurred in highly conserved amino acids, the authors assumed that the alterations were likely pathogenic. In fact, the somatic event suggests that at least the SDHD p.Lys122Arg amino acid change is likely pathogenic, while the *SDHB* alteration remains of unknown significance. Since this is the first animal model that presents spontaneously with PPGL that might be related to *SDHB* and *SDHD* mutations, we have investigated a relatively large series of canine PPGLs by Sanger sequencing for mutations in these genes. In addition, immunohistochemistry was performed for tyrosine hydroxylase, synaptophysin, SDHB, and succinate dehydrogenase subunit A (SDHA), and SNP arrays to identify chromosomal alterations.

2. Results

2.1. Clinical Findings

The canine PPGL immunohistochemistry series included 32 PCCs and 18 PGLs. The average age of the dogs at diagnosis was 11 years for PCCs (ranging from 4 to 16 years) and 9 years for PGLs (ranging from 2 to 11 years). In the PCC group, the distribution of males and females was almost identical (53% male), while the PGL group included more tumors from males (72%). Metastatic behavior was reported in 3% of the dogs with PCCs ($n = 1$) and 11% of the dogs with PGL ($n = 2$).

2.2. Genetic Analyses

Sanger sequencing results are shown in Table 1. Twenty-one PPGLs (20 PCCs and one PGL) with sufficient DNA quality and positive synaptophysin (SYP) or tyrosine hydroxylase (TH) immunohistochemical labeling, were screened for mutations in the *SDHB* and *SDHD* genes. If a tumor had a non-synonymous variant, the presence of this variant was also investigated in corresponding germline DNA.

Three PCCs showed an SDHD (XM_536573) c.365A>G; p.Lys122Arg alteration. In PCC6 and PCC46 the variant was homozygous, while in PCC23 the alteration was heterozygous. Germline DNA was only available for PCC6 and showed the *SDHD* variant in a heterozygous fashion, indicating loss of the wild type (WT) *SDHD* allele in the tumor (Figure 2), which was also confirmed by the loss of heterozygosity analyses for microsatellite markers flanking the *SDHD* gene (Figure 1B). PCC19 showed the previously described *SDHB* (NM_001252217) c.113G>A; p.Arg38Gln alteration, which appeared homozygous in the tumor and corresponding germline DNA of this dog. (Figure 1A)

In addition, genetic screening for *SDHA* mutations was only performed in SDHA immunohistochemically-negative tumor PCC1 (see below Figure 2). Due to the relatively poor quality of the sample it was not possible to obtain *SDHA* DNA sequences of sufficient quality to analyze.

2.3. *Immunohistochemistry*

SYP was positive in 86% of PCCs and 71% of PGLs, while TH was positive in 74% of PCCs and 35% of PGLs. Results of the immunohistochemistry of all tumors are listed in Supplemental Table S1 and illustrated in Figure 1. SDHB immunohistochemistry was performed on all 50 canine PPGLs. PCC1 and PCC6 showed heterogeneous labeling for SDHB, with foci of tumor cells that were immunohistochemically negative for SDHB and areas that were weakly positive. The SDHA labeling for PCC1 also appeared to be negative for the tumor cells in this PCC (Figure 2), while all other tumors were positive. All other PPGLs, as well as the positive control tissues (normal dog adrenals), were immunohistochemically positive, although they did not show the typical granular labeling pattern.

2.4. *SNP Arrays*

Chromosomal alterations were investigated for 11 dog PPGLs by SNP arrays. From those, analysis was not possible for two samples due to high background noise. In addition, three tumors did not show any chromosomal alterations. The chromosomal alterations of the six remaining tumors are listed in Table 2. Furthermore, an illustrative single nucleotide polymorphism (SNP) array result of case PCC20 (logR ratios and b-allele frequencies (BAF)) is depicted in Figure 1C, showing loss of chromosomes 5, 17, 23, 26, 30, and 34. The most frequent genomic alteration was loss of chromosome 5, which occurred in all six dog PPGLs (100%), followed by loss of chromosome 26 in 5/6 dog PPGLs (83%). Chromosome 5 (CanFam3.1) is, for a large part, syntenic to two areas of human chromosome 1 (GRCh38.p3), and to a part of human chromosome 11, including the *SDHD* region, respectively (see Figure 3, Supplemental Table S3). Genomic locations of *SDHA*, *SDHB*, *SDHC*, and *SDHD* are shown in Supplemental Figure S2.

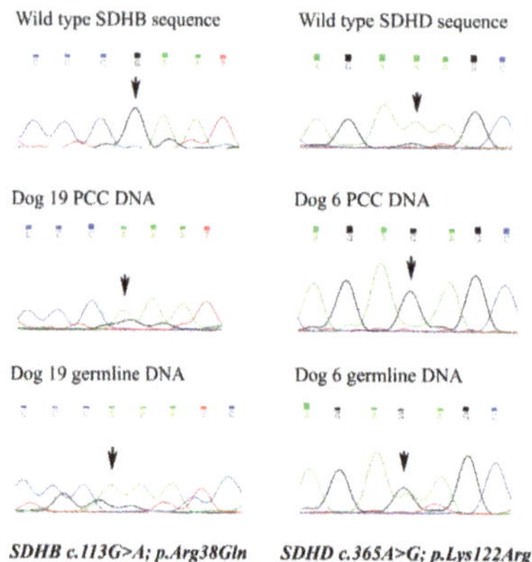

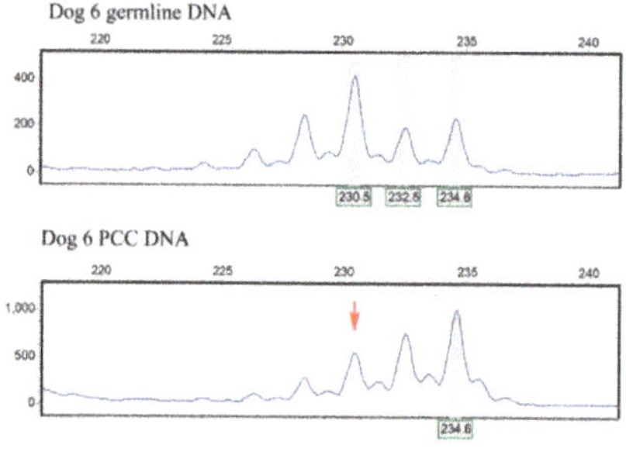

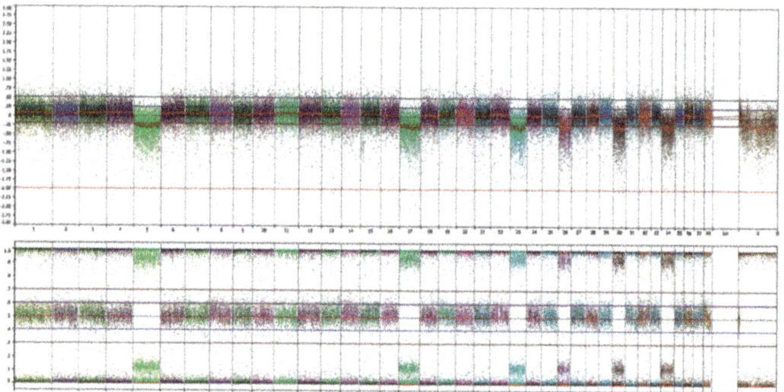

Figure 1. (**A**) In the left panel, succinate dehydrogenase subunit B (*SDHB*) sequences are displayed from healthy reference (upper), PCC19, and corresponding germline DNA. In the right panel, the succinate dehydrogenase subunit D (*SDHD*) sequence is shown from healthy reference, PCC6, and corresponding germline DNA. Note that PCC19 tumor and germline DNA both show the SDHB c.113G>A; p.Arg38Gln variant. PCC6 shows SDHD c.365A>G; p.Lys38Arg in a homozygous fashion in the tumor DNA and heterozygous in the germline DNA, indicating loss of the wild type allele in the tumor. (**B**) Shows loss of heterozygosity of the larger allele in PCC6, confirming the Sanger sequencing results. (**C**) The SNP array result of PCC 20 displays in the upper panel logR ratios, indicating loss of chromosomes 5, 17, 23, 26, 30, and 34. This is also seen in the lower panel by the B-allele frequencies.

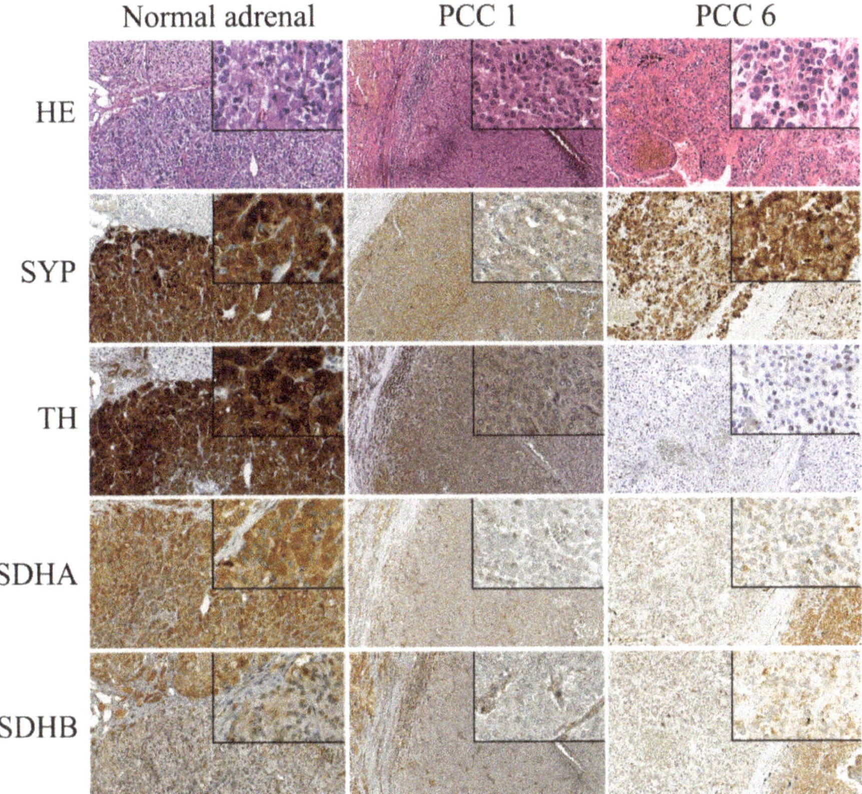

Figure 2. Hematoxylin Eosin staining and immunohistochemistry for synaptophysin (SYP), tyrosine hydroxylase (TH), succinate dehydrogenase subunit A (SDHA) and subunit B (SDHB) of normal dog adrenal, PCC1, and PCC6. Normal adrenal glands were used as positive controls and show strong expression of SYP and tyrosine hydroxylase (TH). PCC1 and 6 label weakly positive for SYP, but for TH only PCC1 shows positive labeling. The normal canine adrenal gland labels positive for SDHA and SDHB, although there is lack of granular labeling, which is characteristic for SDHA and SDHB in human tissues. PCC1 shows labeling of the stromal cells for SDHA and SDHB, which serve as positive control cells, while the PCC cells appear to be heterogeneous weak/negative for SDHB and do not label for SDHA. PCC 6 showed heterogeneous weak expression of SDHB, but there was no difference in labeling intensity between the tumor cells and the normal stromal cells for SDHA. Pictures are at 20× magnification, internal boxes at 40× magnification.

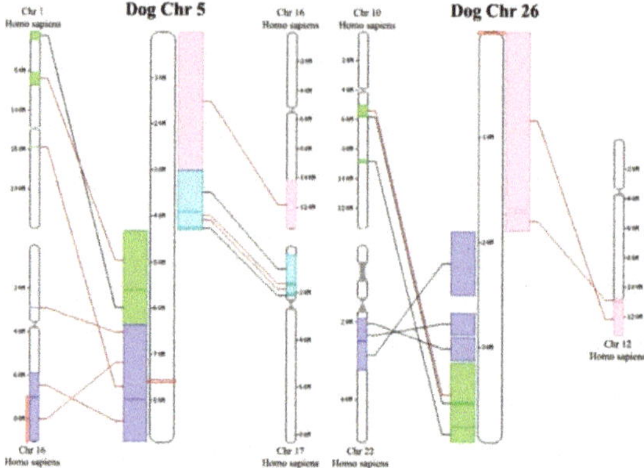

Figure 3. Homology between dog chromosome 5 and 26, and the human genome. It shows the homology between dog chromosome 5 and 26 and several human chromosomes. Of note is that the *SDHD* gene is located on dog chromosome 5 (see Supplemental Figure S2).

Table 1. Variants identified by Sanger Sequencing. SDH-variants that were previously described by Holt et al. [10] as mutations are depicted in bold and italic. If a non-synonymous variation was detected in the tumor, the corresponding germline was investigated for the presence of the variant.

PCC Number	*SDHB* Synonymous	*SDHB* Non-Syn	SDHD Syn	SDHD Non-Syn	Comment
PCC1	p.Y50Y, p.Q164Q, p.A210A		WT		
PCC2	p.Y150Y, p.Q164Q, p.A210A		WT		
PCC3	WT		WT		
PCC4	p.A210A		WT		
PCC5	p.Y150Y, p.Q164Q, p.L188L, p.A210A		WT		
PCC6	p.Y150Y, p.Q164Q, p.A210A		p.A97A	*p.K122R$^{HO/HE}$*	*LOH confirmed*
PCC9	p.Y150Y, p.Q164Q, p.A210A		WT		
PCC10	p.Y150Y, p.Q164Q, p.A210A		WT		
PCC11	p.L188L		WT		
PCC13	p.L188L		WT		
PCC14	p.L188L		WT		
PCC15	p.Y150Y, p.Q164Q, p.L188L, p.A210A		WT		
PCC16	p.L188L		WT		
PCC17	WT		WT		
PCC18	p.L188L		WT		
PCC19	p.Y150Y, p.Q164Q, p.A210A	*p.R38Q$^{HO/HO}$*	WT		*loss Chr. 5*
PCC20	p.L188L		WT		*loss Chr. 5*
PCC21	p.Y150Y, p.Q164Q, p.L188L, p.A210A		WT		
PCC22	p.Y150Y, p.Q164Q, p.L188L, p.A210A		WT		
PCC23	p.Y150Y, p.Q164Q, p.L188L, p.A210A		p.A97A	*p.K122R^{HE}*	
PCC46	NA		WT	*p.K122R^{HO}*	*loss Chr.5*

HO = homozygous in tumor (PCC46); HE = heterozygous in tumor (PCC23); HO/HE = homozygous in variant in tumor, heterogeneous in germline; HO/HO = homozygous variant in both tumor and germline; LOH = loss of heterozygosity in tumor, loss of chromosome 5 detected with the SNP array are indicated in the comments, non-syn = non-synonymous, syn = synonymous.

Table 2. Summary of single nucleotide polymorphism (SNP) array results.

Chromosome	PCC19	PCC20	PCC36 *	PCC37 *	PCC43 *	PCC46 *
2					LOSS	
3					LOSS	
5	LOSS	LOSS	LOSS	LOSS	LOSS	LOSS
7	LOSS			LOSS		LOSS
8					LOSS	
9			GAIN			
12					LOSS	
15					LOSS	
16					LOSS	LOSS
17	LOSS	LOSS				
18					LOSS	
20				LOSS	LOSS	
21					LOSS	
22					LOSS	
23		LOSS				
25					LOSS	
26	LOSS	LOSS	LOSS		LOSS	LOSS
27						
28						
29					LOSS	
30	LOSS	LOSS				
31	LOSS				LOSS	
32	LOSS		LOSS		LOSS	
34	LOSS	LOSS				
35	LOSS				LOSS	

Overview of large chromosomal changes in the informative dog PPGL. * Noisy sample.

3. Discussion

Currently, there is still no curative therapy for patients with metastatic PPGL. In general, malignant behavior occurs in 10% of patients with PPGL. However, patients with *SDHB* germline mutations have a much higher chance of developing distant metastases [11]. Investigating animal models of PPGL could lead to the development and testing of therapies for humans with metastatic PPGL. Thus far, the only animal model that presents with metastatic PCC is a *Pten* KO mouse [12,13]. Since *PTEN* mutations do not play a role in the pathogenesis of human (malignant) PPGL, such models are not the most suitable for the study of human malignant PPGL [8]. A recent study reported that dogs presenting spontaneously with PPGL had potential pathogenic genetic alterations in *SDHB* and *SDHD* [10]. To investigate these results in an independent and larger series we have screened 25 canine PPGLs for mutations and identified one *SDHB* and three non-synonymous *SDHD* genetic alterations, both of which have been described previously [10].

The SDHD p.Lys122Arg variant was identified in three canine PPGLs; once in a heterozygous (PCC23) and twice in a homozygous fashion (PCC6 and PCC46). The corresponding germline DNA from PCC6 showed the variant to be present in a heterozygous fashion, indicating loss of the wild type *SDHD* allele in the tumor DNA. This finding was confirmed by the loss of heterozygosity (LOH) analysis, using microsatellites flanking the *SDHD* gene. Although there was no germline DNA available for PCC46, the homozygous expression of the SDHD p.Lys122Arg variant in the tumor could be explained by the potential loss of the *SDHD* wild type, since the SNP array results showed loss of chromosome 5, which includes the *SDHD* gene. However, this is only speculation, since we cannot confirm the possibility that the *SDHD* variant was heterozygous in the germline DNA, and could also be present as a homozygous SDHD p.Lys122Arg or homozygous wild type.

In addition, another previously described non-synonymous *SDHB* variant [10] was detected in PCC19. This tumor showed the SDHB p.Arg38Gln variant in a homozygous fashion, which was also homozygous in DNA isolated from normal tissue from the same dog. Although the SDHB p.Arg38 is a highly conserved amino acid throughout many species, the fruit fly has a Gln at position 38. Since the variant was already present in a homozygous fashion in the germline, no loss of the *SDHB* locus was seen in the SNP array results. As the p.Arg38Gln amino acid change is probably not deleterious to the function of the protein, we regard this variant as likely benign. However, this should be further investigated functionally.

Sanger sequencing screening of this tumor did not reveal any novel mutations in *SDHB* and *SDHD*. However, mutations could have been missed due to the poor DNA quality, resulting in sequences that could not be analyzed, and due to other driving mechanisms, such as promoter-methylation or large (exon) deletions, which are not detectable by Sanger sequencing [14–16].

The SDHA and SDHB immunohistochemistry appeared to be positive in almost all investigated tumors, with the exception of PCC1 and PCC6. PCC1 also was immunohistochemically negative for SDHA. However, since the positive control tissues (normal dog adrenals) showed homogeneous and not granular cytoplasmic labeling, we suspect that the antibody is not suitable for screening for SDH mutations, as in human PPGL [17,18], and, therefore, no conclusions can be drawn from the SDHA and SDHB immunohistochemistry. In addition, the negative/weak positive SDHA and SDHB labeling could also be due to technical limitations, such as fixation artifacts.

The SNP array results showed large chromosomal alterations in six of the nine PPGLs with informative SNP arrays. The fact that three tumors did not show chromosomal aberrations was most likely due to the low neoplastic cell content of these frozen tissue samples, from which DNA was isolated. From the six tumors that showed chromosomal alterations, loss of chromosome 5 was the most frequent alteration (100%). Canine chromosome 5 shows homology with regions of human chromosome 1p and 11q. Many studies have shown that loss of chromosome 1p and chromosome 11 are frequent events in the pathogenesis of human PPGL [3,19,20]. Our results suggest that there are common genes, located in these homologous chromosomal areas, that might contribute to the pathogenesis of both human and canine PPGL.

4. Materials and Methods

4.1. Patients and Sample Selection

In total, we collected 50 dog PPGLs from 45 dogs (including one case with bilateral tumors), which comprised of 44 formalin-fixed paraffin wax-embedded (FFPE) blocks and six fresh frozen samples (FF), from contributing Veterinary faculties from the University of Bristol, Bristol, United Kingdom (n = 25), Utrecht University, Utrecht, the Netherlands (n = 12), University of Zurich, Zurich, Switzerland (n = 8), and University of Bologna, Bologna, Italy (n = 5). In addition, we also collected three normal canine adrenal glands provided by the Veterinary Faculty of Utrecht University, to be used as positive controls for the immunohistochemistry. In addition, from two dogs, corresponding germline DNA was available (PCC6 and PCC19). All tissue samples were collected during surgery or necropsy examination from pet dogs suffering from PPGL. The owners of the dogs had given permission for the tissues to be used for research purposes. All clinical characteristics including age, breed, and gender are listed in Supplemental Table S1. PPGLs were only considered malignant if distant metastases were present, as for human PPGL. A summary of the current study is shown in Supplemental Figure S1.

4.2. Immunohistochemistry

Immunohistochemistry was performed for all canine samples to confirm the diagnosis of PPGL using markers for synaptophysin (SYP) and tyrosine hydroxylase (TH). SYP and TH were evaluated by Esther Korpershoek and Daphne Dieduksman and scored as positive if there was a weak to strong specific expression in the cytoplasm of all tumor cells. SYP was labeled using the Ventana Benchmark ULTRA automated immunohistochemistry stainer (details available on request), while TH immunohistochemistry was performed as previously described [13]. Since in human PPGL, negative SDHB immunohistochemistry reliably identifies tumors with mutations in *SDHA*, *SDHB*, *SDHC*, or *SDHD*, we also investigated the immunohistochemical expression of SDHB in the canine PPGLs [21]. The peptide to which this SDHB antibody was generated is 99% homologous to the canine peptide; only one of 108 amino acid residues is different. The series of canine PPGLs was also labeled for SDHA, as described previously [17]. Normal dog adrenal glands were used as positive controls for immunohistochemistry. The immunohistochemistry was performed on 5 μm sections using the Ventana automated stainer as described previously [18]. SDHB and SDHA expression was scored as positive if strong expression was observed in all cells, while a tumor was considered as negative if the labeling of the tumor cells was negative or weakly positive compared with the positive granular labeling present in the surrounding endothelial cells, which serve as internal positive controls [17,21].

4.3. Genetic Screening

In total, 24 PPGLs (Supplemental Table S1) that expressed SYP and/or TH immunohistochemically were selected for the genetic screening and one TH/SYP negative PCC was also studied. For the FFPE samples, DNA isolation was performed by manual microdissection, to ensure that the DNA was derived from a high percentage of neoplastic cells. DNA isolation was performed with the DNaesy kit (#69504, Qiagen, Venlo, the Netherlands) according to the manufacturer's protocol. DNA concentrations were measured with the Qubit®dsDNA HS BR assay kit (#Q32850, Thermo Fisher, Waltham, MA, USA) according to the manufacturer's instructions. For the generation of the primers, human *SDHA* (NM_004168), *SDHB* (NM_003000), and *SDHD* (MN_003002) mRNA sequences were aligned with the dog genome (CanFam3.1/canFam3) to identify the exact location and sequences of the genes and exons, enabling the generation of dog-specific primers covering all of the coding sequences. PCR was performed with KAPA2G Hotstart Readymix (#KK5004, Sopachem, Ochten, the Netherlands) for which conditions were optimized per primer pair and are listed, together with the primer sequences, in Supplemental Table S2. In total, 21 DNA samples were of sufficient quality to be screened for mutations. Due to technical limitations, we were unable to investigate exon 1 and 8 of *SDHB*, and exon 1 and 2 of *SDHD*. Sanger sequencing was performed as previously described [17].

4.4. Loss of Heterozygosity

To confirm the loss of the wild type allele in *SDHD*-mutated samples, LOH analysis was performed using two microsatellite markers located upstream and downstream from the dog *SDHD* gene. Primer sequences and PCR conditions are indicated in Supplemental Table S2. Furthermore, PCR was performed as previously described [17].

4.5. SNP Arrays:

To determine the chromosomal alterations present in dog PCC, we performed SNP arrays on 11 canine PPGLs (Table 2). Canine HD Beadchip SNP arrays (#WG-440-1001, Illumina, San Diego, CA, USA) with a high resolution genome-wide coverage (170,000 SNPs; resolution of approximately 15 SNPs per Mb) were performed and analyzed according to standard procedures at the Human Genomics Facility (HuGeF), Erasmus MC, University Medical Center Rotterdam (www.glimdna.org).

Final report output files, containing B-allele frequencies and logR ratios, were generated using Illumina BeadStudio Software. The processed files were accordingly visualized using Nexus Copy Number software package (V7.5; Biodiscovery, El Segundo, CA, USA). The SNP array results were submitted to the Gene Expression Omnibus Database. Noisy samples that clearly showed a drop or gain in B-allele frequencies and logR of entire chromosomes were still included in the analysis, taking into account the risk of missing subtle chromosomal changes.

5. Conclusions

In conclusion, the results of the current study indicate that similar genomic alterations occur in canine and human PPGLs. Although more functional proof is required to classify the pathogenicity for the SDHD p.Lys122Arg variant, our data suggest that this variant could potentially be pathogenic.

Since chromosomal alterations occurred in the dog PPGL at high frequency, affecting chromosomes that are homologous to regions that are also repeatedly lost in human PPGLs, we propose that canine PPGLs are an interesting model for the study of the pathogenesis of human PPGL [22]. More studies are required to identify which common pathways are involved in the pathogenesis of PPGL in both humans and dogs.

Supplementary Materials: The following are available online at http://www.mdpi.com/2072-6694/11/5/607/s1, Figure S1: Summary of study design and results, Figure S2: Genomic locations SDH-related genes in the dog genome according to NCBI Genome Data viewer. Table S1: Clinical data, immunohistochemistry results and gene alterations in dog PPGL, Table S2: Primers, Table S3: Homology overview dog chromosome 5 and 26 with human genome.

Author Contributions: Conceptualization, E.K., S.G., and W.N.M.D.; methodology, A.G.U., A.d.K. and B.E.; software B.E., A.d.K. and A.G.U.; formal analysis, E.K.; investigation, D.F. and H.S.; resources, G.C.M.G., M.J.D., C.E.R., M.H., F.F., and S.G.; data curation, E.K.; writing—original draft preparation, E.K.; writing—review and editing, all; validation, E.K. and D.A.E.R.D.; visualization, E.K., B.E. and N.M.G.K.; supervision, W.D.; project administration, E.K. and D.A.E.R.D.; funding acquisition, E.K. and W.N.M.D.

Funding: This research received no external funding.

Conflicts of Interest: The authors declare no conflict of interest.

References

1. Lenders, J.W.; Eisenhofer, G.; Mannelli, M.; Pacak, K. Phaeochromocytoma. *Lancet* **2005**, *366*, 665–675. [CrossRef]
2. Dahia, P.L. Pheochromocytoma and paraganglioma pathogenesis: Learning from genetic heterogeneity. *Nat. Rev. Cancer* **2014**, *14*, 108–119. [CrossRef] [PubMed]
3. Fishbein, L.; Leshchiner, I.; Walter, V.; Danilova, L.; Robertson, A.G.; Johnson, A.R.; Lichtenberg, T.M.; Murray, B.A.; Ghayee, H.K.; Else, T.; et al. Comprehensive Molecular Characterization of Pheochromocytoma and Paraganglioma. *Cancer Cell* **2017**, *31*, 181–193. [CrossRef] [PubMed]
4. Lenders, J.W.; Duh, Q.Y.; Eisenhofer, G.; Gimenez-Roqueplo, A.P.; Grebe, S.K.; Murad, M.H.; Naruse, M.; Pacak, K.; Young, W.F., Jr. Pheochromocytoma and paraganglioma: An endocrine society clinical practice guideline. *J. Clin. Endocrinol. Metab.* **2014**, *99*, 1915–1942. [CrossRef]
5. Timmers, H.J.; Kozupa, A.; Eisenhofer, G.; Raygada, M.; Adams, K.T.; Solis, D.; Lenders, J.W.; Pacak, K. Clinical presentations, biochemical phenotypes, and genotype-phenotype correlations in patients with succinate dehydrogenase subunit B-associated pheochromocytomas and paragangliomas. *J. Clin. Endocrinol. Metab.* **2007**, *92*, 779–786. [CrossRef] [PubMed]
6. Lepoutre-Lussey, C.; Thibault, C.; Buffet, A.; Morin, A.; Badoual, C.; Benit, P.; Rustin, P.; Ottolenghi, C.; Janin, M.; Castro-Vega, L.J.; et al. From Nf1 to Sdhb knockout: Successes and failures in the quest for animal models of pheochromocytoma. *Mol. Cell. Endocrinol.* **2016**, *421*, 40–48. [CrossRef]
7. Korpershoek, E.; Pacak, K.; Martiniova, L. Murine models and cell lines for the investigation of pheochromocytoma: Applications for future therapies? *Endocr. Pathol.* **2012**, *23*, 43–54. [CrossRef]
8. Van Nederveen, F.H.; Perren, A.; Dannenberg, H.; Petri, B.J.; Dinjens, W.N.; Komminoth, P.; de Krijger, R.R. PTEN gene loss, but not mutation, in benign and malignant phaeochromocytomas. *J. Pathol.* **2006**, *209*, 274–280. [CrossRef]
9. Burnichon, N.; Buffet, A.; Parfait, B.; Letouze, E.; Laurendeau, I.; Loriot, C.; Pasmant, E.; Abermil, N.; Valeyrie-Allanore, L.; Bertherat, J.; et al. Somatic NF1 inactivation is a frequent event in sporadic pheochromocytoma. *Hum. Mol. Genet.* **2012**, *21*, 5397–5405. [CrossRef]
10. Holt, D.E.; Henthorn, P.; Howell, V.M.; Robinson, B.G.; Benn, D.E. Succinate dehydrogenase subunit D and succinate dehydrogenase subunit B mutation analysis in canine phaeochromocytoma and paraganglioma. *J. Comp. Pathol.* **2014**, *151*, 25–34. [CrossRef]
11. Van Hulsteijn, L.T.; Dekkers, O.M.; Hes, F.J.; Smit, J.W.; Corssmit, E.P. Risk of malignant paraganglioma in SDHB-mutation and SDHD-mutation carriers: A systematic review and meta-analysis. *J. Med. Genet.* **2012**, *49*, 768–776. [CrossRef]

12. Korpershoek, E.; Kloosterhof, N.K.; der Made, A.Zi.; Korsten, H.; Oudijk, L.; Trapman, J.; Dinjens, W.N.; de Krijger, R.R. Trp53 inactivation leads to earlier phaeochromocytoma formation in pten knockout mice. *Endocr. Relat. Cancer* **2012**, *19*, 731–740. [CrossRef]
13. Korpershoek, E.; Loonen, A.J.; Corvers, S.; van Nederveen, F.H.; Jonkers, J.; Ma, X.; der Made, A.Zi.; Korsten, H.; Trapman, J.; Dinjens, W.N.; et al. Conditional Pten knock-out mice: A model for metastatic phaeochromocytoma. *J. Pathol.* **2009**, *217*, 597–604. [CrossRef]
14. Bayley, J.P.; Grimbergen, A.E.; van Bunderen, P.A.; van der Wielen, M.; Kunst, H.P.; Lenders, J.W.; Jansen, J.C.; Dullaart, R.P.; Devilee, P.; Corssmit, E.P.; et al. The first Dutch SDHB founder deletion in paraganglioma-pheochromocytoma patients. *BMC Med. Genet.* **2009**, *10*, 34. [CrossRef]
15. Cascon, A.; Montero-Conde, C.; Ruiz-Llorente, S.; Mercadillo, F.; Leton, R.; Rodriguez-Antona, C.; Martinez-Delgado, B.; Delgado, M.; Diez, A.; Rovira, A.; et al. Gross SDHB deletions in patients with paraganglioma detected by multiplex PCR: A possible hot spot? *Genes Chromosomes Cancer* **2006**, *45*, 213–219. [CrossRef]
16. Richter, S.; Klink, B.; Nacke, B.; de Cubas, A.A.; Mangelis, A.; Rapizzi, E.; Meinhardt, M.; Skondra, C.; Mannelli, M.; Robledo, M.; et al. Epigenetic Mutation of the Succinate Dehydrogenase C Promoter in a Patient with Two Paragangliomas. *J. Clin. Endocrinol. Metab.* **2016**, *101*, 359–363. [CrossRef]
17. Korpershoek, E.; Favier, J.; Gaal, J.; Burnichon, N.; van Gessel, B.; Oudijk, L.; Badoual, C.; Gadessaud, N.; Venisse, A.; Bayley, J.P.; et al. SDHA immunohistochemistry detects germline SDHA gene mutations in apparently sporadic paragangliomas and pheochromocytomas. *J. Clin. Endocrinol. Metab.* **2011**, *96*, E1472–E1476. [CrossRef]
18. Papathomas, T.G.; Oudijk, L.; Persu, A.; Gill, A.J.; van Nederveen, F.; Tischler, A.S.; Tissier, F.; Volante, M.; Matias-Guiu, X.; Smid, M.; et al. SDHB/SDHA immunohistochemistry in pheochromocytomas and paragangliomas: A multicenter interobserver variation analysis using virtual microscopy: A Multinational Study of the European Network for the Study of Adrenal Tumors (ENS@T). *Mod. Pathol.* **2015**, *28*, 807–821. [CrossRef]
19. Castro-Vega, L.J.; Letouze, E.; Burnichon, N.; Buffet, A.; Disderot, P.H.; Khalifa, E.; Loriot, C.; Elarouci, N.; Morin, A.; Menara, M.; et al. Multi-omics analysis defines core genomic alterations in pheochromocytomas and paragangliomas. *Nat. Commun.* **2015**, *6*, 6044. [CrossRef]
20. Van Nederveen, F.; Korpershoek, E.; Deleeuw, R.; Verhofstad, A.A.; Lenders, J.W.; Dinjens, W.; Lam, W.; de Krijger, R. Array-CGH in sporadic benign pheochromocytomas. *Endocr. Relat. Cancer* **2009**, *16*, 505–513. [CrossRef]
21. Gaal, J.; van Nederveen, F.H.; Erlic, Z.; Korpershoek, E.; Oldenburg, R.; Boedeker, C.C.; Kontny, U.; Neumann, H.P.; Dinjens, W.N.; de Krijger, R.R. Parasympathetic paragangliomas are part of the Von Hippel-Lindau syndrome. *J. Clin. Endocrinol. Metab.* **2009**, *94*, 4367–4371. [CrossRef] [PubMed]
22. Galac, S.; Korpershoek, E. Pheochromocytomas and paragangliomas in humans and dogs. *Vet. Comp. Oncol.* **2017**, *15*, 1158–1170. [CrossRef] [PubMed]

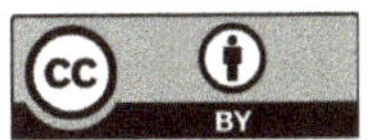

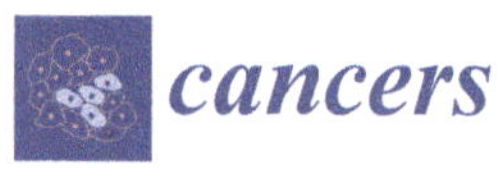 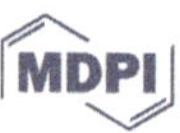

Article

Analysis of Short-term Blood Pressure Variability in Pheochromocytoma/Paraganglioma Patients

Valeria Bisogni [1], Luigi Petramala [1], Gaia Oliviero [1], Maria Bonvicini [1], Martina Mezzadri [1], Federica Olmati [1], Antonio Concistrè [1], Vincenza Saracino [1], Monia Celi [1], Gianfranco Tonnarini [1], Gino Iannucci [2], Giorgio De Toma [3], Antonio Ciardi [4], Giuseppe La Torre [5] and Claudio Letizia [1,*]

1 Department of Translational and Precision Medicine, Unit of Secondary Arterial Hypertension, "Sapienza" University of Rome, Viale del Policlinico 155, 00165 Rome, Italy; valeria.bisogni@hotmail.it (V.B.); luigi.petramala@uniroma1.it (L.P.); gaiaoliviero2@gmail.com (G.O.); bonvimery@gmail.com (M.B.); mezzadri.1615511@studenti.uniroma1.it (M.M.); federica.kolmati@gmail.com (F.O.); antonio.concistre@gmail.com (A.C.); vincenza.saracino@gmail.com (V.S.); celi.monia@gmail.com (M.C.); gianfranco.tonnarini@uniroma1.it (G.T.)

2 Department of Internal Medicine and Medical Specialties, "Sapienza" University of Rome, Viale del Policlinico 155, 00165 Rome, Italy; gino.iannucci@uniroma1.it

3 "Pietro Valdoni" Surgery Department, "Sapienza" University of Rome, Viale del Policlinico 155, 00165 Rome, Italy; giorgio.detoma@uniroma1.it

4 Department of Radiological, Oncological and Anatomy-Pathological Sciences, "Sapienza" University of Rome, Viale del Policlinico 155, 00165 Rome, Italy; antonio.ciardi@uniroma1.it

5 Department of Public Health and Infectious Diseases, "Sapienza" University of Rome, Viale del Policlinico 155, 00165 Rome, Italy; giuseppe.latorre@uniroma1.it

* Correspondence: claudio.letizia@uniroma1.it

Received: 11 April 2019; Accepted: 10 May 2019; Published: 12 May 2019

Abstract: Data on short-term blood pressure variability (BPV), which is a well-established cardiovascular prognostic tool, in pheochromocytoma and paraganglioma (PPGL) patients is still lack and conflicting. We retrospectively evaluated 23 PPGL patients referred to our unit from 2010 to 2019 to analyze 24 h ambulatory blood pressure monitoring (24-h ABPM)-derived markers of short-term BPV, before and after surgical treatment. PPGL diagnosis was assessed according to guidelines and confirmed by histologic examination. The 24-h ABPM-derived markers of short-term BPV included: circadian pressure rhythm; standard deviation (SD) and weighted SD (wSD) of 24-h, daytime, and night-time systolic and diastolic blood pressure (BP); average real variability (ARV) of 24-h, daytime, and night-time systolic and diastolic BP. 7 males and 16 females of 53 ± 18 years old were evaluated. After surgical resection of PPGL we found a significant decrease in 24-h systolic BP ARV (8.8 ± 1.6 vs. 7.6 ± 1.3 mmHg, $p < 0.001$), in 24-h diastolic BP ARV (7.5 ± 1.6 vs. 6.9 ± 1.4 mmHg, $p = 0.031$), and in wSD of 24-h diastolic BP (9.7 ± 2.0 vs 8.8 ± 2.1 mmHg, $p = 0.050$) comparing to baseline measurements. Moreover, baseline 24-h urinary metanephrines significantly correlated with wSD of both 24-h systolic and diastolic BP. Our study highlights as PPGL patients, after proper treatment, show a significant decrease in some short-term BPV markers, which might represent a further cardiovascular risk factor.

Keywords: pheochromocytoma; paraganglioma; hypertension; blood pressure variability; average real variability; weighted standard deviation

1. Introduction

Pheochromocytoma (PHEO) and paraganglioma (PGL), known together as PPGL, are rare and mostly benign neuroendocrine tumors, arising from chromaffin-cells of adrenal medulla and paraganglia of the sympathetic and parasympathetic nervous system, respectively [1]. At least one-third of patients with PPGL have disease-causing germline mutations (i.e., *NF1*, *RET*, *VHL*, *SDHD*,

SDHB, etc.) and subjects with hereditary forms typically show multifocal diseases at younger age than those with sporadic neoplasms [1–4]. The clinical presentation is so variable that PPGLs have been described as "the great masquerades" [5,6]. However, several signs and symptoms are attributed to hemodynamic and metabolic effects of the catecholamines overproduction. One of the most typical manifestations (up to 80% of cases), due to the catecholamine-excess state, is arterial hypertension, either sustained or paroxysmal [5], even though its severity does not seem to depend on the level of circulating catecholamines [6].

Although office blood pressure (BP) values remain the gold standard for the diagnosis of hypertension, the measurement of BP variability (BPV) in addition to office BP, has been demonstrated to have physiopathological and prognostic importance [7,8]. Short-term BPV refers to the BP changes that occur within a day [24 hours (24-h)], and it is influenced by several mechanisms, such as central neural factors, reflex autonomic modulation, changes in the elastic properties of arteries, humoral systems (i.e., insulin, angiotensin II, endothelin-1, bradykinin, and nitric oxide), rheological and mechanical factors [8]. Several studies have shown that higher 24-h BPV, assessed by 24-h ambulatory blood pressure monitoring (24-h ABPM), independently of mean office BP values, is clinically important, as this might increase cardiovascular events, mortality, and hypertension-mediated organ damage [9–14]. Concerning the short-term BPV in PPGL, assessed by 24-h ABPM, only outdated and small studies have been published [15–18] with contrasting results. As higher cardiovascular mortality has been reported in PPGL subjects [19], increased BPV might be a contributor for enhanced cardiovascular morbidity and mortality in this rare disease, besides the known risk factors, such as hypertension, arrhythmias, and altered glucose metabolism [20].

The aim of our study was to analyze changes in the 24-h ABPM-derived short-term BPV markers in patients affected by PPGL, before and after successful treatment by surgical removing of catecholamine-producing tumors.

2. Results

Table 1 shows the baseline characteristics of enrolled patients affected by PPGL. 7 males (30.4%) and 16 females (69.6%), with a median age at the diagnosis of 53 ± 18 years old, were evaluated before and after surgical tumor excision. The main signs and symptoms reported at the first visit are summarized in Table 1; the most frequent were represented by palpitation attacks, headache, sweating crises, and sustained and/or paroxysmal arterial hypertension (in 14 cases), often associated with each other. At the physical examination, we did not find cases of BP decreasing within 3 minutes of standing compared with BP from the sitting or supine position [21]. The most common comorbidities included a past history or current treatment for dyslipidemia (21.7%), coronary artery disease and/or cerebrovascular accidents (17.4%), including transient ischemic attack and ischemic/hemorrhagic stroke. One patient reported a diagnosis of diabetes mellitus type 2 and one patient history of paroxysmal atrial fibrillation.

Most of the patients had an adrenal catecholamine-producing tumor, while two women (8.6%) showed an extra-adrenal catecholamine-producing tumor in the left hypochondrium. One of these, after two years of surgical removal of the pelvic mass, revealed a recurrent form of PPGL disease with discovering a left common carotid tumor. Germline mutations were found in eight patients (34.8%) (Table 1); the most common gene involved was *VHL*, mutated in three brothers affected by von Hipple–Lindau syndrome. We also found two patients with a diagnosis of neurofibromatosis type 1 and mutation of the *NF1* gene. In two sisters we observed a *RET* gene mutation associated with a diagnosis of multiple endocrine neoplasia syndrome (MEN) type 2A. In particular, both of them presented thyroid medullary carcinoma and hyperparathyroidism, but in one patient we found an adrenal PHEO, while in the younger sister the catecholamine-producing tumor was in the left hypochondrium. In only one female, we discovered an *SDHD* gene mutation.

Table 1. Baseline demographic and anthropometric data. Total (n = 23).

Age (Years)	53 ± 18
Males/Females (%)	30.4/69.6
Mean Follow-Up (months)	26 ± 25
Signs and Symptoms (%)	
Hypertension (sustained and/or paroxysmal)	60.8
Palpitation attacks	87.5
Headache	87.5
Sweating	65.2
Syncope	13.0
Orthostatic hypotension	17.4
Chest pain	17.4
Others (i.e., abdominal pain, dizziness, etc.)	21.7
Type of PPGL (%)	
adrenal catecholamine-producing tumor (PHEO)	91.4
extra-adrenal catecholamine-producing tumor (PGL)	8.6
Benign/Malignant form (%)	100/0
Site of Extra-Adrenal Masses (n)	
Abdominal	2
Neck	1
Multifocal forms (n)	1
Germline Mutation	
Total (n, %)	8 (34.8)
NF1 (n)	2
RET (n)	2
VHL (n)	3
SDHD (n)	1
Cigarettes Smoking (%)	
yes	17.4
no	21.7
ex-smokers	13.0
n.a.	47.8
Comorbidities (%)	
Coronary artery disease and/or cerebrovascular accidents	17.4
Atrial fibrillation (history or current)	4.3
Diabetes mellitus	4.3
Dyslipidemia	21.7

Data expressed as mean ± standard deviation unless otherwise specified. PHEO, pheochromocytoma; PGL, paraganglioma; n.a., not available.

Surgical treatment was performed in all cases [22]. Patients with PHEO underwent laparoscopic or laparotomic adrenalectomy and patients with PGL underwent surgical excision of the extra-adrenal mass, leading to complete remission of catecholamines excess based on the normalization of biochemical and clinical features at follow-up. The histologic examination confirmed the diagnosis of PPGL; the specific features were represented by a neoplastic proliferation characterized by small nests or alveolar patterns (Zellballen), in which well-circumscribed nests of round-oval or giant or spindle-shaped nucleated neoplastic cells with eosinophil cytoplasm including catecholamine granules ("salt-and-pepper" pattern). Neoplastic cells were evaluated for chromogranin, neuron-specific enolase (NSE), and synaptophysin and CD56; the proliferation index was analyzed by Ki67 determination. All tumors had benign histological and clinical features.

In Table 2 have been reported clinical and biochemical parameters at baseline compared to follow-up from surgical treatment (mean follow-up: 26 ± 25 months). At the first visit, the levels of 24-h urinary metanephrines were 357.4 ± 190.3 μg/24-h vs. 64.1 ± 30.5 μg/24-h after surgical treatment ($p < 0.001$). Notably, the office systolic BP values were significantly lower after treatment, with a significant reduction of the number of antihypertensive drugs (2.2 ± 1.7 vs. 1.0 ± 1.0, $p = 0.001$). Moreover, we observed a modest improvement in fast glucose levels (99 ± 21 vs. 88 ± 15 mg/dl, $p = 0.05$). On the other hand, we did not find significant regression of hypertension-mediated sub-clinical vascular damage; before treatment, the mean of common carotid intima-media thickness (cIMT) at the Doppler ultrasonography was bilateral >9 mm, without plaques, and it improved only barely at the follow-up. No changes were found in the arterial stiffness variable measured by ankle-brachial index (ABI).

Table 2. Anthropometric, biochemical, and instrumental data at baseline compared to follow-up.

Parameters	Total (n = 23)		
	Baseline	Follow-Up	p
Age (years)	52 ± 18	54 ± 18	0.001
BMI (kg/m2)	23.0 ± 3.4	23.1 ± 3.5	0.875
Waist circumference (cm)	86.7 ± 11.3	88.4 ± 9.0	0.321
Office SBP (mmHg)	147 ± 32	131 ± 16	0.021
Office DBP (mmHg)	85 ± 20	79 ± 10	0.146
Office HR (beats/min)	75 ± 14	70 ± 14	0.754
N. of antihypertensive drugs	2.2 ± 1.7	1.0 ± 1.1	0.001
24-h urinary metanephrines (μg/24-h)	357.4 ± 190.3	64.1 ± 30.5	<0.001
Serum creatinine (mg/dL)	0.83 ± 0.25	0.98 ± 0.43	0.050
Total cholesterol (mg/dL)	217 ± 40	185 ± 27	0.099
LDL cholesterol (mg/dL)	117 ± 37	100 ± 26	0.327
HDL cholesterol (mg/dL)	79 ± 40	63 ± 22	0.034
Triglycerides (mg/dL)	115 ± 52	111 ± 39	0.861
Glycaemia (mg/dL)	99 ± 21	88 ± 15	0.050
Uric acid (mg/dL)	7.5 ± 7.7	4.9 ± 1.4	0.374
Right cIMT (mm)	0.91 ± 0.15	0.88 ± 0.22	0.551
Left cIMT (mm)	0.91 ± 0.15	0.86 ± 0.21	0.086
ABI	1.01 ± 0.19	1.07 ± 0.19	0.786

Data expressed as mean ± standard deviation unless otherwise specified. BMI, body mass index; SBP, systolic blood pressure; DBP, diastolic blood pressure; HR, heart rate; LDL, low-density lipoproteins; HDL, high-density lipoproteins; cIMT, carotid intima-media thickness; ABI, ankle-brachial index.

In Table 3, we summarized data on 24-h ABPM and 24-h ABPM-derived short-term BPV indexes. After surgical treatment, we observed a significant difference in terms of 24-h SBP values, although they were into the normal range and well-controlled after optimization of antihypertensive therapy with α-adrenergic receptor blockers. We did not find significant changes in the circadian BP rhythm, with a systolic dipping of 7.5 ± 8.0 vs. 7.7 ± 6.9 % ($p = 0.80$) and diastolic dipping of 11.7 ± 9.3 vs. 12.3 ± 7.8 % ($p = 0.37$). However, the average real variability (ARV) of both 24-h systolic and diastolic BP components, after surgical treatment, was significantly decreased (8.8 ± 1.6 vs 7.6 ± 1.3 mmHg, $p = 0.001$ and 7.5 ± 1.6 vs 6.9 ± 1.4 mmHg, $p = 0.031$, respectively), as well as the 24-h diastolic weighted SD (wSD) (Table 3). Finally, the 24-h, daytime, and night-time systolic and diastolic BP standard deviation (SD), despite not significant, showed a lowering trend (Table 3). Circadian heart rate variation remained unchanged.

Table 3. 24-h ABPM-derived short-term blood pressure variability (BPV) markers at baseline compared to follow-up after surgical treatment.

Short-Term BPV Markers	Total (*n* = 23)		
	Baseline	Follow-Up	*p*
24-h systolic BP (mmHg)	129 ± 13	115 ± 12	0.002
24-h diastolic BP (mmHg)	73 ± 15	72 ± 9	0.329
24-h heart rate (beats/min)	75 ± 12	78 ± (9)	0.073
Systolic BP dipping (%)	7.5 ± 8.0	7.7 ± 6.9	0.808
Diastolic BP dipping (%)	11.7 ± 9.3	12.3 ± 7.8	0.837
SD of 24-h systolic BP (mmHg)	13.2 ± 4.8	12.2 ± 2.7	0.670
SD of daytime systolic BP (mmHg)	12.4 ± 3.4	11.6 ± 2.7	0.328
SD of night-time systolic BP (mmHg)	10.1 ± 4.0	9.0 ± 3.3	0.348
SD of 24-h diastolic BP (mmHg)	11.3 ± 2.7	10.2 ± 2.3	0.152
SD of daytime diastolic BP (mmHg)	10.3 ± 2.9	9.4 ± 2.5	0.057
SD of night-time diastolic BP (mmHg)	8.4 ± 2.4	7.6 ± 2.9	0.370
SD of 24-h heart rate (beats/min)	10.9 ± 3.6	11.0 ± 4.5	0.852
SD of daytime heart rate (beats/min)	10.7 ± 3.7	10.9 ± 5.0	0.988
SD of night-time heart rate (beats/min)	7.0 ± 2.6	6.7 ± 2.9	0.399
wSD of 24-h systolic BP (mmHg)	11.6 ± 3.1	10.8 ± 2.4	0.173
wSD of 24-h diastolic BP (mmHg)	9.7 ± 2.0	8.8 ± 2.1	0.050
ARV of 24-h systolic BP (mmHg)	8.8 ± 1.6	7.6 ± 1.3	0.001
ARV of 24-h diastolic BP (mmHg)	7.5 ± 1.6	6.9 ± 1.4	0.031

Data expressed as mean ± standard deviation unless otherwise specified. BP, blood pressure; SD, standard deviation; wSD, weighted standard deviation; ARV, average real variability.

A bivariate scatterplot with correlation analysis showed a direct correlation between the mean values of 24-h urinary metanephrines and (i) SD of night-time systolic BP (r = 0.45, $p = 0.022$), (ii) wSD of both 24-h systolic (r = 0.47, $p = 0.009$), and diastolic BP (r = 0.43, $p = 0.019$) performed at baseline. At multivariate analysis, the strongest predictors of 24-h systolic BP wSD were age (β = 0.566, $p = 0.002$) and baseline 24-h urinary metanephrines (β = 0.347, $p = 0.042$). For the 24-h diastolic component of wSD the strongest predictor were the 24-h urinary metanephrines values (β = 0.554, $p = 0.006$).

Lastly, we analyzed the main anthropometric and demographic data of our patients, before and after treatment, distinguishing by gender. We did not observe significant differences in terms of 24-h ABPM-derived short-term BPV indexes.

3. Discussion

Despite their relatively rare incidence in the general population, PPGLs are characterized by high cardiovascular morbidity and mortality [23,24]. The clinical picture associated with increased catecholamines levels, in fact, may vary from asymptomatic tumors (discovered incidentally during examinations performed due to other reasons) to life-threatening complications, such as myocardial infarction, severe heart failure, cardiomyopathy, shock, arrhythmias, and stroke. In a retrospective study, Zelinka et al. [24] observed a relatively high incidence of cardiovascular complications in PPGL subjects, reaching almost 20%. The most prevalent were arrhythmic complications (in about 10% of cases) followed by myocardial ischemia and atherosclerosis, and in about 5% of patients, cerebrovascular accidents [24]. Catecholamines excess can also lead to severe left ventricular hypertrophy. Recently, Olmati et al. presented a case of a young woman with hypertrophic cardiomyopathy secondary to a catecholamine-producing tumor and confirmed by endomyocardial biopsy, in which has been noted severe disarray of cardiomyocytes and ultrastructural evidence of contraction and necrosis of myocytes [25].

Pathogenic mechanisms that link PPGL and cardiovascular complications are multiple but mainly associated to catecholamines overproduction, which leads to increased oxygen consumption, vasoconstriction, cardiac afterload, augmented production of reactive oxygen species, cell hypertrophy through increased protein synthesis, and cardiac remodeling [23]. Arterial hypertension is a consequence of PPGL in up to 80–90% of patients [6] and it may contribute to the development and worsening of the cardiovascular profile, as well as metabolic derangements (i.e. impaired glucose tolerance), which has a reported prevalence of 25 to 75% in PHEO [26].

To evaluate cardiovascular risk in the hypertensive population, the assessment of BPV is a validated screening tool [27,28]. In physiological conditions, the short-, mid-, and long-term BPV variations have been shown to represent an adaptive mechanism to maintain homeostasis. However, sustained increases in BPV over time may also reflect alterations in cardiovascular regulatory mechanisms, which might have prognostic relevance. Clinical and population studies, using non-invasive, intermittent, reading-to-reading over 24-h monitoring provided the evidence that BPV may contribute independently to cardiovascular events prediction, over and beyond average BP [29–31]. Increased BPV has been associated with a higher risk of cardiovascular events, with this prediction depending on the basal risk. In low-to-moderate cardiovascular risk populations, the contribution of BPV to risk stratification has been only marginal [32], whereas in higher-risk patients, as could be those affected by PPGL, increased BPV appeared to have significant prognostic value, which might exceed that of the average BP values. Furthermore, it has been highlighted that in patients with the most common secondary forms of hypertension, such as primary aldosteronism [33], Cushing's syndrome [34], obstructive sleep apnea [35,36], and primary hyperparathyroidism [37], the short-term BPV markers increased compared to essential hypertensive groups and decreased after specific treatments.

In our retrospective study, we evaluated data on 23 patients with a diagnosis of PHEO or PGL underwent surgery. After successfully removing the cause of excessive production of catecholamines the office systolic BP and the number of antihypertensive drugs significantly decreased. Even more important, we found changes in some markers of short-term BPV assessed by 24-h ABPM. In particular, we observed a reduction in ARV of 24-h systolic and diastolic BP. This index focuses on modifications that have been registered over short-time intervals and, thus, corrects some of the limitations of SD, which only reflects the dispersion of BP measurements around the mean [29]. The ARV has been recently demonstrated (i) to be a better estimator of 24-h BPV than other measures of dispersion, (ii) to be more useful for determining therapeutic measures aimed at controlling BPV, (iii) to have greater predictive value than the SD, after adjustment for BP and other clinical factors, for the presence and progression of subclinical organ damage [29], for total and cardiovascular mortality, and fatal combined with nonfatal cerebrovascular events [38]. Therefore, ARV of 24-h systolic and diastolic BP components is crucial to stratify the cardiovascular risk.

In our study, we also discovered a significant correlation between 24-h urinary metanephrines values and wSD of 24-h systolic and diastolic BP at baseline. Moreover, at multivariate analysis, after adjustment for sex and body mass index, the strongest predictors of 24-h systolic and diastolic wSD were the 24-h urinary metanephrines, underlying the feasible role of catecholamines overproduction in the BPV changes. The wSD represents the average of daytime and night-time BP that has been adjusted for the duration of the day and night period to account for day-night BP changes [8] and it allows to exclude the interference of night-time BP fall on overall BPV, and consents a more precise assessment of the clinical value of 24-h BPV [39]. Therefore, together with ARV, the wSD is an index unaffected by day-to-night BP changes and it should be preferred for the BPV evaluation.

According to previous research [40–42], we did not find changes in the systolic and diastolic BP nocturnal fall. However, various causes for the absence of dipping profile are conceivable, including sleep disturbance and psychiatric disorders, which have not been assessed by the anamnestic evaluation in our group of patients. Moreover, despite PPGLs are considered to be a curable cause of hypertension, in the long-term a substantial proportion of patients without recurrence could show higher than suggested nocturnal BP values and/or continue taking antihypertensive agents for BP control. These patients are usually (i) older, (ii) have a family history of hypertension, (iii) show higher BP values at baseline before surgical treatment, (iv) report pre-existing and associated cardiovascular risk factors (such as smoke, dyslipidemia, etc.), and (v) longer disease duration before diagnosis. In particular, referring to the last point, likewise for other forms of secondary hypertension, PPGL might lose the ability to reverse the structural vascular changes associated with secondary hypertension [43].

Lastly, we would point out that, after successful surgical treatment, the metabolic assessment significantly ameliorated with reduction of fasting glucose levels and a decreasing trend in lipid panel variables. These findings are consistent with previously reported results [44,45] and might be implicated in reducing cardiovascular risk in PPGL patients.

In summary, several studies refer to the importance of sympathetic activity and arterial baroreflexes in regulating cardiovascular variability and report other factors, including the vascular response to sympathetic stimuli, which play a role in determining the strength of BP oscillations [46,47]. Therefore, based on our results, we hypothesized that the excessive and pulsatile production of plasma catecholamines and their metabolites might have a pathogenic key role in the BPV changes. As it has been suggested by earlier researches [48,49], two types of mechanisms leading to higher BPV in PPGL patients might be involved: first, the ability of circulating catecholamines to cause rapid BP elevations; second, the high incidence of orthostatic hypotension with normally functioning baroreflex probably related to the tendency to hypovolemia [50] or because of the suppressed central sympathetic outflow [51] as a consequence of the hyperactivation of adrenergic receptors. To support these assumptions, we showed significant changes in ARV of 24-h systolic and diastolic BP and 24-h diastolic BP wSD in patients affected by PPGL after successful surgical tumor excision. These changes might represent, besides well-established and independent risk factors (i.e., hypertension, arrhythmias, and disturbances of glucose metabolism) [1,6], an additional issue for cardiovascular morbidity and mortality in this rare condition. The correlation between 24-h urinary metanephrines and systolic and diastolic wSD and the modifications mentioned above in the blood pressure variability markers at follow-up suggest the potential reversibility of cardiovascular risk by surgery in PPGL.

Thus, we strongly propose considering, in the clinical management of PPGL, as well as in normotensive PPGL subjects, the assessment of short-term 24-h ABPM-derived BPV, which, if increased, might reflect a higher risk of cardiovascular complications.

Limitations and Strengths

Some limitations should be acknowledged. At first, the study used a retrospective design and a small sample of patients, due to the rare occurrence of catecholamine-producing tumors. Secondly, we measured only 24-h urinary metanephrines; we were able to collect plasma catecholamines and plasma metanephrines only in few cases during documented paroxysmal clinical manifestations, and, then, we could not differentiate norepinephrine- from epinephrine-secreting PPGL. Furthermore, in our population, we did not evaluate the tumor size, and we did not have any case of malignant forms; therefore, we did not understand whether the dimension of the mass and its malignant phenotype could influence BPV. Lastly, not all patients were free from other cardiovascular risk factors that could influence BPV indexes, such as smoke that was present in up to 15%, dyslipidemia (in more than 20% of cases), and previous coronary and cerebrovascular accidents.

However, hypertension in PPGLs is very complex with various clinical presentations perhaps due to the desensitization of catecholamine receptors often leading to normotension. In this context, we retain that the assessment of BPV plays a crucial role because of: (i) it allows stratifying the cardiovascular risk in this population; (ii) it could be used as a part of the screening tool of PPGL. Our findings, although only preliminary, consent to speculate a possible role of BPV in the diagnostic workup of PHEO and PGL. ARV and wSD represent better and more accurate estimators of short-term BPV than other measures of dispersion. Their record and analysis might have interesting implications in the complete evaluation and management of patients affected by PPGL, mostly in those with paroxysmal hypertension and/or in those with false-negative laboratory tests, because it may allow discovering an asymptomatic altered cardiovascular profile.

Moreover, changes in BPV markers after specific treatment may contribute to understanding better which mechanisms are implicated in the increase of cardiovascular risk in patients with catecholamine-producing tumors.

4. Materials and Methods

From January 2011 to March 2019, we retrospectively evaluated 23 patients, both of sex and aged ≥18 years old, referred to our Secondary Hypertension Unit, University of Rome "Sapienza," Italy (Figure 1). This study was performed according to the Declaration of Helsinki II and all participants gave informed consent.

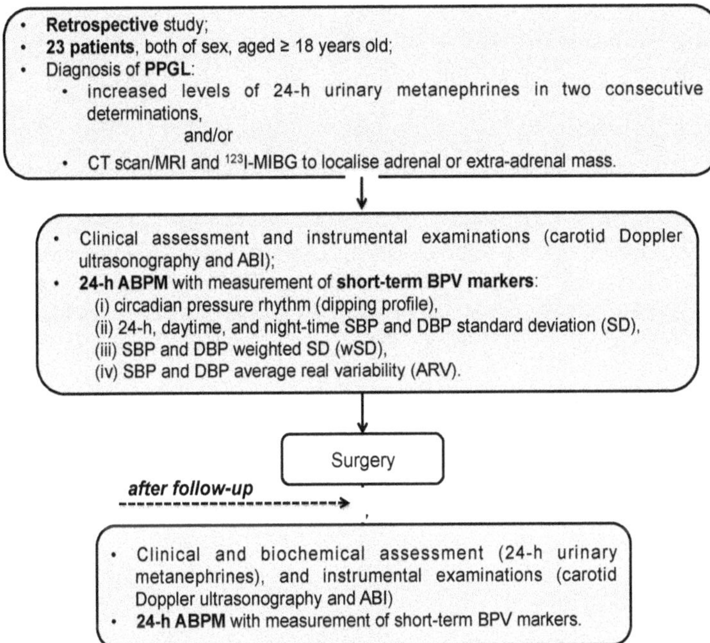

Figure 1. Flow-chart of the study. PPGL, pheochromocytoma and paraganglioma; CT, computed tomography; MRI, magnetic resonance imaging; MIBG, metaiodobenzylguanidine; ABI, ankle-brachial index; SBP, systolic blood pressure; DBP, diastolic blood pressure; SD, standard deviation.

The PPGL diagnosis was performed according to the Endocrine Society Guidelines [1], and the BPV markers were measured agreeing with the most recent recommendations [27], as described below.

All patients underwent genetic testing for the most common familial forms. At baseline and follow-up evaluations, for each patient, we collected data on anthropometric parameters and physical examination (i.e., BMI and waist circumference), past medical history, current treatment, and detailed information on cardiovascular risk (i.e., smoking, dyslipidemia, and previous cardiovascular events). To determinate hypertension-related vascular remodeling we recorded:

(i) Ankle-brachial index (ABI): we measured ABI after a 5 minutes rest in the supine position. The ABI was determined using an automated oscillometric measurement BOSO-ABI system neo (Bosch+Sohn GmbH U. Co. KG, Jungingen, Germany), which allows simultaneous arm-leg BP measurements.
(ii) Carotid Doppler ultrasonography: it determines the common carotid intima-media thickness (calculated from three separate values 1 cm proximal to the common carotid artery bifurcation

in the left and right common carotid arteries), the characteristics of plaques, and the degree of stenosis [52].

4.1. PPGL Diagnosis

The PPGL diagnosis [1] was based on (i) clinical signs and symptoms, such as sustained or paroxysmal arterial hypertension, orthostatic hypotension, tachycardia, diaphoresis, headaches, chest pain, syncope, etc.; (ii) familial history of PPGL with specific involved genetic mutations (e.g., *VHL*, *NF1*, *RET*, *SDHD*, etc.); (iii) 24-h urinary metanephrines (measured by the RIA method; normal range: 20–345 µg/24-h), determined in two consecutive measurements; and/or (iv) abdominal magnetic resonance imaging (MRI) or computed tomography (CT) scan, subsequently confirmed by ^{123}I-metaiodobenzylguanidine (^{123}I-MIBG) scintigraphy, which was performed also in patients with normal values of 24-h urinary metanephrines and/or negative MRI and CT scan but high clinical suspect of PPGL.

4.2. Genetic Analysis

After signing of informed consent, for each patient a blood sample was obtained for the extraction of DNA according to the standardized protocol in the molecular genetics laboratory of our department [5]. DNA was extracted from the peripheral blood leukocytes of each patient with the Nucleospin blood L kit (Macherey-Nagel, Duren, Germany) and analyzed for germline mutations of *RET* (exons 10,11,13,14,15,16), *VHL* (all exons), *SDHD* (all exons), and *SDHB* (all exons). For each gene, coding regions and exon-intron boundaries, polymerase chain reaction (PCR) fragments purified with a commercial kit (PCR purification kit, Qiagen, Milan, Italy) were subject to 2% agarose gel electrophoresis with ethidium bromide staining and subsequently sequenced with a genetic analyzer (ABI PRISM 310, Applied Biosystems, Milan, Italy). For the *NF1* gene was performed a mutation analysis of the 57 exons and flanking intronic regions as well as the untranslated 50 and 30 regions of the *NF1* gene required a redesign of PCR primer pairs in order to exclude amplification of any of the 36 pseudogenes [53]. A germline intragenic mutation scanning was carried out on each of the amplicons using denaturing high-performance liquid chromatography analysis (WAVE analysis system, Transgenomics, Paris, France). Samples displaying abnormal chromatographic patterns were subjected to bidirectional direct sequencing using a MegaBACE500 DNA sequencing machine (Amersham Biosciences, Freiburg, Germany) [5].

4.3. Blood Pressure Variability Assessment

Short-term BPV was assessed by 24-h ABPM using Spacelabs®90207 (SpaceLabs, Snoqualmie, WA, USA), which was carried out as a part of the procedures before diagnosis and after follow-up, in a day separate from the first office visit and after optimization of medical therapy to control BP values.

All data were acquired and analyzed according to the current recommendations [54]. Devices were calibrated periodically with a mercury sphygmomanometer and the arm cuff was positioned on the non-dominant upper limb. The between measurement intervals were 15 minutes (daytime) and 30 minutes (night-time). During each recording, subjects were required to attend at their usual daily activities, only refraining from unusual physical exercise or behavioral challenges. Only recordings rated of sufficient quality, i.e., including at least 70% of valid readings over the 24-h and at least two valid readings per hour during daytime and one valid reading per hour during night-time, were considered for the final analysis. Day and night periods were defined and corrected according to what was reported by the patient in the diary. The average daytime period was finally identified as the interval from 06:00 h to 22:00 h and the night period as the interval from 22:00 h to 06:00 h. For each recording, the mean 24-h, and day- and night-time systolic and diastolic BP have been collected. Moreover, as suggested by previous validation studies [27,55], we identified markers of short-term BPV derived by 24-h ABPM, which included:

(i) Degree of nocturnal BP fall (*dipping* pattern), calculated as [(daytime SBP − night-time SBP)/daytime SBP × 100%] for SBP and [(daytime DBP − night-time DBP)/daytime DBP × 100%] for DBP. Patients were classified as *dippers* if BP falls ≥10% and <20% of daytime average BP or *non-dippers* (fall <10%). Nocturnal BP falls ≥20% and <0% identified *"extreme" dipper* and *"reverse" dipper* subjects.
(ii) Standard deviation (SD) of 24-h, daytime, and night-time SBP and DBP;
(iii) Average of daytime and night-time SD, each weighted for the duration of the day and night periods [24-h "weighted" SD of BP (wSD)], which allows for removing the mathematical interference from night-time BP fall;
(iv) ARV for 24-h SBP and DBP, i.e., the average of the absolute differences between consecutive BP measurements over 24-h, according to a mathematical algorithm: $ARV = 1^{N-1} \sum_{k=1}^{N-1} (BP_{k+1} - BP_k)$, where N denotes the number of valid BP measurements, and k is the order of measurements.

To prevent perioperative cardiovascular complications, during 2–3 weeks before surgery, patients have been treated with α-adrenergic receptor blockers (e.g., doxazosin 2 up to 16 mg daily). Preoperative co-administration of β-adrenergic receptor blockers was performed in patients with uncontrolled BP values and/or tachycardia (e.g., atenolol 50 up to 100 mg daily), only after administration of α-adrenergic receptor blockers [1]. The drugs were well tolerated and no orthostatic hypotension was observed. Moreover, all patients received preoperative volume therapy with intravenously sodium intake. The surgical intervention was performed at the Department of Surgery "Pietro Valdoni."

4.4. Statistical Analysis

Data were expressed as mean and standard deviation (SD). Before statistical analysis, variables that showed a non-Gaussian distribution at Kolmogorov–Smirnov test were transformed to achieve a normal distribution and they were analyzed by non-parametric tests. Categorical variables were compared with Fisher and chi-square tests. Continuous and categorical variables were compared at baseline and follow-up by the Mann–Whitney test. ANOVA with Fisher's Least Significant Difference post-hoc tests was used when needed. Relationships between continuous variables were assessed calculating the Pearson's correlation coefficient. Linear regression models and multivariate analysis were performed to determine the combined effect of several variables on BPV markers. Statistical analysis was performed using SPSS software (version 24 for Mac; IBM®, SPSS®Statistics, Italy) and GraphPad Prism software (version 7.0, GraphPad® Software Inc, San Diego, CA, USA). Significance was set at $p < 0.05$.

5. Conclusions

Our pilot study with its preliminary results demonstrates that (i) successful surgical treatment in patients affected by PPGL is associated with decreasing of two of the most accurate indexes of short-term blood pressure variability, (ii) there is a significant relationship between the weighted standard deviation of 24-h systolic and diastolic BP and 24-h urinary metanephrines. Therefore, it is supposable that the excessive and pulsatile production of plasma catecholamines and their metabolites in PPGLs has a role in the increased BPV markers, which is involved in the increasing of cardiovascular risk. The clinical relevance of our findings relies on the fact that these patients might take particular benefit from surgical removal of the catecholamine-secreting tumor. Moreover, short-term blood pressure variability may be used as a screening tool in the work-up of PPGLs, especially in those cases with high suspicion for which the diagnosis is challenging. Further prospective studies with a larger number of patients free from cardiovascular events and risk factors are necessary to confirm our findings.

Author Contributions: Conceptualization: C.L., V.B., and L.P.; methodology: V.B., G.O., F.O., M.M., and M.B.; software: V.B. and G.O.; validation: C.L., G.L.T., and L.P.; formal analysis: V.B., C.L., and G.L.T.; investigation: V.B., A.C., and V.S.; resources: C.L., A.C., G.D.T.; data curation: G.O., M.M., M.B., F.O., V.S., M.C.; writing—original draft preparation: V.B. and L.P.; writing—review and editing: C.L., L.P., G.I., and G.T.; visualization: L.P.; supervision: C.L. and L.P.; project administration: V.B.; funding acquisition: none.

Funding: This research received no external funding.

Acknowledgments: The authors take responsibility for all aspects of the reliability and freedom from bias of the data presented and their discussed interpretation.

Conflicts of Interest: The authors declare no conflict of interest.

References

1. Lenders, J.W.; Duh, Q.Y.; Eisenhofer, G.; Gimenez-Roqueplo, A.P.; Grebe, S.K.; Murad, M.H.; Naruse, M.; Pacak, K.; Young, W.F., Jr. Endocrine Society. *J. Clin. Endocrinol. Metab.* **2014**, *99*, 1915–1942. [CrossRef]
2. Gimenez-Roqueplo, A.P.; Dahia, P.L.; Robledo, M. An update on the genetics of paraganglioma, pheochromocytoma, and associated hereditary syndromes. *Horm. Metab. Res.* **2012**, *44*, 328–333. [CrossRef]
3. Castinetti, F.; Waguespack, S.G.; Machens, A.; Uchino, S.; Hasse-Lazar, K.; Sanso, G.; Else, T.; Dvorakova, S.; Qi, X.P.; Elisei, R.; et al. Natural history, treatment, and long-term follow up of patients with multiple endocrine neoplasia type 2B: An international, multicentre, retrospective study. *Lancet Diabetes Endocrinol.* **2019**, *7*, 213–220. [CrossRef]
4. Zinnamosca, L.; Petramala, L.; Cotesta, D.; Marinelli, C.; Schina, M.; Cianci, R.; Giustini, S.; Sciomer, S.; Anastasi, E.; Calvieri, S.; et al. Neurofibromatosis type 1 (NF1) and pheochromocytoma: Prevalence, clinical and cardiovascular aspects. *Arch. Dermatol. Res.* **2011**, *303*, 317–325. [CrossRef] [PubMed]
5. Cotesta, D.; Petramala, L.; Serra, V.; Pergolini, M.; Crescenzi, E.; Zinnamosca, L.; De Toma, G.; Ciardi, A.; Carbone, I.; Massa, R.; et al. Clinical experience with pheochromocytoma in a single centre over 16 years. *High Blood Press. Cardiovasc. Prev.* **2009**, *16*, 183–193. [CrossRef] [PubMed]
6. Zelinka, T.; Pacák, K.; Widimský, J., Jr. Characteristics of blood pressure in pheochromocytoma. *Ann. N. Y. Acad. Sci.* **2006**, *1073*, 86–93. [CrossRef]
7. Parati, G.; Ochoa, J.E.; Lombardi, C.; Bilo, G. Assessment and management of blood-pressure variability. *Nat. Rev. Cardiol.* **2013**, *10*, 143–155. [CrossRef] [PubMed]
8. Chadachan, V.M.; Ye, M.T.; Tay, J.C.; Subramaniam, K.; Setia, S. Understanding short-term blood-pressure variability phenotypes: From concept to clinical practice. *Int. J. Gen. Med.* **2018**, *11*, 241–254. [CrossRef] [PubMed]
9. Parati, G.; Pomidossi, G.; Albini, F.; Malaspina, D.; Mancia, G. Relationship of 24 h blood pressure mean and variability to severity of target-organ damage in hypertension. *J. Hypertens.* **1987**, *5*, 93–98. [CrossRef] [PubMed]
10. Mancia, G.; Parati, G. The role of blood pressure variability in end-organ damage. *J. Hypertens. Suppl.* **2003**, *21*, S17–S23. [CrossRef] [PubMed]
11. Parati, G.; Ochoa, J.E.; Bilo, G. Blood pressure variability, cardiovascular risk, and risk for renal disease progression. *Curr. Hypertens. Rep.* **2012**, *14*, 421–431. [CrossRef]
12. Sega, R.; Corrao, G.; Bombelli, M.; Beltrame, L.; Facchetti, R.; Grassi, G.; Ferrario, M.; Mancia, G. Blood pressure variability and organ damage in a general population: Results from the PAMELA study (Pressioni Arteriose Monitorate E Loro Associazioni). *Hypertension* **2002**, *39*, 710–714. [CrossRef] [PubMed]
13. Frattola, A.; Parati, G.; Cuspidi, C.; Albini, F.; Mancia, G. Prognostic value of 24 h blood pressure variability. *J. Hypertens.* **1993**, *11*, 1133–1137. [CrossRef] [PubMed]
14. Sander, D.; Kukla, C.; Klingelhöfer, J.; Winbeck, K.; Conrad, B. Relationship between circadian blood pressure patterns and progression of early carotid atherosclerosis: A 3-year follow-up study. *Circulation* **2000**, *102*, 1536–1541. [CrossRef] [PubMed]
15. Littler, W.A.; Honour, A.J. Direct arterial pressure, heart rate, and electrocardiogram in unrestricted patients before and after removal of a phaeochromocytoma. *Q. J. Med.* **1974**, *43*, 441–449. [PubMed]
16. Van Eps, R.G.S.; van den Meiracker, A.H.; Boomsma, F.; Man in't Veld, A.J.; Schalekamp, M.A. Diurnal variation of blood pressure in patients with catecholamine-producing tumors. *Am. J. Hypertens.* **1994**, *7*, 492–497. [PubMed]

17. Dabrowska, B.; Feltynowski, T.; Wocial, B.; Szpak, W.; Januszewicz, W. Effect of removal of phaeochromocytoma on diurnal variability of blood pressure, heart rhythm and excretion of catecholamines. *J. Hum. Hypertens.* **1990**, *4*, 397–399. [PubMed]
18. Meisel, S.R.; Mor-Avi, V.; Rosenthal, T.; Akselrod, S. Spectral analysis of the systolic blood pressure signal in secondary hypertension: A method for the identification of phaeochromocytoma. *J. Hypertens.* **1994**, *12*, 269–275. [CrossRef] [PubMed]
19. Khorram-Manesh, A.; Ahlman, O.; Nilsson, O.; Friberg, P.; Odén, A.; Stenström, G.; Hansson, G.; Stenquist, O.; Wängberg, B.; Tisell, L.E.; et al. Long-term outcome of a large series of patients surgically treated for pheochromocytoma. *J. Intern. Med.* **2005**, *258*, 55–66. [CrossRef] [PubMed]
20. Lenders, J.W.M.; Eisenhofer, G. Update on Modern Management of Pheochromocytoma and Paraganglioma. *Endocrinol. Metab. (Seoul).* **2017**, *32*, 152–161. [CrossRef] [PubMed]
21. Shibao, C.; Lipsitz, L.A.; Biaggioni, I.; American Society of Hypertension Writing Group. Evaluation and treatment of orthostatic hypotension. *J. Am. Soc. Hypertens.* **2013**, *7*, 317–324. [CrossRef]
22. Cavallaro, G.; Basile, U.; Polistena, A.; Giustini, S.; Arena, R.; Scorsi, A.; Zinnamosca, L.; Letizia, C.; Calvieri, S.; De Toma, G. Surgical management of abdominal manifestations of type 1 neurofibromatosis: Experience of a single center. *Am. Surg.* **2010**, *76*, 389–396.
23. Prejbisz, A.; Lenders, J.W.; Eisenhofer, G.; Januszewicz, A. Cardiovascular manifestations of phaeochromocytoma. *J. Hypertens.* **2011**, *29*, 2049–2060. [CrossRef] [PubMed]
24. Zelinka, T.; Petrák, O.; Turková, H.; Holaj, R.; Strauch, B.; Kršek, M.; Vránková, A.B.; Musil, Z.; Dušková, J.; Kubinyi, J.; et al. High incidence of cardiovascular complications in pheochromocytoma. *Horm. Metab. Res.* **2012**, *44*, 379–384. [CrossRef] [PubMed]
25. Olmati, F.; Petramala, L.; Bisogni, V.; Concistré, A.; Saracino, V.; Oliviero, G.; Bonvicini, M.; Mezzadri, M.; Ciardi, A.; Iannucci, G.; et al. A rare case report of hypertrophic cardiomyopathy induced by catecholamine-producing tumor. *Medicine (Baltimore)* **2018**, *97*, e13369. [CrossRef] [PubMed]
26. Wiesner, T.D.; Blüher, M.; Windgassen, M.; Paschke, R. Improvement of insulin sensitivity after adrenalectomy in patients with pheochromocytoma. *J. Clin. Endocrinol. Metab.* **2003**, *88*, 3632–3636. [CrossRef] [PubMed]
27. Stergiou, G.S.; Parati, G.; Vlachopoulos, C.; Achimastos, A.; Andreadis, E.; Asmar, R.; Avolio, A.; Benetos, A.; Bilo, G.; Boubouchairopoulou, N.; et al. Methodology and technology for peripheral and central blood pressure and blood pressure variability measurement: Current status and future directions-Position statement of the European Society of Hypertension Working Group on blood pressure monitoring and cardiovascular variability. *J. Hypertens.* **2016**, *34*, 1665–1677. [PubMed]
28. Pengo, M.F.; Rossitto, G.; Bisogni, V.; Piazza, D.; Frigo, A.C.; Seccia, T.M.; Maiolino, G.; Rossi, G.P.; Pessina, A.C.; Calò, L.A. Systolic and diastolic short-term blood pressure variability and its determinants in patients with controlled and uncontrolled hypertension: A retrospective cohort study. *Blood Press.* **2015**, *24*, 124–129. [CrossRef]
29. Mena, L.J.; Felix, V.G.; Melgarejo, J.D.; Maestre, G.E. 24-Hour Blood Pressure Variability Assessed by Average Real Variability: A Systematic Review and Meta-Analysis. *J. Am. Heart Assoc.* **2017**, *6*, e006895. [CrossRef] [PubMed]
30. Hansen, T.W.; Thijs, L.; Li, Y.; Boggia, J.; Kikuya, M.; Björklund-Bodegård, K.; Richart, T.; Ohkubo, T.; Jeppesen, J.; Torp-Pedersen, C.; et al. International Database on Ambulatory Blood Pressure in Relation to Cardiovascular Outcomes Investigators. Prognostic value of reading-to-reading blood pressure variability over 24 h in 8938 subjects from 11 populations. *Hypertension* **2010**, *55*, 1049–1057. [CrossRef] [PubMed]
31. Palatini, P.; Reboldi, G.; Beilin, L.J.; Casiglia, E.; Eguchi, K.; Imai, Y.; Kario, K.; Ohkubo, T.; Pierdomenico, S.D.; Schwartz, J.E.; et al. Added predictive value of night-time blood pressure variability for cardiovascular events and mortality: The Ambulatory Blood Pressure-International Study. *Hypertension* **2014**, *64*, 487–493. [CrossRef] [PubMed]
32. Mancia, G.; Facchetti, R.; Parati, G.; Zanchetti, A. Visit-to-visit blood pressure variability, carotid atherosclerosis, and cardiovascular events in the European Lacidipine Study on Atherosclerosis. *Circulation* **2012**, *126*, 569–578. [CrossRef]
33. Grillo, A.; Bernardi, S.; Rebellato, A.; Fabris, B.; Bardelli, M.; Burrello, J.; Rabbia, F.; Veglio, F.; Fallo, F.; Carretta, R. Ambulatory Blood Pressure Monitoring-Derived Short-Term Blood Pressure Variability in Primary Aldosteronism. *J. Clin. Hypertens. (Greenwich)* **2015**, *17*, 603–608. [CrossRef] [PubMed]

34. Rebellato, A.; Grillo, A.; Dassie, F.; Sonino, N.; Maffei, P.; Martini, C.; Paoletta, A.; Fabris, B.; Carretta, R.; Fallo, F. Ambulatory blood pressure monitoring-derived short-term blood pressure variability is increased in Cushing's syndrome. *Endocrine* **2014**, *47*, 557–563. [CrossRef]
35. Marrone, O.; Bonsignore, M.R. Blood-pressure variability in patients with obstructive sleep apnea: Current perspectives. *Nat. Sci. Sleep* **2018**, *10*, 229–242. [CrossRef] [PubMed]
36. Bilo, G.; Pengo, M.F.; Lombardi, C.; Parati, G. Blood pressure variability and obstructive sleep apnea. A question of phenotype? *Hypertens. Res.* **2019**, *42*, 27–28. [CrossRef]
37. Concistrè, A.; Grillo, A.; La Torre, G.; Carretta, R.; Fabris, B.; Petramala, L.; Marinelli, C.; Rebellato, A.; Fallo, F.; Letizia, C. Ambulatory blood pressure monitoring-derived short-term blood pressure variability in primary hyperparathyroidism. *Endocrine* **2018**, *60*, 129–137. [CrossRef] [PubMed]
38. Mena, L.J.; Maestre, G.E.; Hansen, T.W.; Thijs, L.; Liu, Y.; Boggia, J.; Li, Y.; Kikuya, M.; Björklund-Bodegård, K.; Ohkubo, T.; et al. International Database on Ambulatory Blood Pressure in Relation to Cardiovascular Outcomes (IDACO) Investigators. How many measurements are needed to estimate blood pressure variability without loss of prognostic information? *Am. J. Hypertens.* **2013**, *27*, 46–55. [CrossRef]
39. Bilo, G.; Giglio, A.; Styczkiewicz, K.; Caldara, G.; Kawecka-Jaszcz, K.; Mancia, G.; Parati, G. How to improve the assessment of 24 h blood pressure variability. *Blood Press. Monit.* **2005**, *10*, 321–323. [CrossRef]
40. Padfield, P.L.; Jyothinagaram, S.G.; McGinley, I.M.; Watson, D.M. Reversal of the relationship between heart rate and blood pressure in phaeochromocytoma: A non-invasive diagnostic approach? *J. Hum. Hypertens.* **1991**, *5*, 501–504.
41. Spieker, C.; Barenbrock, M.; Rahn, K.H.; Zidek, W. Circadian blood pressure variations in endocrine disorders. *Blood Press.* **1993**, *2*, 35–39. [CrossRef] [PubMed]
42. Middeke, M.; Schrader, J. Nocturnal blood pressure in normotensive subjects and those with white coat, primary, and secondary hypertension. *Br. Med. J.* **1994**, *308*, 630–632. [CrossRef] [PubMed]
43. Plouin, P.F.; Chatellier, G.; Fofol, I.; Corvol, P. Tumor Recurrence and Hypertension Persistence After Successful Pheochromocytoma Operation. *Hypertension* **1997**, *29*, 1133–1139. [CrossRef]
44. McCullagh, E.P.; Engel, W.J. Pheochromocytoma with hypermetabolism: Report of two cases. *Ann. Surg.* **1942**, *116*, 61–75. [CrossRef] [PubMed]
45. Petrák, O.; Haluzíková, D.; Kaválková, P.; Štrauch, B.; Rosa, J.; Holaj, R.; Brabcová Vránková, A.; Michalsky, D.; Haluzík, M.; Zelinka, T.; et al. Changes in energy metabolism in pheochromocytoma. *J. Clin. Endocrinol. Metab.* **2013**, *98*, 1651–1658. [CrossRef] [PubMed]
46. Malpas, S.C. Neural influences on cardiovascular variability: Possibilities and pitfalls. *Am. J. Physiol. Heart Circ. Physiol.* **2002**, *282*, H6–H20. [CrossRef]
47. Thrasher, T.N. Baroreceptors and the long-term control of blood pressure. *Exp. Physiol.* **2004**, *89*, 331–335. [CrossRef] [PubMed]
48. Bravo, E.; Tagle, R. Pheochromocytoma: State-of-the-art and future prospects. *Endocr. Rev.* **2003**, *24*, 539–553. [CrossRef]
49. Zelinka, T.; Strauch, B.; Petrák, O.; Holaj, R.; Vranková, A.; Weisserová, H.; Pacák, K.; Widimský, J., Jr. Increased blood pressure variability in pheochromocytoma compared to essential hypertension patients. *J. Hypertens.* **2005**, *23*, 2033–2039. [CrossRef]
50. Munakata, M.; Aihara, A.; Imai, Y.; Noshiro, T.; Ito, S.; Yoshinaga, K. Altered sympathetic and vagal modulations of the cardiovascular system in patients with pheochromocytoma: Their relations to orthostatic hypotension. *Am. J. Hypertens.* **1999**, *12*, 572–580. [CrossRef]
51. Levenson, J.A.; Safar, M.E.; London, G.M.; Simon, A.C. Haemodynamics in patients with phaeochromocytoma. *Clin. Sci. (Lond.)* **1980**, *58*, 349–356. [CrossRef] [PubMed]
52. Aboyans, V.; Ricco, J.B.; Bartelink, M.E.L.; Björck, M.; Brodmann, M.; Cohnert, T.; Collet, J.P.; Czerny, M.; De Carlo, M.; Debus, S.; et al. 2017 ESC Guidelines on the Diagnosis and Treatment of Peripheral Arterial Diseases, in collaboration with the European Society for Vascular Surgery (ESVS). *Eur. Heart J.* **2018**, *39*, 763–816. [CrossRef]
53. Neumann, H.P.; Bausch, B.; McWhinney, S.R.; Bender, B.U.; Gimm, O.; Franke, G.; Schipper, J.; Klisch, J.; Altehoefer, C.; Zerres, K.; et al. Germ-line mutations in nonsyndromic pheochromocytoma. *N. Engl. J. Med.* **2002**, *346*, 1459–1466. [CrossRef] [PubMed]

54. O'Brien, E.; Asmar, R.; Beilin, L.; Imai, Y.; Mallion, J.M.; Mancia, G.; Mengden, T.; Myers, M.; Padfield, P.; Palatini, P.; et al. European Society of Hypertension recommendations for conventional, ambulatory and home blood pressure measurement. *J. Hypertens.* **2003**, *21*, 821–848. [CrossRef] [PubMed]
55. Mena, L.; Pintos, S.; Queipo, N.V.; Aizpúrua, J.A.; Maestre, G.; Sulbarán, T.J. A reliable index for the prognostic significance of blood pressure variability. *J. Hypertens.* **2005**, *23*, 505–511. [CrossRef]

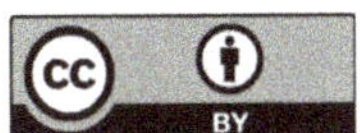

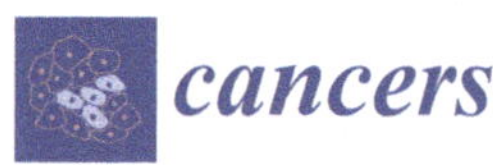
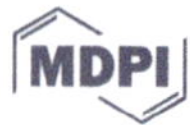

Article

Efficacy and Safety of Ablative Therapy in the Treatment of Patients with Metastatic Pheochromocytoma and Paraganglioma

Jacob Kohlenberg [1], Brian Welch [2], Oksana Hamidi [3], Matthew Callstrom [2], Jonathan Morris [2], Juraj Sprung [4], Irina Bancos [1,*] and William Young, Jr. [1]

1 Division of Endocrinology, Diabetes, Metabolism, and Nutrition, Mayo Clinic, 200 First Street SW, Rochester, MN 55905, USA; Kohlenberg.Jacob@mayo.edu (J.K.); Wyoung@mayo.edu (W.Y.J.)
2 Department of Radiology, Mayo Clinic, 200 First Street SW, Rochester, MN 55905, USA; Welch.Brian@mayo.edu (B.W.); Callstrom.Matthew@mayo.edu (M.C.); Morris.Jonathan@mayo.edu (J.M.)
3 Division of Endocrinology and Metabolism, University of Texas Southwestern Medical Center, 5323 Harry Hines Blvd., Dallas, TX 75390, USA; Oksana.Hamidi@utsouthwestern.edu
4 Department of Anesthesiology, Mayo Clinic, 200 First Street SW, Rochester, MN 55905, USA; Sprung.Juraj@mayo.edu
* Correspondence: Bancos.Irina@mayo.edu

Received: 12 January 2019; Accepted: 5 February 2019; Published: 7 February 2019

Abstract: Metastatic pheochromocytoma and paraganglioma (PPGL) are incurable neuroendocrine tumors. The goals of treatment include palliating symptoms and reducing tumor burden. Little is known about the use of radiofrequency ablation (RFA), cryoablation (CRYO), and percutaneous ethanol injection (PEI) to treat metastatic PPGL. We performed a retrospective study of patients age 17 years and older with metastatic PPGL who were treated with ablative therapy at Mayo Clinic, USA, between June 14, 1999 and November 14, 2017. Our outcomes measures were radiographic response, procedure-related complications, and symptomatic improvement. Thirty-one patients with metastatic PPGL had 123 lesions treated during 42 RFA, 23 CRYO, and 4 PEI procedures. The median duration of follow-up was 60 months (range, 0–163 months) for non-deceased patients. Radiographic local control was achieved in 69/80 (86%) lesions. Improvement in metastasis-related pain or symptoms of catecholamine excess was achieved in 12/13 (92%) procedures. Thirty-three (67%) procedures had no known complications. Clavien-Dindo Grade I, II, IV, and V complications occurred after 7 (14%), 7 (14%), 1 (2%), and 1 (2%) of the procedures, respectively. In patients with metastatic PPGL, ablative therapy can effectively achieve local control and palliate symptoms.

Keywords: radiofrequency ablation; cryoablation; percutaneous ethanol injection; neuroendocrine tumor; minimally invasive procedure; percutaneous ablation

1. Introduction

Pheochromocytoma (PHEO) and paraganglioma (PGL) are rare neuroendocrine tumors that arise from the adrenal medulla and autonomic paraganglia, respectively. The incidence in the United States is 500 to 1600 cases per year [1]. While the majority of PHEO and PGL (PPGL) do not metastasize, 2–13% of PHEO and 2.4–50% of PGL are metastatic [2–4]. PPGL are considered metastatic when nodal or distant metastases are identified [5].

Patients with metastatic PPGL most frequently present with manifestations of catecholamine excess [6]. However, patients also present with symptoms from tumor-related mass effect or incidentally following imaging performed for an unrelated indication [6]. The natural history of metastatic PPGL is highly variable: for some patients it progresses rapidly, but others have prolonged survival [6]. Patients with metastatic PPGL have a median overall survival of 24.6 years and a 5-year mortality rate of 37% [6,7]. There are no differences in disease-specific mortality between metastatic PHEO and PGL [6].

A number of localized and systemic therapies are currently used to treat patients with metastatic PPGL; however, none of the options is curative. The goals of treatment are to reduce manifestations of catecholamine excess, palliate metastasis-related pain, and improve prognosis by treating lesions likely to progress and become symptomatic.

Given the rarity of metastatic PPGL, many of its treatment options have not been extensively studied. In particular, little is known regarding the use of thermal and chemical ablation to treat metastatic PPGL. Therefore, the objectives of this study were to investigate the efficacy and safety of radiofrequency ablation (RFA), cryoablation (CRYO), and percutaneous ethanol injection (PEI) in the treatment of patients with metastatic PPGL. In this study, we found that ablative therapy can be successfully used in patients with metastatic PPGL to achieve radiographic local control, palliate metastasis-related pain, and reduce symptoms of catecholamine excess. We also found that the majority of patients treated with ablation did not experience any procedure-related adverse effects.

2. Results

2.1. Patient Demographics and Clinical Presentation

All ablations were performed between June 14, 1999 and November 14, 2017. Thirty-one patients ($n = 22$, 71% women) with metastatic PPGL ($n = 24$, 77% with PGL, and $n = 7$, 23% with PHEO) underwent treatment of metastatic lesions with RFA, CRYO, or PEI (Table 1).

Table 1. Baseline clinical characteristics of patients with metastatic pheochromocytoma and paraganglioma treated with ablative therapy. Categorical data presented as absolute and relative frequencies (percentages). Continuous data presented as median (minimum–maximum range). * B symptoms include fevers, chills, night sweats, weight loss, and anorexia. Abbreviations: mm, millimeter; *NF1*, neurofibromatosis type 1; PGL, paraganglioma; PHEO, pheochromocytoma; *SDHB*, succinate dehydrogenase subunit B; and *SDHD*, succinate dehydrogenase subunit D.

Characteristics	Data, Number (Percent or Range)
N	31
Female sex, *n* (%)	22 (71%)
Primary tumor, *n* (%)	
PGL	24 (77%)
PHEO	7 (23%)
Genetic status, *n* (%)	
SDHB positive	17 (74%)
SDHD positive	1 (4%)
NF1 positive	1 (4%)
Sporadic	4 (17%)
No genetic testing performed	8
Age at primary tumor diagnosis, years (range)	27 (8–72)
Mode of primary tumor discovery, *n* (%)	
Symptoms of catecholamine excess	12 (39%)
Symptoms of tumor-related mass effect	9 (29%)
Incidental discovery on imaging	5 (16%)
Symptoms of catecholamine excess + tumor mass effect	2 (6%)
Hypervascular right tonsillar mass	1 (3%)
Syncope with neck rotation	1 (3%)
B symptoms *	1 (3%)
Unknown	1
Primary tumor location, *n* (%)	
Abdomen/pelvis	31 (76%)
Skull base and neck	7 (17%)
Thorax	3 (7%)

Table 1. *Cont.*

Characteristics	Data, Number (Percent or Range)
Primary tumor hormonal status, *n* (%)	
Functional	19 (83%)
Non-functional	4 (17%)
Unknown	8
Primary tumor size, mm (range)	55.5 (10–190)
Surgical resection of the primary tumor, *n* (%)	32 (94%)
Age at diagnosis of metastatic disease, years (range)	38 (12–77)
Time to diagnosis of metastatic disease, years (range)	4 (0–53)
Metachronous metastases, *n* (%)	23 (74%)
Location of metastases, *n* (%)	
Osseous	27 (90%)
Abdomen	23 (74%)
Thorax	13 (42%)
Pelvis	10 (33%)
Neck	3 (10%)
Brain	1 (3%)
Metastases per patient, *n* (range)	>5 (1–>5)
Treatment with systemic therapy, *n* (%)	14 (45%)

2.2. Ablation Sessions

Thirty-one patients underwent a total of 69 ablation sessions to treat 123 metastatic lesions. Of the 123 metastatic lesions, 114 were treated with percutaneous ablation and 9 were ablated intra-operatively. A total of 42 RFA, 23 CRYO, and 4 PEI were performed. Seven patients underwent more than one type of ablation during the same session (e.g., RFA of one lesion immediately followed by CRYO of a separate lesion) for a total of 57 procedural sessions (Table 2).

Table 2. Therapeutic approaches and outcomes in patients with metastatic pheochromocytoma and paraganglioma. Categorical data presented as absolute and relative frequencies (percentages). Continuous data presented as median (minimum–maximum range). Abbreviations: mm, millimeter.

Variable	Data
Total lesions ablated, *n*	123
Total procedural sessions, *n*	57
Ablation sessions per patient, *n* (range)	1 (1–8)
Total ablation sessions, *n* (%)	69
Radiofrequency ablation	42 (61%)
Cryoablation	23 (33%)
Percutaneous ethanol injection	4 (6%)
Location of ablated lesions, *n* (%)	
Osseous	63 (51%)
Hepatic	54 (44%)
Abdominal/pelvic, non-hepatic	6 (5%)
Lesions ablated per patient, *n*	3 (1–15)
Size of ablated lesions, mm (range)	
Osseous	15.5 (3–65)
Hepatic	15 (4–47)
Abdominal/pelvic, non-hepatic	21.5 (16–36)
Metastases treated at the time of ablation, *n* (%)	
Not all present metastases treated	35 (76%)
All present metastases treated	11 (24%)
Unknown	11
Technical success for each ablated lesion, *n* (%)	
Achieved	94 (94%)
Not achieved	6 (6%)
Unknown	19

2.3. Ablation Session Indications

Manifestations of catecholamine excess were present prior to 18 (37.5%) procedural sessions and absent prior to 30 (62.5%) procedural sessions (Figure 1). Eleven (22%) procedural sessions were performed to treat 17 painful lesions (Figure 2). Five of the ablated lesions were in high-risk anatomic locations, for example an osseous lesion in close proximity to the spinal cord. In general, ablation was performed to achieve local oncologic control and to mitigate the risks associated with local tumor progression.

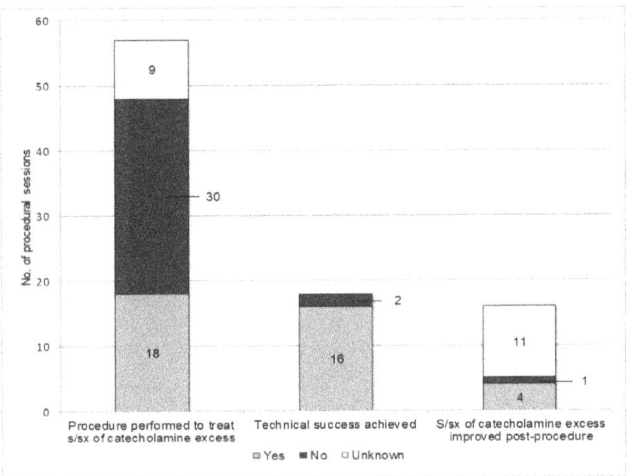

Figure 1. Outcomes of ablations performed to treat manifestations of catecholamine excess in patients with metastatic pheochromocytoma and paraganglioma. Eighteen procedures were performed to treat patients with manifestations of catecholamine excess. Technical success was achieved in 16 of those procedures, after which five patients had known symptom outcomes. Of those five, four patients had improvement in symptoms of catecholamine excess following ablation. Abbreviations: s/sx, signs and symptoms.

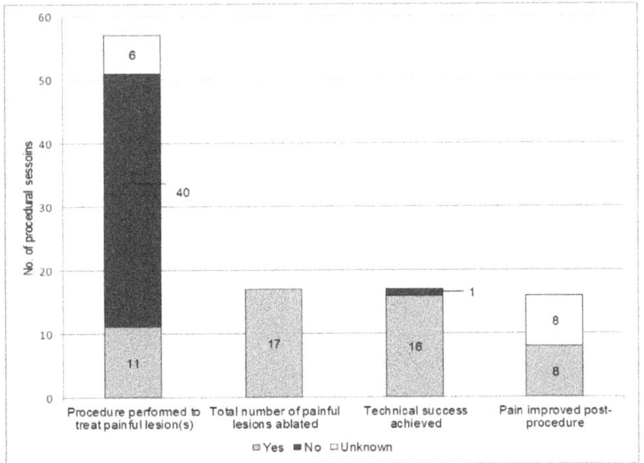

Figure 2. Outcomes of ablations performed to treat pain in patients with metastatic pheochromocytoma and paraganglioma. Eleven procedures were performed to treat a total of 17 painful metastases. Technical success was achieved for 16 of the ablated metastases. Of those lesions, all eight patients with symptom follow-up post procedure had improvement in pain.

2.4. Pre-Ablation Adrenergic Blockade

Functioning metastases were targeted in 31 (63%) of the 49 procedural sessions that had a known pre-ablation biochemical status. Of these, 5 (16%) had an adrenergic biochemical phenotype, 25 (81%) had a noradrenergic biochemical phenotype, and 1 (3%) was dopaminergic only.

Of the 31 procedural sessions performed to treat functioning metastases, α-adrenergic blockade was given prior to 29 (97%), β-adrenergic blockade was given prior to 27 (87%), and the tyrosine hydroxylase inhibitor—metyrosine—was given prior to 23 (74%). Of the 26 procedural sessions performed to treat metastases with a non-functioning or unknown hormonal status, α-adrenergic blockade was given prior to 10 (50%), β-adrenergic blockade was given prior to 4 (20%), and metyrosine was given prior to 1 (5%). The purpose of pre-ablation adrenergic blockade was to reduce hemodynamic variability due to catecholamine release during the procedure.

We initiated α-adrenergic blockade generally 7–14 days pre-ablation, with phenoxybenzamine the most frequent medication prescribed. For patients with heart rates persistently greater than 80 beats/minute, we administered β-adrenergic blockade 2–5 days before ablation. Adrenergic blockade was titrated to effect and if patients remained hypertensive, a calcium channel blocker was added. Metyrosine therapy was used in patients with anticipated significant catecholamine release who were not controlled with α-adrenergic blockade. The initiation of metyrosine was based on clinical judgment and was often prescribed for patients undergoing ablation of multiple lesions during the same procedural session, patients with significantly elevated catecholamines and metanephrines, and patients who had significant hemodynamic variability during previous ablation sessions. Metyrosine was administered orally in the form of 250 milligram (mg) capsules. The Mayo Clinic protocol for short-term metyrosine preparation for patients already taking α-adrenergic blockade is to start metyrosine 4 days pre-ablation at a dose of 250 mg 4 times daily (QID) and up-titrate as tolerated to 500 mg QID 3 days pre-ablation, 750 mg QID 2 days pre-ablation, and 1000 mg QID the day prior to ablation, with the last dose (1000 mg) given on the morning of the ablation.

2.5. Ablated Lesions

A total of 123 lesions were ablated, with a median of 3 ablated lesions per patient (range, 1–15). Of the 123, 63 (51%) were osseous and 54 (44%) were hepatic. Six (5%) were abdominal/pelvic non-hepatic lesions including 4 retroperitoneal lesions, 1 abdominal lymph node, and 1 peri-urethral soft tissue metastasis (Table 2).

2.6. Technical Success

Technical success was achieved in 94 (94%) of the ablated lesions. For 19 lesions, the status of technical success was unknown due to lack of post-ablation imaging. Four lesions were not assessed for technical success because the patient died during the ablation (Table 2).

2.7. Radiographic Outcomes

Of the 123 ablated lesions, 80 (65%) were included in radiographic outcomes analysis. Of the 43 excluded lesions, 37 lacked post-procedural imaging (many patients were referred solely for therapy and received post-ablation care elsewhere) and technical success was not achieved for 6. Overall, local control was accomplished in 69 (86%) of the ablated lesions (Table 3).

Fourteen (45%) of the 31 patients were treated with systemic therapy, including cytotoxic chemotherapy, molecularly targeted therapy, and radiolabeled somatostatin analogs. Several of these patients had ablations performed while receiving systemic therapy (Table 1). Overall, local control was achieved in 36 (78%) lesions that were ablated in patients who had received systemic therapy at any time during the disease course.

For lesions with local control, the median total duration of follow-up was 26 months (range, 2–163 months) after ablation. With the exception of 1 peri-urethral soft tissue lesion, all metastases treated with CRYO were osseous lesions.

Table 3. Radiographic outcomes of ablated metastases in patients with metastatic pheochromocytoma and paraganglioma. Categorical data presented as absolute and relative frequencies (percentages). Continuous data presented as median (minimum–maximum range). * One patient underwent cryoablation (CRYO) and percutaneous ethanol injection (PEI) of a single osseous lesion (right humerus) during the same procedural session. Since this lesion was treated with two ablative modalities during the same procedural session, it was excluded from analysis.

All Ablated Metastases			
Variable			**Data**
Local control, *n* (%)			69/80 (86%)
Radiofrequency ablation			44/51 (86%)
Cryoablation			24/28 (86%)
Percutaneous ethanol injection			1/2 (50%)
Local control, *n* (%)			69/80 (86%)
Patients treated with systemic therapy			36/46 (78%)
Patients not treated with systemic therapy			33/34 (97%)
Duration of follow-up for ablated lesions with local control, months (range)			26 (2–163)
Progression for ablated lesions, *n* (%)			11/80 (14%)
Radiofrequency ablation			7/51 (14%)
Cryoablation			4/28 (14%)
Percutaneous ethanol injection			1/2 (50%)
Time to progression, months (range)			16 (6–69)
Osseous and hepatic metastases treated with radiofrequency ablation and cryoablation			
	Osseous	**Hepatic**	***p* value**
N	45	32	
Local control, *n* (%)	37/45 (82%)	30/32 (94%)	0.14
Radiofrequency ablation	14/19 (74%)	30/32 (94%)	0.04
Cryoablation	23/26 (88%)*	0/0 (0%)	
Progression, *n* (%)	8/45 (18%)	2/32 (6%)	0.14
Radiofrequency ablation	5/19 (26%)	2/32 (6%)	0.04
Cryoablation	3/26 (12%)*	0/0 (0%)	

Of 80 ablated lesions, 11 (14%) progressed at a median of 16 months (range, 6–69 months) (Table 3). All 11 lesions that progressed occurred in only 5 patients. Of the patients who underwent technically successful hepatic ablations, additional hepatic metastases developed outside the area of ablation in 10 (67%) instances at a median of 16 months (range, 2–24 months) following ablation.

2.8. Symptom Outcomes

Technical success was achieved for 16 of the 17 painful metastases that were ablated. Symptom response to ablation was documented for 8 (50%) of the 16 lesions with technical success. Of those 8, all (100%) had improvement in pain following ablation (Figure 2).

Of the 18 procedural sessions performed to treat manifestations of catecholamine excess, 13 were excluded from symptom outcome analysis due to either lack of technical success, simultaneous resection of the primary tumor, intra-ablation death, or unknown post-procedural symptoms. Of the remaining 5 procedural sessions, symptoms of catecholamine excess improved following 4 (80%) (Figures 1 and 3).

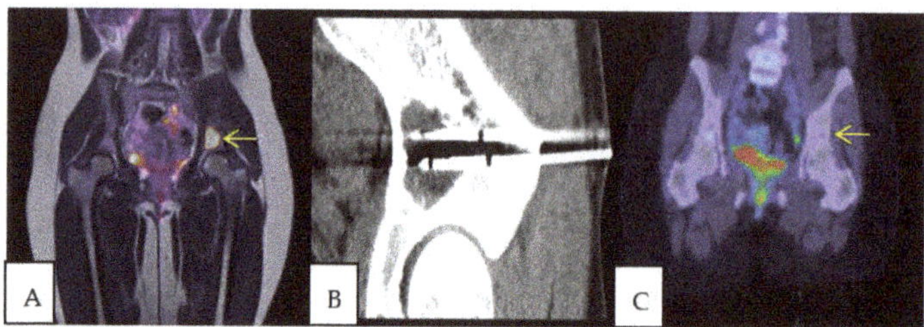

Figure 3. A 17 year old female with widely metastatic paraganglioma underwent CRYO and radiofrequency ablation (RFA) of multiple osseous lesions to palliate symptoms of catecholamine excess and achieve local control. Pre-ablation PET/MRI demonstrated a fluorodeoxyglucose (FDG) avid lesion involving the supraacetabular left ilium (**A**). Two cryoablation needles were placed into the lesion and the iceball encompassed the metastasis (**B**). At 20 months post procedure, PET/CT demonstrated no evidence of residual hypermetabolic paraganglioma in the supraacetabular left ilium (**C**). Additionally, following ablation her symptoms of catecholamine excess improved and she reduced the dose of her chronic adrenergic blockade.

2.9. Ablation Session Complications

No complications occurred following 33 (67%) procedural sessions. Clavien–Dindo Grade I minor complications occurred following 7 (14%) procedural sessions and included transient fever, persistent ablation site pain, and minor bleeding not requiring intervention. Grade II complications developed following 7 (14%) procedural sessions and the most common intervention for these patients was intravenous blood pressure medications. Overall, overnight continuous hemodynamic monitoring for labile hemodynamics was required following 6 procedural sessions. One patient had a Grade IV complication following RFA of four metastatic lesions within the retroperitoneum. He initially did well post-ablation but approximately one week later developed gastrointestinal bleeding and required surgery although the sites of gastrointestinal bleeding were not suspected to be directly related to his ablation procedure. One patient had a Grade V complication and died from a likely argon gas embolism during CRYO of 4 osseous lesions (Table 4).

Table 4. Procedure-related complications and long-term mortality data of patients with metastatic pheochromocytoma and paraganglioma treated with ablative therapy. Procedural session complications were graded according to the revised Clavien–Dindo classification system. Categorical data presented as absolute and relative frequencies (percentages). Continuous data presented as median (minimum–maximum range). Abbreviations: PPGL, pheochromocytoma and paraganglioma.

Complication and Mortality Rates	Data, Number (Percent or Range)
Procedural session complication rate, *n* (%)	
No complication	33 (67%)
Grade I	7 (14%)
Grade II	7 (14%)
Grade III	0
Grade IV	1 (2%)
Grade V	1 (2%)
Long-term patient outcomes	
Deceased secondary to metastatic PPGL, *n* (%)	10 (32%)
Time from ablation session to death, months (range)	
Session 1 (n = 10)	63.5 (2–133)
Session 2 (n = 4)	68.5 (8–113)
Session 3 (n = 3)	52 (51–89)
Session 4 (n = 2)	21 (0–42)
Session 5 (n = 2)	17.5 (0–35)
Session 6 (n = 1)	26
Alive at time of last follow-up, *n* (%)	21 (68%)
Time from ablation session 1 to most recent follow-up, months (range)	60 (0–163)

2.10. Long-Term Outcomes

Of the 31 patients, 10 (32%) died secondary to metastatic PPGL (median age at death, 53.5 years; range, 31–75 years) and 21 (68%) were alive at the time of last follow-up (median 60 months; range, 0–163 months) (Table 4). Of the 14 patients treated with systemic therapy, 7 (50%) died secondary to metastatic PPGL.

3. Discussion

In this study, we described the indications, efficacy, and safety of thermal and chemical ablation in the treatment of patients with metastatic PPGL. We found that the main indications for ablation therapy were to palliate metastasis-related pain, reduce manifestations of catecholamine excess, stabilize metastases in high-risk anatomic locations, and achieve local oncologic control to prevent risks associated with local tumor progression. We found that 94% of ablations were technically successful, and radiographic local control was achieved following 86% of those ablations. Ablative therapy was also successful in reducing metastasis-related pain and treating manifestations of catecholamine excess. Overall, ablative therapy was safe for the majority of patients. However, complications were noted after one third of procedures. Most of these complications were minor with no long-term sequelae. However, there was 1 ablation-related death.

In our study, the most common indication for ablation therapy was to achieve local control. Overall, radiographic outcomes were similar for type of ablation (CRYO versus RFA) and location of metastases (osseous versus hepatic). Of the lesions treated with thermal ablation, osseous metastases were treated with both RFA and CRYO, while hepatic metastases were treated only with RFA. We found that for metastases treated with RFA, radiographic local control was achieved more frequently for hepatic lesions (94%) than osseous lesions (74%). In contrast to hepatic lesions, osseous lesions can be more challenging to ablate because of their location and the propagation of thermal energy in the bony matrix. Further, it is easier to visualize and confirm complete treatment of hepatic metastases than osseous metastases because of the inherent differences between the two environments.

Local control was achieved in 78% of ablated lesions in patients who received systemic therapy at any time during the disease course. In contrast, local control was achieved in 97% of ablated lesions in patients who never received systemic therapy. This suggests that patients requiring systemic therapy have more aggressive disease that is more likely to ultimately progress. However, ablative therapy can still be an effective means to achieve local control in lesions in high risk anatomic locations in patients who require systemic therapy.

The previously published literature on ablative therapy for the treatment of metastatic PPGL is limited to single patient reports and small case series, which makes it challenging to compare our findings [8–11]. However, there is suggestion that interventional radiology techniques may delay the development of serious skeletal-related events in patients with metastatic PPGL [12].

Regarding radiographic response to ablation, prior studies used different definitions of local control than our study. For example, in a case series of 6 patients with metastatic PHEO treated with RFA, complete ablation was achieved in six of the seven ablated metastatic lesions at a mean follow-up of 12.3 months [10]. In this report, complete ablation was defined as a lack of enhancement within the ablation zone on follow-up CT [10]. Moreover, in a previous report from our institution, local control was defined as the absence of metastases in the treated region and was observed in 15 of 27 (56%) ablated lesions.

However, in our current study of 31 patients who had 123 lesions ablated, we defined local control as either no evidence of disease in the area of ablation or decreased tumor burden in the area of ablation when compared to pre-ablation imaging. Our definition of local control was chosen for several reasons—most significantly to provide a clinically meaningful classification. PPGL are known to have a slow response to therapy: following successful treatment, a residual mass is often present on imaging [13]. However, this alone does not represent treatment failure because imaging findings that indicate local control of PPGL following treatment include decreased tumor enhancement and decreased tumor size [13]. Additionally, since metastatic PPGL is incurable, the goal of therapy is to reduce tumor burden to palliate symptoms and intervene early when a patient has lesions expected to progress and become symptomatic.

Only 14% of the 80 technically successful ablated lesions had radiographic progression at a median of 16 months (range, 6–69 months) after ablation. Due to the limited number of technically successful ablations with subsequent radiographic progression, we were not able to identify predictors of lesion progression following ablation.

Our results suggest that ablative therapy can be a successful treatment modality to improve metastasis-related pain and symptoms of catecholamine excess, although the sample size is limited. Of the 8 painful lesions that had technically successful ablations and available follow-up, ablation led to improvement in metastasis-related pain in all cases. Of the 5 technically successful procedural sessions with available follow-up that were performed to treat manifestations of catecholamine excess, improvement in symptoms of catecholamine excess occurred in four (80%). Given the limited number of patients with available follow-up data who had ablations performed to treat manifestations of catecholamine excess, we did not analyze biochemical response following ablation. Excluding the prior case series from our institution, other published studies did not report on symptom outcome for patients with metastatic PPGL who were treated with ablative therapy [8–11].

With regard to procedure-related complications, we found that for the majority of patients, treatment of metastatic PPGL with ablative therapy was safe. No complications were noted following 33 (67%) procedural sessions with available follow-up, and 7 (14%) procedural sessions had only Clavien–Dindo Grade 1 complications. One patient did have a Grade IV complication; however the gastrointestinal bleeding was noted at multiple sites so it is unclear if this complication was directly caused by the RFA. Additionally, one patient died due to a rare complication of a suspected argon gas embolism during CRYO of 4 osseous lesions.

Unsurprisingly, cardiovascular monitoring for labile post-ablation hemodynamics was required following 6 (12%) procedural sessions. However, there were no long-term sequelae for these patients. Even with pre-ablation adrenergic blockade and metyrosine, significant release of catecholamines can occur during ablation. Therefore, it is essential for patients with functioning metastases to be treated carefully with pre-ablation adrenergic blockade and/or metyrosine and to have appropriate anesthesia care intra- and post-ablation.

Our study has several strengths and limitations. Some of the patients in our study were referred only for ablation and had post-ablation follow-up elsewhere, and therefore unknown long-term outcomes. However, the retrospective study design allowed us to have a relatively large sample size of patients, given the rarity of metastatic PPGL. The retrospective study design also allowed us to follow patients for many years post-ablation, which was particularly valuable for determining long-term radiographic response to treatment. A potential bias in our cohort was the treatment of patients within a single tertiary-care setting. In general, there is a number of local and systemic treatment combinations available to treat metastatic PPGL and selection of therapy is often based on the experience of the individual clinician and the practice at a specific institution. Ultimately, our cohort of patients was heterogeneous in regard to the aggressiveness and extent of disease, functional classification, and treatment with therapies in addition to ablation. The heterogeneity of our cohort reflects the population of patients with metastatic PPGL and the radiographic, symptom, and safety outcomes of our study are generalizable to patients with metastatic PPGL.

4. Materials and Methods

4.1. Patient Demographics and Clinical Presentation

To study the efficacy and safety of RFA, CRYO, and PEI in the treatment of patients with metastatic PPGL, we retrospectively reviewed medical records of a consecutive cohort of patients with metastatic PPGL. We only included patients who provided authorization to use their health records for research purposes. These patients were evaluated in the Mayo Clinic System, USA, between June 14, 1999 and November 14, 2017. The study was approved by the Institutional Review Board of Mayo Clinic, Rochester, MN (the IRB number for this project: 13-004137).

4.2. Subjects

The Mayo Clinic PPGL database was reviewed to identify patients with metastatic PPGL who were treated with RFA, CRYO, or PEI. Of the 273 patients identified with metastatic disease, 31 (11%) were treated with at least one thermal or chemical ablation. All of these patients treated with ablation were 17 years or older at the time of ablation. The medical records were reviewed to assess each patient's clinical presentation, biochemical data, imaging results, procedural reports, pathology, and response to ablation. Of note, a Mayo Clinic case series published in 2011 examined 10 patients who had 47 metastatic lesions ablated with RFA, CRYO, or PEI [8]. Our study included patients from this original Mayo Clinic case series [8].

4.3. Disease-Related Definitions

For the purposes of this study, metastatic disease was defined according to the 2017 World Health Organization criteria [5]. A patient was considered to have synchronous metastatic disease if metastases were diagnosed within three months of the primary tumor's discovery. Metachronous metastatic disease was defined as the development of metastases at least 3 months after the primary tumor was diagnosed. PPGL tumors were defined as functional when plasma or urine total or fractioned catecholamines or metanephrines were above the upper limit of normal for each value's reference range. Tumors producing excess epinephrine or metanephrine were defined as adrenergic. Tumors producing excess norepinephrine or normetanephrine were defined as noradrenergic. Tumors with excess dopamine production were defined as dopaminergic. Biochemical evaluation was only included in data analysis if it was completed within three months prior to each ablation session.

4.4. Thermal and Chemical Ablation Overview

Our ablation procedural technique and protocol have been previously described [14–16]. All procedures were performed with patients under general anesthesia. Hepatic ablations at Mayo Clinic were performed with RFA or PEI. PEI was only utilized for hepatic lesions when a lesion was not amenable to thermal treatment due to close proximity to central bile ducts (<1 cm). All extra-osseous RFA treatments were performed with an impedance-based internally cooled RFA device (Cool-tip^{TM}, Medtronic/Covidien, Dublin, Ireland). The STAR tumor ablation system (DFINE, San Jose, CA, USA) was used for all RFAs in the spine and bone. All CRYO treatments were performed using the Precise Cryoablation System (Galil Medical, Yokneam, Israel) or Endocare Cryotherapy System (Healthtronics, Irvine, CA, USA). The decision to use CRYO or RFA for osseous lesions was based on operator preference and consideration of patient safety.

Protective maneuvers to mitigate the risk of injury to adjacent structures were employed based on operator preference and tumor location. Hydrodissection using normal saline or sterile water was used when the bowel or skin necessitated movement for complete ablation. Computed tomography (CT) myelography was performed during spinal ablation when precise visualization of the spinal cord and adjacent nerve roots were needed. Neurophysiologic monitoring via motor or somatosensory evoked potentials by the Department of Neurology was utilized on a case-by-case basis when a tumor was closely associated with the spine or major peripheral nerves. CT and/or ultrasound guidance was utilized for probe placement: the number of probes and duration of treatment was based on tumor size, tumor location, and operator preference. CT utilizing a Siemens Somatom Sensation open 40-slice system (Siemens AG, Munich, Germany) was used for peri-procedural monitoring of treatment.

4.5. Radiographic Outcomes Definitions

For the purpose of this study, RFA, CRYO, and PEI were considered technically successful if the ablation defect encompassed the index tumor with no intra- or peri-tumoral enhancement on imaging performed within three months after the ablation, typically CT or MRI. Additionally, for lesions treated with CRYO, the ablation was considered technically successful if the ice ball completely encompassed the metastatic lesion during the ablation.

Post-ablation imaging was compared to pre-ablation imaging to determine each tumor's radiographic response to therapy. Radiographic local control was assessed using the most recent post-ablation follow-up imaging study. Radiographic local control was defined as no evidence of disease in the area of ablation or decreased tumor burden in the area of ablation compared to pre-ablation imaging. A lesion was considered to have radiographic progression if tumor burden in the area of ablation increased or was stable compared to pre-ablation imaging. The same radiologist assessed the imaging studies to determine if there was local control or progression.

4.6. Symptom Outcomes

The two symptom outcomes studied were (1) post-ablation improvement in manifestations of catecholamine excess and (2) metastasis-related pain. A patient was considered to have manifestations of catecholamine excess if a provider attributed any number of symptoms (hypertension, headaches, anxiety, palpitations, paroxysmal spells, etc.) to the patient's metastatic PPGL. Clinical notes were reviewed following ablation to determine if manifestations of catecholamine excess and metastasis-related pain improved following treatment. Symptom improvement was considered a categorical variable (improved/not improved).

4.7. Procedural Complications

Procedural complications were graded using the revised Clavien–Dindo classification system. This system defines a complication as any deviation from the normal postoperative course [17]. A Grade I complication does not require intervention outside of basic therapeutic regimens such as analgesics or anti-emetics [17]. A Grade II complication requires pharmacologic treatment with medications other than those allowed for a Grade I complication [17]. A Grade III complication requires a procedural intervention [17]. A Grade IV complication is a life-threatening event, and a Grade V complication is death [17].

4.8. Statistical Analysis

The data were summarized using descriptive statistics. Continuous data were presented as median and minimum–maximum range. Categorical data were presented as absolute and relative frequencies (percentages). For categorical variables, the reported frequencies (percentages) only included known outcomes unless otherwise stated. Associations between categorical variables were assessed using the chi-square test. p values less than 0.05 were considered significant. Data were analyzed using JMP software, version 10 (SAS, Cary, NC, USA).

5. Conclusions

For patients with metastatic PPGL, ablation therapy with RFA, CRYO, or PEI should be considered in the following circumstances: (1) to palliate painful abdominal/pelvic or osseous metastases when there are a limited number of culprit lesions; (2) to reduce symptoms of catecholamine excess secondary to functioning abdominal/pelvic or osseous metastases when the bulk of the disease burden can be targeted with ablation; and, (3) to achieve radiographic local control and halt progression of abdominal/pelvic or osseous metastases that are likely to cause morbidity with continued growth. Due to the rarity of metastatic PPGL and the multi-disciplinary approach required to treat patients with this disease, the patient's best interest is served by having ablative procedures performed in high volume centers. Given the potential for serious procedure-related complications, shared decision making between clinicians and patients regarding the risks and benefits of ablative therapy is essential.

Author Contributions: Conceptualization, J.K., I.B., and W.Y.J.; Methodology, B.W., M.C., J.M., J.S., I.B, and W.Y.J.; Verification, J.K., B.W., and O.H.; Formal analysis, J.K., I.B., and W.Y.J.; Investigation, J.K., B.W., O.H., M.C., J.M., J.S., I.B., and W.Y.J.; Writing—original draft preparation, J.K., B.W.; Writing—review and editing, J.K., B.W., O.H., M.C., J.M., J.S., I.B., and W.Y.J.; Visualization, J.K., B.W., I.B., and W.Y.J.; Supervision, I.B., and W.Y.J.; Project administration, J.K., I.B., and W.Y.J.

Funding: This research received no external funding.

Conflicts of Interest: The authors declare no conflict of interest.

References

1. Chen, H.; Sippel, R.S.; O'Dorisio, M.S.; Vinik, A.I.; Lloyd, R.V.; Pacak, K. The North American Neuroendocrine Tumor Society consensus guideline for the diagnosis and management of neuroendocrine tumors: Pheochromocytoma, paraganglioma, and medullary thyroid cancer. *Pancreas* **2010**, *39*, 775–783. [CrossRef] [PubMed]
2. Bravo, E.L. Pheochromocytoma: New concepts and future trends. *Kidney Int.* **1991**, *40*, 544–556. [CrossRef] [PubMed]
3. Plouin, P.F.; Chatellier, G.; Fofol, I.; Corvol, P. Tumor recurrence and hypertension persistence after successful pheochromocytoma operation. *Hypertension* **1997**, *29*, 1133–1139. [CrossRef] [PubMed]
4. Goldstein, R.E.; O'Neill, J.A., Jr.; Holcomb, G.W., 3rd; Morgan, W.M., 3rd; Neblett, W.W., 3rd; Oates, J.A.; Brown, N.; Nadeau, J.; Smith, B.; Page, D.L.; et al. Clinical experience over 48 years with pheochromocytoma. *Ann. Surg.* **1999**, *229*, 755–764. [CrossRef] [PubMed]
5. Tischler, A.S.; de Krijger, R.R.; Gill, A.; Kawashima, A.; Kimura, N.; Komminoth, P.; Papathomas, T.G.; Thompson, L.D.R.; Tissier, F.; Williams, M.D.; et al. *Tumours of the Adrenal Medulla and Extra-Adrenal Paraganglia*, 4th ed.; International Agency for Research on Cancer: Lyon, France, 2017; Volume 10, pp. 184–185.
6. Hamidi, O.; Young, W.F., Jr.; Iniguez-Ariza, N.M.; Kittah, N.E.; Gruber, L.; Bancos, C.; Tamhane, S.; Bancos, I. Malignant Pheochromocytoma and Paraganglioma: 272 Patients Over 55 Years. *J. Clin. Endocrinol. Metab.* **2017**, *102*, 3296–3305. [CrossRef] [PubMed]
7. Hamidi, O.; Young, W.F., Jr.; Gruber, L.; Smestad, J.; Yan, Q.; Ponce, O.J.; Prokop, L.; Murad, M.H.; Bancos, I. Outcomes of patients with metastatic phaeochromocytoma and paraganglioma: A systematic review and meta-analysis. *Clin. Endocrinol.* **2017**, *87*, 440–450. [CrossRef] [PubMed]
8. McBride, J.F.; Atwell, T.D.; Charboneau, W.J.; Young, W.F., Jr.; Wass, T.C.; Callstrom, M.R. Minimally invasive treatment of metastatic pheochromocytoma and paraganglioma: Efficacy and safety of radiofrequency ablation and cryoablation therapy. *J. Vasc. Interv. Radiol.* **2011**, *22*, 1263–1270. [CrossRef] [PubMed]
9. Mamlouk, M.D.; vanSonnenberg, E.; Stringfellow, G.; Smith, D.; Wendt, A. Radiofrequency ablation and biopsy of metastatic pheochromocytoma: emphasizing safety issues and dangers. *J. Vasc. Interv. Radiol.* **2009**, *20*, 670–673. [CrossRef] [PubMed]
10. Venkatesan, A.M.; Locklin, J.; Lai, E.W.; Adams, K.T.; Fojo, A.T.; Pacak, K.; Wood, B.J. Radiofrequency ablation of metastatic pheochromocytoma. *J. Vasc. Interv. Radiol.* **2009**, *20*, 1483–1490. [CrossRef] [PubMed]
11. Pacak, K.; Fojo, T.; Goldstein, D.S.; Eisenhofer, G.; Walther, M.M.; Linehan, W.M.; Bachenheimer, L.; Abraham, J.; Wood, B.J. Radiofrequency ablation: A novel approach for treatment of metastatic pheochromocytoma. *J. Natl. Cancer Inst.* **2001**, *93*, 648–649. [CrossRef] [PubMed]
12. Gravel, G.; Leboulleux, S.; Tselikas, L.; Fassio, F.; Berraf, M.; Berdelou, A.; Ba, B.; Hescot, S.; Hadoux, J.; Schlumberger, M.; et al. Prevention of serious skeletal-related events by interventional radiology techniques in patients with malignant paraganglioma and pheochromocytoma. *Endocrine* **2018**, *59*, 547–554. [CrossRef] [PubMed]
13. Mukherji, S.K.; Kasper, M.E.; Tart, R.P.; Mancuso, A.A. Irradiated paragangliomas of the head and neck: CT and MR appearance. *AJNR* **1994**, *15*, 357–363. [PubMed]
14. Atwell, T.D.; Carter, R.E.; Schmit, G.D.; Carr, C.M.; Boorjian, S.A.; Curry, T.B.; Thompson, R.H.; Kurup, A.N.; Weisbrod, A.J.; Chow, G.K.; et al. Complications following 573 percutaneous renal radiofrequency and cryoablation procedures. *J. Vasc. Interv. Radiol.* **2012**, *23*, 48–54. [CrossRef] [PubMed]

15. Welch, B.T.; Callstrom, M.R.; Carpenter, P.C.; Wass, C.T.; Welch, T.L.; Boorjian, S.A.; Nichols, D.A.; Thompson, G.B.; Lohse, C.M.; Erickson, D.; et al. A single-institution experience in image-guided thermal ablation of adrenal gland metastases. *J. Vasc. Interv. Radiol.* **2014**, *25*, 593–598. [CrossRef] [PubMed]
16. Welch, B.T.; Callstrom, M.R.; Morris, J.M.; Kurup, A.N.; Schmit, G.D.; Weisbrod, A.J.; Lohse, C.M.; Kohli, M.; Costello, B.A.; Olivier, K.R.; et al. Feasibility and oncologic control after percutaneous image guided ablation of metastatic renal cell carcinoma. *J. Urol.* **2014**, *192*, 357–363. [CrossRef] [PubMed]
17. Dindo, D.; Demartines, N.; Clavien, P.A. Classification of surgical complications: A new proposal with evaluation in a cohort of 6336 patients and results of a survey. *Ann. Surg.* **2004**, *240*, 205–213. [CrossRef] [PubMed]

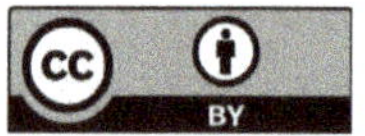

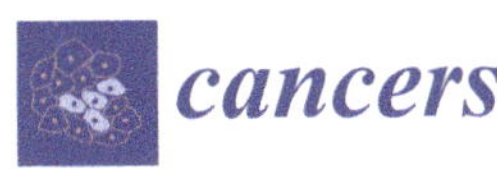

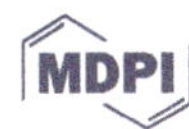

Article

RNA-Sequencing Analysis of Adrenocortical Carcinoma, Pheochromocytoma and Paraganglioma from a Pan-Cancer Perspective

Joakim Crona [1,2,*], Samuel Backman [3], Staffan Welin [1], David Taïeb [4], Per Hellman [3], Peter Stålberg [3], Britt Skogseid [1] and Karel Pacak [2]

1 Department of Medical Sciences, Uppsala University, Akademiska Sjukhuset ing 78, 75185 Uppsala, Sweden; staffan.welin@medsci.uu.se (S.W.); britt.skogseid@medsci.uu.se (B.S.)

2 Section on Medical Neuroendocrinology, Eunice Kennedy Shriver National Institute of Child Health and Human Development, National Institutes of Health, 10 Center Drive, Building 10, Room 1E-3140, Bethesda, MD 20892, USA; karel@mail.nih.gov

3 Department of Surgical Sciences, Uppsala University, Akademiska Sjukhuset ing 70, 75185 Uppsala, Sweden; samuel.backman@surgsci.uu.se (S.B.); per.hellman@surgsci.uu.se (P.H.); peter.stalberg@surgsci.uu.se (P.S.)

4 Department of Nuclear Medicine, La Timone University Hospital, European Center for Research in Medical Imaging, Aix Marseille Université, 13385 Marseille, France; David.TAIEB@ap-hm.fr

* Correspondence: joakim.crona@medsci.uu.se; Tel.: +46-186-118-630

Received: 30 October 2018; Accepted: 13 December 2018; Published: 15 December 2018

Abstract: Adrenocortical carcinoma (ACC) and pheochromocytoma and paraganglioma (PPGL) are defined by clinicopathological criteria and can be further sub-divided based on different molecular features. Whether differences between these molecular subgroups are significant enough to re-challenge their current clinicopathological classification is currently unknown. It is also not fully understood to which other cancers ACC and PPGL show similarity to. To address these questions, we included recent RNA-Seq data from the Cancer Genome Atlas (TCGA) and Therapeutically Applicable Research to Generate Effective Treatments (TARGET) datasets. Two bioinformatics pipelines were used for unsupervised clustering and principal components analysis. Results were validated using consensus clustering model and interpreted according to previous pan-cancer experiments. Two datasets consisting of 3319 tumors from 35 disease categories were studied. Consistent with the current classification, ACCs clustered as a homogenous group in a pan-cancer context. It also clustered close to neural crest derived tumors, including gliomas, neuroblastomas, pancreatic neuroendocrine tumors, and PPGLs. Contrary, some PPGLs mixed with pancreatic neuroendocrine tumors or neuroblastomas. Thus, our unbiased gene-expression analysis of PPGL did not overlap with their current clinicopathological classification. These results emphasize some importances of the shared embryological origin of these tumors, all either related or close to neural crest tumors, and opens for investigation of a complementary categorization based on gene-expression features.

Keywords: pheochromocytoma; paraganglioma; adrenocortical carcinoma; adrenal tumor; pan-cancer analysis; neural crest; neuroendocrine

---

1. Introduction

The adrenal gland is derived from two components that are developmentally and physiologically distinct: Cells of the adrenal cortex are derived from mesoderm and are characterized by steroid metabolism. Neuroectodermally derived adrenal medulla is encircled by the adrenal cortex and contains neuroendocrine (chromaffin) cells synthesizing catecholamines [1]. These characteristics are retained in adrenal neoplasms that are classified accordingly by the World Health Organization into tumors of the adrenal cortex and tumors of chromaffin cells of the adrenal medulla and extra-adrenal paraganglia (PPGL) [2]. Molecular techniques further stratifies these tumors into distinct categories [3,4]. The adrenal cortex derived adrenocortical carcinoma (ACC) is separated into three subgroups; cluster of clusters 1–3 with differences in steroid differentiation, cell proliferation, DNA methylation and spectrum of genetic driver events [5,6]. Similarly, PPGLs are separated into 4 groups named after their molecular characteristics: pseudohypoxia related to succinate dehydrogenase or *VHL/EPAS1* disturbances, wnt-altered and kinase-signaling pathways [7–9].

New approaches and methods for analysis of molecular pan-cancer datasets may obtain novel insights into the characteristics of a wide range of neoplasms in a single experiment. Their results can be used to test whether the current clinicopathological classification of a particular tumor remains relevant on a molecular level [10,11]. Current state of the art and views suggest that a majority of tumor types categorize accordingly to their established clinicopathological classifications in such pan-cancer analyses [11]. However, an alternative scenario where new molecular analyses proposed a new disease categorization has been shown for some cancers [12]. One example is esophageal carcinoma where the squamous cell subtype resembled squamous cell carcinomas of other organs, whereas the esophageal adenocarcinoma clustered with gastric adenocarcinoma [12]. Thus, we hypothesized that the differences between subgroups of ACC and PPGL could be significant enough to support an updated classification of these tumors. One example could be the pronounced pseudohypoxia phenotype that is shared among some PPGLs and other neural crest tumors. We used a pan-cancer analysis, that allowed for an unbiased clustering of tumors based on gene expression data, to test this hypothesis.

2. Results

2.1. Aim 1: To Determine if ACC and PPGL Show Integrity in a Transcriptomic Pan-Cancer Context

To address whether the current clinicopathological classification of ACC and PPGL remains relevant in a transcriptomic pan-cancer context, we performed unsupervised clustering and principal component analyses. RNA-seq data from 3319 tumor samples of 35 different categories from the Cancer Genome Atlas (TCGA) and Therapeutically Applicable Research to Generate Effective Treatments (TARGET) (Figure 1A, Table 1) were included.

Cases were grouped by TCGA tumor category and genes with high variability between tumor categories were extracted. Dendrograms of unsupervised clustering showed integrity of both ACC and PPGL which formed two separate clusters (Supplementary Figures S1A–C and S2). In the second series of experiments we analyzed the dataset on a per sample basis. Genes with a variable expression in-between 3319 cases were selected and analyzed with unsupervised clustering. The pan-cancer dendrogram recapitulated previous findings described by Hoadley et al. including clustering accordingly to organ (e.g., kidney, gastrointestinal tract) and cell of origin (e.g., squamous cell cluster) (Supplementary Figure S3A–C) [10,11]. Except for a few outliers, ACC remained a homogenous group whereas PPGL mixed with pancreatic neuroendocrine tumors (PNETs) in 2 out of 3 unsupervised clustering experiments (Figure 1B, Supplementary Figure S3A–C). In order to investigate the robustness of these results, we designed a second bioinformatics pipeline that used different software for sample selection, identification of genes with variable expression and unsupervised clustering. These results validated that ACC formed one homogenous cluster whereas a group of kinase signaling PPGL mixed with a group of neuroblastoma (NBL) (Supplementary Figure S4A,B). Inspection of the clustering dendrogram revealed sub-separation of ACC Cluster of Clusters 1 (COC1) from COC2 and 3. In PPGL, kinase signaling tumors separated either gradually (bioinformatics pipeline 1) and distinctively (bioinformatics pipeline 2) from pseudohypoxic and wnt-altered tumors (Figure 1, Supplementary Figure S4A).

Table 1. Samples included from the Cancer Genome Atlas (TCGA) and Therapeutically Applicable Research To Generate Effective Treatments (TARGET). TCGA official nomenclature is shown in parentheses. *n*, number of cases included; ref, reference.

Cohort	Cohort, Full Name	*n*	Reference
ACC	Adrenocortical carcinoma	78	[5]
BLCA	Bladder urothelial carcinoma	100	[13,14]
BRCA	Breast invasive carcinoma	100	[15]
CESC	Cervical squamous cell carcinoma and Endocervical adenocarcinoma	100	[16]
CHOL	Cholangiocarcinoma	44	[17]
COAD	Colon adenocarcinoma	100	[18]
DLBC	Lymphoid neoplasm diffuse large B-cell lymphoma	47	
ESCA	Esophageal carcinoma	100	[12]
GBM	Glioblastoma multiforme	100	[19,20]
HNSC	Head and neck squamous cell carcinoma	100	[21]
KICH	Kidney chromophobe	88	[22]
KIRC	Kidney renal clear cell carcinoma	100	[23]
KIRP	Kidney renal papillary cell carcinoma	100	[24]
LAML	Acute myeloid leukemia	100	[25]
LGG	Brain Lower Grade Glioma	100	[19,26]
LIHC	Liver hepatocellular carcinoma	100	[27]
LUAD	Lung adenocarcinoma	100	[28]
LUSC	Lung squamous cell carcinoma	100	[29]
MESO	Mesothelioma	85	
OV	Ovarian serous cystadenocarcinoma	100	[30]
PAAD	Pancreatic adenocarcinoma	100	[31]
PNET (PAAD)	Pancreatic neuroendocrine tumor	8	[31]
PPGL (PCPG)	Pheochromocytoma and paraganglioma	179	[9]
PRAD	Prostate adenocarcinoma	100	[32]
READ	Rectum adenocarcinoma	100	[18]
SARC	Sarcoma	100	[33]
SKCM	Skin cutaneous melanoma	100	[34]
STAD	Stomach adenocarcinoma	100	[35]
TGCT	Testicular germ cell tumors	100	[36]
THCA	Thyroid carcinoma	100	[37]
THYM	Thymoma	100	[38]
UCEC	Uterine corpus endometrial Carcinoma	100	[39]
UCS	Uterine carcinosarcoma	55	[40]
UVM	Uveal melanoma	79	[41]
NBL	Neuroblastoma	156	[42]
Total		3319	

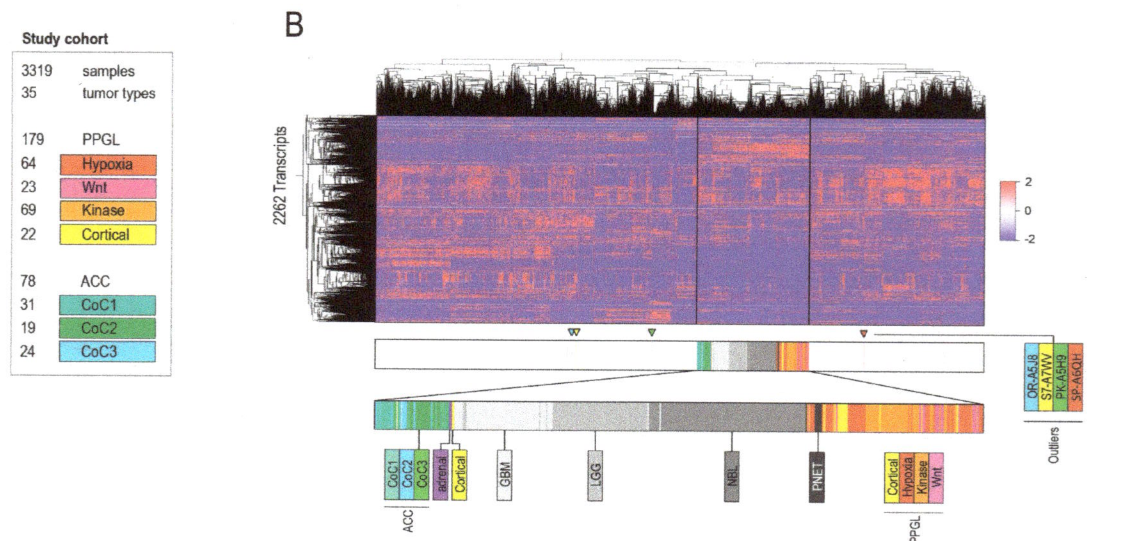

Figure 1. Pan-cancer dataset and transcriptomic classification. (**A**) Pan-cancer analysis dataset and pipeline. Results from bioinformatics pipeline 1. (**B**) Unsupervised hierarchal clustering of RNA-seq data from 3319 TCGA and TARGET samples annotated for cancer type processed by bioinformatics pipeline 1. Abbreviations; ACC, Adrenocortical Carcinoma; GBM, Glioblastoma Multiforme; LGG, Brain Lower Grade Glioma Neuroblastoma; PNET, Pancreatic Neuroendocrine Tumor; PPGL, Pheochromocytoma and Paraganglioma; Cortical, Cortical Admixture PPGL; Hypoxia, Pseudohypoxic PPGL; Kinase; Kinase signaling PPGL and Wnt, wnt-altered PPGL.

Detailed Analysis of ACC and PPGL Outliers

ACC and PPGL samples that clustered outside their disease group in both bioinformatics pipelines were carefully examined. There was one ACC, OR-A5J8, of sarcomatoid type with 100% purity that clustered among sarcomas (SARC). It showed a cortical differentiation score of 7.9, 4th lowest among ACCs (Figure 2). Analysis of all ACCs and all SARCs available in TCGA that showed that OR-A5J8 clustered to the SARC group (Supplementary Figure S5A–C). The second sarcomatoid ACC available in the TCGA dataset clustered among ACCs.

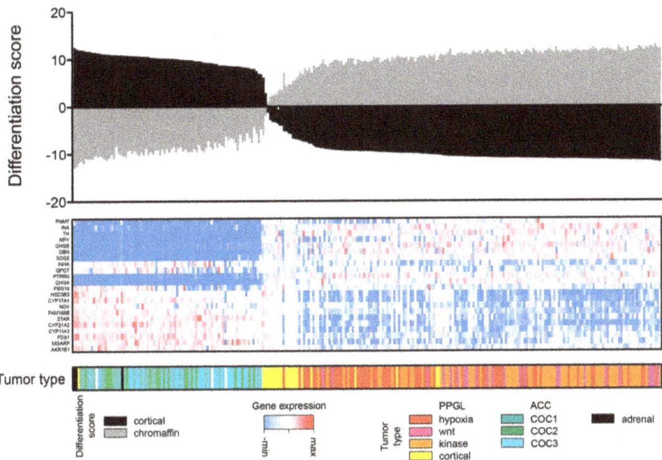

Figure 2. Chromaffin and cortical cell differentiation. Cortical and chromaffin cell differentiation of adrenocortical carcinoma (ACC), pheochromocytoma and paraganglioma (PPGL) and adrenal gland samples. Each column represents a unique sample that was ordered according to cortical cell differentiation. From above: differentiation scores for adrenal cortex (black) and adrenal medulla (grey). Middle; heatmap with expression values of genes representing chromaffin cells (upper half) and cortical cells (bottom half). Bottom: annotation of sample type accordingly to PPGL and ACC molecular subtypes. COC, Cluster of Clusters; Cortical, Cortical Admixture PPGL; Hypoxia, Pseudohypoxic PPGL; Kinase; Kinase signaling PPGL and Wnt, wnt-altered PPGL.

One PPGL mixed into the ACC cluster: TT-A6YO of the cortical admixture subgroup with 66% purity. It had a cortical differentiation score of 12 (higher than all ACCs) and a chromaffin differentiation score of −12 (lower than all PPGLs). In TCGA, this sample was noted to have cortical cells through histopathological analysis [9]. Two additional PPGLs clustered outside the main group, both were pheochromocytomas of the cortical admixture subgroup (one had admixture of adrenocortical cells by histopathology) and their tumor purity was 54 and 100%, respectively. Cortical differentiation score was 6.1 and −3.5, respectively (2nd and 8th highest among PPGL). Chromaffin differentiation score was −5.9 and 2.9, respectively (2nd and 8th lowest among PPGL). Thus, we have concluded that sample misclassification and infiltration of non-tumor cells are two likely explanations for samples that consistently clustered outside ACC or PPGL main groups (Figure 2).

PNETs (bioinformatics pipeline 1, Section 4.1) and NBL (bioinformatics pipeline 2, Section 4.2) infiltrated the PPGL group (Figure 2, Supplementary Figures S3A–C and S4A,B). Inspection of samples that clustered outside PPGL main group in one of two bioinformatics pipelines revealed a pattern with enrichment of either dopamine secreting thoracic PPGL with metastatic disease (bioinformatics pipeline 1) or kinase signaling PPGL (bioinformatics pipeline 2).

2.2. Aim 2: To Identify with Which Cancers ACC and PPGL Show Similarities

Adrenocortical carcinoma, glioblastoma multiforme (GBM), low grade glioma (LGG), NBL, PNET, and PPGL clustered together in the 6 of the 8 experiments performed in the bioinformatics pipelines (Supplementary Figures S1A–C, S2, S3A–C and S4A,B). The relative associations within this group of tumors varied between the different experiments. To exclude that the inclusion of ACC and PPGL molecular subtypes skewed the results of the per-TCGA tumor category analysis, unsupervised clustering was repeated without separation of ACC and PPGL into molecular subgroups. This experiment showed similar results (Supplementary Figures S6A–C and S7). We also investigated whether a signal of adrenocortical cells in PPGL could influence the outcome and thus, we removed all pheochromocytomas. Unsupervised clustering showed that ACC remained among neural crest tumors (Supplementary Figure S8). Consensus clustering experiments validated an ACC, GBM, LGG, NBL, PNET, and PPGL cluster that also included skin cutaneous melanoma (SKCM) and uveal melanoma (UVM) (Figure 3A,B, Supplementary Figure S9A–C). As the number of permitted clusters was increased, this cluster was partitioned into: (1) GBM, LGG, NBL, PNET, and PPGL as well as (2) ACC, SKCM and UVM (Figure 3B). These results overlapped previous pan-cancer findings where PPGL grouped together with either GBM and LGG or NBL [11].

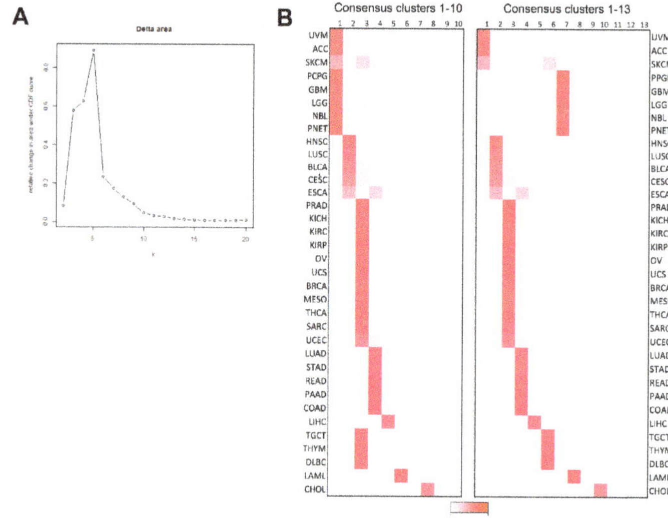

Figure 3. Pan-cancer consensus clustering. Unsupervised consensus clustering of 3319 TCGA and TARGET samples annotated for their specific cancer type. (**A**), Delta CDF plot with information on the additional explanatory power provided through increasing the number of clusters. Y-axis, relative change in the area under CDF curve and y-axis; *k*, the number of consensus clusters. (**B**), Proportion of cases assigned to the different clusters ranging from 0% (white) to 100% (red) in both 10 and 13 clusters. X-axis, consensus cluster numbers and y-axis, a cancer type.

The clustering of ACCs to neural crest tumors was an unexpected finding lacking an obvious explanation [11,43]. In order to identify the gene expression profile that drove these results, we have identified transcripts that were able to discriminate ACC, GBM, LGG, NBL, PNET, and PPGL from the remaining tumors. A total of 78 transcripts showed an AUC of >0.9. Fifteen of these fulfilled the following criteria: 2-fold higher expression in ACC compared to remaining tumors (pan-cancer minus GBM, LGG, NBL, PNET and PPGL) and no less than 0.1-fold difference in expression compared to GBM, LGG, NBL, PNET, and PPGL. Of these 15 genes, 14 had lower expression in ACC compared to neural crest tumors (Supplementary Table S1a). There were no shared molecular hallmarks between

ACC to the group of GBM, LGG, PNET, and PPGL detectable through annotation with gene-ontology information (Supplementary Table S1b).

A Separate Pan-Glioma-Neuroendocrine Tumor Cluster Analysis

In the previous analyses we found that GBM, LGG, NBL, PNET, and PPGL form a group of tumors with overlapping transcriptomic profiles. We further analyzed this neural crest group using unsupervised clustering and principal component analysis after removal cortical admixture PPGLs (total $n = 152$) to reduce signal from non-chromaffin cells. To balance the size of the different groups, GBM and LGG were restricted to 150 samples each. Results showed a separation into two clusters, one consisting of low and high grade gliomas and a second including NBL, PNET, and PPGL (Figure 4, Supplementary Figures S10A–C and S11A–C).

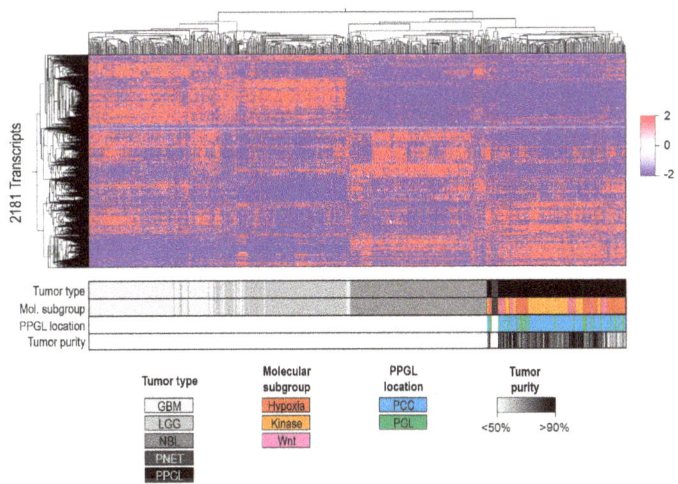

Figure 4. Pan-glioma-neuroendocrine tumors cluster. Unsupervised clustering of RNA-seq data of GBM ($n = 150$), LGG ($n = 150$), NBL ($n = 156$), PNET ($n = 8$) and PPGL (cortical admixture excluded, $n = 152$) processed by bioinformatics pipeline 1.

3. Discussion

In this study we used a pan-cancer model to investigate the degree of overlap between unbiased gene-expression clustering to the current clinicopathological classifications of ACC and PPGL. A second aim was to investigate which other cancer types these two diseases show similarity to. We found that ACC was a homogenous transcriptomic group that showed a surprising association with neural crest derived tumors. PPGLs mixed with either pancreatic NETs or NBL. In addition, it also clustered together with GBM and LGG as well as ACC.

The unique aspect of this study is the combination of two datasets that together has a high number of samples from many different tumor types. The included data provides a very comprehensive characterization of gene expression that has the highest standard for quality control. Specifically, we used the publically available TCGA and TARGET resources to include 3319 tumor samples originating from 35 different tumor types. The most important and novel aspect came from merging a large number of NBLs (TARGET cohort) with other neural crest tumors, including GBM, LGG, PNET, and PPGL (TCGA cohort).

Our first aim was to determine whether findings from an unsupervised clustering of a pan-cancer gene expression dataset overlapped current clinocopathological classifications of ACC and PPGL. Through eight different unsupervised clustering experiments as well as principal component analysis and consensus clustering, we found that both ACCs and PPGLs were relatively homogenous groups of diseases, but that PPGLs mixed with either NBLs or PNETs. As such, our unbiased clustering based on gene expression features did not fully overlap with the current clinicopathological classification of PPGL. This was similar to previous findings related to pancreatic and small intestinal NETs, where clustering by gene expression data revealed mixing of a minority of tumors independently of their primary location [44]. Future studies aggregating NETs from many different primary sites could be used to test whether this group of diseases could use gene-expression data to form a complementary classification.

Our second aim was to identify with which tumor types either ACC or PPGL transcriptomes show similarities to. Our findings corroborate previous pan-cancer studies that identified similarities between PPGLs to both NBLs as well as to low and high grade gliomas (GBMs and LGGs) on the transcriptomic level [11,43]. However the associations of ACC to these cancers differed from a recent pan-cancer study where ACC clustered together with chromophobe renal cancer [11]. We failed to identify a distinct gene expression signature that drove clustering of ACCs to the neural crest group in our experiments. Our conclusion from these observations is that ACC, in relative terms, is more similar to neural crest tumors than other entities included in this pan-cancer study. However, in absolute terms, the similarities between ACC and neural crest tumors are likely not strong. We must note that although the cortical cell has its unique features related to steroid synthesis and metabolism, certain aspects of the ACC genetic landscape overlaps with that of neural crest tumors. This includes presence of both telomerase activation and alternative lengthening of telomeres due to ATRX or DAXX truncation as well as somatic or germline driver mutations in *MEN1* [5,6,45,46]. Another interesting conclusion from this study is that ACC did not cluster with tumors originating from gonadal cells (ovarian serous cystadenocarcinoma and testicular germ cell tumors) with which it shares its developmental origin. This improved knowledge of disease relationships may ultimately be used to motivate cautious extrapolation of results from more extensively studied diseases such as GBM, LGG, and NBL to a rare tumor type such as PPGL that lacks both representative disease models and curative systemic treatment options.

Our analysis validated previous findings in pan-cancer studies including separation tumors accordingly to organ (kidney, gastrointestinal adenocarcinomas etc.) and cell of origin (squamous cell cancers, including separation of esophageal carcinoma). But when interpreting our results some weaknesses should be acknowledged: only one group of neoplasms derived from adrenal cortex (ACC) was included compared to four different diagnoses and 5-fold higher number of samples of GBM, LGG, NBL, PNET and PPGL. Another weakness is that the transcriptomic data was generated from tissue homogenates that do not allow for separation of tumor and non-tumoral cells. Third, our method for transcript selection is likely to select gene expression patterns that are specific to cell-of-origin. As show by Creighton et al., cell-of-origin specific transcripts can be filtered out using an alternative bioinformatics strategy, resulting in a separation according to disease driving mechanisms and a very different clustering of tumors [47]. Finally, our study used only one class of molecular data. As already demonstrated in a pan-cancer analysis of >10000 tumors included in the TCGA consortium, a pan-molecular analysis have the potential to provide additional insights [11].

4. Methods

TCGA and TARGET datasets are well suited for comparative studies due to (1) the high number of samples across different disease categories, and (2) the extraordinary standardization in data generation including tissue collection, genome analysis as well as bioinformatics processing. All cases were annotated accordingly to established clinicopathological classifications used in the TCGA and TARGET cohorts (Table 1). ACCs and PPGLs were further annotated accordingly to the molecular classifications proposed in the respective TCGA projects [5,9]. We selected mRNA expression as a proxy of tissue biology due to the gene-specific correlation between mRNA and protein levels [48]. This study falls under an approval from the regional Ethics Committee in Uppsala (544/2015).

4.1. Bioinformatics Pipeline 1

4.1.1. Sample Selection and Annotation

Publicly available level 3 data; RNA-seq V2 and clinical annotations available through TCGA and TARGET consortiums were downloaded 2017-08-23 from Genomics Data Commons https://gdc.cancer.gov (Table 1). In the pan-cancer experiments each cohort was restricted to a maximum of 100 samples in order to limit the size for the dataset and to balance the relative weight in-between subgroups. All samples were included for two cohorts; PPGLs (n = 179) and NBL (n = 156). A total of 8 samples with histopathology of neuroendocrine tumors were included from the pancreatic ductal adenocarcinoma project and annotated as PNET [31]. Samples from primary tumors (01A) were prioritized. For RNA-seq analysis FPKM normalized files were selected and annotated on a per transcript basis for further analysis. Cases were annotated by (1) TCGA tumor type, and (2) sample type (primary tumor, metastasis or normal tissue). Molecular clusters defined by primary TCGA publications were used; ACC, cluster of clusters 1–3; and PPGL, pseudohypoxia, wnt-altered, kinase signaling, and cortical admixture [5,9]. ACC samples without any molecular subtype had a COC value randomly assigned; PPGL samples without a molecular subtype were assigned identical value of tumor samples available from the same patient. Tumor purity values were extracted from the primary publications for PPGL and ACC [5,9]. Three samples from normal adrenal was available through the PPGL cohort and annotated as "Adrenal" [9].

4.1.2. Unsupervised Clustering

Files were imported into the Subio Platform version v1.21.5074 (Subio Inc, Kagoshima, Japan, https://www.subioplatform.com). FPKM transcript counts were subjected to Log2 normalization and genes with low expression values (mean FPKM < 1) were discarded. Genes with high standard deviation of expression in-between (1) TCGA categories, or (2) individual samples were selected for further analysis, three different datasets with different standard deviation thresholds was used for each unsupervised clustering experiment. Unsupervised clustering was performed using a Spearman test as the distance metric. Subio Platform raw data figures were imported into Microsoft PowerPoint (Microsoft Inc, Redmond, WA, USA) and edited for improved readability.

4.2. Bioinformatics Pipeline 2

4.2.1. Sample Selection and Annotation

FPKM and raw count files release 10.0 were downloaded between 2018-02-05 and 2018-02-08 from https://gdc.cancer.gov. Cohort size and annotation was performed identical to previous experiments: all NBL, PNET and PPGL samples were included. ACC that were not assigned to a COC in the original publication were assigned as N/A. For other cohorts, a maximum of 100 samples were selected through a random process that was independent to previous experiments.

4.2.2. Unsupervised Clustering

Sample based clustering: All genes with an index of dispersion (variance/mean) with at least 60 were included. This cutoff was arbitrarily selected to obtain an appropriate number of genes. Values were log2-transformed, using an offset of 1 in order to avoid errors for any samples with FPKM-values of 0 for any of the included genes. A heatmap was generated and clustering based on the Euclidean distance was performed using the heatmap.2 function in the *gplots* R package [49–51].

TCGA category-based clustering: The mean expression of each of the included genes in each tumor type was calculated on the basis of the selected samples and heatmap generation and clustering was performed as described.

4.3. Consensus Clustering

The dataset comprising 2262 genes identified through extraction of mRNAs with a high variance in expression in-between samples through bioinformatics pipeline 1 was used. Consensus clustering was performed using the *ConsensusClusterPlus* R package [52]. One thousand iterations were performed with a sample inclusion probability of 0.8 and an item inclusion probability of 1. The number of clusters was selected based on inspection of the Delta CDF plot.

4.4. Interpretation of Results

Supported by the findings of Hoadley et al. [10] we considered two principle outcomes of the experiments: (1) Concordance between the clinicopathological/anatomic and molecular classification if ACC and PPGL cluster into two homogenous groups, or (2) discordance if ACC or PPGL cluster with other tumor types into intermixed groups or if ACC or PPGL are separated across multiple different clusters.

4.5. Multidimensional Scaling Plots

The raw count files of the included samples were processed with the *voom* function in the *limma* R package. Multidimensional scaling-plots were generated using the *plotMDS* function and the *ggplot2* R package.

4.6. Adrenal Medulla and Cortex Differentiation Scores

A dataset of 2262 genes identified through extraction of mRNAs with a high deviance in expression through bioinformatics pipeline 1 was used to select transcripts that were previously identified as preferentially expressed in either adrenal cortex or medulla from the proteinatlas.org [53]. Twenty-two transcripts were selected, 11 from adrenal medulla and 11 from adrenal cortex. The dataset was analyzed using Gene Set Enrichment Analysis version 9.09 on the gene pattern platform (https://genepattern.broadinstitute.org) [54,55]. Samples were normalized to log-scale and analyzed with default settings.

4.7. Identification of Transcripts Shared between Cancer Types

The dataset comprising 2262 genes identified through extraction of mRNAs with a high deviance in expression through bioinformatics pipeline 1 was used. Genes with area under the Receiver Operating Characteristic (ROC) curve (Harrell's C-statistic) of >0.9 for ACC, GBM, LGG, PPGL, NBL, and PNET versus remaining tumor types were selected. Difference between median gene expression value in ACC compared to (1) GBM, LGG, NBL, PNET and PPGL, and (2) remaining tumors were determined. Genes with fold change in ACC of <0.1 (compared to GBM, LGG, NBL, PNET and PPGL) and <2 (compared to remaining tumor types) were excluded. Remaining genes were annotated for overlapping gene ontology annotations version 2018-05-07 (https://www.ebi.ac.uk/QuickGO/).

5. Conclusions

ACC was a homogenous molecular group that showed a surprising association with neural crest derived tumors. PPGL mixed with both pancreatic NETs and NBL. Thus, the unbiased gene-expression analysis did not fully overlap with current clinicopathological classification of these tumors. In line with previous results, PPGL clustered together with other neural crest derived neoplasms.

Supplementary Materials: The following are available online at http://www.mdpi.com/2072-6694/10/12/518/s1, Figure S1: Bioinformatics pipeline 1. Unsupervised hierarchal clustering based on transcriptome data from 35 TCGA tumor categories with adrenal tumors annotated accordingly to molecular subtype, Figure S2: Bioinformatics pipeline 2. 1975 transcripts selected. Unsupervised clustering of 35 TCGA tumor categories with adrenal tumors annotated accordingly to molecular subtype, Figure S3: Bioinformatics pipeline 1. Unsupervised hierarchal clustering of 3319 samples annotated for TCGA tumor category with selected tumors annotated accordingly to molecular subtype, Figure S4: (A) Bioinformatics pipeline 2. 1975 transcripts selected. Unsupervised hierarchal clustering of 3319 samples annotated for TCGA tumor category with selected tumors annotated accordingly to molecular subtype. (B) Bioinformatics pipeline 2. Principal component analysis of 3319 samples with selected tumors annotated for TCGA or TARGET tumor category, Figure S5: Bioinformatics pipeline 1. Unsupervised hierarchal clustering of all ACC and SARC samples available in the TCGA database, Figure S6: Bioinformatics pipeline 1. Unsupervised clustering of 35 TCGA tumor categories as well as 8 PAAD samples annotated as PNET, Figure S7: Bioinformatics pipeline 2. 1975 transcripts selected. Unsupervised clustering of 35 TCGA tumor categories as well as 8 PAAD samples annotated as PNET, Figure S8: Bioinformatics pipeline 1. Unsupervised hierarchal clustering based on transcriptome data from 35 TCGA tumor categories with adrenal tumors annotated accordingly to molecular subtype. All samples in the PPGL cohort labeled as pheochromocytoma were removed, Figure S9: Consensus matrices of unsupervised cluster of cluster classification of 3319 TCGA and TARGET samples, Figure S10: Bioinformatics pipeline 1. Unsupervised hierarchal clustering of all PPGL as well as 8 PAAD samples annotated as PNET, Figure S11: Unsupervised hierarchal clustering of GBM, LGG, NBL, PNET and PPGL (minus cortical admixture subgroup), Table S1a: Genes preferentially expressed in Adrenocortical carcinoma (ACC) as well in as neural crest tumors (glioblastoma, low grade glioma, neuroblastoma, pancreatic neuroendocrine tumor and pheochromocytoma and paraganglioma), Table S1b: Go-enrichment analysis of genes co-expressed in Adrenocortical carcinoma (ACC) and glioma (glioblastoma and low grade glioma) and neuroendocrine tumors (neuroblastoma, pancreatic neuroendocrine tumor and pheochromocytoma and paraganglioma).

Author Contributions: Conceptualization, J.C. and K.P.; Formal analysis, J.C., S.B., B.S. and K.P.; Funding acquisition, J.C., S.W., P.H., P.S., B.S. and K.P.; Methodology, J.C. and S.B.; Supervision, K.P.; Validation, S.B. and D.T.; Visualization, J.C. and K.P.; Writing – original draft, J.C. and K.P.; Writing – review & editing, J.C., S.B., S.W., D.T., P.H., P.S., B.S. and K.P.

Funding: This study was funded by Lions Cancerforskningsfond Uppsala, Svenska Endokrinologföreningen, the Paradifference foundation and by the National Cancer Institute and the *Eunice Kennedy Shriver* National Institute of Child Health and Human Development. JCs research position is funded by Akademiska Sjukhuset, Uppsala.

Acknowledgments: We acknowledge the Cancer Genome Atlas and Therapeutically Applicable Research to Generate Effective Treatments consortiums as well as its collaborators for the outstanding datasets used in this study.

Conflicts of Interest: J.C. received lecture honoraria from Novartis. Other authors declare no conflict of interest.

Abbreviations

Abbrev.	Defination
TCGA	the Cancer Genome Atlas
TARGET	Therapeutically Applicable Research to Generate Effective Treatments
ACC	Adrenocortical carcinoma
PPGL	pheochromocytoma and paraganglioma
PNET	pancreatic neuroendocrine tumor
NBL	Neuroblastoma
COC	Cluster of Clusters
BRCA	Breast invasive carcinoma
BLCA	Bladder urothelial carcinoma
CESC	Cervical squamous cell carcinoma and Endocervical adenocarcinoma
CHOL	Cholangiocarcinoma
COAD	Colon adenocarcinoma
DLBC	Lymphoid neoplasm diffuse large B-cell lymphoma
ESCA	Esophageal carcinoma
GBM	Glioblastoma multiforme
KICH	Kidney chromophobe

KIRC	Kidney renal clear cell carcinoma
KIRP	Kidney renal papillary cell carcinoma
LAML	Acute myeloid leukemia
LGG	Brain Lower Grade Glioma
LIHC	Liver hepatocellular carcinoma
LUAD	Lung adenocarcinoma
LUSC	Lung squamous cell carcinoma
MESO	Mesothelioma
OV	Ovarian serous cystadenocarcinoma
PAAD	Pancreatic adenocarcinoma
PRAD	Prostate adenocarcinoma
READ	Rectum adenocarcinoma
SARC	Sarcoma
SKCM	Skin cutaneous melanoma
STAD	Stomach adenocarcinoma
HNSC	Head and neck squamous cell carcinoma
TGCT	Testicular germ cell tumors
THCA	Thyroid carcinoma
THYM	Thymoma
UCEC	Uterine corpus endometrial Carcinoma
UCS	Uterine carcinosarcoma
UVM	Uveal melanoma

References

1. Kölliker, R.V. *Handbuch der Braunschweig Gewebelehre der Menschen;* Druck und Verlag von Freidrich Vieweg und Sohn: Braunschweig, Germany, 1855.
2. Lloyd, R.V.; Osamura, R.Y.; Kloppel, G.; Rosai, J. *WHO Classification of Tumours: Pathology and Genetics of Tumours of Endocrine Organs;* IARC: Lyon, France, 2017.
3. Akerstrom, T.; Carling, T.; Beuschlein, F.; Hellman, P. Genetics of adrenocortical tumours. *J. Intern. Med.* **2016**, *280*, 540–550. [CrossRef] [PubMed]
4. Crona, J.; Taieb, D.; Pacak, K. New Perspectives on Pheochromocytoma and Paraganglioma: Toward a Molecular Classification. *Endocr. Rev.* **2017**, *38*, 489–515. [CrossRef] [PubMed]
5. Zheng, S.; Cherniack, A.D.; Dewal, N.; Moffitt, R.A.; Danilova, L.; Murray, B.A.; Lerario, A.M.; Else, T.; Knijnenburg, T.A.; Ciriello, G.; et al. Comprehensive Pan-Genomic Characterization of Adrenocortical Carcinoma. *Cancer Cell* **2016**, *29*, 723–736. [CrossRef] [PubMed]
6. Assie, G.; Letouze, E.; Fassnacht, M.; Jouinot, A.; Luscap, W.; Barreau, O.; Omeiri, H.; Rodriguez, S.; Perlemoine, K.; Rene-Corail, F.; et al. Integrated genomic characterization of adrenocortical carcinoma. *Nat. Genet.* **2014**, *46*, 607–612. [CrossRef] [PubMed]
7. Flynn, A.; Benn, D.; Clifton-Bligh, R.; Robinson, B.; Trainer, A.H.; James, P.; Hogg, A.; Waldeck, K.; George, J.; Li, J.; et al. The genomic landscape of phaeochromocytoma. *J. Pathol.* **2014**, *236*, 78–89. [CrossRef] [PubMed]
8. Castro-Vega, L.J.; Letouze, E.; Burnichon, N.; Buffet, A.; Disderot, P.H.; Khalifa, E.; Loriot, C.; Elarouci, N.; Morin, A.; Menara, M.; et al. Multi-omics analysis defines core genomic alterations in pheochromocytomas and paragangliomas. *Nat. Commun.* **2015**, *6*, 6044. [CrossRef] [PubMed]
9. Fishbein, L.; Leshchiner, I.; Walter, V.; Danilova, L.; Robertson, G.; Johnson, A.R.; Lichtenberg, T.M.; Murray, B.A.; Ghayee, H.K.; Else, T.; et al. Comprehensive Molecular Characterization of Pheochromocytoma and Paraganglioma. *Cancer Cell* **2017**, *31*, 1–13. [CrossRef]
10. Hoadley, K.A.; Yau, C.; Wolf, D.M.; Cherniack, A.D.; Tamborero, D.; Ng, S.; Leiserson, M.D.; Niu, B.; McLellan, M.D.; Uzunangelov, V.; et al. Multiplatform analysis of 12 cancer types reveals molecular classification within and across tissues of origin. *Cell* **2014**, *158*, 929–944. [CrossRef] [PubMed]
11. Hoadley, K.A.; Yau, C.; Hinoue, T.; Wolf, D.M.; Lazar, A.J.; Drill, E.; Shen, R.; Taylor, A.M.; Cherniack, A.D.; Thorsson, V.; et al. Cell-of-Origin Patterns Dominate the Molecular Classification of 10,000 Tumors from 33 Types of Cancer. *Cell* **2018**, *173*, 291–304. [CrossRef]

12. Cancer Genome Atlas Research Network. Integrated genomic characterization of oesophageal carcinoma. *Nature* **2017**, *541*, 169–175. [CrossRef] [PubMed]
13. Robertson, A.G.; Kim, J.; Al-Ahmadie, H.; Bellmunt, J.; Guo, G.; Cherniack, A.D.; Hinoue, T.; Laird, P.W.; Hoadley, K.A.; Akbani, R.; et al. Comprehensive Molecular Characterization of Muscle-Invasive Bladder Cancer. *Cell* **2017**, *171*, 540–556. [CrossRef] [PubMed]
14. Cancer Genome Atlas Research Network. Comprehensive molecular characterization of urothelial bladder carcinoma. *Nature* **2014**, *507*, 315–322. [CrossRef] [PubMed]
15. Ciriello, G.; Gatza, M.L.; Beck, A.H.; Wilkerson, M.D.; Rhie, S.K.; Pastore, A.; Zhang, H.; McLellan, M.; Yau, C.; Kandoth, C.; et al. Comprehensive Molecular Portraits of Invasive Lobular Breast Cancer. *Cell* **2015**, *163*, 506–519. [CrossRef] [PubMed]
16. Cancer Genome Atlas Research Network. Integrated genomic and molecular characterization of cervical cancer. *Nature* **2017**, *543*, 378–384. [CrossRef] [PubMed]
17. Farshidfar, F.; Zheng, S.; Gingras, M.C.; Newton, Y.; Shih, J.; Robertson, A.G.; Hinoue, T.; Hoadley, K.A.; Gibb, E.A.; Roszik, J.; et al. Integrative Genomic Analysis of Cholangiocarcinoma Identifies Distinct IDH-Mutant Molecular Profiles. *Cell Rep.* **2017**, *18*, 2780–2794. [CrossRef] [PubMed]
18. Cancer Genome Atlas Network. Comprehensive molecular characterization of human colon and rectal cancer. *Nature* **2012**, *487*, 330–337. [CrossRef] [PubMed]
19. Ceccarelli, M.; Barthel, F.P.; Malta, T.M.; Sabedot, T.S.; Salama, S.R.; Murray, B.A.; Morozova, O.; Newton, Y.; Radenbaugh, A.; Pagnotta, S.M.; et al. Molecular Profiling Reveals Biologically Discrete Subsets and Pathways of Progression in Diffuse Glioma. *Cell* **2016**, *164*, 550–563. [CrossRef]
20. Brennan, C.W.; Verhaak, R.G.; McKenna, A.; Campos, B.; Noushmehr, H.; Salama, S.R.; Zheng, S.; Chakravarty, D.; Sanborn, J.Z.; Berman, S.H.; et al. The somatic genomic landscape of glioblastoma. *Cell* **2013**, *155*, 462–477. [CrossRef]
21. Cancer Genome Atlas Network. Comprehensive genomic characterization of head and neck squamous cell carcinomas. *Nature* **2015**, *517*, 576–582. [CrossRef]
22. Davis, C.F.; Ricketts, C.J.; Wang, M.; Yang, L.; Cherniack, A.D.; Shen, H.; Buhay, C.; Kang, H.; Kim, S.C.; Fahey, C.C.; et al. The somatic genomic landscape of chromophobe renal cell carcinoma. *Cancer Cell* **2014**, *26*, 319–330. [CrossRef]
23. Cancer Genome Atlas Network. Comprehensive molecular characterization of clear cell renal cell carcinoma. *Nature* **2013**, *499*, 43–49. [CrossRef] [PubMed]
24. Linehan, W.M.; Spellman, P.T.; Ricketts, C.J.; Creighton, C.J.; Fei, S.S.; Davis, C.; Wheeler, D.A.; Murray, B.A.; Schmidt, L.; Vocke, C.D.; et al. Comprehensive Molecular Characterization of Papillary Renal-Cell Carcinoma. *N. Engl. J. Med.* **2016**, *374*, 135–145. [CrossRef] [PubMed]
25. Ley, T.J.; Miller, C.; Ding, L.; Raphael, B.J.; Mungall, A.J.; Robertson, A.; Hoadley, K.; Triche, T.J., Jr.; Laird, P.W.; Baty, J.D.; et al. Genomic and epigenomic landscapes of adult de novo acute myeloid leukemia. *N. Engl. J. Med.* **2013**, *368*, 2059–2074. [CrossRef] [PubMed]
26. Brat, D.J.; Verhaak, R.G.; Aldape, K.D.; Yung, W.K.; Salama, S.R.; Cooper, L.A.; Rheinbay, E.; Miller, C.R.; Vitucci, M.; Morozova, O.; et al. Comprehensive, Integrative Genomic Analysis of Diffuse Lower-Grade Gliomas. *N. Engl. J. Med.* **2015**, *372*, 2481–2498. [CrossRef] [PubMed]
27. Ally, A.; Balasundaram, M.; Carlsen, R.; Chuah, E.; Clarke, A.; Dhalla, N.; Holt, R.A.; Jones, S.J.; Lee, D.; Ma, Y.; et al. Comprehensive and Integrative Genomic Characterization of Hepatocellular Carcinoma. *Cell* **2017**, *169*, 1327–1341. [CrossRef] [PubMed]
28. Cancer Genome Atlas Research Network. Comprehensive molecular profiling of lung adenocarcinoma. *Nature* **2014**, *511*, 543–550. [CrossRef] [PubMed]
29. Cancer Genome Atlas Research Network. Comprehensive genomic characterization of squamous cell lung cancers. *Nature* **2012**, *489*, 519–525. [CrossRef]
30. Cancer Genome Atlas Research Network. Integrated genomic analyses of ovarian carcinoma. *Nature* **2011**, *474*, 609–615. [CrossRef]
31. Raphael, B.J.; Hruban, R.H.; Aguirre, A.J.; Moffitt, R.A.; Yeh, J.J.; Stewart, C.; Robertson, A.G.; Cherniack, A.D.; Gupta, M.; Getz, G.; et al. Integrated Genomic Characterization of Pancreatic Ductal Adenocarcinoma. *Cancer Cell* **2017**, *32*, 185–203. [CrossRef]
32. Abeshouse, A.; Ahn, J.; Akbani, R.; Ally, A.; Amin, S.; Andry, C.D.; Annala, M.; Aprikian, A.; Armenia, J.; Arora, A.; et al. The Molecular Taxonomy of Primary Prostate Cancer. *Cell* **2015**, *163*, 1011–1025. [CrossRef]

33. Cancer Genome Atlas Research Network. Comprehensive and Integrated Genomic Characterization of Adult Soft Tissue Sarcomas. *Cell* **2017**, *171*, 950–965. [CrossRef]
34. Akbani, R.; Akdemir, K.C.; Aksoy, B.A.; Albert, M.; Ally, A.; Amin, S.B.; Arachchi, H.; Arora, A.; Auman, J.T.; Ayala, B.; et al. Genomic Classification of Cutaneous Melanoma. *Cell* **2015**, *161*, 1681–1696. [CrossRef] [PubMed]
35. Cancer Genome Atlas Research Network. Comprehensive molecular characterization of gastric adenocarcinoma. *Nature* **2014**, *513*, 202–209. [CrossRef] [PubMed]
36. Shen, H.; Shih, J.; Hollern, D.P.; Wang, L.; Bowlby, R.; Tickoo, S.K.; Thorsson, V.; Mungall, A.J.; Newton, Y.; Hegde, A.M.; et al. Integrated Molecular Characterization of Testicular Germ Cell Tumors. *Cell Rep.* **2018**, *23*, 3392–3406. [CrossRef] [PubMed]
37. Agrawal, N.; Akbani, R.; Aksoy, B.A.; Ally, A.; Arachchi, H.; Asa, S.L.; Auman, J.T.; Balasundaram, M.; Balu, S.; Baylin, S.B.; et al. Integrated genomic characterization of papillary thyroid carcinoma. *Cell* **2014**, *159*, 676–690. [CrossRef]
38. Radovich, M.; Pickering, C.R.; Felau, I.; Ha, G.; Zhang, H.; Jo, H.; Hoadley, K.A.; Anur, P.; Zhang, J.; McLellan, M.; et al. The Integrated Genomic Landscape of Thymic Epithelial Tumors. *Cancer Cell* **2018**, *33*, 244–258. [CrossRef] [PubMed]
39. Kandoth, C.; Schultz, N.; Cherniack, A.D.; Akbani, R.; Liu, Y.; Shen, H.; Robertson, A.G.; Pashtan, I.; Shen, R.; Benz, C.C.; et al. Integrated genomic characterization of endometrial carcinoma. *Nature* **2013**, *497*, 67–73. [CrossRef] [PubMed]
40. Cherniack, A.D.; Shen, H.; Walter, V.; Stewart, C.; Murray, B.A.; Bowlby, R.; Hu, X.; Ling, S.; Soslow, R.A.; Broaddus, R.R.; et al. Integrated Molecular Characterization of Uterine Carcinosarcoma. *Cancer Cell* **2017**, *31*, 411–423. [CrossRef]
41. Robertson, A.G.; Shih, J.; Yau, C.; Gibb, E.A.; Oba, J.; Mungall, K.L.; Hess, J.M.; Uzunangelov, V.; Walter, V.; Danilova, L.; et al. Integrative Analysis Identifies Four Molecular and Clinical Subsets in Uveal Melanoma. *Cancer Cell* **2017**, *32*, 204–220. [CrossRef] [PubMed]
42. Wei, J.S.; Kuznetsov, I.B.; Zhang, S.; Song, Y.K.; Asgharzadeh, S.; Sindiri, S.; Wen, X.; Patidar, R.; Nagaraj, S.; Walton, A.; et al. Clinically Relevant Cytotoxic Immune Cell Signatures and Clonal Expansion of T Cell Receptors in High-risk MYCN-not-amplified Human Neuroblastoma. *Clin. Cancer Res.* **2018**. [CrossRef] [PubMed]
43. Szabo, P.M.; Pinter, M.; Szabo, D.R.; Zsippai, A.; Patocs, A.; Falus, A.; Racz, K.; Igaz, P. Integrative analysis of neuroblastoma and pheochromocytoma genomics data. *BMC Med. Genomics* **2012**, *5*, 48. [CrossRef] [PubMed]
44. Alvarez, M.J.; Subramaniam, P.S.; Tang, L.H.; Grunn, A.; Aburi, M.; Rieckhof, G.; Komissarova, E.V.; Hagan, E.A.; Bodei, L.; Clemons, P.A.; et al. A precision oncology approach to the pharmacological targeting of mechanistic dependencies in neuroendocrine tumors. *Nat. Genet.* **2018**, *50*, 979–989. [CrossRef] [PubMed]
45. Scarpa, A.; Chang, D.K.; Nones, K.; Corbo, V.; Patch, A.M.; Bailey, P.; Lawlor, R.T.; Johns, A.L.; Miller, D.K.; Mafficini, A.; et al. Whole-genome landscape of pancreatic neuroendocrine tumours. *Nature* **2017**, *543*, 65–71. [CrossRef] [PubMed]
46. Job, S.; Draskovic, I.; Burnichon, N.; Buffet, A.; Cros, J.; Lepine, C.; Venisse, A.; Robidel, E.; Verkarre, V.; Meatchi, T.; et al. Telomerase activation and ATRX mutations are independent risk factors for metastatic pheochromocytoma and paraganglioma. *Clin. Cancer Res.* **2018**. [CrossRef] [PubMed]
47. Chen, F.; Zhang, Y.; Gibbons, D.L.; Deneen, B.; Kwiatkowski, D.J.; Ittmann, M.; Creighton, C.J. Pan-Cancer Molecular Classes Transcending Tumor Lineage Across 32 Cancer Types, Multiple Data Platforms, and over 10,000 Cases. *Clin. Cancer Res.* **2018**, *24*, 2182–2193. [CrossRef] [PubMed]
48. Edfors, F.; Danielsson, F.; Hallstrom, B.M.; Kall, L.; Lundberg, E.; Ponten, F.; Forsstrom, B.; Uhlen, M. Gene-specific correlation of RNA and protein levels in human cells and tissues. *Mol. Syst. Biol.* **2016**, *12*, 883. [CrossRef] [PubMed]
49. Warnes, G.R.; Bolker, B.; Bonebakker, L.; Gentleman, R.; Huber, W.; Liaw, A.; Lumley, T.; Maechler, M.; Magnusson, A.; Moeller, S.; et al. gplots: Various R Programming Tools for Plotting Data. R package version 3.0.1. Available online: https://CRAN.R-project.org/package=gplots (accessed on 26 March 2018).
50. R Core Team. R: A Language and Environment for Statistical Computing. Available online: https://www.R-project.org/ (accessed on 26 March 2018).
51. RStudio Team. RStudio: Integrated Development for R. Available online: http://www.rstudio.com/ (accessed on 26 March 2018).
52. Wilkerson, M.D.; Hayes, D.N. ConsensusClusterPlus: A class discovery tool with confidence assessments and item tracking. *Bioinformatics* **2010**, *26*, 1572–1573. [CrossRef]

53. Bergman, J.; Botling, J.; Fagerberg, L.; Hallstrom, B.M.; Djureinovic, D.; Uhlen, M.; Ponten, F. The Human Adrenal Gland Proteome Defined by Transcriptomics and Antibody-Based Profiling. *Endocrinology* **2017**, *158*, 239–251. [CrossRef]
54. Subramanian, A.; Tamayo, P.; Mootha, V.K.; Mukherjee, S.; Ebert, B.L.; Gillette, M.A.; Paulovich, A.; Pomeroy, S.L.; Golub, T.R.; Lander, E.S.; et al. Gene set enrichment analysis: A knowledge-based approach for interpreting genome-wide expression profiles. *Proc. Natl. Acad. Sci. USA* **2005**, *102*, 15545–15550. [CrossRef]
55. Barbie, D.A.; Tamayo, P.; Boehm, J.S.; Kim, S.Y.; Moody, S.E.; Dunn, I.F.; Schinzel, A.C.; Sandy, P.; Meylan, E.; Scholl, C.; et al. Systematic RNA interference reveals that oncogenic KRAS-driven cancers require TBK1. *Nature* **2009**, *462*, 108–112. [CrossRef]

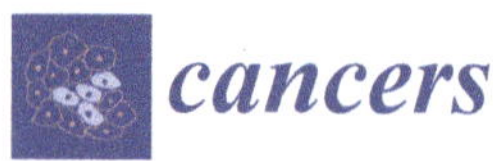
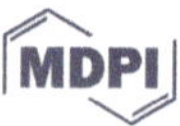

Review

Malignant Pheochromocytomas/Paragangliomas and Ectopic Hormonal Secretion: A Case Series and Review of the Literature

Anna Angelousi [1,*], Melpomeni Peppa [2], Alexandra Chrisoulidou [3], Krystallenia Alexandraki [4], Annabel Berthon [5], Fabio Rueda Faucz [5], Eva Kassi [1,6] and Gregory Kaltsas [4]

1 Department of Internal Medicine, Unit of Endocrinology, National and Kapodistrian University of Athens, Laiko hospital, Goudi, 11527 Athens, Greece; evakassis@gmail.com
2 Endocrine Unit, 2nd Department of Internal Medicine Propaedeutic, Research Institute and Diabetes Center, National and Kapodistrian University of Athens, Attikon University Hospital, 12462 Haidari, Greece; moly6592@yahoo.com
3 Unit of Endocrinology, Theagenio Cancer Hospital, 2 Al Simeonidi Str., 54007 Thessaloniki, Greece; a.chrisoulidou@gmail.com
4 1st Department of Propaedeutic Internal Medicine, National and Kapodistrian University of Athens, Laiko hospital, Goudi, 11527 Athens, Greece; alexandrakik@gmail.com (K.A.); gkaltsas@endo.gr (G.K.)
5 Section on Endocrinology and Genetics, Eunice Kennedy Shriver National Institute of Child Health and Human Development, National Institutes of Health, Bethesda, MD 20892, USA; annabel.berthon@nih.gov (A.B.); fabio.faucz@pucpr.br (F.R.F.)
6 Department of Biological Chemistry, Medical School, National and Kapodistrian University of Athens, Goudi, 11527 Athens, Greece
* Correspondence: a.angelousi@gmail.com; Tel.: +30-6978167876

Received: 3 April 2019; Accepted: 17 May 2019; Published: 24 May 2019

Abstract: Malignant pheochromocytomas (PCs) and paragangliomas (PGLs) are rare neuroendocrine neoplasms defined by the presence of distant metastases. There is currently a relatively paucity of data regarding the natural history of PCs/PGLs and the optimal approach to their treatment. We retrospectively analyzed the clinical, biochemical, imaging, genetic and histopathological characteristics of fourteen patients with metastatic PCs/PGLs diagnosed over 15 years, along with their response to treatment. Patients were followed-up for a median of six years (range: 1–14 years). Six patients had synchronous metastases and the remaining developed metastases after a median of four years (range 2–10 years). Genetic analysis of seven patients revealed that three harbored succinate dehydrogenase subunit B/D gene (SDHB/D) mutations. Hormonal hypersecretion occurred in 70% of patients; normetanephrine, either alone or with other concomitant hormones, was the most frequent secretory component. Patients were administered multiple first and subsequent treatments including surgery (n = 12), chemotherapy (n = 7), radionuclide therapy (n = 2) and radiopeptides (n = 5). Seven patients had stable disease, four had progressive disease and three died. Ectopic hormonal secretion is rare and commonly encountered in benign PCs. Ectopic secretion of interleukin-6 in one of our patients, prompted a literature review of ectopic hormonal secretion, particularly from metastatic PCs/PGLs. Only four cases of metastatic PC/PGLs with confirmed ectopic secretion of hormones or peptides have been described so far.

Keywords: metastatic OR malignant pheochromocytoma; paraganglioma; ectopic secretion; IL-6; normetanephrines

1. Introduction

Malignant pheochromocytomas (PCs) and paragangliomas (PGLs) are rare neuroendocrine tumors with an incidence of less than 1/1,000,000, defined by the presence of metastatic disease in non-chromaffin tissues without considering recurrent or locally invasive tumors [1–3]. The WHO Endocrine Tumor Classification 4th Edition (2017) [4] prompted the new concept that all PGLs have some metastatic potential and assigned an International Classification of Diseases for Oncology (ICD-O)-3 (malignant tumors) for all PGLs, surpassing the previous categories of benign and malignant tumors in favor of an approach based on risk stratification [4].

Long-term follow-up has shown that PCs/PGLs exhibit a 15–20% 10-year probability of recurrence and up to 20% malignancy rate [5]. In the presence of metastatic disease, a wide 5-year survival rate range, from 40 to 77%, has been described, as well as a heterogeneous progression free survival (PFS) ranging from 4 to 36 months following various therapeutic modalities [6–8]. Synchronous metastases at initial diagnosis are encountered in 10% in PCs and 34% in PGLs but can occur up to 20 years after initial diagnosis with the most common metastatic sites being regional lymph nodes, bone (50%), liver (50%) and lung (30%) [9,10].

Although surgical removal is the mainstay of treatment of PCs/PGLs, further risk stratification regarding their malignant potential is required to define the follow-up protocols after complete resection [9]. A number of histopathological scores have been developed to denote the malignant potential of these neoplasms such as the Adrenal Pheochromocytoma and Paraganglioma (GAPP) Score used to evaluate the malignant potential of both PCs and sympathetic PGLs, and the Pheochromocytoma of the Adrenal Gland Scaled Score (PASS) used to evaluate the malignant potential of PCs only, although it exhibits a relatively low predictive value (sensitivity 50% and specificity 45%) [11,12]. Besides these scores, a number of clinical characteristics and biomarkers have also been proposed to predict the metastatic potential of PCs/PGLs including younger age at presentation [5,13,14], larger sized (>5 cm) tumors [5,15], extra-adrenal location of the neoplasm [5], and higher circulating norepinephrine levels [5,15,16]. However, the majority of these markers exhibit a relatively low positive predictive value. Currently the presence of inactivating mutations of the succinate dehydrogenase subunit B (*SDHB*) gene is strongly associated with the development of metastatic PCs and PGLs [17].

The natural history of patients with malignant PCs/PGLs is divergent as approximately half of the patients with metastatic PCs/PGLs have stable disease (SD) one year after diagnosis without any therapeutic intervention [18,19]. Although the timing of further therapeutic interventions for metastatic PCs/PGLs has not been clearly defined, further therapeutic options for symptomatic patients in the presence of progressive disease include cytoreductive surgery, systemic chemotherapy (using either the combination of cyclophosphamide, vincristine, and dacarbazine (CVD) or temozolomide) and/or ^{131}I- metaiodobenzylguanidine (^{131}I-MIBG) [20]. Recently, some data have also emerged for the activity of peptide receptor radionuclide therapies (PRRTs) that bind to somatostatin receptors expressed by such neoplasms [19]. Percutaneous ablation has also been used as a minimally invasive local treatment option [20].

Ectopic secretion of bioactive compounds (hormones or peptides) from PCs or PGLs is rare; approximately 1.3% of all PCs may produce ectopic adrenocorticotropic hormone (ACTH) secretion; in rare cases, ectopically secreted corticotropin releasing hormone (CRH) may also occur [21]. Case reports have also described the production of parathyroid hormone related-peptide (PTHrP), vasoactive intestinal peptide (VIP), vasopressin, growth hormone releasing hormone (GHRH), insulin, somatostatin, aldosterone, renin, interleukin-6 (IL-6), and neuropeptide Y. However, the majority of ectopic secretion is encountered in non-metastatic PCs/PGLs, whereas there is paucity of data regarding its prevalence in metastatic PCs/PGLs.

In this study, we retrospectively analyzed the clinical, biochemical, radiological and genetic features of patients with metastatic PCs/PGs, along with the therapeutic modalities employed and their response to various treatments. These data were compared with the currently existing data on metastatic PCs/PGLs, focusing on the ectopic secretion of biologically active compounds from metastatic PCs/PGLs.

2. Results

2.1. Epidemiological and Clinicopathological Data

Fourteen patients with a median age of 45 years (interquartile range (IQR): 30) were included in the present study; seven patients with metastatic PCs, six with metastatic PGLs and one with both PC and PGL. The median follow-up period was six years (range: 1–14, IQR: 10 years) (Table 1). Half of the patients (50%) presented with synchronous metastases (5 PGLs, 2 PCs); 69% of all cases developed metastases in the distal lymph nodes (cervical and abdominal); 46% in the liver, 23% in the bones and 15% in the lung. In one patient with a bladder PGL, metastases were found in the aortopulmonary window and the heart (substantiated by dedicated cardiac magnetic resonance imaging (MRI)). The remainder of the patients developed metastases after a median time of four years from diagnosis (range 0.8–10 years, IQR = 8) in the liver, lung, distal lymph nodes and vertebrae.

Table 1. Epidemiological and clinicopathological characteristics of the studied population.

Characteristics	
Number (PC)	14 (7)
Female sex, n (%)	8 (57%)
Median age (IQR), years	45 (30)
Size primary tumor (cm)	4.25 (4)
Sychronous/ Metachronous metastases	7/7
Functionality n, (%)	10 (71%)
-normetanephrines	3
-metanephrine	0
-normetanephrines and metanephrines	4
-dopamine	1
-normetanephrine and dopamine	1
-normetanephrines. metanephrnes, dopamine	1
Functional imaging	
-Octreoscan (positive, %)	4/7 (57%)
-^{68}Gallium labelled octreotide (positive, %)	3/3 (100%)
-^{18}F-FGD-PET (positive, %)	9/11 (82%)
-^{131}I-MIBG (positive, %)	8/10 (80%)
Follow-up, median (IQR, range), years	6 (10, 1–14)
Treatment (any line)	
-Surgery	12 (86%)
-PRTTs (^{131}I-MIBG or ^{17}Lu-Dotate)	5 (35%)
-Chemotherapy	7 (50%)
-Radiotherapy	2 (14%)
Genetic status (n)	7
-SDHB+	2/7
-SDHD+	1/7
Mortality	3 (21%)

Abbreviations: PC: pheochromocytoma, IQR: interquartile range, PRRTs: peptide receptor radionuclide therapy, SDHB/D: succinate dehydrogenase subunit B/D.

Ten patients (71%) had functional tumors; three had normetanephrine hypersecretion, four had concomitant normetanephrine and metanephrine secretion, one had only dopamine secretion, one had normetanephrine and dopamine secretion, and one had normetanephrine, metanephrine and dopamine secretion. All patients presented with relevant symptoms attributed to hormonal hypersecretion, or symptoms due to compression of nearby tissues, except two cases in whom the diagnosis was made incidentally (Table 1).

In nine patients, the diagnosis of malignant PC/PGL and radiological follow-up was performed with MRI, which showed increased signal intensity in the T2-weighted sequence, whereas in the remaining five patients, initial diagnosis as well as radiological follow-up were performed with computed tomography (CT). ^{131}I-MIBG was performed and found to be positive in eight out of ten patients. Octreoscan was performed in seven patients showing increased uptake in the primary tumor and metastases in four, ^{68}Gallium-Labeled (1,4,7,10-tetraazacyclododecane-*N,N′,N″,N‴*-tetraacetic acid)-1-NaI3-octreotide(^{68}Ga-DOTANOC) was performed in three patients and showed increased uptake in all, whereas ^{18}F-fluorodeoxyglucose positron emission tomography (^{18}F-FDG PET) was positive in nine out of eleven patients (Table 1).

The median size of the neoplasms was 4.25 cm (IQR: 4). Histological confirmation was performed in 12 patients and all patients with PCs had a PASS > 6 (Table 2). All tumors were positive for chromogranin and synaptophysin immunostaining. The mean Ki-67% proliferative indices of the primary and metastatic sites were 11 ± 3.8% and 44 ± 7%, respectively. Three tumors out of five showed intense immunochemical staining for somatostatin receptor 2, with two of them also staining for somatostatin receptor 5 (Table 2).

Table 2. Tumors' (PCs and PGLs) characteristics.

Characteristics	N (%)
Primary tumor location, n (%)	
-PC	7 (50%)
-PGL	6 (46%)
bladder PGL	1
para-aortic PGL	2
paravertebral PGL	1
abdominal PGL	2
-PCs + PGLs	1
Primary tumor size, mm (median, IQR)	4.25, 4
Location of metastases	
-lymph nodes (abdominal/cervical)	9 (69%)
-liver	6 (46%)
-lung	2 (15%)
-bones	3 (23%)
Metastases per patient	>2 (1–4)
Histopathological data	
-Ki-67 (mean ± SD)	11 ± 3.8%
-PASS	7.75
-SSTR2,5(positive/total (n))	(3/5)

Abbreviations: PC: pheochromocytoma, PGL: paraganglioma, SD: standard variation, PASS: Pheochromocytoma of the Adrenal Gland Scaled Score, SSTR 2,5: somatostatin receptor (2, 5).

Out of seven patients tested for germline mutations, two had *SDHB* mutations and one had a *SDHD* mutation (Table 1). One patient with a *SDHB* mutation had a functional left PC, secreting normetanephrine and dopamine. It was treated initially by surgery but developed metastases in the vertebrae after six years. The second was a female patient with concomitant presence of PC and multiple abdominal PGLs that were non-secretory. The patient with the *SDHD* mutation was a female with a functional bladder PGL secreting dopamine and multiple PGLs in the cervical spine, the aorto-pulmonary window and the carotid.

2.2. Treatment and Outcome

As first line treatment, nine patients underwent radical surgical resection of the primary tumor (all R0), four patients were treated with chemotherapy (cisplatin/etoposide or capecitabin/temozolomide) and one with ^{131}I-MIBG. Three patients exhibited SD until the last follow-up and no further treatment was needed: the first was treated with ^{131}I-MIBG and the two others with surgical resection of the primary and metastases. One patient who was treated with chemotherapy died from the disease and the remaining ten developed progressive disease (PD) and received second line treatment. Two patients were treated with chemotherapy (cisplatin/etoposide), one of whom died, three with radionuclides (^{131}I-MIBG (n = 1), ^{177}Lu-DOTATE (n = 2)), three with repeated surgical resection and two with local radiotherapy. Four patients developed SD after second line treatment (two had been treated with PRRT, the third with surgical debulking and the fourth with radiotherapy), whereas the remaining five developed PD; two had no further treatment and were followed-up. Three patients received third line treatment; two with temozolomide (one died after three cycles) and the third with chemotherapy (cisplatin/etoposide) and subsequently with ^{131}I-MIBG (4th line treatment). Overall, at the end of the follow-up period, seven patients exhibited SD (50%), three (2 PGLs, 1PCs) died (21%) and four developed PD (29%). Patients with PCs developed PD after a median time of 4.14 years (IQR: 3.38) following initial treatment, whereas patients with PGL developed PD after a median time of 1.6 years (IQR: 1.03) (p = 0.8). Median overall survival (OS) for PGLs was 14 years (IQR: 11.7) (Figure 1a,b).

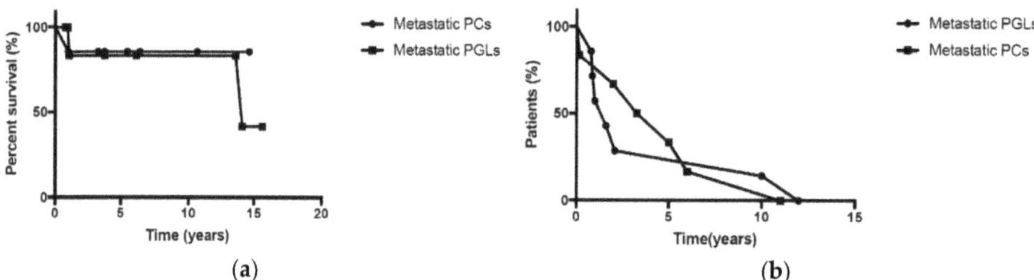

Figure 1. (**a**). Overall survival (OS) of malignant pheochromocytomas (PCs) and paragangliomas (PGL) (median OS for PGLs = 14 years, IQR: 11.7) (**b**) Median progression free survival (PFS) until the presence of the first or new metastases: malignant PCs: 4.14 years (IQR: 3.38) and PGLs: 1.6 years (IQR: 1.03) (p = 0.8). Abbreviations: MPCs: metastatic pheochromocytoma, MPGLs: metastatic paragangliomas, IQR: interquartile range.

2.3. Ectopic Secretion and Review of the Literature

One patient with non-functional PGLs and synchronous metastases to the vertebrae and muscles developed pyrexia not attributed to an infectious state and that was resistant to anti-inflammatory drugs. IL-6 levels were measured and were found to be elevated at 236 pg/mL (normal values < 7). Besides blood analysis, immunohistochemical staining confirmed the higher cytoplasmic expression of IL-6 in the paraffin-embedded tissue of the patient's PGL compared to PC tissue of a patient without fever (control tissue), which showed weaker staining. Following surgical debulking, the pyrexia improved but recurred due to PD and the patient was treated with chemotherapy (cisplatin and etoposide) and temozolomide, but died one year after the initial diagnosis. A systematic review of the literature revealed seventy-six relevant English language articles, mainly case reports, addressing ectopic secretion of bioactive compounds of PC/PGLs over the last 30 years (Figure 2).

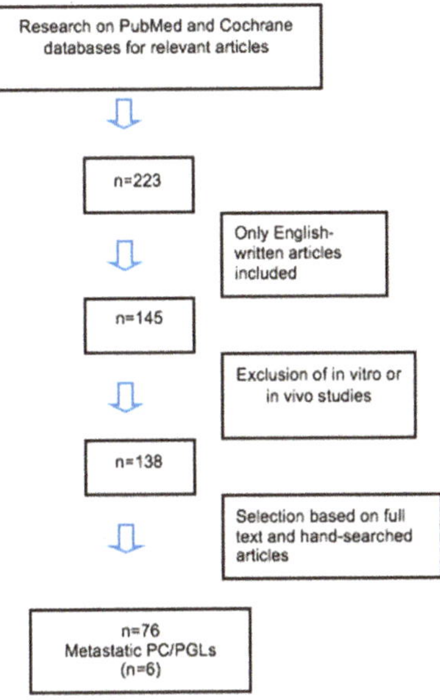

Figure 2. Flow diagram.

A total of 150 cases (Table 3) with ectopic secretion from PCs/PGLs have been reported (data presented in Table 3). ACTH secretion accounted for 33% of all cases (n = 49), whereas CRH, VIP, vasopressin, PTH, renin, aldosterone, insulin or somatostatin, GHRH, and neuropeptide Y secretion have also been described [16,21–98]. IL-6 secretion has already been reported in 40 cases with PCs/PGLs (Table 3). Only four case reports with confirmed ectopic secretion from metastatic PCs/PGLs have been described (data presented in Table 4). In particular, regarding metastatic PCs, one secreted ACTH and another one secreted PTHrP. For metastatic PGLs, one secreted ACTH and another secreted ACTH and IL-6. There was one case of PC with suspicion of IL-6 secretion without laboratory confirmation and a PGL with suspicion of IL-b and tumor necrosis factor (TNF) secretion without biochemical confirmation. In all cases, patients with IL-6 ectopic secretion presented with pyrexia resistant to any treatment, which resolved after surgical debulking of the tumor (Table 4).

Table 3. Ectopically secreted bioactive compounds from PCs/PGLs based on the literature.

Hormone	No of Cases	PCs	PGLs	Malignant (n)	References
Total	150	137	13	5	
-ACTH	49	43	6	2 (1PC, 1PGLs)	[21–51]
-CRH	8	6	2	0	[52–59]
-VIP	6	6	0	0	[33,60–62]
-Vasopressin	1	1	0	0	[57]
-Calcium	1	1	0	0	[63]
-IL-6	40	39	1	1	[64–77]
-PTH/PTHrp	17	17	0	1	[78–82]
-Calcitonin	5	5	0	0	[33,83–85]
-GH/GHRH	7	6	1	0	[86–90]
-Insuline/IGF-1	1	0	1	0	[91]
-Somatostatin	1	1	0	0	[92]
-Aldosterone	1	1	0	0	[33]

Table 3. *Cont.*

Hormone	No of Cases	PCs	PGLs	Malignant (n)	References
-Renin	2	2	0	0	[33,93]
-CRH and ACTH	2	1	1	0	[59,94]
-CRH or ACTH and vasopressin	2	2	0	0	[57,58]
-IL b	1	1	0		[95]
-ACTH and IL-6	1	0	1	1	[76]
-Calcitonin and VIP	3	3	0	0	[33,63,83]
-PTH and aldosterone	1	1	0	0	[96]
-Neuropeptide Y	1	1	0	0	[16]

Abbreviations: PCs: pheochromocytomas, PGLs: paragangliomas, ACTH: adrenocorticotropic hormone, CRH: corticotropin-releasing hormone, VIP: vasoactive intestinal peptide, IL-6: interleukin-6, PTH: parathormone, PTHrp: parathyroid hormone related-peptide, GH: growth hormone, GHRH: growth hormone releasing hormone, IGF-1:insulin growth factor-1. IL-b: interleukin b.

Table 4. Ectopic secretion of bioactive compounds from malignant PCs/PGLs based on the literature.

References	Number	PCs/PGLs	Metastases	Ectopic Secretion	Treatment
Kakudo K, et al. 1984 [25]	Case report (n = 1)	PC	Liver, lungs, bones, lymph nodes	ACTH (blood and tissue)	Surgery
Teno et al. 1996 [97]	Case report (n = 1)	PC	Bones	Suspicion of IL-6 but not measured	External Radiation
Tutal E et al. 2017 [30]	Case report (n = 1)	Renal PGL	Lymph nodes	ACTH (blood and tissues)	Surgery
Omura M et al. 1994 [75]	Case report (n = 1)	Cervical PGL	Bones	ACTH, IL-6 (blood and tumor)	Surgery and chemotherapy
Mutabagani KH et al. 1999 [98]	Case report (n = 1)	Mediastinal PGL	Liver	Anemia (probably Il-1 and anti-TNF secretion but never measured)	Surgery and hepatic arterial chemoembolization
Bridgewater JA et al. 1993 [80]	Case report (n = 1)	PC	Left para-aortic lymph node	PTHrp (blood and tissue)	Surgical resection

Abbreviations: PCs: pheochromocytomas, PGLs: paragangliomas, ACTH: adrenocorticotropic hormone, IL-6: interleukin-6, PTHrp: parathyroid hormone related-peptide, anti-TNF A: anti-tumor necrosis factor A.

3. Discussion

In the present study we present our experience from a series of 14 malignant PCs/PGLs treated with multiple therapeutic modalities. Three patients (2 PGLs, 1PC) died as result of the disease after a median follow-up of six years. Despite multiple therapeutic modalities, seven out of eleven patients (63%) exhibited PD; patients with PGLs appear to have more rapid PD (1.16 years) compared to patients with PCs (4 years), although due to the relatively small number of patients included, this was not statistically significant. One of the patients with a metastatic PGL presented with refractory pyrexia due to ectopic secretion of IL-6, confirmed by elevated IL-6 levels in the serum and histological confirmation of IL-6 protein expression in the tissue. Systematic review of the literature showed that although ectopic secretion of IL-6 is relatively common in benign PCs/PGLs, only one further case of metastatic PGL with confirmed IL-6 and ACTH secretion has been reported [75].

In a recent large study including 330 PCs/PGLs, the incidence of metastatic PCs/PGLs was 6.9% [99]. The risk of metastases was associated with an age at diagnosis ≤35 years (hazard ratio [HR] 2.74, [95% Confidence Interval (CI) 1.19–6.35), tumor size ≥6.0 cm (HR 2.43, 95% CI 1.06–5.56), extra-adrenal location (HR 2.73, 95% CI 1.10–7.40), and tumor producing only normetamephrine (HR 2.96, 95% CI (1.30–6.76)) [100]. In our series the median age of 45 years was higher, yet similar, to the mean age (41 ± 17 years old) of the metastatic group of the previous study. The median size of the primary tumor was smaller (4.25 cm), whereas the hormonal profile was similar, showing that secretion of norepinephrine was the predominant secretory component.

Epinephrine-secreting tumors, either alone or with norepinephrine, originate exclusively from the adrenal gland [10]. Norepinephrine-secreting PGLs are tumors in which norepinephrine only or norepinephrine plus dopamine are produced; 50% of PCs and 100% of PGLs are of this type [10]. In our series 64% of the patients with malignant PCs/PGLs (3 with PGLs, 5 with PCs, 1 with a PC and PGL) had either norepinephrine secreting PCs/PGLS or norepinephrine in combination with epinephrine or dopamine. Previous studies are in line with these data, reporting that the metastatic ratio is twice as high in norepinephrine-secreting PCs compared to epinephrine-secreting PCs [10]. Norepinephrine-secreting PGLs lack phenylethanolamine N-methyltransferase, the enzyme that converts ormetanephrine to metanephrine and are considered less differentiated than adrenaline-producing (metanephrine) tumors [10]. In addition, dopamine hypersecretion is considered a feature of immaturity and a marker for metastatic PGLs [15]. Dopamine-secreting PGLs are typically non-symptomatic; it has been reported that the plasma level of methoxytyramine, the O-methylated metabolite of dopamine, is 4.7-fold higher in patients with metastases than in those without, suggesting its use as a potential biomarker [100].

Only half of our patients showed uptake in octreoscan, whereas 82% exhibited increased uptake in ^{18}F-FDG-PET and 80% in ^{131}I-MIBG. Data in the literature have shown that ^{131}I-MIBG and ^{18}F-FDG-PET exhibit higher sensitivity than octreoscan [101]. However, it subsequently became apparent that the sensitivity of ^{68}Ga- 1,4,7,10-tetraazacyclododecane-1,4,7,10-tetraacetic acid (DOTA) tyrosine-3-octreotate (DOTATATE)-PET/CT imaging in patients with PCs/PGLs seems to be higher than that of ^{131}I-MIBG scintigraphy and ^{18}F-FDG-PET in mapping metastatic PCs/PGLs [101–104]. In our series, three cases out of five (one PC and two PGLs) showed immunochemical expression of somatostatin receptor 2, and in two of them this was concomitant with receptor 5.

Currently, there are no systemic therapies approved by the European Medicines Agency or the US Food and Drug Administration (FDA) for patients with metastatic PCs/PGLs [17,18]. Surgical resection or debulking is the gold standard of treatment. Other treatment options for non-operable tumors are limited to chemotherapy (CVD) with relatively low response rates (complete response in 4%, partial response in 37% and SD in 14%) and inappropriately high toxicity [105–107]. Nevertheless, chemotherapy is considered part of the initial management in patients with metastatic *SDHB*-related PGLs (median of 20.5 cycles) [107]. Lately there is increased interest in the use of PRRT in malignant PCs/PGLs [108,109]. Recent studies including patients with metastatic PCs/PGLs treated with ^{90}Y-DOTATATE or ^{177}Lu-DOTATATE have shown a mean progression free survival (PFS) (36% had PD and 50% SD) and OS of 39 and 61 months, respectively, compared to conventional ^{131}I-MIBG treatment (mean PFS: 14 months and OS: 23 months) [110,111]. In our series, three patients with metastatic PCs/PGLs were treated with ^{131}I-MIBG and two with ^{177}Lu-DOTATATE either as first, second, third or fourth line treatment; two of them developed PD and three SD during the last follow-up, whereas the median PFS was 3.5 years (range: 0.05–11.8, IQR = 7.3), which is the longest compared to the other therapeutic modalities employed. These data appear encouraging although larger series are required.

One of our patients with a non-functional malignant PGL presented with pyrexia resistant to any treatment due to IL-6 ectopic secretion. Ectopic secretion of hormones or peptides, from PCs/PGLs is rare (approximately 1% of all PCs), encountered mostly in non-malignant and non-genetic cases. It is probable that ectopic secretion of bioactive compounds from these tumors is often overloooked or clinical manifestations are masked by the hypersecretion of catecholamines. The most frequent ectopically-secreted hormone is ACTH, mostly reported in benign PCs [21–51]. Ectopic secretion of hormones or peptides from malignant PCs/PGLs has been reported even more scarcely. In particular, only four cases of metastatic PCs/PGLs with biochemically or immunohistochemically confirmed ectopic secretion of hormones or peptides have been described in the English literature so far [25,30,75,80]. In two other cases of malignant PCs/PGLs, ectopic secretion has been suspected but not confirmed biologically or immunohistochemically [97,98].

IL-6 ectopic secretion has already been reported in 40 cases of PCs/PGLs, however only one of them, a case of cervical PGL, was metastatic [64–77]. The reason for the high level of IL-6 expression in PCs/PGLs is unclear. It has been suggested that IL-6 over-production can be either ascribed directly to the tumor or indirectly accounted for by tumoral production of the high circulating norepinephrine levels [74]. However, the presence of IHC expression of IL-6 protein in the PGL tissue of our patient with ectopic IL-6 secretion is more in favor of IL-6 synthesis and secretion by the PGL neoplastic cells.

4. Methods

4.1. Patients

In this retrospective study, data were obtained from three Greek Endocrine Units; the Endocrine Unit of Laiko Hospital (n = 11) and the Endocrine Unit of Attiko Hospital (n = 2) of the National and Kapodistrian University of Athens and the Theagenio Hospital in Thessaloniki (n = 1). The medical records of patients with metastatic PCs/PGLs over a period of 20 years (1998–2018) were reviewed by two independent researchers (Anna Angelousi and Krystallenia Alexandraki) in order to collect the clinico-pathological characteristics of these patients along with imaging and biochemical findings. In addition, the therapeutic response to the various utilized treatments was also recorded.

The study protocol was approved by the Ethics or Audit Committees of all participating centers. All patients gave informed consent according to the Declaration of Helsinki and Good Clinical Practice guidelines. Informed consent was obtained from patients' relatives in the case of death. The ethical code number is AP 450 and the date of decision of approval from the ethical committee of the "General Laiko" hospital of Athens is 8 April 2019.

Patients with the following criteria were included in our study: (i) histopathological and/or biochemical and/or imaging confirmation of the diagnosis of primary PCs/PGLs and distant metastases; (ii) available data during the follow-up period. Exclusion criteria included: (i) benign PCs/PGLs; (ii) patients with documented venous or loco-regional or proximal lymph node spread only. For the systematic review of the literature, ectopic secretion was defined as ectopic production, involving the synthesis and secretion of bioactive compounds (peptides or hormones) from benign or malignant tumors that do not normally synthesize and secrete these particular compounds.

4.2. Review of the Literature on Ectopic Hormonal Secretion

To identify studies and determine their eligibility, a systematic review was conducted in the PubMed and Cochrane Databases. Search terms included the following: "pheochromocytoma OR metastatic pheochromocytoma", "paraganglioma OR metastatic paraganglioma", "paraneoplastic syndrome", "ectopic secretion", "IL-6". The above keywords were also combined with the Boolean operators AND and OR. Two of the authors (Anna Angelousi and Eva Kassi) independently examined all potentially eligible titles and abstracts. Full manuscripts were obtained as necessary to finalize eligibility. Reference lists of eligibility studies were also searched through to identify additional studies. Only English language papers were selected. Studies with hormonal ectopic secretion from tumors other than PCs/PGLs were also excluded as well as in vitro studies. Seventy-six articles were finally included (Figure 2).

4.3. Hormonal Secretion

All patients had 24 h urinary metanephrine and normetanephrine levels measured by high-performance liquid chromatography. IL-6 levels were measured with High–Performance Liquid Chromatography (HPLC) (Bio-Rad, Athens, Greece).

4.4. Imaging

All patients underwent conventional imaging with either CT or MRI along with functional imaging including ^{131}I-MIBG, ^{111}In-pentetreotide (Octreoscan) and ^{68}Gallium labelled octreotide, or

^{18}F-fluorodeoxyglucose positron emission tomography (^{18}F-FDG PET). In all patients primary tumor and metastases were detected and followed-up with conventional imaging (five patients with CT and nine with MRI). In addition, all patients had at least one form of functional imaging.

4.5. Statistical Analyses

All statistical analyses were conducted using GraphPad Prism Version 6 for Mac OS X (GraphPad Software, La Jolla, California, USA). Quantitative values are reported as median (interquartile range (IQR) and/or 25–75% range) or mean ± standard deviation (SD), and categorical variables as percentages. Overall survival (OS) was defined by time from diagnosis of PCs/PGLs to death by any cause. Progression free survival (PFS) was defined from the time of the initiation of a specific treatment to presence of new metastases or progression of the existing ones (according to Response Evaluation Criteria in Solid Tumors (RECIST)). OS and PFS were estimated using Kaplan–Meier curves. Comparison of the PFS and OS between patients with metastatic PCs and patients with metastatic PGLs was performed using the Wilcoxon test (GraphPad Software, La Jolla, California, USA) A p value < 0.05 was considered significant.

5. Conclusions

Malignant PCs/PGLs are a rare entity that can metastasize many years after surgical resection of the primary tumor, even 10 years after the initial diagnosis as in our case. In our series metastatic PGLs appear to have more rapid PD (1.16 years) compared to patients with PCs (4 years). Available treatments are, so far, non-curative; further research is needed to evaluate therapies with novel mechanisms of action. PRRT seems to improve the outcome of our patients with metastatic PCs/PGLs, resulting in longer PFS, but should be studied in larger clinical trials. Ectopic secretion of a number of bioactive compounds from PCs/PGLs is rare and becomes extremely rare in malignant ones according to the literature. However, it could be overlooked and should always be considered, especially when patients present with unusual symptoms that cannot be totally attributed to catecholamine hypersecretion.

Author Contributions: Conceptualization, G.K. and A.A.; Methodology, E.K.; Software, A.A.; Validation E.K. and K.A.; Formal Analysis, A.A., Data Curation, A.A., K.A., A.B., F.R.F.; Writing—Original Draft Preparation, A.A., G.K., M.P., A.C., Writing—Review & Editing, A.A., E.K., G.K., M.P., A.C.

Funding: The authors declare no funding.

Conflicts of Interest: The authors declare no conflict of interest.

References

1. Lenders, J.; Eisenhofer, G.; Mannelli, M.; Pacak, K. Phaeochromocytoma. *Lancet* **2005**, *366*, 665–675. [CrossRef]
2. Chrisoulidou, A.; Kaltsas, G.; Ilias, I.; Grossman, A.B. The diagnosis and management of malignant phaeochromocytoma and paraganglioma. *Endocr. Relat. Cancer* **2007**, *14*, 569–585. [CrossRef]
3. International Agency for Research on Cancer (IRAC). *WHO Classification of Tumors of Endocrine Organs*; World Health Organization: Lyon, France, 2017.
4. Tischler, A.S.; de Krijger, R.R. Phaeochromocytoma. In *WHO Classification of Tumors of Endocrine Organs*, 4th ed.; Lloyd, R.V., Osamura, R.Y., Kloppel, G., Eds.; IARC Press: Lyons, France, 2017; pp. 183–189.
5. Ayala-Ramirez, M.; Feng, L.; Johnson, M.M.; Ejaz, S.; Habra, M.A.; Rich, T.; Busaidy, N.; Cote, G.J.; Perrier, N.; Phan, A.; et al. Clinical risk factors for malignancy and overall survival in patients with pheochromocytomas and sympathetic paragangliomas: Primary tumor size and primary tumor location as prognostic indicators. *J. Clin. Endocrinol. Metab.* **2011**, *96*, 717–725. [CrossRef]
6. Huang, K.H.; Chung, S.D.; Chen, S.C.; Chueh, S.C.; Pu, Y.S.; Lai, M.K.; Lin, W.C. Clinical and pathological data of 10 malignant pheochromocytomas: Long-term follow up in a single institute. *Int. J. Urol.* **2007**, *14*, 181–185. [CrossRef] [PubMed]
7. Prejbisz, A.; Lenders, J.W.; Eisenhofer, G.; Januszewicz, A. Mortality associated with phaeochromocytoma. *Horm. Metab. Res.* **2013**, *45*, 154–158. [CrossRef]

8. Amar, L.; Lussey-Lepoutre, C.; Lenders, J.W.; Djadi-Prat, J.; Plouin, P.F.; Steichen, O. Management of endocrine disease: Recurrence or new tumors after complete resection of pheochromocytomas and paragangliomas: A systematic review and meta-analysis. *Eur. J. Endocrinol.* **2016**, *175*, 135–145. [CrossRef]
9. Bravo, E.L.; Tagle, R. Pheochromocytoma: State-of-the-art and future prospects. *Endocr. Rev.* **2003**, *24*, 539–553. [CrossRef] [PubMed]
10. Kimura, N.; Takekoshi, K.; Naruse, M. Risk Stratification on Pheochromocytoma and Paraganglioma from Laboratory and Clinical Medicine. *J. Clin. Med.* **2018**, *7*, 242. [CrossRef]
11. Mlika, M.; Kourda, N.; Zorgati, M.M.; Bahri, S.; Ben Ammar, S.; Zermani, R. Prognostic value of Pheochromocytoma of the Adrenal Gland Scaled Score (Pass score) tests to separate benign from malignant neoplasms. *Tunis Med.* **2013**, *91*, 209–215. [PubMed]
12. Kim, K.Y.; Kim, J.H.; Hong, A.R.; Seong, M.W.; Lee, K.E.; Kim, S.J.; Kim, S.W.; Shin, C.S.; Kim, S.Y. Disentangling of malignancy from benign pheochromocytomas/paragangliomas. *PLoS ONE* **2016**, *11*, e0168413. [CrossRef] [PubMed]
13. Zelinka, T.; Musil, Z.; Dušková, J.; Burton, D.; Merino, M.J.; Milosevic, D.; Widimský, J.; Pacak, K. Metastatic pheochromocytoma: Does the size and age matter? *Eur. J. Clin. Investig.* **2011**, *41*, 1121–1128. [CrossRef] [PubMed]
14. Hamidi, O.; Young, W.F.; Iñiguez-Ariza, N.M.; Kittah, N.E.; Gruber, L.; Bancos, C.; Tamhane, S.; Bancos, I. Malignant Pheochromocytoma and Paraganglioma: 272 Patients Over 55 Years. *J. Clin. Endocrinol. Metab.* **2017**, *102*, 3296–3305. [CrossRef] [PubMed]
15. Van der Harst, E.; de Herder, W.W.; de Krijger, R.R.; Bruining, H.A.; Bonjer, H.J.; Lamberts, S.W.; van den Meiracker, A.H.; Stijnen, T.H.; Boomsma, F. The value of plasma markers for the clinical behaviour of phaeochromocytomas. *Eur. J. Endocrinol.* **2002**, *147*, 85–94. [CrossRef]
16. Plouin, P.F.; Chatellier, G.; Grouzmann, E.; Azizi, M.; Denolle, T.; Comoy, E.; Corvol, P. Plasma neuropeptide Y and catecholamine concentrations and urinary metanephrine excretion in patients with adrenal or ectopic phaeochromocytoma. *J. Hypertens.* **1991**, *9*, 272–273.
17. Toledo, R.; Jimenez, C. Recent advances in the management of malignant pheochromocytoma and paraganglioma: Focus on tyrosine kinase and hypoxia-inducible factor inhibitors. *F1000Res.* **2018**, *30*, 7. [CrossRef]
18. Hescot, S.; Leboulleux, S.; Amar, L.; Vezzosi, D.; Borget, I.; Bournaud-Salinas, C.; de la Fouchardiere, C.; Libé, R.; Do Cao, C.; Niccoli, P.; et al. French Group of Endocrine and Adrenal Tumors (Groupe des Tumeurs Endocrines-REseau NAtional des Tumeurs ENdocrines and COrtico-MEdullo Tumeurs Endocrines Networks Neuroendocrine Tumors. NCCN Guidelines. 2017. Available online: http://www.NCCN.org (accessed on 2 May 2019).
19. Mak, I.Y.F.; Hayes, A.R.; Khoo, B.; Grossman, A. Peptide Receptor Radionuclide Therapy as a Novel Treatment for Metastatic and Invasive Phaeochromocytoma and Paraganglioma. *Neuroendocrinology* **2019**, 12. [CrossRef]
20. McBride, J.F.; Atwell, T.D.; Charboneau, W.J.; Young, W.F.; Wass, T.C.; Callstrom, M.R. Minimally invasive treatment of metastatic pheochromocytoma and paraganglioma: Efficacy and safety of radiofrequency ablation and cryoablation therapy. *J. Vasc. Interv. Radiol.* **2011**, *22*, 1263–1270. [CrossRef]
21. Ballav, C.; Naziat, A.; Mihai, R.; Karavitaki, N.; Ansorge, O.; Grossman, A.B. Mini-review: Pheochromocytomas causing the ectopic ACTH syndrome. *Endocrine* **2012**, *42*, 69–73. [CrossRef]
22. Lois, K.B.; Santhakumar, A.; Vaikkakara, S.; Mathew, S.; Long, A.; Johnson, S.J.; Peaston, R.; Neely, R.D.G.; Richardson, D.L.; Graham, J.; et al. Phaeochromocytoma and ACTH-dependent cushing's syndrome: Tumor secretion can mimic pituitary cushing's disease. *Clin. Endocrinol. (Oxf.)* **2016**, *84*, 177–184. [CrossRef] [PubMed]
23. Araujo Castro, M.; Palacios García, N.; Aller Pardo, J.; Izquierdo Alvarez, C.; Armengod Grao, L.; Estrada García, J. Ectopic Cushing syndrome: Report of 9 cases. *Endocrinol. Diabetes Nutr.* **2018**, *65*, 255–264. [CrossRef] [PubMed]
24. Sakuma, I.; Higuchi, S.; Fujimoto, M.; Takiguchi, T.; Nakayama, A.; Tamura, A.; Kohno, T.; Komai, E.; Shiga, A.; Nagano, H.; et al. Cushing Sndrome Due to ACTH-Secreting Pheochromocytoma, Aggravated by Glucocorticoid-Driven Positive-Feedback Loop. *J. Clin. Endocrinol. Metab.* **2016**, *101*, 841–846. [CrossRef]
25. Kakudo, K.; Uematsu, K.; Matsuno, Y.; Mitsunobu, M.; Toyosaka, A.; Okamoto, E.; Fukuchi, M. Malignant pheochromocytoma with ACTH production. *Acta Pathol. Jpn.* **1984**, *34*, 1403–1410. [CrossRef] [PubMed]

26. Brenner, N.; Kopetschke, R.; Ventz, M.; Strasburger, C.J.; Quinkler, M.; Gerl, H. Cushing's syndrome due to ACTH-secreting pheochromocytoma. *Can. J. Urol.* **2008**, *15*, 3924–3927.
27. Otsuka, F.; Miyoshi, T.; Murakami, K.; Inagaki, K.; Takeda, M.; Ujike, K.; Ogura, T.; Omori, M.; Doihara, H.; Tanaka, Y.; et al. An extra-adrenal abdominal pheochromocytoma causing ectopic ACTH syndrome. *Am. J. Hypertens.* **2005**, *18*, 1364–1368. [CrossRef]
28. Beaser, R.S.; Guay, A.T.; Lee, A.K.; Silverman, M.L.; Flint, L.D. An adrenocorticotropic hormone-producing pheochromocytoma: Diagnostic and immunohistochemical studies. *J. Urol.* **1986**, *135*, 10–13. [CrossRef]
29. Chen, H.; Doppman, J.L.; Chrousos, G.P.; Norton, J.A.; Nieman, L.K.; Udelsman, R. Adrenocorticotropic hormone-secreting pheochromocytomas: The exception to the rule. *Surgery* **1995**, *118*, 988–994. [CrossRef]
30. Tutal, E.; Yılmazer, D.; Demirci, T.; Cakır, E.; Gültekin, S.S.; Celep, B.; Topaloğlu, O.; Çakal, E. A rare case of ectopic ACTH syndrome originating from malignant renal paraganglioma. *Arch. Endocrinol. Metab.* **2017**, *61*, 291–295. [CrossRef] [PubMed]
31. Apple, D.; Kreines, K. Cushing's syndrome due to ectopic ACTH production by a nasal paraganglioma. *Am. J. Med. Sci.* **1982**, *283*, 32–35. [CrossRef]
32. Dahir, K.M.; Gonzalez, A.; Revelo, M.P.; Ahmed, S.R.; Roberts, J.R.; Blevins, L.S., Jr. Ectopic adrenocorticotropic hormone hypersecretion due to a primary pulmonary paraganglioma. *Endocr. Pract.* **2004**, *10*, 424–428. [CrossRef] [PubMed]
33. Kirkby-Bott, J.; Brunaud, L.; Mathonet, M.; Hamoir, E.; Kraimps, J.L.; Trésallet, C.; Amar, L.; Rault, A.; Henry, J.F.; Carnaille, B. Ectopic hormone-secreting pheochromocytoma: A francophone observational study. *World J. Surg.* **2012**, *36*, 1382–1388. [CrossRef] [PubMed]
34. Alvarez, P.; Isidro, L.; González-Martín, M.; Loidi, L.; Arnal, F.; Cordido, F. Ectopic adrenocorticotropic hormone production by a noncatecholamine secreting pheochromocytoma. *J. Urol.* **2002**, *167*, 2514–2515. [CrossRef]
35. White, A.; Ray, D.W.; Talbot, A.; Abraham, P.; Thody, A.J.; Bevan, J.S. Cushing's syndrome due to phaeochromocytoma secreting the precursors of adrenocorticotropin. *J. Clin. Endocrinol. Metab.* **2000**, *85*, 4771–4775. [CrossRef]
36. Loh, K.C.; Gupta, R.; Shlossberg, A.H. Spontaneous remission of ectopic Cushing's syndrome due to pheochromocytoma: A case report. *Eur. J. Endocrinol.* **1996**, *135*, 440–443. [CrossRef]
37. Terzolo, M.; Alì, A.; Pia, A.; Bollito, E.; Reimondo, G.; Paccotti, P.; Scardapane, R.; Angeli, A. Cyclic Cushing's syndrome due to ectopic ACTH secretion by an adrenal pheochromocytoma. *J. Endocrinol. Investig.* **1994**, *17*, 869–874. [CrossRef]
38. Mendonça, B.B.; Arnhold, I.J.; Nicolau, W.; Avancini, V.A.; Boise, W. Cushing's syndrome due to ectopic ACTH secretion by bilateral pheochromocytomas in multiple endocrine neoplasia type 2A. *N. Engl. J. Med.* **1988**, *319*, 1610–1611.
39. Schroeder, J.O.; Asa, S.L.; Kovacs, K.; Killinger, D.; Hadley, G.L.; Volpé, R. Report of a case of pheochromocytoma producing immunoreactive ACTH and beta-endorphin. *J. Endocrinol. Investig.* **1984**, *7*, 117–121. [CrossRef]
40. Van Brummelen, P.; Van Hooff, J.P.; Van Seters, A.P.; Giard, R.W. Ectopic ACTH production by a functioning phaeochromocytoma. *Neth. J. Med.* **1982**, *25*, 237–241.
41. Spark, R.F.; Connolly, P.B.; Gluckin, D.S.; White, R.; Sacks, B.; Landsberg, L. ACTH secretion from a functioning pheochromocytoma. *N. Engl. J. Med.* **1979**, *301*, 416–418. [CrossRef]
42. Thomas, T.; Zender, S.; Terkamp, C.; Jaeckel, E.; Manns, M.P. Hypercortisolaemia due to ectopic adrenocorticotropic hormone secretion by a nasal paraganglioma: A case report and review of the literature. *BMC Res. Notes* **2013**, *19*, 331. [CrossRef]
43. Serra, F.; Duarte, S.; Abreu, S.; Marques, C.; Cassis, J.; Saraiva, M. Cushing's syndrome due to ectopic ACTH production by a nasal paraganglioma. *Endocrinol. Diabetes Metab. Case Rep.* **2013**, *2013*, 130038. [CrossRef]
44. Folkestad, L.; Andersen, M.S.; Nielsen, A.L.; Glintborg, D. A rare cause of Cushing's syndrome: An ACTH-secreting phaeochromocytoma. *BMJ Case Rep.* **2014**, *8*, 2014. [CrossRef] [PubMed]
45. Li, X.G.; Zhang, D.X.; Li, X.; Cui, X.G.; Xu, D.F.; Li, Y.; Gao, Y.; Yin, L.; Ren, J.Z. Adrenocorticotropic hormone-producing pheochromocytoma: A case report and review of the literature. *Chin. Med. J.* **2012**, *125*, 1193–1196.

46. Bernardi, S.; Grimaldi, F.; Finato, N.; De Marchi, S.; Proclemer, A.; Sabato, N.; Bertolotto, M.; Fabris, B. A pheochromocytoma with high adrenocorticotropic hormone and a silent lung nodule. *Am. J. Med. Sci.* **2011**, *342*, 429–432. [CrossRef] [PubMed]
47. Nijhoff, M.F.; Dekkers, O.M.; Vleming, L.J.; Smit, J.W.; Romijn, J.A.; Pereira, A.M. ACTH-producing pheochromocytoma: Clinical considerations and concise review of the literature. *Eur. J. Intern. Med.* **2009**, *20*, 682–685. [CrossRef] [PubMed]
48. Van Dam, P.S.; van Gils, A.; Canninga-van Dijk, M.R.; de Koning, E.J.; Hofland, L.J.; de Herder, W.W. Sequential ACTH and catecholamine secretion in a phaeochromocytoma. *Eur. J. Endocrinol.* **2002**, *147*, 201–206. [CrossRef] [PubMed]
49. Lieberum, B.; Jaspers, C.; Munzenmaier, R. ACTH-producing paraganglioma of the paranasal sinuses. *HNO* **2003**, *51*, 328–331. [CrossRef]
50. Forman, B.H.; Marban, E.; Kayne, R.D.; Passarelli, N.M.; Bobrow, S.N.; Livolsi, V.A.; Merino, M.; Minor, M.; Farber, L.R. Ectopic ACTH syndrome due to pheochromocytoma: Case report and review of the literature. *Yale J. Biol. Med.* **1979**, *52*, 181–189.
51. Inoue, M.; Okamura, K.; Kitaoka, C.; Kinoshita, F.; Namitome, R.; Nakamura, U.; Shiota, M.; Goto, K.; Ohtsubo, T.; Matsumura, K.; et al. Metyrapone-responsive ectopic ACTH-secreting pheochromocytoma with a vicious cycle via a glucocorticoid-driven positive-feedback mechanism. *Endocr. J.* **2018**, *65*, 755–767. [CrossRef]
52. Eng, P.H.K.; Tan, L.H.C.; Wong, K.S.; Cheng, C.W.; Fok, A.C.K.; Khoo, D.H.C. Cushing's syndrome in a patient with a corticotropin-releasing hormone-producing pheochromocytoma. *Endocr. Pr.* **1999**, *5*, 84–87.
53. Ruggeri, R.M.; Ferraù, F.; Campennì, A.; Simone, A.; Barresi, V.; Giuffrè, G.; Tuccari, G.; Baldari, S.T.F. Immunohistochemical localization and functional characterization of somatostatin receptor subtypes in a corticotropin releasing hormone- secreting adrenal phaeochromocytoma: Review of the literature and report of a case. *Eur. Histochem.* **2009**, *53*, 1–6. [CrossRef]
54. Bayraktar, F.; Kebapcilar, L.; Kocdor, M.A.; Asa, S.L.; Yesil, S.; Canda, S.; Demir, T.; Saklamaz, A.; Seçil, M.; Akinci, B.; et al. Cushing's syndrome due to ectopic CRH secretion by adrenal pheochromocytoma accompanied by renal infarction. *Exp. Clin. Endocrinol. Diabetes* **2006**, *114*, 444–447. [CrossRef] [PubMed]
55. Jessop, D.S.; Cunnah, D.; Millar, J.G.; Neville, E.; Coates, P.; Doniach, I.; Besser, G.M.R.L. A phaeochromocytoma presenting with Cushing's syndrome associated with increased concentrations of circulating corticotrophin-releasing factor. *J. Endocrinol.* **1987**, *113*, 133–138. [CrossRef] [PubMed]
56. O'Brien, T.; Young, W.F., Jr.; Davila, D.G.; Scheithauer, B.W.; Kovacs, K.; Horvath, E.; Vale, W.; van Heerden, J.A. Cushing's syndrome associated with ectopic production of corticotrophin-releasing hormone, corticotrophin and vasopressin by a phaeochromocytoma. *Clin. Endocrinol.* **1992**, *37*, 460–467. [CrossRef]
57. Iwayama, H.; Hirase, S.; Nomura, Y.; Ito, T.; Morita, H.; Otake, K.; Okumura, A.; Takagi, J. Spontaneous adrenocorticotropic hormone (ACTH) normalisation due to tumor regression induced by metyrapone in a patient with ectopic ACTH syndrome: Case report and literature review. *BMC Endocr. Disord.* **2018**, *18*, 19. [CrossRef] [PubMed]
58. Willenberg, H.S.; Feldkamp, J.; Lehmann, R.; Schott, M.; Goretzki, P.E.; Scherbaum, W.A. A case of catecholamine and glucocorticoid excess syndrome due to a corticotropin-secreting paraganglioma. *Ann. N. Y. Acad. Sci.* **2006**, *1073*, 52. [CrossRef] [PubMed]
59. Hashimoto, K.; Suemaru, S.; Hattori, T.; Sugawara, M.; Ota, Z.; Takata, S.; Hamaya, K.; Doi, K.; Chrétien, M. Multiple endocrine neoplasia with Cushing's syndrome due to paraganglioma producing corticotropin-releasing factor and adrenocorticotropin. *Acta Endocrinol. (Cph.)* **1986**, *113*, 189–195. [CrossRef]
60. Sackel, S.G.; Manson, J.E.; Harawi, S.J.; Burakoff, R. Watery diarrhea syndrome due to an adrenal pheochromocytoma secreting vasoactive intestinal polypeptide. *Dig. Dis. Sci.* **1985**, *30*, 1201–1207. [CrossRef] [PubMed]
61. Cooperman, A.M.; Desantis, D.; Winkelman, E.; Farmer, R.; Eversman, J.; Said, S. Watery diarrhea syndrome. Two unusual cases and further evidence that VIP is a humoral mediator. *Ann. Surg.* **1978**, *187*, 325–328. [CrossRef]
62. Herrera, M.F.; Stone, E.; Deitel, M.; Asa, S.L. Pheochromocytoma producing multiple vasoactive peptides. *Arch. Surg.* **1992**, *127*, 105–108. [CrossRef]
63. Stewart, A.F.; Hoecker, J.L.; Mallette, L.E.; Segre, G.V.; Amatruda, T.T., Jr.; Vignery, A. Hypercalcemia in pheochromocytoma. Evidence for a novel mechanism. *Ann. Intern. Med.* **1985**, *102*, 776–779. [CrossRef]

64. Suzuki, K.; Miyashita, A.; Inoue, Y.; Iki, S.; Enomoto, H.; Takahashi, Y.; Takemura, T. Interleukin-6-producing pheochromocytoma. *Acta Haematol.* **1991**, *85*, 217–219. [CrossRef]
65. Takagi, M.; Egawa, T.; Motomura, T.; Sakuma-Mochizuki, J.; Nishimoto, N.; Kasayama, S.; Hayashi, S.; Koga, M.; Yoshizaki, K.; Yoshioka, T.; et al. Interleukin-6 secreting phaeochromocytoma associated with clinical markers of inflammation. *Clin. Endocrinol. (Oxf.)* **1997**, *46*, 507–509. [CrossRef]
66. Shimizu, C.; Kubo, M.; Takano, K.; Takano, A.; Kijima, H.; Saji, H.; Katsuyama, I.; Sasano, H.; Koike, T. Interleukin-6 (IL-6) producing phaeochromocytoma: Direct IL-6 suppression by non-steroidal anti-inflammatory drugs. *Clin. Endocrinol. (Oxf.)* **2001**, *54*, 405–410. [CrossRef]
67. Tokuda, H.; Hosoi, T.; Hayasaka, K.; Okamura, K.; Yoshimi, N.; Kozawa, O. Overexpression of protein kinase C-delta plays a crucial role in interleukin-6-producing pheochromocytoma presenting with acute inflammatory syndrome: A case report. *Horm. Metab. Res.* **2009**, *41*, 333–338. [CrossRef]
68. Fukumoto, S.; Matsumoto, T.; Harada, S.; Fujisaki, J.; Kawano, M.; Ogata, E. Pheochromocytoma with pyrexia and marked inflammatory signs: A paraneoplastic syndrome with possible relation to interleukin-6 production. *J. Clin. Endocrinol. Metab.* **1991**, *73*, 877–881. [CrossRef]
69. Minetto, M.; Dovio, A.; Ventura, M.; Cappia, S.; Daffara, F.; Terzolo, M.; Angeli, A. Interleukin-6 producing pheochromocytoma presenting with acute inflammatory syndrome. *J. Endocrinol. Investig.* **2003**, *26*, 453–457. [CrossRef]
70. Kang, J.M.; Lee, W.J.; Kim, W.B.; Kim, T.Y.; Koh, J.M.; Hong, S.J.; Huh, J.R.J.Y.; Chi, H.S.; Kim, M.S. Systemic inflammatory syndrome and hepatic inflammatory cell infiltration caused by an interleukin-6 producing pheochromocytoma. *Endocr. J.* **2005**, *52*, 193–198. [CrossRef]
71. Salahuddin, A.; Rohr-Kirchgraber, T.; Shekar, R.; West, B.; Loewenstein, J. Interleukin-6 in the fever and multiorgan crisis of pheochromocytoma. *Scand. J. Infect. Dis.* **1997**, *29*, 640–642. [CrossRef]
72. Nagaishi, R.; Akehi, Y.; Ashida, K.; Higuchi-Tubouchi, K.; Yokoyama, H.; Nojiri, T.; Aoki, M.; Anzai, K.; Nabeshima, K.; Tanaka, M.; et al. Acute inflammatory syndrome and intrahepatic cholestasis caused by an interleukin-6-producing pheochromocytoma with pregnancy. *Fukuoka Igaku Zasshi* **2010**, *101*, 10–18.
73. Ciacciarelli, M.; Bellini, D.; Laghi, A.; Polidoro, A.; Pacelli, A.; Bottaccioli, A.G.; Palmaccio, G.; Stefanelli, F.; Clemenzi, P.; Carini, L.; et al. IL-6-Producing, Noncatecholamines Secreting Pheochromocytoma Presenting as Fever of Unknown Origin. *Case Rep. Med.* **2016**, *2016*, 3489046. [CrossRef]
74. Yarman, S.; Soyluk, O.; Altunoglu, E.; Tanakol, R. Interleukin-6-producing pheochromocytoma presenting with fever of unknown origin. *Clinics (Sao Paulo)* **2011**, *66*, 1843–1845. [CrossRef]
75. Omura, M.; Sato, T.; Cho, R.; Iizuka, T.; Fujiwara, T.; Okamoto, K.; Tashiro, Y.; Chiba, S.; Nishikawa, T. A patient with malignant paraganglioma that simultaneously produces adrenocorticotropic hormone and interleukin-6. *Cancer* **1994**, *74*, 1634–1639. [CrossRef]
76. Garbini, A.; Mainardi, M.; Grimi, M.; Repaci, G.; Nanni, G.; Bragherio, G. Pheochromocytoma and hypercalcemia due to ectopic production of parathyroid hormone. *N. Y. State J. Med.* **1986**, *86*, 25–27. [CrossRef]
77. Cheng, X.; Zhang, M.; Xiao, Y.; Li, H.; Zhang, Y.; Ji, Z. Interleukin-6-producing pheochromocytoma as a new reason for fever of unknown origin: A retrospective study. *Endocr. Pract.* **2018**, *24*, 507–511. [CrossRef]
78. Shanberg, A.M.; Baghdassarian, R.; Tansey, L.A.; Bacon, D.; Greenberg, P.; Perley, M. Pheochromocytoma with hypercalcemia: Case report and review of literature. *J. Urol.* **1985**, *133*, 258–259. [CrossRef]
79. Mune, T.; Katakami, H.; Kato, Y.; Yasuda, K.; Matsukura, S.; Miura, K. Production and secretion of parathyroid hormone-related protein in pheochromocytoma: Participation of an alpha-adrenergic mechanism. *J. Clin. Endocrinol. Metab.* **1993**, *76*, 757–762.
80. Bridgewater, J.A.; Ratcliffe, W.A.; Bundred, N.J.; Owens, C.W. Malignant phaeochromocytoma and hypercalcaemia. *Postgrad. Med. J.* **1993**, *69*, 77–79. [CrossRef]
81. Kimura, S.; Nishimura, Y.; Yamaguchi, K.; Nagasaki, K.; Shimada, K.; Uchida, H. A case of pheochromocytoma producing parathyroid hormone-related protein and presenting with hypercalcemia. *J. Clin. Endocrinol. Metab.* **1990**, *70*, 1559–15563. [CrossRef]
82. Fairhurst, B.J.; Shettar, S.P. Hypercalcaemia and phaeochromocytoma. *Postgrad. Med. J.* **1981**, *57*, 459–460. [CrossRef]
83. Kanamori, A.; Suzuki, S.; Suzuki, Y.; Abe, Y.; Takada, I.; Fujita, Y.; Yajima, Y.; Okabe, H.; Kameya, T.; Yamaguchi, K. A case of pheochromocytoma associated with hypercalcitoninemia and ectopic production of many peptide hormones. *Nippon Naika GakkaiZasshi* **1986**, *75*, 1610–1615. [CrossRef]

84. Heath, H., 3rd; Edis, A.J. Pheochromocytoma associated with hypercalcemia and ectopic secretion of calcitonin. *Ann. Intern. Med.* **1979**, *91*, 208–210. [CrossRef]
85. Kalager, T.; Glück, E.; Heimann, P.; Myking, O. Phaeochromocytoma with ectopic calcitonin production and parathyroid cyst. *Br. Med. J.* **1977**, *2*, 21. [CrossRef]
86. Vieira Neto, L.; Taboada, G.F.; Corrêa, L.L.; Polo, J.; Nascimento, A.F.; Chimelli, L.; Rumilla, K.; Gadelha, M.R. Acromegaly secondary to growth hormone-releasing hormone secreted by an incidentally discovered pheochromocytoma. *Endocr. Pathol.* **2007**, *18*, 46–52. [CrossRef]
87. Saito, H.; Sano, T.; Yamasaki, R.; Mitsuhashi, S.; Hosoi, E.; Saito, S. Demonstration of biological activity of a growth hormone-releasing hormone-like substance produced by a pheochromocytoma. *Acta Endocrinol. (Cph.)* **1993**, *129*, 246–250. [CrossRef]
88. Sano, T.; Saito, H.; Yamazaki, R.; Kameyama, K.; Ikeda, M.; Hosoi, E.; Hizawa, K.; Saito, S. Production of growth hormone-releasing factor in pheochromocytoma. *N. Engl. J. Med.* **1984**, *311*, 1520.
89. Roth, K.A.; Wilson, D.M.; Eberwine, J.; Dorin, R.I.; Kovacs, K.; Bensch, K.G.; Hoffman, A.R. Acromegaly and pheochromocytoma: A multiple endocrine syndrome caused by a plurihormonal adrenal medullary tumor. *J. Clin. Endocrinol. Metab.* **1986**, *63*, 1421–1426. [CrossRef]
90. Ghazi, A.A.; Amirbaigloo, A.; Dezfooli, A.A.; Saadat, N.; Ghazi, S.; Pourafkari, M.; Tirgari, F.; Dhall, D.; Bannykh, S.; Melmed, S.; et al. Ectopic acromegaly due to growth hormone releasing hormone. *Endocrine* **2013**, *43*, 293–302. [CrossRef]
91. Uysal, M.; Temiz, S.; Gul, N.; Yarman, S.; Tanakol, R.; Kapran, Y. Hypoglycemia due to ectopic release of insulin from a paraganglioma. *Horm. Res.* **2007**, *67*, 292–295. [CrossRef]
92. Hirai, H.; Midorikawa, S.; Suzuki, S.; Sasano, H.; Watanabe, T.; Satoh, H. Somatostatin-secreting Pheochromocytoma Mimicking Insulin-dependent Diabetes Mellitus. *Intern. Med.* **2016**, *55*, 2985–2991. [CrossRef]
93. Kaslow, A.M.; Riquier-Brison, A.; Peti-Peterdi, J.; Shillingford, N.; HaDuong, J.; Venkatramani, R.; Gayer, C.P. An ectopic renin-secreting adrenal corticoadenoma in a child with malignant hypertension. *Physiol. Rep.* **2016**, *4*, 5. [CrossRef]
94. Wang, F.; Tong, A.; Li, C.; Cui, Y.; Sun, J.; Song, A.; Li, Y. AZD8055 inhibits ACTH secretion in a case of bilateral ACTH-secreting pheochromocytoma. *Oncol. Lett.* **2018**, *16*, 4561–4566. [CrossRef]
95. Chung, C.H.; Wang, C.H.; Tzen, C.Y.; Liu, C.P. Intrahepatic cholestasis as a paraneoplastic syndrome associated with pheochromocytoma. *J. Endocrinol. Investig.* **2005**, *28*, 175–179. [CrossRef]
96. Bernini, M.; Bacca, A.; Casto, G.; Carli, V.; Cupisti, A.; Carrara, D.; Farnesi, I.; Barsotti, G.; Naccarato, A.G.; Bernini, G. A case of pheochromocytoma presenting as secondary hyperaldosteronism, hyperparathyroidism, diabetes and proteinuric renal disease. *Nephrol. Dial. Transplant.* **2011**, *26*, 1104–1107. [CrossRef]
97. Teno, S.; Tanabe, A.; Nomura, K.; Demura, H. Acutely exacerbated hypertension and increased inflammatory signs due to radiation treatment for metastatic pheochromocytoma. *Endocr. J.* **1996**, *43*, 511–516. [CrossRef]
98. Mutabagani, K.H.; Klopfenstein, K.J.; Hogan, M.J.; Caniano, D.A. Metastatic paraganglioma and paraneoplastic-induced anemia in an adolescent: Treatment with hepatic arterial chemoembolization. *J. Pediatr. Hematol. Oncol.* **1999**, *21*, 544–547. [CrossRef]
99. Cho, Y.Y.; Kwak, M.K.; Lee, S.E.; Ahn, S.H.; Kim, H.; Suh, S.; Kim, B.J.; Song, K.H.; Koh, J.M.; Kim, J.H.; et al. A clinical prediction model to estimate the metastatic potential of pheochromocytoma/paraganglioma: ASES score. *Surgery* **2018**, *164*, 511–517. [CrossRef]
100. Eisenhofer, G.; Tischler, A.; de Krijger, R.R. Diagnostic tests and biomarkers for pheochromocytoma and extra-adrenal paraganglioma: From routine laboratory methods to disease stratification. *Endocr. Pathol.* **2012**, *23*, 4–14. [CrossRef]
101. Maurice, J.B.; Troke, R.; Win, Z.; Ramachandran, R.; Al-Nahhas, A.; Naji, M.; Dhillo, W.; Meeran, K.; Goldstone, A.P.; Martin, N.M.; et al. A comparison of the performance of ^{68}Ga-DOTATATE PET/CT and ^{123}I-MIBG SPECT in the diagnosis and follow-up phaeochromocytoma and paraganglioma. *Eur. J. Nucl. Med. Mol. Imaging* **2012**, *39*, 1266–1270. [CrossRef]
102. Tan, T.H.; Hussein, Z.; Saad, F.F.; Shuaib, I.L. Diagnostic Performance of (68)Ga-DOTATATE PET/CT, (18)F-FDG PET/CT and (131)I-MIBG Scintigraphy in Mapping Metastatic Pheochromocytoma and Paraganglioma. *Nucl. Med. Mol. Imaging* **2015**, *49*, 143–151. [CrossRef]

103. Mundschenk, J.; Unger, N.; Schulz, S.; Höllt, V.; Schulz, S.; Steinke, R.; Lehnert, H. Somatostatin receptor subtypes in human pheochromocytoma: Subcellular expression pattern and functional relevance for octreotide scintigraphy. *J. Clin. Endocrinol. Metab.* **2003**, *88*, 5150–5157. [CrossRef]
104. Niemeijer, N.D.; Alblas, G.; van Hulsteijn, L.T.; Dekkers, O.M.; Corssmit, E.P. Chemotherapy with cyclophosphamide, vincristine and dacarbazine for malignant paraganglioma and pheochromocytoma: Systematic review and meta-analysis. *Clin. Endocrinol. (Oxf.)* **2014**, *81*, 642–651. [CrossRef]
105. Van Hulsteijn, L.T.; Niemeijer, N.D.; Dekkers, O.M.; Corssmit, E.P. (131)I-MIBG therapy for malignant paraganglioma and phaeochromocytoma: Systematic review and meta-analysis. *Clin. Endocrinol. (Oxf.)* **2014**, *80*, 487–501. [CrossRef] [PubMed]
106. Ayala-Ramirez, M.; Feng, L.; Habra, M.A.; Rich, T.; Dickson, P.V.; Perrier, N.; Phan, A.; Waguespack, S.; Patel, S.; Jimenez, C. Clinical benefits of systemic chemotherapy for patients with metastatic pheochromocytomas or sympathetic extra-adrenal paragangliomas: Insights from the largest single-institutional experience. *Cancer* **2012**, *118*, 2804–28012. [CrossRef] [PubMed]
107. Jawed, I.; Velarde, M.; Därr, R.; Wolf, K.I.; Adams, K.; Venkatesan, A.M.; Balasubramaniam, S.; Poruchynsky, M.S.; Reynolds, J.C.; Pacak, K.; et al. Continued Tumor Reduction of Metastatic Pheochromocytoma/Paraganglioma Harboring Succinate Dehydrogenase Subunit B Mutations with Cyclical Chemotherapy. *Cell Mol. Neurobiol.* **2018**, *38*, 1099–1106. [CrossRef] [PubMed]
108. Forrer, F.; Riedweg, I.; Maecke, H.R.; Mueller-Brand, J. Radiolabeled DOTATOC in patients with advanced paraganglioma and pheochromocytoma. *Q. J. Nucl. Med. Mol. Imaging* **2008**, *52*, 334–340.
109. Van Essen, M.; Krenning, E.P.; Kooij, P.P.; Bakker, W.H.; Feelders, R.A.; de Herder, W.W.; Wolbers, J.G.; Kwekkeboom, D.J. Effects of therapy with [177Lu-DOTA, Tyr3]octreotate in patients with paraganglioma, meningioma, small cell lung carcinoma, and melanoma. *J. Nucl. Med.* **2006**, *47*, 1599–1606. [PubMed]
110. Nastos, K.; Cheung, V.T.F.; Toumpanakis, C.; Navalkissoor, S.; Quigley, A.M.; Caplin, M.; Khoo, B. Peptide Receptor Radionuclide Treatment and (131)I-MIBG in the management of patients with metastatic/progressive phaeochromocytomas and paragangliomas. *J. Surg. Oncol.* **2017**, *115*, 425–434. [CrossRef] [PubMed]
111. Kong, G.; Grozinsky-Glasberg, S.; Hofman, M.S.; Callahan, J.; Meirovitz, A.; Maimon, O.; Pattison, D.A.; Gross, D.J.; Hicks, R.J. Efficacy of Peptide Receptor Radionuclide Therapy for Functional Metastatic Paraganglioma and Pheochromocytoma. *J. Clin. Endocrinol. Metab.* **2017**, *102*, 3278–3287. [CrossRef]

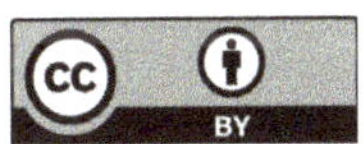

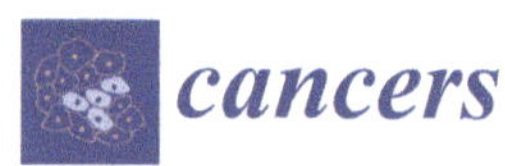
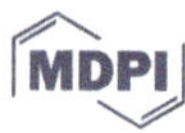

Article

Favorable Outcome in Patients with Pheochromocytoma and Paraganglioma Treated with ^{177}Lu-DOTATATE

Achyut Ram Vyakaranam [1,*], Joakim Crona [2], Olov Norlén [3], Dan Granberg [2], Ulrike Garske-Román [1,4], Mattias Sandström [1], Katarzyna Fröss-Baron [2], Espen Thiis-Evensen [5], Per Hellman [3] and Anders Sundin [1]

1 Section of Radiology, Molecular Imaging, Department of Surgical Sciences, Uppsala University, Akademiska Sjukhuset, SE-751 85 Uppsala, Sweden
2 Department of Medical Sciences, Uppsala University, Uppsala University Hospital, SE-751 85 Uppsala, Sweden
3 Section of Endocrine Surgery, Department of Surgical Sciences, Uppsala University, Uppsala University Hospital, SE-751 85 Uppsala, Sweden
4 Department of Nuclear Medicine, Sahlgrenska University Hospital, SE-413 45 Gothenburg, Sweden
5 Department of Gastroenterology, Oslo University Hospital, Rikshospitalet, 0372 Oslo, Norway
* Correspondence: achyutram.vyakaranam@surgsci.uu.se

Received: 10 June 2019; Accepted: 26 June 2019; Published: 28 June 2019

Abstract: Peptide receptor radiotherapy (PRRT) with ^{177}Lu-DOTATATE has emerged as a promising therapy for neuroendocrine tumors (NETs). This retrospective cohort study aimed to assess the outcome of PRRT for 22 patients with histopathologically confirmed pheochromocytoma (PCC) and paraganglioma (PGL), of which two were localized and 20 metastatic. Radiological response utilized response evaluation criteria in solid tumors 1.1 and toxicity was graded according to common terminology criteria for adverse events version 4. Median 4 (range 3–11) 7.4 GBq cycles of ^{177}Lu-DOTATATE were administered as first-line therapy (n = 13) or because of progressive disease (n = 9). Partial response (PR) was achieved in two and stable disease (SD) in 20 patients. The median overall survival (OS) was 49.6 (range 8.2–139) months and median progression-free survival (PFS) was 21.6 (range 6.7–138) months. Scintigraphic response >50% was achieved in 9/19 (47%) patients. Biochemical response (>50% decrease) of chromogranin A was found in 6/15 (40%) patients and of catecholamines in 3/12 (25%) patients. Subgroup analysis showed Ki-67 <15% associated with longer OS (p = 0.013) and PFS (p = 0.005). PRRT as first-line therapy was associated with increased OS (p = 0.041). No hematological or kidney toxicity grade 3–4 was registered. ^{177}Lu-DOTATATE therapy was associated with favorable outcome and low toxicity. High Ki-67 (≥15%) and PRRT received because of progression on previous therapy could constitute negative predictive factors for OS.

Keywords: pheochromocytoma; paraganglioma; ^{177}Lu-DOTATATE; peptide receptor radiotherapy; PRRT; neuroendocrine tumor; NET; PCC; PGL

---

1. Introduction

Pheochromocytomas (PCCs) and paragangliomas (PGLs) are rare tumors arising from enterochromaffin cells in adrenal medulla and autonomous ganglia [1]. Up to 70% of PCC and PGL have either germ line or somatic mutations in established disease-driver genes [2,3]. The five-year overall survival (OS) rate of patients with metastatic tumors ranges from 40 to 77% [4]. Surgery is the preferred therapy and may cure or allow a long-term remission in patients with resectable disease [5]. The oncologic treatment arsenal consists of local and systemic radiotherapy as well as systemic chemotherapy; the most commonly used systemic treatment is iodine-131-labeled meta-iodo-benzyl-guanidine (^{131}I-MIBG) followed by chemotherapy with cyclophosphamide, vincristine, and dacarbazine [6–8].

In neuroendocrine tumors (NETs), peptide receptor radiotherapy (PRRT) with lutetium-177 (^{177}Lu)- and yttrium-90 (^{90}Y)-labeled somatostatin analogs, such as tyrosine octreotide (TOC) and octreotate (TATE), has become frequently used. Predominantly, ^{177}Lu-DOTATATE has been utilized, but also ^{90}Y-DOTATOC, with favorable results in NETs [9–11]. Furthermore, encouraging results of PRRT have been shown in small cohorts of PCC/PGL patients treated with ^{90}Y- DOTATOC [9,12] and with ^{177}Lu-DOTATATE [13–16]. In one study, 20 patients received ^{177}Lu-DOTATATE, of whom nine also underwent concomitant chemotherapy with fluorouracil as a radiosensitizer, which in 14 evaluable patients (RECIST 1.1) resulted in disease control ((partial response (PR) + stable disease (SD)) in 12/14 (86%) patients with 39 months median OS [14]. In a second study, ^{177}Lu-DOTATATE was combined with capecitabine in 25 patients and in 21 evaluable patients achieving disease control, that is, 21/25 (84%) patients, with median 32 months PFS [15]. A third larger ^{177}Lu-DOTATATE study included 12 PCC/PGL patients, of whom eight were evaluable (RECIST 1.1) showing disease control (PR + SD) in 6/8 (75%) with 52 months estimated mean OS [16]. ^{90}Y-DOTATOC was administered to 28 PCC/PGL patients with disease control (PR + SD) in 71% [12] and in 11 PCC and 28 PGL patients, who were included in a larger PRRT study, radiological response was achieved in 4/11 (36%) of PCC and 3/28 (11%) of PGL patients with mean 32 and 82 months OS, respectively [9].

In our center, we have performed PRRT with ^{177}Lu-DOTATATE since 2005, initially applying the treatment protocol developed by the Rotterdam group [10], administering 4 cycles of 7.4 GBq ^{177}Lu-DOTATATE (maximum activity 29.6 GBq). By developing a method for normal organ dosimetry, based on uptake measurements on single photon emission computed tomography/computed tomography (SPECT/CT) performed during PRRT, we were able to more accurately estimate the absorbed radiation doses to the kidneys and bone marrow [17,18]. Since 2007, we have therefore instead applied a dosimetry-guided protocol by which PRRT may be individualized for each patient in order to administer as many cycles as possible until reaching 23 Gy absorbed dose to the kidneys or 2 Gy to bone marrow [17,18].

So far, we have treated approximately 800 patients with various NET types. In a prospective study including 200 of these patients with mixed NET types who underwent dosimetry-guided PRRT, because of disease progression or as first-line therapy, tumor response was achieved in 24% and disease control (complete response (CR) + PR + SD) in 96% with 27 months median progression-free survival in all patients, 33 months in those in whom the absorbed dose to the kidneys reached 23 Gy and 15 months in those in whom it did not [19]. In the present study, we retrospectively describe the outcome from treatment with ^{177}Lu-DOTATATE in a relatively large group of patients with PCC/PGL.

2. Results

Twenty-two patients with PCC and PGL undergoing ^{177}Lu-DOTATATE between 2005 and 2018 were identified and included in the study.

2.1. Baseline Patient Characteristics

Baseline patient characteristics are shown in Table 1. There were 22 patients (13 men / 9 women) median age 60 years (range 24–80) at the start of therapy, nine had pheochromocytoma and 13 harbored paraganglioma. Ki-67 index was available for 18 patients and the median result was 11% (range 1–30). Except for PCCs (n = 9), the primary tumor localization for the PGLs was retroperitoneum (n = 7), neck (n = 2), and one PGL each in the liver, kidney, urinary bladder, and cauda equina. All tumors except the two PGLs in the neck were metastatic, predominantly to regional retroperitoneal lymph nodes and with distant metastases to bone and liver.

Table 1. Baseline patient characteristics.

Pat. No.	Age at PRRT Start	Sex	Tumor Type	Primary Tumor Localization	Ki-67 Index	Genotype	Indication for PRRT	Metastases	Previous Therapy			
									Surgery	RT	^{131}I-MIBG	ChT
1	61	F	PGL	Retroperitoneum	5%	*SDHB*	Sympt	Retroper lgll, Liver, Bone	+	+	-	-
2	33	F	PGL	Urinary bladder	10%	*SDHD*	NA	Mediast lgll, Neck, Heart	+	-	-	-
3	24	M	PGL	Retroperitoneum	<2%	Sporadic	Sympt	Retroper lgll, Bone	+	+	+	-
4	67	M	PGL	Aortic bifurcation	15%	*SDHB*	PD	Bone	-	+	+	-
5	53	F	PCC		2%	Sporadic	Sympt	Liver	+	-	-	-
6	25	M	PGL	Retroperitoneum	NA, 4/10HPF	NA	PD	Bone	+	+	-	+
7	56	M	PCC		12%	NA	PD	Retroper lgll, Bone	+	+	-	-
8	71	F	PGL	Liver	25%	Sporadic	NA	Bone	+	-	-	-
9	70	F	PGL	Kidney	20%	NA	PD	Bone	+	+	+	-
10	25	M	PGL	Retroperitoneum	25%	*SDHB*	NA	Liver, Bone, Lung	-	-	-	-
11	56	F	PCC		30%	*NF1*	PD	Liver, Bone	+	-	-	-
12	59	F	PGL	Retroperitoneum	NA	NA	PD	Bone, Mediastinal lgll	+	+	+	-
13	55	M	PCC		22%	NA	Sympt	Bone	-	+	-	-
14	65	F	PGL	Cauda equina	13%	Sporadic	PD	0	+	+	-	-
15	62	M	PCC		<1%	NA	Sympt	Liver, Bone, Lung	+	+	-	-
16	67	M	PGL	Aortic bifurcation	5%	NA	PD	Liver, Bone	+	-	-	-
17	80	M	PCC		<1%	*SDHA*	Sympt	Retroper lgll. Liver, Lung, Bone	+	-	+	-
18	39	F	PCC		3%	*SDHB*	NA	Retroper and mediastinal lgll, Lung	-	+	-	-
19	72	M	PCC		1%	NA	NA	Liver, Bone	+	-	-	-
20	63	M	HNPGL	Bilateral neck	NA	*SDHD*	Sympt	0	-	+	-	-
21	79	M	PCC		NA	*NF1*	PD	Bone	+	+	+	-
22	31	M	HNPGL	Bilateral neck	NA	NA	Sympt	Liver, Bone	-	+	-	-

F, female; M, male; PCC, pheochromocytoma; PGL, paraganglioma; HNPGL, head and neck paraganglioma; NA, not available; Sympt, symptomatic; Retroper lgll, Retroperitoneal lymph node metastases; Mediast lgll, Mediastinal lymph node metastases: RT, Radiotherapy; ChT, Chemotherapy.

Genetic syndromes were identified based on information from diagnostic DNA sequencing and interpretation available in the medical records. A diagnosis of neurofibromatosis type 1 was also considered from clinical criteria. Nine patients had a genetic syndrome, *SDHB* or *SDHD*-related PGL in seven, neurofibromatosis type 1 in two, four patients were classified as sporadic cases, and genetic testing had not been performed in nine patients. At baseline, chromogranin A was elevated in 15 patients, normal in four, and missing in three patients. Plasma/Urinary (P/U)-catecholamines and their metabolites were normal in 10 patients and elevated in 12. In these 12 patients, normetanephrine was elevated in all, metanephrines in two patients, and methoxytyramine in four. Ten patients experienced catecholamine-related symptoms, which for two patients worsened during PRRT. The patients underwent PRRT because of tumor progression on previous therapies (n = 9) or as first-line treatment (n = 13). First-line therapy, in eight patients, was administered because of symptomatic disease and for five patients the indication for treatment was not documented in the patient records. The primary tumor was unresectable in three patients because of proximity to vital structures and in three patients due to tumor size (Table 1). Seven patients were previously included in a prospective dosimetry-tailored PRRT study of 200 patients [19]. Eight patients were alive, 11 were deceased, and three patients were lost to follow-up.

2.2. *Treatment and Toxicity*

The PRRT data and registered toxicity are shown in Table 2. Dosimetry-tailored PRRT was performed in 19/22 patients and the first 3/22 patients received PRRT according to a standard four-cycle protocol. The patients received between 3 and 8 cycles of ^{177}Lu-DOTATATE during their first treatment. Upon progression, five patients received salvage therapy with another 2 to 4 cycles. Including salvage therapy, between 3 and 11 cycles were administered. Five patients received 3 cycles, seven patients received 4 cycles, five patients 5 cycles, two patients 2, and one patient each received 7, 10, and 11 cycles, respectively. The median amount of ^{177}Lu-DOTATATE activity per cycle was 7.4 GBq and the median total administered activity (including salvage therapy) was 29.6 (range 22.2–81.4) GBq. The reasons to stop PRRT were 23 Gy dose to the kidneys reached (n = 17), use of a four-cycle PRRT protocol (n = 3), and progressive disease (n = 2). Hematological side effects occurred in 16/22 (73%) patients, all classified as grades 1 (n = 10) or 2 (n = 6) (Table 3). No kidney toxicity was observed.

2.3. *Therapy Outcome and Response Assessment*

Median follow-up time was 32 (range 8–139) months. Median overall survival (OS) was 49.6 (range 8.2–139) months (Figure 1A) and median PFS was 21.6 (range 6.7–138) months (Figure 1B). Response rates are summarized in Table 3. The median best response on CT according to RECIST 1.1 (%) across the cohort was −10% (range 0 to −65%). The time to best response was median 14.4 months (range 4.7 to 128 months). Best response was partial response (PR) in two patients and the remaining 20 patients reached stable disease (SD), whereas no complete response (CR) was found.

Table 2. Number of administered ^{177}Lu-DOTATATE cycles and hematological toxicity.

Patient No.	No. PRRT Cycles First Treatment	No. PRRT Cycles Salvage Treatment	No. PRRT Cycles in Total	Hematological Toxicity		
				Trbc Toxicity Grade	RBC Toxicity Grade	WBC Toxicity Grade
1	3		3	0	1	1
2	4		4	0	0	0
3	4		4	0	2	0
4	4		4	0	0	0
5	4	3	7	0	0	2
6	4		4	0	0	0
7	6	4	10	0	1	0
8	4		4	0	0	2
9	3		3	0	0	0
10	8	3	11	0	0	2
11	3		3	1	1	0
12	5		5	0	2	0
13	6		6	0	1	0
14	3	2	5	0	2	0
15	4		4	0	0	0
16	5		4	0	0	0
17	5		4	0	1	0
18	4	2	6	0	1	0
19	3		3	1	0	1
20	5		5	0	1	0
21	3		3	0	1	0
22	4		4	0	1	1
Sum	94	14	108	$n = 2$ grade 1	$n = 9$ grade 1 $n = 3$ grade 2	$n = 3$ grade 1 $n = 3$ grade 2

PRRT, peptide receptor radiotherapy; Trbc, thrombocytes; RBC, red blood cell; WBC, white blood cell.

Table 3. Response rates for peptide receptor radiotherapy (PRRT) with ^{177}Lu-DOTATATE in 22 patients with pheochromocytoma or paraganglioma (PCC/PGL).

Patient No.	NM Response ≥50%	Best Response RECIST 1.1 (%)	Best Response RECIST 1.1 (Category)	Time to BR RECIST 1.1 (Months)	OS (Months)	PFS (Months)	Catecholamine Response	CgA Response
1	NA	−17	SD	6.7	86.8	6.7	−48% *	NA
2	NA	0	SD	128.4	138.2	138.2	Normal	Normal
3	NA	0	SD	45.2	139.2	53	−43% *	−61
4	Yes	−13	SD	4.7	8.2	8.2	Normal	−21
5	Yes	−18	SD	15.2	109.4	22.5	−28%	−35
6	No	0	SD	6.5	21.6	21.6	Normal	Normal
7	Yes	−2	SD	15.0	49.6	27	−38% *	−5
8	Yes	0	SD	12.0	37.3	16.7	Normal	−51
9	No	−14	SD	11.3	19.2	5.6	−14%	164
10	No	−29	SD	13.8	54.1	18.8	Normal	−85
11	No	−15	SD	9.8	16.5	11.8	Normal	NA
12	Yes	−65	PR	10.5	15.6	14.6	−81%	−15
13	No	−6	SD	15.6	18.8	18.3	−43%	−52
14	Yes	−18	SD	15.0	41.3	38.9	Normal	Normal
15	Yes	−50	PR	9.5	14	12.7	−29%	−6
16	Yes	−6	SD	15.8	55.6	39.1	315%	138
17	No	−7	SD	20.0	45.4	28	−53%	−56
18	No	0	SD	8.2	26.4	26.4	Normal	−14
19	Yes	0	SD	32.8	46.2	38.8	−13%	−55
20	No	−7	SD	15.5	15.6	15.6	Normal	Normal
21	No	−15	SD	16.4	24.9	22.3	−89% *	−1
22	No	−15	SD	8.6	11.9	8.6	Normal	Normal

NM response, response on scintigraphy during PRRT; NA, not available; PR, partial response; SD, stable disease; PD, progressive disease; BR, best response; OS, overall survival; PFS, progression-free survival; CgA, chromogranin A; Normal, within or not higher than 10% above the upper reference value. Catecholamines were measured in plasma except *, in urine.

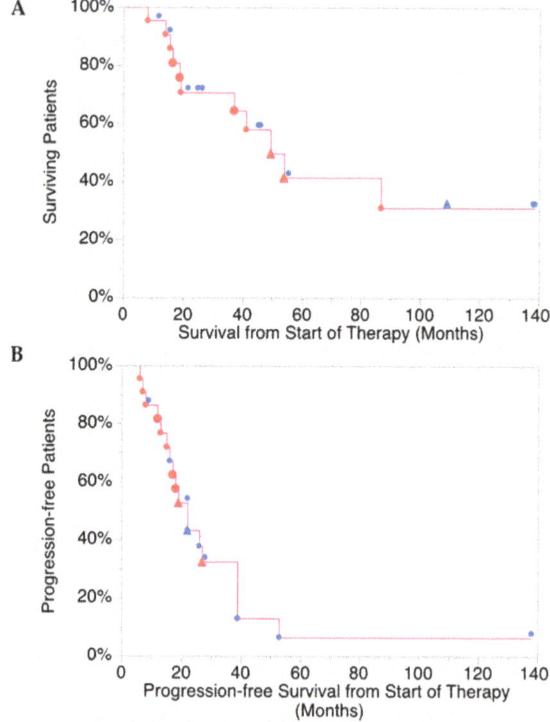

Figure 1. (**A**) Kaplan–Meier analysis of overall survival, median 49.6 (range 8.2–139) months and (**B**) progression-free survival, median 21.6 (range 6.7–138) months. Blue symbols, patient alive; red symbols, patient deceased. Triangles, patient received salvage therapy.

In the 9 patients who were progressive at PRRT start, 1 achieved PR and 8 SD with response according to RECIST1.1 median −14% (range −56 to 0%), as compared to 13 patients who received PRRT as first-line therapy of whom 12 achieved SD and 1 PR with RECIST1.1 response median −16% (range −50 to 0%).

Response on ^{177}Lu-DOTATATE-SPECT/CT and whole-body scans was seen in 14/19 (74%) patients and the visually rated decrease in tumor accumulation, as compared to scintigraphy during the first cycle, was median 50% (range 20–65%), resulting in a response rate PR in nine (47%), SD in eight (42%) and progressive disease (PD) in two (11%) patients.

The biochemical response data are shown in Table 3. P/U-catecholamines were available for all patients and were normal in 10/22 (45%). Catecholamine response with >50% reduction was found in 3/12 evaluable patients (25%), >25–50% decrease in 6/12 (50%), >0–25% reduction in 2/12 (17%), and biochemical progression in 1/12 (8%). The biochemical response was consistent with the morphological response rate on computed tomography or magnetic resonance imaging (CT/MRI) (RECIST 1.1), except in one radiologically stable patient who showed biochemical progression and in one patient with partial remission in whom the P/U-catecholamines showed a mere 29% decrease.

Chromogranin A was normal in 5/20 (25%) patients and not available in 2 patients. Biochemical response with >50% reduction of chromogranin A was achieved in 6/15 evaluable patients (40%), >25–50% decrease in 1/15 (7%), >0–25% reduction in 6/15 (40%), and biochemical progression was found in 2 patients (13%). The biochemical response was consistent with the morphological response rate on CT/MRI (RECIST 1.1), except in two radiologically stable patients who showed biochemical progression.

A conflicting biochemical result was found in only one patient with a clear increase of chromogranin A, whereas the catecholamines decreased somewhat in this radiologically stable patient. Of 10 patients with catecholamine-related symptoms during PRRT, these symptoms worsened in 2 patients, improved in 4, and were stable in 4.

The results of two patients with non-metastatic HNPGLs (Nos. 20 and 22, Table 1) were analyzed separately. They did not undergo primary tumor resection because of their tumor's size and proximity to vital organs/tissue but, previous to PRRT, they had received external radiation radiotherapy. Patient 20 had an SDHD mutation, whereas the other patient was not tested for a genetic profile. Both patients received PRRT as first-line therapy with 4 and 5 cycles, respectively, and achieved −17% and −15% tumor decrease according to RECIST 1.1, resulting in stable disease and 15.6 and 8.6 months PFS and 15.6 and 11.9 months OS, respectively.

2.4. Predictors of Outcome

An arbitrary threshold of Ki-67 index 15% was selected as a cut-off. Ki-67 <15% compared to Ki-67 ≥15% ($p = 0.013$) and PRRT received as first-line therapy compared to PPRT received because of tumor progression ($p = 0.041$) were associated with longer OS (Figure 2A,B). Tumor type (PCC or PGL), visual response on scintigraphy (≥50%), biochemical response, number of cycles, administered activity, and previous therapies (surgery, radiotherapy, chemotherapy, ^{131}I-MIBG) were factors unrelated to OS. The genetic profile, available for only 15/22 patients, did not allow for analysis as possible predictors of survival.

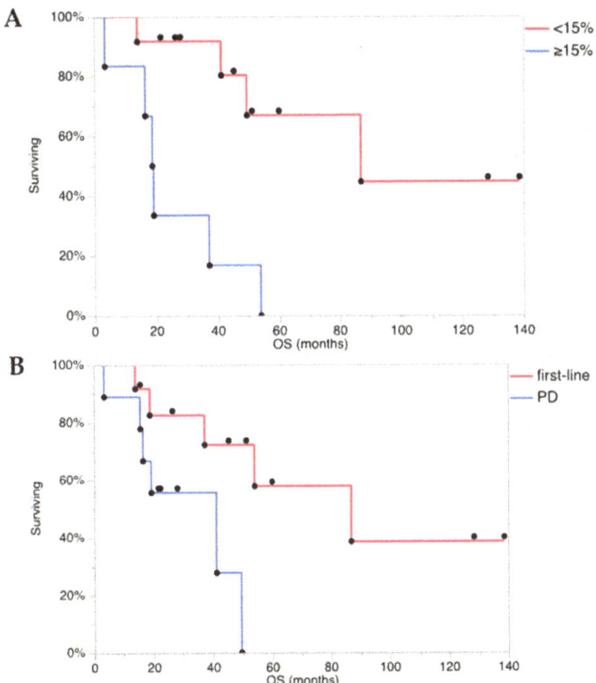

Figure 2. (**A**) Ki-67 index <15% in the Kaplan–Meier analysis was found as a positive predictive factor for OS (Log rank test $p = 0.013$). Out of 18 analyzed patients, 6 had Ki-67 index ≥15% and 12 <15%. Seven patients received PRRT as first-line therapy and 11 because of progressive disease. (**B**) In addition, PRRT administered as first-line treatment, and not because of progressive disease (PD), was found as a positive predictive factor for OS (Log rank test $p = 0.41$). All 22 patients were analyzed and PRRT was administered as first-line therapy in 13 patients and because of progressive disease in 9.

Ki-67 <15% (p = 0.005) was associated with longer PFS, whereas PRRT received as first-line therapy, tumor type, visual response on scintigraphy (≥50%), biochemical response, number of cycles, administered activity, and previous therapies (surgery, radiotherapy, chemotherapy, ^{131}I-MIBG) were all factors unrelated to PFS.

3. Discussion

We studied the outcome after ^{177}Lu-DOTATATE administration in 22 patients with PCC and PGL. Consistent with the results in several reports on PRRT with ^{177}Lu-DOTATATE in gastro-entero-pancreatic NETs and lung NETs, the outcome in our patients with PCC and PGL was favorable with disease stabilization in 20 patients and PR in 2 subjects. We observed a median OS of 49.6 (range 8.2–139) months and a median PFS of 21.6 (range 6.7–138) months. Corresponding to two recently published ^{177}Lu-DOTATATE studies in small groups of PCC/PGL patients, we had similar duration of follow-up, median 32 (8–139) months, in comparison to the publication by Kong et al. [14] reporting 28 (range 5–74) months follow-up for 14 patients and Yadav et al. [15] who followed 25 patients median 30 (15–96) months after PRRT combined with 1250 mg/m^2 capecitabine (days 0 to 14 of each cycle). Our follow-up, however, allowed for the calculation of OS, whereas median OS was not reached in the other studies [14,15].

The median PFS 39 months, in the study by Kong et al. and 32 months PFS reported by Yadav et al. were both, however, longer than in the present study (21.6 months). Disease control (PR + SD) according to RECIST 1.1. was achieved in all of our patients as compared to 21/25 (84%) patients and 12/14 (86%) in the two previous reports [14,15], and notably, 11 of our patients were still alive at the time of evaluation. Four of our patients were progression-free between 9 and 138 months. Another ^{177}Lu-DOTATATE study, including 12 PGL patients during a median 13 (range 4–30) months follow-up, achieved SD in five and PD in four of nine evaluable patients [13]. In a larger ^{177}Lu-DOTATATE therapy study, on mainly high grade (G3) gastroenteropancreatic and lung NETs, 12 patients with PCC/PGL were included of whom eight were evaluable [16]. PRRT resulted in four PR, two SD, and two PD, but in this study the survival data were instead reported as estimated mean OS 51.8 (95% CI 39.8–63.8) months and PFS 31.4 (95% CI 20.3–42.4) months, outcomes which however are difficult to compare to the present results.

A problem potential with utilizing ^{90}Y-DOTATOC is the toxicity, as in the study by Imhof et al. [9], who reported transient grade 3–4 myelosuppression in 142/1109 (13%) patients, but in particular kidney toxicity, with severe permanent renal impairment in 102/1109 (9%) patients. Interestingly, no hematological and kidney toxicity greater than grade 1 was experienced by Forrer et al. in 28 patients with surgical incurable PCC/PGL who underwent PRRT with ^{90}Y-DOTATOC [12]. With ^{177}Lu-DOTATATE, we experienced no kidney toxicity and only grade 1 (n = 10) and 2 (n = 6) hematological toxicity. Similarly, Yadav et al., who combined ^{177}Lu-DOTATATE with capecitabine, reported 3/25 (12%) patients who developed grade 1 lymphopenia, but no other hematological toxicity, and no kidney toxicity [15]. Additionally, Kong et al., who in half of their patients combined ^{177}Lu-DOTATATE with fluorouracil, reported mainly grade 2 lymphopenia. However, they also experienced 4/20 (20%) patients with grade 3 lymphopenia. Renal impairment in two of their patients was considered attributed to underlying disease processes [14]. In the larger study by Demirci et al., in 186 patients with mixed NET types, toxicity data for the subgroup of 12 patients with PCC/PGL are not reported. Grade 1 or 2 hematological toxicity was however found in 148/186 (80%) of patients but also 2 (1%) with grade 3 toxicity [16]. No severe kidney toxicity was noted.

The fact that the first three patients were treated according to the original Rotterdam protocol, with four PRRT cycles, and that the remaining patients were instead subjected to a change in protocol where the number of cycles were based on dosimetry, leads to a large variation in the number of administered PRRT cycles and the present results must be interpreted accordingly.

The biochemical responses, regarding chromogranin A and catecholamines, were consistent in all evaluable patients except one in whom a clear increase of chromogranin A was found, whereas the catecholamines decreased somewhat in this radiologically stable patient. Chromogranin A response differed slightly from that of the morphological response rate according to RECIST 1.1. (CT/MRI). Thus, biochemistry indicated PD in two patients with SD on CT/MRI but, in the remaining patients, the biochemical and morphological responses were in agreement. Similarly, the catecholamine response was consistent with the morphological response rate, except in one radiologically stable patient who showed biochemical progression and in one patient with partial remission in whom a mere 29% catecholamine decrease was noted.

Better chromogranin A response was reported by Yadav et al. with >25% reduction in 11/24 (46%) patients of whom >50% reduction was found in 7/24 (29%) [15]. This was also the case in the study by Kong et al. who, out of 14 evaluable patients, found 10/14 (71%) with >25% reduction of chromogranin A, of whom 8/14 (57%) had >50% biochemical response [14]. With ^{90}Y-DOTATOC, biochemical responses were reported in 2/11 (18%) and 4/28 (14%) PCC and PGL patients, respectively [9]. We found less biochemical response regarding catecholamines than for chromogranin A. A similar degree of catecholamine response was found by Kong et al., who for 7 patients reported >50% decrease of plasma metanephrine in 1 patient, 25% to 50% reduction in 4 patients, and biochemical increase in 2 patients, and with fairly similar biochemical response figures regarding plasma normetanephrine [14].

Ten of our patients had catecholamine-related symptoms, which in two were aggravated during PRRT, including the development of hypertensive crisis. These symptoms and signs were, however, present already at baseline and it is difficult to confidently determine whether the worsening of symptoms was a consequence of PRRT, or represented fluctuations of catecholamine levels due to the disease itself.

The response to ^{177}Lu-DOTATATE therapy was also assessed during each PRRT cycle by scintigraphy, including both whole-body scans and SPECT/CT, whereby a visual rating of the tumor uptake is made for each cycle in relation to the first. In this evaluation, we found response (≥50%) in 9/19 (47%) of our patients who underwent dosimetry and for whom scintigraphic examinations were available. Another means for therapy monitoring was applied by Kong et al., who utilized ^{68}Ga-DOTATATE-PET/CT and reported a similar fraction of responding patients (8/17, 47%) [14].

^{131}I-MIBG therapy constitutes the mainstay in radionuclide therapy of PCC/PGL, and which five of our patients had previously undergone. With ^{177}Lu/^{90}Y-DOTATATE/TOC therapy, the tumors need to show sufficient somatostatin receptor expression on imaging, usually Krenning grade 3 or 4 (higher than that of the liver) or at lease grade 2 (similar to that of the liver) in order to be eligible for PRRT. Correspondingly, the tumors on ^{123}I-MIBG scintigraphy need to show sufficient uptake for the patient to qualify for ^{131}I-MIBG therapy. A problem with ^{123}I-MIBG in PCC/PGL patients is that the uptake in general is high, resulting in excellent sensitivity on ^{123}I-MIBG scintigraphy for diagnosing disease on a patient basis. However, ^{123}I-MIBG scintigraphy has shown reduced sensitivity in extra-adrenal, multiple, or hereditary PGLs (52–75%) associated with von Hippel Lindau syndrome as well as *SDHB*-related PGLs and patients with metastatic disease in whom ^{123}I-MIBG scintigraphy may underestimate the extent of disease. The sensitivity of ^{123}I-MIBG scintigraphy is particularly low in head and neck PGLs (HNPGL) (18–50%) [20]. Consequently, the low tumor accumulation on ^{123}I-MIBG scintigraphy disqualifies many of these patients for ^{131}I-MIBG therapy. Our patients underwent both ^{123}I-MIBG scintigraphy and somatostatin receptor scintigraphy, and first-line therapy was chosen based on these results. In the case of inhomogeneous expression, the tracer with the most favorable distribution was applied for subsequent therapy (Figure 3). In addition, patient No. 3 had a mosaic expression for the two tracers, which resulted in treatment with both, consecutively. One lesion without any uptake was treated with additional external beam radiation.

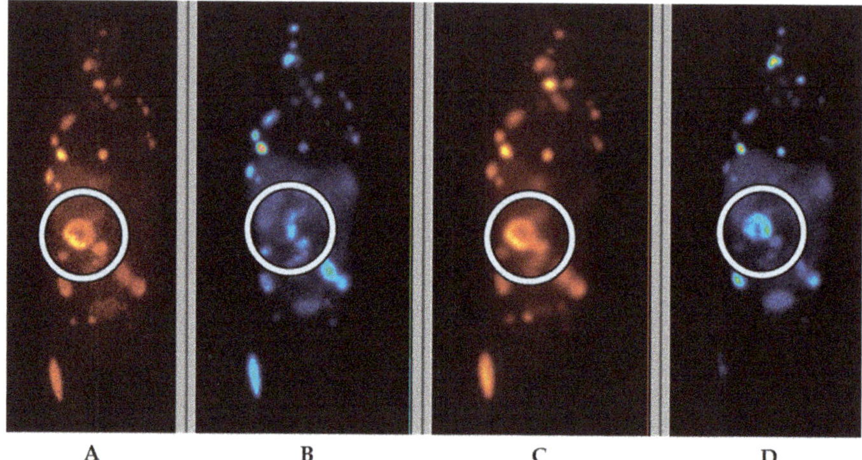

Figure 3. Frontal planar scintigraphy images in patient No. 4, in whom the primary PCC had higher uptake on ^{123}I-MIBG scintigraphy (**A**) than on somatostatin receptor scintigraphy (OctreoScan™) (**B**). After one cycle of ^{131}I-MIBG (**C**) scintigraphy during therapy) an upregulation of somatostatin receptors was noted and further therapy was given with ^{177}Lu-DOTA-octreotate (**D**) scintigraphy during therapy).

The concept of Ki-67 proliferation index as a predictive marker of response to treatment in patients with NET in general, and in NET patients treated with ^{177}Lu-DOTATATE in particular, is well established and part of clinical routine. In PCC and PGL, Ki-67 index is, however, not validated as a predictive marker. Interestingly, we found such a correlation and Ki-67 ≥15% was shown to be a predictor for worse OS and PFS. Another negative predictor for OS, but not for PFS, was found to be PRRT undertaken because of progression on previous therapy, and not started as a first-line treatment. We were however unable to show any predictive value for tumor type (PCC or PGL), visual response on scintigraphy, or previous therapies (surgery, radiotherapy, chemotherapy, ^{131}I-MIBG), which were all factors unrelated to OS and PFS. Most probably, because of the small number of observations, neither was the patients' genetical profile or disease stage useful as predictors of survival.

In three of our patients, the PGL was located in the cauda equina, liver, and kidney, respectively. Although PGL in these anatomical positions are extremely uncommon, they were, because of previously published reports on PGLs in these sites, regarded as primary tumors. It can of course not be confidently excluded that these tumors represented metastases from an undiagnosed PGL with unknown primary location.

4. Materials and Methods

This was a retrospective cohort study of patients treated at the Department of Nuclear Medicine, Uppsala University Hospital, Uppsala, Sweden. All patients receiving ^{117}Lu-DOTATATE therapy between 2005 and 2018 were screened for inclusion using information available through the digital radiological information and picture archive and retrieval systems (RIS-PACS). The study was approved by the local ethics committee, and written informed consent was obtained from all individual patients since 2010 (No. 2009-320). Before 2010, patients were admitted after giving their informed consent on a single-patient basis for compassionate use with individual permission of the Swedish Medical Products Agency.

Clinical, biochemical, and radiological imaging follow-up data were retrieved from the RIS-PACS and from the hospital's digital patient record system. Survival was analyzed for Swedish patients

($n = 15$), based on entries to the national health registry accessed on 5 April 2019. For international patients, the referring center was contacted for an updated follow-up.

Inclusion criteria for PRRT were patients with pheochromocytoma or paraganglioma confirmed by histopathological examination, and a tumor uptake higher than that of the normal liver (Krenning scores 3 and 4) on somatostatin receptor scintigraphy (SRS), life expectancy > 3 months, white blood cell count (WBC) > 3.0×10^9/L, platelet count > 100×10^9/L, bilirubin < 40 μmol /L, albumin > 25 g/L, ASAT and ALAT less than 5 times upper limit, creatinine < 110 μmol/L or, if higher, GFR (cystatin-C) > 50 mL/min/1.73 m^2. Exclusion criteria were pregnancy, tumors amenable to surgery or locoregional ablation, and inability to stay isolated for 24 h.

4.1. PRRT Treatment Protocol

Chemotherapy and targeted therapy were stopped at least one month before the treatment start. Therapy monitoring utilized intravenously contrast-enhanced computed tomography (CT) or magnetic resonance imaging (MRI) performed according to clinical NET imaging protocols within one month before PRRT, in connection with every second cycle, 3 months after the end of treatment, and thereafter every 3–6 months until tumor progression.

Three patients were treated according to the original Rotterdam PRRT protocol with 4 cycles × 7.4 GBq ^{177}Lu-DOTATATE [10] and 19 patients underwent dosimetry-guided PRRT [19], whereby as many cycles as possible were administered with an intended interval of 6 to 8 weeks between cycles up to 23 Gy to the kidneys or 2 Gy to bone marrow, or other reasons to stop therapy occurred.

Dosimetry for solid organs and bone marrow was calculated as previously described in detail [17,18]. For solid organs, dosimetry was based on the small volume method performed on single photon emission tomography with low dose CT performed together with single photon computed emission tomography (SPECT/CT) at 1, 4, and 7 days after therapy. Volumes of interest (4 mL) were drawn in representative regions with homogeneous uptake. The activity concentrations were fitted to a mono-exponential function. For complete bone marrow dosimetry, the blood activity was calculated from integrated blood activity curves derived from blood samples at 0.5, 1, 2.5, 4, 8, and 24 h and complemented with tissue activity measurements on whole-body scans at 1, 4, and 7 days after start of therapy. Complete dosimetry was performed during the first cycle, after delay, in the instance of large changes in tumor volume, and at least at every fourth cycle. For all other cycles, a short dosimetry protocol used SPECT/CT over the abdomen and a whole-body scan at 24 h.

The peptide was a kind gift from Prof. Eric Krenning, ^{177}Lu was purchased (IDB, Holland BV, Baarle-Nassau, The Netherlands) and labeling was performed in-house. Kidney protection comprised 2 L amino acid mixture (Vamin 14 gN/L electrolyte-free, Kabi Fresenius) i.v. over 8 h, starting 30 m before treatment. I.v. antiemetics was given 1 h before therapy (8 mg of betamethasone and 8 mg of ondansetron or 250 μg of palonosetron).

4.2. Evaluations

White blood cell (WBC) count was checked before each cycle and had to be >3×10^9/L, granulocytes >1.5×10^9/L, and platelets >100×10^9/L. If these criteria were not met within 6 months, PRRT was stopped. In occasional instances, the interval between cycles was prolonged, alternatively the administered activity per cycle was decreased by 30%, rather than delaying the treatment. Plasma chromogranin A as well as plasma/urinary metanephrines or catecholamines were collected in connection with every cycle. In order to monitor side effects, routine blood tests (complete blood count, liver enzymes, electrolytes, and creatinine) were performed every second week on an outpatient basis. CT/MRI was performed within one month before PRRT start, before every second treatment cycle, 3 months after the last treatment, and thereafter at least every 6 months.

4.3. *Response Assessment*

CT/MRI results were assessed according to RECIST 1.1. [21] to determine the best tumor response (%) (BR%) and response category (complete response (CR), partial response (PR), stable disease (SD), and progressive disease (PD)) and the time to BS from start of PRRT. The progression-free survival (PFS) and overall survival (OS) were calculated.

Biochemical tumor response of P-chromogranin A and P/U-catecholamines was registered in four categories, namely, decrease >50%, decrease >25–50%, decrease >0–25%, or increase >50%, as compared to baseline values.

SPECT/CT and whole-body scans and SPECT during each cycle were evaluated by a specialist in nuclear medicine, whereby the overall decrease in tumor uptake (%) on scans performed during each PRRT cycle was assessed in relation to that of the first cycle. PR was defined as ≥50% decrease and PD was registered in the case of pronounced increase in tumor accumulation or appearance of new tumor lesions.

4.4. *Toxicity*

Toxicity was reported using the Common Terminology Criteria for Adverse Events version 4.0, and toxicities grade 1 to 4 were reported from the start of treatment until 3 months after the last treatment.

4.5. *Statistical Analysis*

Univariate correlation to PFS and OS was performed with JMP 13.1.0 (SAS Institute Inc., Cary, NC, USA) using the Kaplan–Meier log rank test. Possible predictive factors for OS and PFS were tested in the Kaplan–Meier analysis by dichotomization. Multivariate analysis was excluded due to the limited sample number.

5. Conclusions

In conclusion, PRRT with ^{177}Lu-DOTATATE was associated with a favorable outcome and low toxicity. High Ki-67 (≥15%) and PRRT received because of progression on previous therapy were negative predictive factors for OS.

Author Contributions: Conceptualization, A.S. and P.H.; Methodology, A.S. and M.S.; Validation, A.R.V., A.S., U.G.-R., and J.C.; Formal Analysis, A.R.V. and A.S.; Investigation, A.R.V. and A.S.; Data Curation, A.R.V., K.F.-B., U.G.-R., M.S., and A.S.; Writing—Original Draft Preparation, A.R.V. and A.S.; Writing—Review and Editing, A.R.V., A.S., P.H., O.N., U.G.-R., D.G., and E.T.-E.; Supervision, A.S. and J.C.

Funding: This research received no external funding.

Conflicts of Interest: J.C. received lecture honoraria from Novartis and educational honoraria from NET Connect (funded by Ipsen). A.S. received lecture honoraria from Ipsen. Other authors declare no potential conflicts of interests.

References

1. Lenders, J.W.; Eisenhofer, G.; Mannelli, M.; Pacak, K. Phaeochromocytoma. *Lancet* **2005**, *366*, 665–675. [CrossRef]
2. Fishbein, L.; Leshchiner, I.; Walter, V.; Danilova, L.; Robertson, A.G.; Johnson, A.R.; Lichtenberg, T.M.; Murray, B.A.; Ghayee, H.K.; Else, T.; et al. Cancer Genome Atlas Research Network, Pacak K, Nathanson KL, Wilkerson MD. Comprehensive Molecular Characterization of Pheochromocytoma and Paraganglioma. *Cancer Cell.* **2017**, *31*, 181–193. [CrossRef] [PubMed]
3. Crona, J.; Lamarca, A.; Ghosal, S.; Welin, S.; Skogseid, B.; Pacak, K. Genotype-phenotype correlations in pheochromocytoma and paraganglioma. *Endocr. Relat. Cancer* **2019**. [CrossRef]

4. Hamidi, O.; Young, W.F., Jr.; Gruber, L.; Smestad, J.; Yan, Q.; Ponce, O.J.; Prokop, L.; Murad, M.H.; Bancos, I. Outcomes of patients with metastatic phaeochromocytoma and paraganglioma: A systematic review and meta-analysis. *Clin. Endocrinol.* **2017**, *87*, 440–450. [CrossRef] [PubMed]
5. Lenders, J.W.; Duh, Q.Y.; Eisenhofer, G.; Gimenez-Roqueplo, A.P.; Grebe, S.K.; Murad, M.H.; Naruse, M.; Pacak, K.; Young, W.F., Jr. Endocrine Society. Pheochromocytoma and paraganglioma: An endocrine society clinical practice guideline. *J. Clin. Endocrinol. Metab.* **2014**, *99*, 1915–1942. [CrossRef]
6. Gonias, S.; Goldsby, R.; Matthay, K.K.; Hawkins, R.; Price, D.; Huberty, J.; Damon, L.; Linker, C.; Sznewajs, A.; Shiboski, S.; et al. Phase II study of high-dose [131I] metaiodobenzylguanidine therapy for patients with metastatic pheochromocytoma and paraganglioma. *J. Clin. Oncol.* **2009**, *27*, 4162–4168. [CrossRef]
7. Huang, H.; Abraham, J.; Hung, E.; Averbuch, S.; Merino, M.; Steinberg, S.M.; Pacak, K.; Fojo, T. Treatment of malignant pheochromocytoma/paraganglioma with cyclophosphamide, vincristine, and dacarbazine: Recommendation from a 22-year follow-up of 18 patients. *Cancer* **2008**, *113*, 2020–2028. [CrossRef]
8. Joshua, A.M.; Ezzat, S.; Asa, S.L.; Evans, A.; Broom, R.; Freeman, M.; Knox, J.J. Rationale and evidence for sunitinib in the treatment of malignant paraganglioma/pheochromocytoma. *J. Clin. Endocrinol. Metab.* **2009**, *94*, 5–9. [CrossRef]
9. Imhof, A.; Brunner, P.; Marincek, N.; Briel, M.; Schindler, C.; Rasch, H.; Mäcke, H.R.; Rochlitz, C.; Müller-Brand, J.; Walter, M.A. Response, survival, and long-term toxicity after therapy with the radiolabelled somatostatin analogue [90Y-DOTA]-TOC in metastasised neuroendocrine cancers. *J. Clin. Oncol.* **2011**, *29*, 2416–2423. [CrossRef]
10. Kwekkeboom, D.J.; Bakker, W.H.; Kam, B.L.; Teunissen, J.J.; Kooij, P.P.; de Herder, W.W.; Feelders, R.A.; van Eijck, C.H.; de Jong, M.; Srinivasan, A.; et al. Treatment of patients with gastro-entero-pancreatic (GEP) tumours with the novel radiolabelled somatostatin analogue [(177)Lu-DOTA(0), Tyr(3)] octreotate. *Eur. J. Nucl. Med. Mol. Imaging* **2003**, *30*, 417–422. [CrossRef]
11. Brabander, T.; van der Zwan, W.A.; Teunissen, J.J.M.; Kam, B.L.R.; Feelders, R.A.; de Herder, W.W.; van Eijck, C.H.J.; Franssen, G.J.H.; Krenning, E.P.; Kwekkeboom, D.J. Long-Term Efficacy, Survival, and Safety of [^{177}Lu-DOTA^0, Tyr^3] octreotate in Patients with Gastroenteropancreatic and Bronchial Neuroendocrine Tumors. *Clin. Cancer Res.* **2017**, *23*, 4617–4624. [CrossRef] [PubMed]
12. Forrer, F.; Riedweg, I.; Maecke, H.R.; Mueller-Brand, J. Radiolabeled DOTATOC in patients with advanced paraganglioma and pheochromocytoma. *Q. J. Nucl. Med. Mol. Imaging* **2008**, *52*, 334–340. [PubMed]
13. Van Essen, M.; Krenning, E.P.; Kooij, P.P.; Bakker, W.H.; Feelders, R.A.; de Herder, W.W.; Wolbers, J.G.; Kwekkeboom, D.J. Effects of therapy with [177Lu-DOTA0, Tyr3] octreotate in patients with paraganglioma, meningioma, small cell lung carcinoma, and melanoma. *J. Nucl. Med.* **2006**, *47*, 1599–1606.
14. Kong, G.; Grozinsky-Glasberg, S.; Hofman, M.S.; Akhurst, T.; Meirovitz, A.; Maimon, O.; Krausz, Y.; Godefroy, J.; Michael, M.; Gross, D.J.; et al. Highly favourable outcomes with peptide receptor radionuclide therapy (PRRT) for metastatic rectal neuroendocrine neoplasia (NEN). *Eur. J. Nucl. Med. Mol. Imaging* **2019**, *46*, 718–727. [CrossRef] [PubMed]
15. Yadav, M.P.; Ballal, S.; Bal, C. Concomitant ^{177}Lu-DOTATATE and capecitabine therapy in malignant paragangliomas. *EJNMMI Res.* **2019**, *9*, 13. [CrossRef]
16. Demirci, E.; Kabasakal, L.; Toklu, T.; Ocak, M.; Şahin, O.E.; Alan-Selcuk, N.; Araman, A. 177Lu-DOTATATE therapy in patients with neuroendocrine tumours including high-grade (WHO G3) neuroendocrine tumours: Response to treatment and long-term survival update. *Nucl. Med. Commun.* **2018**, *39*, 789–796. [CrossRef]
17. Sandström, M.; Garske, U.; Granberg, D.; Sundin, A.; Lundqvist, H. Individualized dosimetry in patients undergoing therapy with (177) Lu-DOTA-D-Phe (1)-Tyr (3)-octreotate. *Eur. J. Nucl. Med. Mol. Imaging* **2010**, *37*, 212–225. [CrossRef]
18. Sandström, M.; Garske-Román, U.; Granberg, D.; Johansson, S.; Widström, C.; Eriksson, B.; Sundin, A.; Lundqvist, H.; Lubberink, M. Individualized dosimetry of kidney and bone marrow in patients undergoing 177Lu-DOTA-octreotate treatment. *J. Nucl. Med.* **2013**, *54*, 33–41. [CrossRef]
19. Garske-Román, U.; Sandström, M.; Fröss Baron, K.; Lundin, L.; Hellman, P.; Welin, S.; Johansson, S.; Khan, T.; Lundqvist, H.; Eriksson, B.; et al. Prospective observational study of ^{177}Lu-DOTA-octreotate therapy in 200 patients with advanced metastasized neuroendocrine tumours (NETs): Feasibility and impact of a dosimetry-guided study protocol on outcome and toxicity. *Eur. J. Nucl. Med. Mol. Imaging* **2018**, *45*, 970–988. [CrossRef]

20. Taïeb, D.; Timmers, H.J.; Hindié, E.; Guillet, B.A.; Neumann, H.P.; Walz, M.K.; Opocher, G.; de Herder, W.W.; Boedeker, C.C.; de Krijger, R.R.; et al. European Association of Nuclear Medicine. EANM 2012 guidelines for radionuclide imaging ofmphaeochromocytoma and paraganglioma. *Eur. J. Nucl. Med. Mol. Imaging* **2012**, *39*, 1977–1995. [CrossRef]
21. Eisenhauer, E.A.; Therasse, P.; Bogaerts, J.; Schwartz, L.H.; Sargent, D.; Ford, R.; Dancey, J.; Arbuck, S.; Gwyther, S.; Mooney, M.; et al. New response evaluation criteria in solid tumours: Revised RECIST guideline (version 1.1). *Eur. J. Cancer* **2009**, *45*, 228–247. [CrossRef] [PubMed]

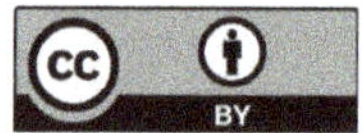

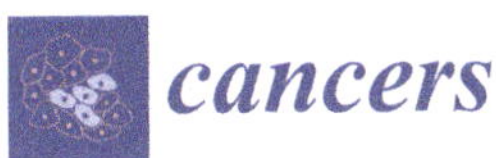

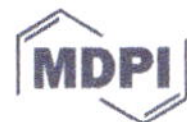

Review

Intricacies of the Molecular Machinery of Catecholamine Biosynthesis and Secretion by Chromaffin Cells of the Normal Adrenal Medulla and in Pheochromocytoma and Paraganglioma

Annika M.A. Berends [1,*], Graeme Eisenhofer [2], Lauren Fishbein [3], Anouk N.A. van der Horst-Schrivers [1], Ido P. Kema [4], Thera P. Links [1], Jacques W.M. Lenders [5,6] and Michiel N. Kerstens [1]

1 Department of Endocrinology, University of Groningen, University Medical Center Groningen, 9700 RB Groningen, The Netherlands
2 Department of Clinical Chemistry and Laboratory Medicine and Department of Medicine III, University Hospital Carl Gustav Carus, Technical University Dresden, 01069 Dresden, Germany
3 Division of Endocrinology, Metabolism and Diabetes and Division of Biomedical Informatics and Personalized Medicine, Department of Medicine, University of Colorado School of Medicine, University of Colorado Cancer Center, Aurora, CO 80045, USA
4 Department of Laboratory Medicine, University of Groningen, University Medical Center Groningen, 9700 RB Groningen, The Netherlands
5 Department of Medicine III, University Hospital Carl Gustav Carus, Technical University Dresden, 01307 Dresden, Germany
6 Department of Internal Medicine, Radboud University Medical Center, 6525 GA Nijmegen, The Netherlands
* Correspondence: m.a.berends@umcg.nl

Received: 22 June 2019; Accepted: 12 July 2019; Published: 6 August 2019

Abstract: The adrenal medulla is composed predominantly of chromaffin cells producing and secreting the catecholamines dopamine, norepinephrine, and epinephrine. Catecholamine biosynthesis and secretion is a complex and tightly controlled physiologic process. The pathways involved have been extensively studied, and various elements of the underlying molecular machinery have been identified. In this review, we provide a detailed description of the route from stimulus to secretion of catecholamines by the normal adrenal chromaffin cell compared to chromaffin tumor cells in pheochromocytomas. Pheochromocytomas are adrenomedullary tumors that are characterized by uncontrolled synthesis and secretion of catecholamines. This uncontrolled secretion can be partly explained by perturbations of the molecular catecholamine secretory machinery in pheochromocytoma cells. Chromaffin cell tumors also include sympathetic paragangliomas originating in sympathetic ganglia. Pheochromocytomas and paragangliomas are usually locally confined tumors, but about 15% do metastasize to distant locations. Histopathological examination currently poorly predicts future biologic behavior, thus long term postoperative follow-up is required. Therefore, there is an unmet need for prognostic biomarkers. Clearer understanding of the cellular mechanisms involved in the secretory characteristics of pheochromocytomas and sympathetic paragangliomas may offer one approach for the discovery of novel prognostic biomarkers for improved therapeutic targeting and monitoring of treatment or disease progression.

Keywords: PPGL; catecholamines; adrenomedullary function

---

1. Introduction

The adrenal medulla occupies the central portion of the adrenal gland and accounts for about 10% of total adrenal gland volume [1]. The adrenal medulla is essentially a specialized sympathetic ganglion releasing hormones in response to neural input and therefore is an integral part of the autonomic nervous system [2,3]. The adrenomedullary chromaffin cells are embryologically derived from migrating neural crest cells that develop into sympathoadrenal progenitors [4,5]. These sympathoadrenal progenitor cells also give rise to the chromaffin cells present in the sympathetic chain and prevertebral paraganglia. During adrenal organogenesis, close interactions between its two components, medulla and cortex, are necessary for differentiation, morphogenesis, and survival of the adrenal gland. This cortical–chromaffin crosstalk remains important for physiological regulation of adrenal hormone biosynthesis in adult life and also is relevant for the pathogenesis of various adrenal gland disorders [6–9]. One of the histological infrastructural requirements for this crosstalk is the centripetally directed arterial blood flow from adrenal cortex to medulla. In addition, cortical cells are diffusely present in the adrenal medulla and, conversely, chromaffin cells are intermixed with cortical cells within all three zones of the adrenal cortex [10].

The principal function of the adrenal medulla is the biosynthesis and the secretion into the circulation of the catecholamine epinephrine [6,11]. Epinephrine has a crucial role in the "fight-or-flight" response, which allows an organism to adapt to stressful conditions. The acute rise in epinephrine in response to physical or psychological stress stimuli results in hemodynamic and metabolic effects that modulate various functions such as blood pressure, cardiac output, and blood glucose by acting on cells expressing α- and β- adrenergic receptors [12,13]. Under basal conditions, however, epinephrine functions as a circulating metabolic hormone, and it is the norepinephrine secreted by sympathetic nerves acting immediately in the vicinity of exocytotic secretion that is the catecholamine mainly regulating cardiovascular function. The norepinephrine that escapes re-uptake processes to enter the circulation has negligible impact on the cardiovascular system. Nevertheless, both norepinephrine and epinephrine secreted by pheochromocytomas in excessive amounts directly into the circulation can have profound effects on cardiovascular function, with further impacts of co-secreted peptides. From a clinical perspective, these tumors are the most important disease of the adrenal medulla. Chromaffin cell tumors may also arise in extra-adrenal sympathetic paraganglia, in which case they are termed sympathetic paragangliomas [14–16].

A cardinal feature of chromaffin cell tumors is their capacity to produce and secrete excessive amounts of catecholamines, which may evoke signs and symptoms such as paroxysmal hypertension, sweating, and tachycardia. The hypersecretion of catecholamines may cause acute, life-threatening blood pressure elevations and arrhythmias and is associated with a significantly increased rate of cardiovascular morbidity and mortality [17–20].

Pheochromocytomas and sympathetic paragangliomas are rare neuroendocrine tumors with respective reported annual incidences of 0.46 and 0.11 per 100,000 individuals [21]. Detected incidence of pheochromocytomas has doubled during the past two decades, most likely a result of changes in diagnostic practices leading to earlier detection. The cornerstone of biochemical diagnosis of a pheochromocytoma or a sympathetic paraganglioma is the demonstration of elevated plasma or urinary concentrations of metanephrine, normetanephrine, or 3-methoxytyramine, i.e., the O-methylated metabolites of epinephrine, norepinephrine, or dopamine, respectively [22]. Several anatomical and functional imaging studies are available for localization of the tumor, after which curative treatment by surgical resection can be offered [23].

Pheochromocytomas and paragangliomas are highly heterogeneous neuro-endocrine tumors with regards to possible anatomic location, genetic context, symptomatology, metastatic potential, and the degree of catecholamine release. Genetic mutations play a critical role in tumorigenesis and affect various metabolic pathways, which also result in different mutation-dependent biochemical phenotypes [3,24–26].

In recent years, our knowledge of the genotype–phenotype interrelationship and metabolomics of these intriguing neuro-endocrine tumors has expanded rapidly. Nevertheless, there are still several areas of uncertainty. For instance, in the absence of metastases, it is difficult to predict whether a pheochromocytoma or a paraganglioma will demonstrate a benign or a malignant clinical course [16]. There are no clear-cut pathological markers to establish malignancy with certainty at first presentation. Also, there is no straightforward relationship between the biochemical phenotype of a pheochromocytoma or sympathetic paraganglioma and the associated signs or symptoms [3]. In the present review, we aim to provide a detailed picture of the pathways involved in catecholamine production and secretion in normal adrenomedullary chromaffin cells. We also visit what is known about the molecular perturbations in catecholamine biosynthesis and secretion in pheochromocytoma and sympathetic paraganglioma. Improved understanding of these mechanisms at the molecular level might provide insight into associated pathological complications, clarify highly variable presentations, and aid in identification of new diagnostic or therapeutic strategies for personalized care.

2. Adrenomedullary Function

2.1. Biosynthesis of Catecholamines

Adrenomedullary catecholamine biosynthesis starts with uptake of the nonessential amino acid L-tyrosine by the chromaffin cell. L-tyrosine is obtained from food sources or is derived from the essential amino acid phenylalanine through the activity of phenylalanine hydroxylase, which is mainly expressed in liver, kidney, and pancreas [27,28]. L-tyrosine is transported into the cytoplasm of the adrenal chromaffin cell by the membrane bound L-type amino acid transporter system (LAT1 and LAT2) [29,30]. Catecholamine biosynthesis involves the sequential activity of four enzymes: tyrosine hydroxylase (TH), aromatic L-amino acid decarboxylase (AADC), dopamine β-hydroxylase (DBH), and phenylethanolamine-*N*-methyltransferase (PNMT). Except for DBH, all these enzymes are localized in the cytoplasm of the chromaffin cell (Figure 1). The end products of this biosynthetic route are dopamine, norepinephrine, or epinephrine, depending on intracellular enzyme expression. Epinephrine is mainly produced by the adrenomedullary chromaffin cells (>95%) and functions as a hormone released directly into the bloodstream. In contrast, circulating norepinephrine is mainly derived from overflow of the neurotransmitter from sympathetic nerve endings with adrenomedullary chromaffin cell production providing usually a less than 10% contribution [11,13,31].

2.1.1. Tyrosine Hydroxylase

The initial and rate limiting step in catecholamine biosynthesis is the conversion of L-tyrosine to L-3,4-dihydroxyphenylalanine (L-DOPA) by tyrosine hydroxylase (TH, EC 1.14.16.2, molecular mass of approximately 240 kDa) [32,33]. Locations of catecholamine biosynthesis are therefore dependent on the expression of TH, which is largely confined to postganglionic sympathetic nerve endings and adrenal and extra-adrenal chromaffin cells. In the adrenal medulla, this enzyme has a Km of 2×10^{-5} mol/L [27]. For this specific hydroxylation step, TH requires tetrahydrobiopterin, molecular oxygen, and Fe^{2+} as cofactors. Tetrahydrobiopterin is synthesized from guanosine triphosphate (GTP) and serves as a donor for hydrogen atoms to maintain TH in a reduced and active state [27,34]. The human *TH* gene is located at chromosome 11p15.5 and contains 13 exons [35], with four isoforms produced by alternative mRNA splicing.

Regulation of TH activity is an important way to control catecholamine biosynthesis. This is a complex process encompassing multiple modes of regulation. Short-term post-transcriptional mechanisms include feedback inhibition by catecholamines, enzyme phosphorylation and dephosphorylation, as well as ubiquitination. Long-term regulation mainly involves transcriptional mechanisms [36]. The ubiquitin–proteasome pathway is thought to be involved in the degradation of TH [37]. Catecholamines exert negative feedback control through oxidation of tetrahydrobiopterin to pteridine, thereby preventing the formation of TH in its reduced active state [27]. In addition, catecholamines act as competitive antagonists of tetrahydrobiopterin at the active site of the catalytic domain of TH [27]. Short-term regulation of TH activity is also achieved by a mechanism of phosphorylation and dephosphorylation of one or more of the four serine residues at the regulatory site of TH. Phosphorylation is catalyzed by multiple kinases (e.g., PKA, PKC, CaMKII, MAPKAP-K2,

ERK1, ERK2, MSK1, PRAK) and results in release from the feedback inhibition by catecholamines, thereby stimulating enzyme activity.

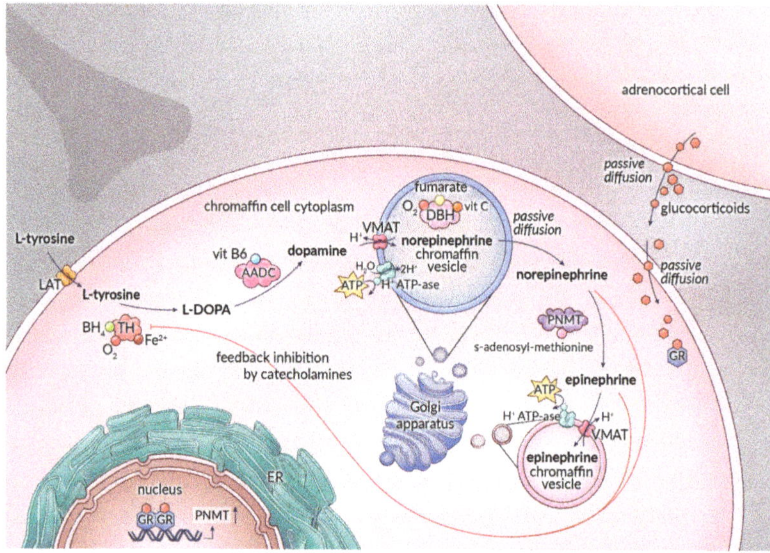

Figure 1. The catecholamine biosynthetic pathway in an adrenomedullary chromaffin cell or a pheochromocytoma cell. Norepinephrine and epinephrine are stored in separate chromaffin storage vesicles. Abbreviations: LAT: L-type amino acid transporter; TH: tyrosine hydroxylase; L-DOPA: L-3,4-dihydroxyphenylalanine; AADC: aromatic L-amino acid decarboxylase; DBH: dopamine β-hydroxylase; PNMT: phenylethanolamine-N-methyltransferase; BH4: tetrahydrobiopterin; 02: molecular oxygen; VitB6: pyridoxalphosphate; VitC: ascorbate; VMAT: vesicular monoamine transporters; GR: glucocorticoid receptor.

Dephosphorylation by phosphatase PP2A, and to a lesser extent by PP2C, restores catecholaminergic inhibition of the TH enzyme [36]. This negative feedback is mediated via alpha2-adrenergic or D2-dopaminergic receptors, which activate cyclic adenosine monophosphate (cAMP) or Ca^{2+}/calmodulin-dependent protein phosphatases [27]. Prolonged stimulation of catecholamine biosynthesis results in induction of TH protein synthesis through several cAMP dependent pathways activating *TH* gene transcription [27,34,36,38–40].

Given the importance of its activity to catecholamine synthesis and the complexity of its regulation, TH has gained great interest in many fields of biomedical research. Recent studies, for example, have demonstrated the presence of several TH polymorphisms in the general population, some of which appear associated with increased norepinephrine levels and elevated blood pressure [35,41].

2.1.2. Aromatic L-Amino Acid Decarboxylase

The next step in catecholamine biosynthesis is the decarboxylation of L-DOPA to dopamine by cytosolic aromatic L-amino acid decarboxylase (AADC; EC 4.1.1.28). For this conversion, pyridoxalphosphate (vitamin B6) is required as a cofactor [27,42]. AADC is a 100 kDa homodimeric protein encoded by a single gene located at chromosome 7p12.1 with a Km of 4×10^{-4} mol/L [42,43]. The calculated Km greatly exceeds the endogenous concentration of L-DOPA, which means that the AADC enzyme is not fully saturated, and the rate at which dopamine can be synthesized is therefore limited by the availability of L-DOPA as a substrate [42]. The AADC enzyme has a wide tissue distribution and is not specific for chromaffin cells [42,44].

Short-term regulation of AADC enzyme activity by a previously postulated mechanism involving cAMP or phosphorylation by protein kinases seems to play no significant role in the regulation of the catecholamine biosynthetic pathway in situ [42,45]. The added value of AADC enzyme upregulation by modulation of gene expression for physiological demands to increase catecholamine production in postganglionic sympathetic nerve endings remains questionable [45–47].

2.1.3. Dopamine β-hydroxylase

In adrenal chromaffin cells, dopamine is further catalyzed to norepinephrine by dopamine β-hydroxylase (DBH; EC 1.14.17.1). Because of the intravesicular location of DBH, dopamine first must be translocated into norepinephrine storage vesicles by vesicular monoamine transporters (VMATs) [11]. The intravesicular conversion of dopamine represents the final step in the biosynthesis of norepinephrine. DBH, a mixed-function oxidase, is a 290 kDa copper protein with a Km of 8.4×10^{-4} mol/L and utilizes molecular oxygen, fumarate, and L-ascorbic acid as its main cofactors [27,48,49]. These requirements for L-ascorbic acid and fumarate are not specific. Catechol (i.e., pyrocatechol or 1,2 dihydroxybenzene) seems to be a weak substitute for L-ascorbic acid and other activating anions, such as acetate and chloride, which can replicate the effects of fumarate at least partially [27,48,50–52].

In humans, DBH is encoded by a gene located at chromosome 9q34.2. Increased catecholamine biosynthesis in response to stress is associated with increased levels of mRNAs encoding catecholamine synthesizing enzymes. In adrenomedullary chromaffin cells, this response to stress is rapid, especially for TH and PNMT [39]. Previous studies also revealed upregulation of adrenal *DBH* gene expression by various transcriptional mechanisms in response to prolonged or repeated stressors [39,53]. However, in contrast to *TH*, short or intermediate duration of stress does not result in a significant increase of *DBH* mRNA [39].

2.1.4. Phenylethanolamine-*N*-Methyltransferase

Norepinephrine formed in the chromaffin vesicles diffuses passively into the cytosol, where it is converted to epinephrine by the enzyme phenylethanolamine-*N*-methyl transferase (PNMT; EC 2.1.1.28) [11,24]. PNMT, which has a predicted molecular weight of 30.9 kDa and a Km of 9.2×10^{-6} mol/L, requires *S*-adenosylmethionine as a methyl donor and cosubstrate [27,54,55]. PNMT is not substrate specific and also is involved in the biosynthesis of other *N*-methylated trace amines [11,27]. Expression of PNMT is controlled by glucocorticoid receptor-mediated mechanisms, acting in concert with several other transcription factors such as Egr-1, AP2, Sp1, and MAZ [6,39,56,57]. The proximity of adrenocortical cells to the adrenal medulla guarantees high circulating glucocorticoid levels, which cross the chromaffin cell membrane through passive diffusion. Glucocorticoid binds to the intracytoplasmatic glucocorticoid receptor, and the receptor–hormone complex migrates to the cell nucleus and binds to the glucocorticoid response element of the promoter region of the *PNMT* gene located on chromosome 17q12, activating gene transcription [7,58,59]. This explains why the adrenal gland is the body's most important source of epinephrine, whereas the expression of extra-adrenal PNMT is limited to a small number of neurons in the central nervous system and to a subset of cardiomyocytes [6,60,61].

2.1.5. Co-Secreted Products

Chromaffin cells of the adrenal medulla synthesize a large variety of other substances, such as neurotransmitters, enzymes, peptides, and proteins, which are also stored in chromaffin vesicles and co-secreted along with catecholamines [62–64]. Over the past decades, the components of this vesicular cocktail have been studied in great detail (Table 1).

Table 1. Overview of the co-secreted products of chromaffin vesicles with description of their function in normal adrenal medulla and reported alterations in pheochromocytoma and paraganglioma (PPGL).

Component	Function in Human Adrenal Medulla	Reported Alterations in PPGL
Granins		
Chromogranin A–C [65–77]	Role in vesiculogenesis, vesicle protein stability, hormone storage within vesicles. Sorting proteins in the regulated secretory pathway. Precursor protein for several peptides; chromogranin A (vasostatin I–II, catestatin, cateslytin, chromacin, chromofungin, pancreastatin, parastatin, WE-14, EL35), chromogranin B (secretolytin), chromogranin C (secretoneurin, EM66, manserin).	Higher plasma levels of chromogranin A and B are reported in PPGL compared to healthy volunteers. Chromogranin C mRNA was overexpressed in PPGL compared to non-tumoral chromaffin tissue. Higher expression of chromogranin A and B in *RET* associated PPGL compared to *VHL* associated PPGL at both the mRNA and protein levels. Downregulation of chromogranin B and chromogranin C observed to be associated with malignant behavior.
Secretogranins III–VII [78–87]	Secretogranin III (syn. 1B1075) not found in adrenal medulla. Presence of secretogranin IV (syn. HISL-19), V (syn. 7B2), VI (syn. NESP55) and VII (VGF) reported in human adrenal medulla, exact function still mainly unknown. Proposed role of secretogranin VII (syn. VGF) in the regulation of energy homeostasis.	More pronounced immunoreactivity of secretogranin IV in malignant PPGL compared to benign PPGL. Significantly higher plasma levels of secretogranin V in PPGL compared to age-matched normal subjects. Secretogranin VI immunoreactivity found in PPGL with no differences between benign and malignant tumors. Variable proVGF-immunoreactive fragments are observed in human PPGL.
Glycoproteins		
Glycoprotein I–V [88–90]	Glycoprotein I, i.e., DBH, catalyzes the conversion of dopamine into norepinephrine. Glycoprotein IV, i.e., the H^+-ATP-ase subunit M45, provides the driving force for vesicular uptake of catecholamines by VMAT.	High expression levels of glycoprotein I (DBH) are reported in PPGL.
Prohormone processing enzymes		
Aminopeptidase B (Ap-B) [91]	Exopeptidase involved in final conversion of proenkephalin to enkephalin.	Association of Ap-B with the secretory machinery is suggested in rat pheochromocytoma (PC12) cells.
Aspartic Proteinase [92]	Contributes to enkephalin precursor cleaving activity.	Unknown
Carboxypeptidase E (CPE) [93,94]	Role in peptide processing and sorting of prohormones.	High expression of CPE mRNA are reported. Elevated expression correlated with tumor growth and metastasis in pheochromocytomas. CPE promotes survival of pheochromocytoma (PC12) cells under nutrient starvation and hypoxic conditions by upregulation of pro-survival genes possibly by activation of the ERK1/2 pathway.
Cathepsin L [95,96]	Endopeptidase involved in proteolysis of proenkephalin into (Met)enkephalin. Proprotein convertase for biosynthesis of NPY and catestatin.	Unknown
Prohormone convertase 1/3 and 2 [73,78,97]	Conversion of chromogranin C into secretoneurin and EM66.	*PC1* and *PC2* mRNA expression levels are significantly higher in benign and malignant PPGL compared to normal adrenal medulla. mRNA expression and protein levels of *PC1* and *PC2* is 3–4 times higher in benign tumors compared to malignant tumors.
Tissue-Type Plasminogen Activator (t-PA) [98,99]	Participation in plasmin-dependent processing of bioactive peptides including chromogranin A and indirectly modulate chromogranin A release (negative-feedback loop).	Marked expressions of t-PA mRNA are reported in human pheochromocytomas.

Table 1. *Cont.*

Component	Function in Human Adrenal Medulla	Reported Alterations in PPGL
Granins		
Inhibitors of endogenous proteases		
Endopin 1–2 [100]	Endopin 1 inhibits trypsin-like serine proteases. Endopin 2 inhibits papain-like cysteine proteases, including cathepsin L, as well as the serine protease elastase.	Unknown
Transmitter peptides		
Adrenomedullin [65,101–105]	Increases blood flow in the adrenal gland. Increases catecholamine release. Induces systemic vasodilation. Increases natriuresis.	High plasma levels are reported, especially in PPGL patients with high blood pressure.
Bombesin [106–108]	Modulation of stress response. Paracrine regulatory effects on growth, structure and function of the adrenal cortex.	Highly variable immunoreactivity in pheochromocytomas and paragangliomas. An association between clinically malignant PPGL and lower expression of bombesin is postulated.
Calcitonin Gene-Related Peptide [109,110]	Vasodilatation, enhances aldosterone and corticosterone release by adrenocortical cells.	Slightly elevated levels are reported.
Catestatin, Cateslytin [111,112]	Inhibits release of catecholamines, chromogranin A, NPY, and ATP by acting as noncompetitive antagonist of the nicotinic receptor.	Unknown
EM66 (via PACAP) [73,113,114]	Derivate from chromogranin C (syn. secretogranin II). Synthesis and secretion regulated by PACAP. Paracrine regulation of steroidogenic cells in the adrenal gland.	Elevated in PPGL. Higher levels of EM66 reported in benign vs. malignant PPGL.
Natriuretic peptides (ANP, BNP, CNP) [102,115,116]	Autocrine/paracrine inhibition of catecholamine secretion via the ANF-R2 receptor subtype. Inhibition of aldosterone production by a direct action on the adrenal cortex both in vivo and in vitro.	Elevated in PPGL patients with high blood pressure.
Neuropeptide Y (NPY) [65,76,101,117–122]	Increases catecholamine biosynthesis (stimulates *TH* gene expression) and secretion. Potentiates catecholamine induced vasoconstriction.	Influence on tumorigenesis and stimulation of neoangiogenesis is described. High levels of NPY mRNA have been found in benign tumors, whereas its plasma levels are elevated in patients with malignant PPGL. Significantly lower expression level of NPY in *VHL* associated PPGL compared to other hereditary and sporadic PPGL is reported.
Neurotensin [123,124]	Not detected in human adrenal medulla. Various central and peripheral effects have been postulated in bovine, cat and rat, e.g., hypotension, hypothermia, analgesia.	Neurotensin has rarely been demonstrated in human PPGL.
Opioid peptides (enkephalins, endorphins) [96,117,125–128]	Decrease catecholamine release via binding G_i protein coupled receptor resulting in inhibition of Ca^{2+} channels Analgesia, enhancement of immune reaction.	Enkephalin decreases norepinephrine release in human pheochromocytomas. Different enkephalins (i.e., (Met)enkephalin, (Leu)enkephalin) are observed in human pheochromocytomas. Expression of (Met) enkephalin and (Leu)enkephalin is highly variable compared to normal adrenal medulla. Possible association between malignant PPGL and lower expression of enkephalins.
PACAP [40,63,101,117,129,130]	Induces transcription and stimulates activity of TH, DBH, and PNMT Stimulates expression and secretion of several other peptides e.g., brain natriuretic peptide, enkephalins, EM66, and secretoneurin.	High mRNA expression of PACAP and PAC1-R in PPGL reported. Comparable expression levels in benign and metastatic PPGL found in a relatively small series.
Secretoneurin (via PACAP) [131–133]	Derivate from chromogranin C (syn. secretogranin II). Synthesis and secretion regulated by PACAP. Role in angiogenesis and modulation of inflammatory response by chemoattractant effects on monocytes, eosinophils, fibroblasts, vascular smooth muscle cells, and endothelial cells.	Unknown

Table 1. *Cont.*

Component	Function in Human Adrenal Medulla	Reported Alterations in PPGL
Transforming Growth Factor β [134–136]	Role in regulation of chromaffin cell proliferation and differentiation. Reduction of TGF β has been shown to increase proliferation of chromaffin cell in vivo.	Unknown
Granins		
Vasostatins [137–139]	The N-terminal fragment of chromogranin A Inhibition of endothelin-induced vasoconstriction Antibacterial and antifungal activity.	Unknown
Anti-bacterial/anti-fungal peptides		
Chromacin P, G and PG [140]	Antibacterial activity against Gram positive bacteria.	Unknown
Secretolytin [141]	Antibacterial activity against Gram positive bacteria.	Unknown
Ubifungin [142]	Antifungal activity.	Unknown
Other minor components		
Ascorbic acid [143]	Regulation of DBH activity.	Unknown
Coenzyme A glutathione disulfide [144]	Vasoconstriction, modulation of AngII effects.	Unknown
Ions (Ca^{2+}, Na^{+}, K^{+}, Mg^{2+}, Cl^{-}) [145]	Regulation of exocytosis.	Unknown
Galanin [81,146,147]	Stimulation of norepinephrine and glucocorticoid secretion.	Immunoreactivity in human PPGL. Higher levels reported in PPGL compared to normal adrenal medulla. Variable expression; galanin was predominantly found in noradrenergic pheochromocytoma cells. Induction of apoptosis in PC12 cells. Inhibition of dopamine secretion in pheochromocytoma cells.
Nucleotides (ATP, ADP, GTP) [148]	Formation of intravesicular complex with catecholamines, buffer function, decreases intravesicular osmotic pressure, neuromodulation.	Unknown
Substance P [149–153]	Inhibition of nicotinic acetylcholine receptor mediated catecholamine release. Vasodilation.	Variable immunoreactivity demonstrated in human pheochromocytomas. Elevated plasma levels in minority of patients.
Vasoactive intestinal polypeptide [154–156]	Stimulation of catecholamine release, stimulation of steroid secretion.	Few cases described of human PPGL with concomitant excessive VIP secretion.

Abbreviations: ANF-R2, atrial natriuretic factor receptor subtype 2; AngII, angiotensin II; CGA, Chromogranin A; CGB, Chromogranin B; CGC, Chromogranin C; DBH, dopamine β-hydroxylase; HISL-19, human islet cell antigen 19; NESP55, neuroendocrine secretory protein 55; NPY, Neuropeptide Y; PACAP, pituitary adenylate cyclase-activating polypeptide; PAC1-R, PACAP-preferring receptor; PC, Prohormone-Converting Enzymes; TH, tyrosine hydroxylase.

Among these substances, chromogranin A and the trophic and secretion stimulating peptides pituitary adenylate cyclase-activating polypeptide (PACAP), neuropeptide Y (NPY), and adrenomedullin (AM) have gained the most attention because of their endocrine, paracrine, and autocrine effects, their importance for vesiculogenesis, and their possible roles in neoplastic chromaffin cell proliferation, differentiation, and survival, as further discussed below [62–65,101,113,129,157].

2.2. *Storage and Secretion of Catecholamines*

2.2.1. Storage and Vesicular Transmembrane Dynamics

In adrenomedullary chromaffin cells, catecholamines are stored in specialized vesicles. The bidirectional vesicular–cytosolic exchange of catecholamines is a dynamic process of active uptake into these chromaffin storage vesicles and passive leakage from vesicles into the cytosol [3]. After synthesis, dopamine and epinephrine are actively transported from the cytosol into chromaffin storage vesicles by vesicular monoamine transporters (VMAT1 and VMAT2) [158,159]. The driving force for this active transport is provided by an ATP-dependent vesicular membrane proton pump that maintains a transvesicular hydrogen ion (H^+) electrochemical gradient by acidifying the vesicle matrix. Vesicular uptake for catecholamines via VMAT is accompanied by exchange of an H+ ion from the vesical matrix towards the cytosol [62,160] (Figure 1).

2.2.2. Characteristics of Chromaffin Storage Vesicles

Chromaffin storage vesicles are highly specialized organelles of the chromaffin cells for storage and exocytosis. These membrane-bound electron-dense organelles originate from the Golgi network and are 150 to 350 nm in diameter. Each adrenomedullary chromaffin cell contains about 12,000 to 30,000 of these vesicles, corresponding (on average) to 13.5% of the cytoplasmic cell volume [63,65].

The adrenal medulla of some species harbors two distinct populations of chromaffin cells, which either produce epinephrine or norepinephrine depending on the presence or the absence of PNMT [3,11,63]. The proportion of epinephrine versus norepinephrine producing chromaffin cells in the adrenal medulla varies between species, but the adrenergic phenotype usually predominates [3,6,62,63,161]. This is particularly so in humans, where most chromaffin cells appear to have mixed function [6,11,62,161,162]. Nevertheless, there are clear ultrastructural differences between epinephrine and norepinephrine-containing vesicles when studied by electron microscopy. Epinephrine-containing vesicles are round or elongated in shape and demonstrate fine granular, medium-density vesicles with a characteristic narrow and uniform peripheral halo, whereas norepinephrine-containing vesicles demonstrate a high density and homogeneous content with a limiting membrane, which may be separated from the matrix constituents by a prominent lucent halo.

The mechanisms initiating and regulating the biogenesis of chromaffin vesicles are largely unknown. It is believed that structural proteins of the granin family, in particular chromogranin A, have an important role in vesiculogenesis, providing structural domains that drive chromaffin vesicle formation in the Golgi network. Furthermore, the ability of chromogranin A to bind catecholamines is thought to regulate stability of the vesicle by reducing osmotic pressure, thereby preventing vesicles from bursting; it is also thought to protect catecholamines against enzymatic degradation until secretion is warranted [27,63,65].

After the formation of chromaffin vesicles, maturation continues with catecholamine synthesis and storage not occurring until late in vesicle formation [63]. Fully matured chromaffin vesicles remain in the chromaffin cell until stimulation for exocytosis [63,65].

The molecular composition of chromaffin vesicles is complex. Besides catecholamines, intravesicular contents include a diverse mixture of peptides, proteases, enzymes, and granins (chromogranins, secretogranins) with a multiplicity of functions (Table 1). The high concentration of regulatory and modulating peptides and proteins reflects broad endocrine, paracrine, and autocrine functions of adrenomedullary chromaffin vesicles. The physiological processes modulated by these constituents not only involve the fine-tuning of catecholamine biosynthesis and secretion but also encompass various analgesic, immunomodulatory, antimicrobial, and anti-inflammatory responses to cell stress [62,63].

2.2.3. Secretion and Re-Uptake of Catecholamines

After exocytosis of storage vesicles and secretion of catecholamines into the bloodstream, norepinephrine and epinephrine are removed from the circulation by neural and extra-neuronal monoamine transporters and are inactivated by metabolizing enzymes [163]. The re-uptake mechanism through the norepinephrine transporter (NET) by catecholamine synthesizing cells is only relevant in sympathetic postganglionic and central nervous system neurons and provides rapid termination of the neurotransmitter signal at the postsynaptic membrane and enables recycling of catecholamines for re-release. NET is not only located presynaptically but also at several extraneuronal sites, including the adrenal medulla [31,163,164]. The precise function of the NET in the adrenal gland is, however, not entirely clear. A detailed discussion of reuptake as well as pre- and postsynaptic effects of catecholamines is beyond the scope of the current review, and for further reading, we refer to the literature [163,165,166].

2.3. *Regulation of Adrenomedullary Activity*

2.3.1. Stimulus-Dependent Exocytosis in Adrenal Chromaffin Cells

Exocytosis of chromaffin storage vesicles is a tightly controlled process. Under basal conditions, only a few secretory vesicles are released into the circulation, resulting in a catecholamine secretion rate in the order of nanograms per minute [117]. Toxic effects of excessive chronic catecholamine release such as in heart failure, pulmonary edema, and malignant hypertension have been reported from incessant circulating catecholamine concentrations of 10^{-6} mol/L or more, corresponding to the release of 5% of all adrenomedullary chromaffin vesicles [167]. In acute stress situations, the amount of released vesicles from the total adrenal gland can be temporarily greatly increased, with plasma catecholamine concentrations reaching up to 60 times more than normal [117,167]. Well-known stimuli that activate the exocytotic process are hypoglycaemia, hypovolemia, hypotension, hypoxemia, and severe pain or emotional distress [3].

The rather complex mechanisms regulating chromaffin cell exocytotic machinery are executed at neuronal and non-neuronal levels [145,167–169]. It is thought that each adrenomedullary chromaffin cell receives its own individual neuronal and non-neuronal input [167].

At a neuronal level, adrenomedullary chromaffin cells are innervated by the cholinergic preganglionic sympathetic fibers of the splanchnic nerve. One single chromaffin cell can receive input by up to five synapses [170]. Acetylcholine released by these nerve endings predominantly binds to nicotinic receptors on the chromaffin cell, resulting in membrane depolarization with subsequent calcium influx followed by stimulation of exocytosis and catecholamine secretion. Cholinergic receptors of the muscarinic type are also expressed on the chromaffin cell, but their contribution to catecholamine secretion is less important. Further enhancement of the stimulation–secretion coupling is provided by propagation of the secretion signal via gap junctions between chromaffin cells formed by connexins, which are specific proteins involved in cell-to-cell communication. This intercellular communication can be upregulated in stressful conditions [170]. Besides acetylcholine, splanchnic nerve terminals also contain PACAP as a neurotransmitter. This neuropeptide is not only stored in chromaffin vesicles and co-secreted with catecholamines but also acts as an important neurotransmitter at the splanchnic medullary synapse, where it activates the PACAP-preferring receptor (PAC1-R) on the postsynaptic membrane of the chromaffin cell. Laboratory experiments have shown that PACAP is only released at high frequencies of nerve stimulation, which is the firing rate occurring in stress conditions. In contrast to the acetylcholine evoked catecholamine secretion, adrenomedullary stimulation by PACAP is not susceptible to desensitization, which ensures robust catecholamine release under conditions of continuous stress (Figure 2) [40,130].

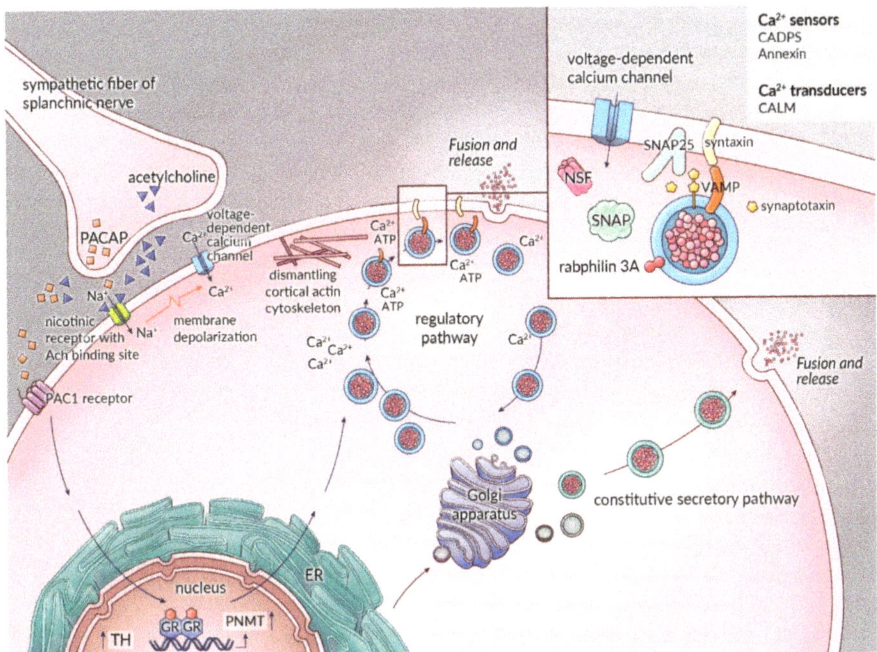

Figure 2. Schematic overview of the stimulation–secretion coupling in the adrenomedullary chromaffin cell with the multiple functionally definable stages and the different secretory pathways. Abbreviations: ER: endoplasmic reticulum; Ach: acetylcholine; VAMP: vesicle-associated membrane protein; SNAP: synaptosomal-associated protein; NSF: N-ethylmaleimide Soluble Factor proteins; CADPS: Ca^{2+} dependent secretion activator; CALM: calmodulin; PACAP: pituitary adenylate cyclase-activating polypeptide; PAC1 receptor: PACAP-preferring receptor; GR: glucocorticoid receptor.

Non-neuronal regulation of exocytosis occurs predominantly through autocrine or paracrine routes. As a result, cellular catecholamine secretion is partially under the influence of the exocytotic activity of neighboring chromaffin cells [167]. Furthermore, both lipopolysaccharide and cytokine receptors were recently demonstrated on chromaffin cells, pointing towards a role of the adrenal medulla in the complex regulation of the inflammatory stress response [40].

In general, the exocytotic secretion of vesicular contents of adrenomedullary chromaffin cells can be achieved via regulated and constitutive secretory pathways. The regulated secretory pathway provides the principle mechanism responsible for controlled release of catecholamines and is calcium-dependent and responsive to both neuronal and non-neuronal input. In contrast, the constitutive secretory pathway, which is calcium-independent, is mainly unresponsive to neuronal and non-neuronal input. The principal function of the constitutive secretory pathway is thought to be the transport of proteins and macromolecules to the cell surface for purposes of membrane maintenance and support of the extracellular matrix. In addition, this pathway may also contribute to basal release of catecholamines (Figure 2) [145,169].

2.3.2. Neuronal Regulation of the Calcium-Dependent Catecholamine Secretory Pathway

In recent years, considerable progress has been made in unravelling the complex molecular background and the functional elements of the highly regulated exocytotic machinery in adrenomedullary chromaffin cells (Figure 2) [145,171,172]. Release of acetylcholine by the splanchnic nerve activates the nicotinic receptor on chromaffin cells, resulting in opening of the ionophoric part of the receptor protein, thereby allowing the entry of extracellular sodium (Na^+) and calcium (Ca^{2+}). This generates a small membrane depolarization, resulting in the opening of voltage dependent Na^+ channels. The subsequent Na^+ influx results in a large membrane depolarization, which opens various types of voltage dependent Ca^{2+} channels [167].

The distribution of the different calcium channel subtypes is species specific. The P/Q-type calcium channel predominates in human adrenomedullary chromaffin cells [167,171,172]. As a consequence of elevated intracellular Ca^{2+} concentrations, the exocytotic machinery and the regulatory components for vesicular exocytosis are activated, which occurs through a pathway consisting of secretory vesicle recruitment, docking, priming, and fusion with the plasma membrane. Priming is the process in which secretory vesicles become fusion competent [167,172]. First, Ca^{2+} influx leads to dismantling of the cortical actin cytoskeleton of the chromaffin cell, a dynamic network of numerous cytoplasmic proteins located on the inner face of the chromaffin cell membrane [173]. Although this can be activated without Ca^{2+}, this is mainly an ATP and a Ca^{2+} dependent step, as are recruitment, tethering, and docking of the vesicles.

Fusion, release, and retrieval of vesicles can be triggered by Ca^{2+} in the absence of ATP [145,174]. Various soluble and membrane-bound proteins are involved in the complex protein–protein interactions underlying membrane trafficking and fusion. Key components of this process are *N*-ethylmaleimide soluble factor proteins (soluble cytosolic NSF), soluble NSF attachment proteins (SNAPs), and soluble NSF attachment receptor proteins (SNAREs). The vesicle-associated membrane protein (VAMP or synaptobrevin) and the calcium binding protein synaptotagmin are SNAREs located at the secretory vesicle membrane. The synaptosomal-associated protein 25 (SNAP-25) and syntaxin are SNAREs acting on the chromaffin cell plasma membrane [145,167,172]. The complex formed by chromaffin vesicle SNAREs (VAMP, synaptotagmin), the chromaffin cell membrane SNAREs (syntaxin, SNAP-25), and the cytosolic proteins (NSF) is thought to provide the primary molecular machinery responsible for the docking and the fusion of synaptic vesicles at the chromaffin cell plasma membrane (Figure 2) [174]. Furthermore, it is believed that NSF and SNAPs have multiple sites of actions on SNARE proteins. Besides pre-docking actions and their function as molecular chaperones in SNARE priming, they also act on SNAREs post-fusion to facilitate vesicle retrieval and allow recycling of empty vesicles [145,167,172,174].

Apart from NSF, SNAPs, and SNAREs, several other proteins are involved in calcium triggered exocytosis. Proposed candidates are the stabilizing protein Munc18-1, the calcium transducer calmodulin (CALM), the Ca^{2+} dependent secretion activator (CAPS), rabphilin, and annexins [169,172,174]. Rabphilin3A is a small GTP-ase, which acts as a molecular switch, thereby determining the sensitivity of secretory vesicles for docking and fusion. Overexpression of rabphilin3A has been found to inhibit exocytosis in adrenomedullary chromaffin cells and probably protects against spontaneous exocytosis under basal conditions [175]. Annexins have the ability to form cross-links between secretory vesicles and the plasma membrane by a functional interplay with SNAREs during exocytosis [145,169,176–178].

2.3.3. Non-Neuronal Regulation of Catecholamine Secretion

Along with catecholamines, the adrenal medulla synthesizes and releases numerous enzymes, peptides, and proteins that exert various trophic and neurotransmitter activities, which provide fine-tuning of catecholamine synthesis and secretion in an autocrine and a paracrine manner [62–65,101,111,113,117,118,129,157] (Table 1). We discuss here in more detail neuropeptide Y (NPY), adrenomedullin (AM), PACAP, and the secretion-inhibiting peptide catestatin [101,111,117,118,129]. These peptides modulate chromaffin cell function through a variety of membrane receptors, the vast majority of which belong to the family of G protein-coupled receptors (GPCRs) [117].

Neuropeptide Y is a 36-amino acid neuropeptide, which is widely and abundantly distributed in the brain and the sympathetic nervous system, including the human adrenal medulla. Several NPY receptors (i.e., Y1, Y2, Y4, and Y5) are expressed in the adrenal gland, indicating that NPY exerts local autocrine effects. It has been shown that NPY is able to stimulate catecholamine secretion by inducing TH expression and increasing intracellular calcium [63,101,117,118,129,179].

Adrenomedullin (AM) is a 52-amino acid peptide originally isolated from a human pheochromocytoma and also is present at high concentrations in the normal adrenal medulla [101,117,129]. AM demonstrates autocrine and paracrine effects through binding to the adrenomedullin receptor (ADMR), the receptor dog cDNA (RDC1), and the calcitonin receptor-like receptor (CRLR), which results in augmentation of the adrenal blood flow and stimulation of catecholamine release. In addition, the endocrine effects of AM include systemic vasodilatation and stimulation of natriuresis [63,101,117,129].

As previously mentioned, PACAP not only acts as a neurotransmitter released by the splanchnic nerve but is also co-secreted with catecholamines, exerting its effects by binding to the PACAP-preferring receptor (PAC1-R) and VIP/PACAP receptors (VPAC1-R and VPAC2-R), the former representing the predominant receptor in chromaffin cells (Figure 2) [101,117,129]. PACAP, a neuropeptide of 27 or 38 amino acids, enhances catecholamine secretion by induction of transcription as well as stimulating the activity of the biosynthetic enzymes TH, DBH, and PNMT [101]. In normal adrenal medullary chromaffin cells, PACAP also stimulates the expression and the secretion of several other peptides, such as brain natriuretic peptide, enkephalins, EM66, and secretoneurin, which in turn exert their own individual autocrine/paracrine effects on catecholamine secretion [40,63,101,117,129,130].

Catestatin is a biologically active peptide fragment derived from proteolytic chromogranin A cleavage [63]. Catestatin acts mainly as a noncompetitive nicotinic cholinergic antagonist, thus providing a strong negative feedback inhibition of catecholamine secretion [111,112].

3. Pheochromocytoma and Paraganglioma

From a genetic perspective, pheochromocytomas and paragangliomas (PPGL) have one of the richest hereditary backgrounds among all neoplasms. At least 35—perhaps up to 40%—of all PPGL harbor a germline pathogenic variant in one of the several susceptibility genes [180–184]. Initial gene expression profiling studies by Dahia et al. in 2005 [185] revealed two cluster groups, designated cluster 1 and cluster 2, that reflected respective activation of pseudohypoxia and kinase signaling pathways. Those different gene expression signatures matched closely to those reported in an earlier study for norepinephrine- versus epinephrine-producing sporadic tumors and tumors from patients with von-Hippel Lindau (VHL) syndrome and multiple endocrine neoplasia type 2 (MEN2) [186]. The molecular characterization from The Cancer Genome Atlas (TCGA) project has more recently provided a sophisticated molecular taxonomy of PPGL, which divides these neuroendocrine tumors into groups with similar pathogenesis and molecular biology and provides an up-to-date framework (Figure 3) [187–189]. The recent identification of newly recognized somatic mutations in the driver genes, *Cold shock domain-containing E1 (CSDE1)* and *Mastermind-like transcriptional coactivator 3 (MAML3)*, could add a third cluster—i.e., the Wnt altered group [187]—to the original classification of Dahia et al. of 2005 [185]. This cluster 3 is associated with an abnormal activation of the Wnt-signaling pathway.

Cluster 1, the pseudohypoxia group, can be subdivided into a tricarboxylic acid (TCA) cycle- and a *VHL/EPAS1* related group. The TCA cycle-related subgroup consists of germline pathogenic variants in genes encoding fumarate hydratase *(FH)* or one of the succinate dehydrogenase *(SDH)* subunits A, B, C, D, or the complex assembly factor 2 (AF2). Germline pathogenic variants in *Malate Dehydrogenase 2 (MDH2)* and somatic mutations in *Isocitrate Dehydrogenase type 2 (IDH2)* genes also can be categorized in this subgroup [190,191]. The *VHL/EPAS1*-related subgroup consists of germline and somatic pathogenic variants in the genes *VHL* and *EPAS1* [encoding the hypoxia inducible factor 2α (HIF2α) protein] [192]. In addition, it was proposed that mutations in genes encoding prolyl hydroxylase 1 (*PHD1*, also known as egl nine homolog 2; *EGLN2*) and iron regulatory protein 1 *(IRP1)* should also be considered as members of this subgroup [193].

Pseudohypoxia *15-20% PPGL*	**Wnt signaling** *5-10% PPGL*	**Kinase signaling** *50-60% PPGL*
Driver genes	Driver genes	Driver genes
TCA cycle + *Germline 100%* FH, MDH2, SDHx *TCA cycle -* *Germline 25%* VHL, PHD1, IRP1, EPAS1	*Germline 0%* CSDE1, MAML3	*Germline 20%* RET, NF1, MAX, TMEM127, HRAS
Biochemical	Biochemical	Biochemical
NE DA NMN/3-MT VMAT high no PNMT NE NMN VMAT high no PNMT	NE (E) NMN/MN VMAT low PNMT low	E NMN/MN PNMT high
Location	Location	Location
Adrenal, extra-adrenal	Adrenal	Adrenal
Chromaffin cell type	Chromaffin cell type	Chromaffin cell type
Immature, dedifferentiated exocytotic machinery	Intermediate	Mature, differentiated exocytotic machinery
Signs and symptoms	Signs and symptoms	Signs and symptoms
Sustained HT, constipation, sweating, headache	Mixed	Paroxysmal HT, flushing, palpitations
Secretory pathway	Secretory pathway	Secretory pathway
Constitutive pathway	Not known	Regulatory pathway
Metastatic disease risk	Metastatic disease risk	Metastatic disease risk
+	+/-	-
Future diagnostic options	Future diagnostic options	Future diagnostic options
Metabolic profiling Hypoxia imaging	Not known	Not known
Future treatment options	Future treatment options	Future treatment options
Methylome: TCA-cycle + = hypermethylation: demyelination azacytidine/decitabine **Metabolome:** TCA-cycle + glutaminase inhibitor (phase I) **Hypoxiome:** HIF1α/2α inhibitors and VEGF inhibition **Receptor targeted therapy:** SDHx: peptide receptor radionuclide therapy ^{90}Y or ^{177}LU somatostatin analogue (DOTATATE): targeted cytotoxic	Not known	**Influencing kinase pathway:** RET1: Tyrosine kinase inhibitors NF1: MEK inhibitors

Figure 3. The Pseudohypoxia group (cluster I) divided into two subgroups: tricarboxylic acid (TCA) cycle related, containing germline pathogenic variants in succinate dehydrogenase subunits *SDHA*, *SDHB*, *SDHC*, and *SDHD* as well as *SDHAF2 (SDHx)*, assembly factor for the succinate dehydrogenase

complex, and *FH*, a second enzyme in the tricarboxylic acid (TCA) cycle. The second subgroup: *VHL/EPAS1*—related with somatic and germline pathogenic variants. Pathogenic variants in three additional genes encoding for malate dehydrogenase 2 *(MDH2)*, prolyl hydroxylase 1 (*PHD1*, also known as egl nine homolog 2; *EGLN2*), and iron regulatory protein 1 *(IRP1)* were not included previously in the molecular classification by TCGA but were recently discovered. Based on their signaling pathways, it is believed that these new genes should be included as part of the cluster I pseudohypoxia group because *MDH2* is part of to the TCA cycle and both *PDH1* and *IRP1* belong to the *VHL/EPAS1* related subgroup. Cluster I is characterized by the expression of genes involved in the "hypoxic response", resulting in a "pseudo-hypoxic" phenotype with uncontrolled expression of HIF1α regulated genes such as VEGF. HIF1α regulates the transcription of genes associated with tumorigenesis and angiogenesis. *Wnt altered signaling group (cluster III)* consists of newly recognized somatic mutations in *CSDE1* as well as somatic gene fusions affecting *MAML3*. This group exclusively consists of somatic mutations that activate the Wnt pathway, which is not activated under normal conditions. Wnt signaling and therefore increased expression of β-catenin is associated with a poorer prognosis and a higher metastatic potential of tumors. There is still much unknown about this group. *Kinase signaling group (Cluster II)* consists of germline or somatic pathogenic variants in the driver genes *RET*, *NF1*, *TMEM127*, *MAX*, and *HRAS*. This cluster is characterized by an increased activation of the MAP kinase and the P13K/AKT pathways, which results in an increased expression of genes involved in protein synthesis, kinase signaling, endocytosis, and preservation of differentiated/mature chromaffin cell catecholamine biosynthetic machinery. *MAX* mutated tumors are an exception, since they show an intermediate catecholamine biochemical phenotype with detectable expression of PNMT and some production of epinephrine. *MAX* is a distinct sub-cluster of the kinase signaling group and was recently proposed to be possibly redivided in a new group, the cortical admixture group [187–189,193].

Cluster 2 related mutations are associated with abnormal kinase signaling pathways and include germline or somatic pathogenic variants in genes encoding for rearranged-during-transfection *(RET)*, neurofibromin *(NF1)*, transmembrane protein 127 *(TMEM127)*, MYC-associated factor X *(MAX)*, and Harvey rat sarcoma proto-oncogene *(H-RAS)* [193,194].

Each of these clusters is associated with unique downstream signaling pathways, which correspond to certain clinical features and offer potential targets for future diagnostic, therapeutic, and prognostic purposes (Figure 3).

The hallmark of pheochromocytomas and sympathetic paragangliomas is their ability to secrete catecholamines in an uncontrolled fashion compared to normal adrenomedullary chromaffin cells. Unlike normal adrenomedullary chromaffin cells, chromaffin tumor cells are not innervated, and catecholamine secretion is therefore not stimulated by the previously described neuronal stimuli [195]. Theoretically, and as discussed below, the hypersecretion of catecholamines could be explained by various perturbations of the molecular machinery involved in their biosynthesis, secretion, and metabolism.

3.1. *Increased Biosynthesis of Catecholamines*

The most obvious explanation for the hypersecretion of catecholamines by pheochromocytomas is the increased number of cells able to produce and secrete catecholamines. There are limited data on the tissue concentration of catecholamines in normal adrenal medulla as compared with pheochromocytoma, demonstrating either no difference or a higher content of epinephrine in the latter [88,195]. At the cellular level, there is evidence of an upregulation of expression and activity of the biosynthetic enzymes. In particular, Jarrot et al. [89] described in 1977 that the activity of TH, AADC, and DBH was enhanced in human pheochromocytoma compared to normal human adrenal medulla tissue specimens. These early observations were subsequently supported by several immunohistochemical studies [196–201].

Isobe et al. demonstrated that pheochromocytoma cells contained increased levels of mRNA encoding *TH*, *AADC*, and *DBH* compared to normal adrenal medulla [88]. They also found a strong positive correlation between *TH* mRNA concentration and total catecholamine content in pheochromocytomas that was absent in normal adrenal medulla tissue. Moreover, they found lower concentrations of *PNMT* mRNA in pheochromocytoma compared to normal adrenal medulla [88], which might be explained, in part, by lower concentrations of cortisol reaching tumor tissues [88,202]. Of interest, Kimura et al. [196] demonstrated that PNMT immunoreactivity was limited to the mixed epinephrine and norepinephrine producing pheochromocytomas, and tumor cells with PNMT tended to be located close to the adrenal cortex.

All above referenced studies involving comparisons of pheochromocytoma tissue with normal adrenal medulla must be interpreted cautiously since it is difficult to isolate normal adrenal medullary from cortical tissue and thereby establish true differences between normal and tumor cells [203]. What is clear is that catecholamine contents of pheochromocytoma or paraganglioma tumor tissue are highly variable, both in terms of total amounts and relative content of norepinephrine and epinephrine [195,199,204]. Most tumors produce relatively low amounts of dopamine, but there are exceptions, usually isolated paragangliomas presumably lacking significant expression of DBH [205–207].

3.1.1. Relationship between Genotype and Catecholamine Biochemical Phenotype

Mutation-dependent differentiation of the chromaffin progenitor cells influences the expression of the biosynthetic enzymes, which leads to distinct phenotypic features of the tumors [206]. Three biochemical phenotypes can be distinguished, i.e., noradrenergic, adrenergic, and dopaminergic, based on the main catecholamines that are produced. Typical pheochromocytomas produce both norepinephrine and epinephrine in variable proportions. A small subset of PPGL is biochemically silent, and almost all of these are paragangliomas [208,209].

The two gene expression clusters (cluster 1 and 2) described earlier are not only characterized by distinct patterns of gene activation but also distinct catecholamine biochemical phenotypes [186,207,210]. Cluster 2 tumors due to somatic and/or germline *NF1*, *RET*, *TMEM127*, *MAX*, and *HRAS* pathogenic variants, which are characterized by activated kinase and protein translation signaling pathways, almost always originate in the adrenals and produce epinephrine due to expression of PNMT. They have more mature catecholamine secretory pathways and phenotypic features [186,207,210] and also tend to develop later in life than tumors due to cluster 1 mutations.

In contrast, cluster 1 tumors with the pseudohypoxic phenotype due to germline pathogenic variants of *VHL*, *SDHx*, *FH*, and somatic mutations of *EPAS1* (HIF2α) occur with variable frequencies at extra-adrenal or adrenal locations and show negligible epinephrine production due to near absent expression of PNMT [186,187,207,210]. This is also independent of their adrenal or extra-adrenal locations due to hypermethylation of the *PNMT* promoter [211]. The underlying pseudohypoxic phenotype of cluster 1 tumors is due to HIF stabilization, and it appears that it is the stabilization of HIF2α that is more important than that of HIF1α for the distinct phenotypic features of cluster 1 compared to cluster 2 chromaffin cell tumors [186,212–215]. Indeed, HIF2α was identified in 2004 as a key differentially expressed gene, which is more highly expressed in noradrenergic tumors compared to adrenergic tumors, where its expression is essentially absent [186]. Mechanistic studies by Qin et al. [215] showed that expression and the stabilization of HIF2α in chromaffin cells that normally expressed PNMT and produced epinephrine resulted in complete suppression of steroid-induced induction of PNMT. Since HIF2α is expressed transiently in chromaffin progenitors during embryogenesis [216–218], it is possible that HIF2α stabilization may promote a noradrenergic rather than an adrenergic phenotype. This concept is supported by findings that transgenic mice with mutations that stabilize HIF2α are characterized by adrenals that express less PNMT and produce more norepinephrine than epinephrine compared to adrenals of wild type mice [219].

Thus, it seems that cluster 1 adrenal tumors arise from chromaffin progenitors in which both transcriptional expression of HIF2α and stabilization of the translated HIF2α protein blocks the effects of steroids produced locally by cortical cells, explaining why these tumors in the end do not produce epinephrine. Such influences occurring during embryogenesis could also be responsible for the younger age of presentation of patients with cluster 1 compared to cluster 2 tumors as well as their propensity for a multifocal presentation [211].

The effect of HIF2α to block steroid induced expression of PNMT and other genes is suggested to involve a mechanism involving the MYC/MAX complex and MYC-mediated control of gene transcription [215]. A role of MAX is indicated by the demonstration that, in rat PC12 pheochromocytoma cells, which lack a functional *MAX* gene, re-expression of MAX facilitates return of steroid-induced PNMT expression. In contrast, silencing MAX in pheochromocytoma cells that express PNMT results in attenuated steroid-induced PNMT [215]. This provides a potential point of intersection for almost all upstream tumor susceptibility genes and also explains the catecholamine biochemical phenotype of MAX-mutated pheochromocytomas, which express some PNMT and produce some epinephrine, though in amounts that lie in between cluster 1 and cluster 2 tumors [207,220].

3.1.2. Relationship between Genotype and Catecholamine Secretory Pathways

The two distinct genetic clusters seem to be not only associated with differences in biochemical profile but also with variations in secretory processes. For example, data derived from microarrays and proteomics have shown reduced expression of various components of the regulated secretory pathway (e.g., SNAP25, syntaxin, rabphilin 3A, annexin) in *VHL*-related pheochromocytomas compared to *RET*-related pheochromocytomas [169]. In addition, the rate constant for baseline catecholamine secretion was found to be 20-fold higher in *VHL*- than in *RET*-related pheochromocytoma. Moreover, only in *RET*-mutated tumors catecholamine, secretion was shown to be responsive to glucagon. These observations suggest that catecholamine secretion in *VHL*-associated pheochromocytomas exhibits more constitutive-like continuous secretory characteristics, whereas in *RET*-associated pheochromocytomas, secretion still is constrained by expression of many components of the regulated secretory pathway. Thus, differences in the molecular machinery underlying catecholamine exocytosis may explain the more paroxysmal nature of symptoms and signs in patients with MEN2 as compared to those with the VHL syndrome. In addition, it was demonstrated that the expression of *VMAT1* mRNA was significantly higher in pheochromocytomas from VHL compared to MEN2 patients [164,189]. In addition, higher levels of *VMAT1* correlated with lower tumor tissue contents of catecholamines and lower numbers of catecholamine containing vesicles, which likely reflects the higher turnover of catecholamines in noradrenergic *VHL*-related compared to adrenergic pheochromocytomas [164].

3.2. Alterations in Chromaffin Cell Pathways Associated with Metastatic Pheochromocytoma and Paraganglioma

3.2.1. Clinical Features and Risk Factors

The majority of PPGLs are characterized by a benign clinical course. In 10–15% of cases, however, metastases are present at diagnosis or will develop during follow-up. The most common metastatic sites for chromaffin cell tumors are local lymph nodes, bone, liver, and lung [221]. At the moment, there are no discriminative histopathological features by which the biological behavior of a pheochromocytoma or a paraganglioma can be assessed or predicted reliably [222–225]. Therefore, the most recent WHO Classification of Endocrine Organs states that all chromaffin cell tumors are considered to have metastatic potential for which long-term follow-up of patients is required, even after successful resection of a pheochromocytoma or a paraganglioma [221].

Several clinical risk factors have been identified that confer an increased risk for development of metastatic disease. Large size (in general > 5 cm) and extra-adrenal location of the primary tumor are associated with metastatic disease [226–230]. Although representing about 20% of the chromaffin cell tumors, sympathetic paragangliomas are the primary source for about 60% of cases with metastatic PPGL [229].

Germline pathogenic variants of the *SDHB* gene are present in a relatively high frequency of 8–10% in patients with a PPGL [184]. Large cohort studies targeted at the genotype–phenotype relationship have shown that, in particular carriers of an *SDHB* germline, pathogenic variants have an increased risk of metastatic PPGL [184,230–232]. Typical *SDHB* related PPGLs occur at a younger age and arise more frequently in extra-adrenal locations [233]. A possible increased predisposition to metastatic disease has been suggested for rare germline pathogenic variants in *FH* [234], *SLC25A11* [235], *SDHA*, and *TMEM127* [236], although the number of cases is quite low, making the association difficult to confirm.

In addition to size and location of the PPGL and the presence of certain germline mutations, the risk of metastatic disease is also increased in association with certain alterations in the biochemical profile [237]. In particular, plasma concentrations of dopamine and its metabolite 3-methoxytyramine are significantly higher in patients with metastatic PPGL compared to those with non-metastatic disease [237,238]. Most patients with metastatic PPGLs demonstrate a noradrenergic profile with elevated plasma levels of both norepinephrine and normetanephrine, with concomitant lack of or negligible relative increases in plasma concentrations of epinephrine and metanephrine compared to subjects without metastatic disease [237,239]. In a relatively large series of patients with metastatic PPGL, only a minority (11%) of patients had an adrenergic phenotype. Of note, none of these patients had a *SDHB*-related pheochromocytoma or paraganglioma [240]. The biochemical profile has also been linked to prognosis, as it was shown that patients with elevated plasma levels of dopamine and norepinephrine had a faster progression of their disease [239].

3.2.2. Molecular Alterations in SDHx-Related PPGL and Their Effect on Catecholamine Biosynthesis

The SDH complex is a hetero-tetrameric mitochondrial enzyme that consists of two catalytic subunits (SDHA and SDHB) and two membrane-anchoring subunits (SDHC and SDHD). SDH catalyzes the oxidation of succinate to fumarate in the TCA cycle and transfers electrons to the ubiquinone (coenzyme Q) pool in the respiratory chain. SDH assembly factor (SDHAF) is required for the flavination of SDHA, an essential step in formation of the SDH complex.

SDH deficiency leads to the accumulation of succinate, which has structural similarity to 2-ketoglutarate. Succinate is therefore able to act as a competitive inhibitor of 2-ketogluarate-dependent dioxygenases, which include prolyl hydroxylase domain proteins (PHDs), ten-eleven translocation (TET) enzymes, and jumonji-domain histone demethylases (JmjC) demethylases [241,242]. This results in hypermethylation of CpG (cytosine preceding guanine) islands, regions within the genome that are common in promoter sites rich in CpG dinucleotides. Succinate is a typical example of an oncometabolite, a metabolite that abnormally accumulates in cancer cells as a result of a defective gene encoding the corresponding enzyme, thereby modifying signaling pathways and epigenetic regulation mechanisms. In the study by Letouzé et al. [211], the level of hypermethylation was significantly higher in *SDHB* compared to other *SDHx* mutated tumors. Of interest, it was shown that succinate:fumarate ratios were higher in tumor tissue derived from patients with a *SDHB* pathogenic variant as compared from those with a *SDHC/D* pathogenic variant [243]. This suggests that functional activity of the SDH complex is most disrupted in the case of mutations of the SDHB subunit, resulting in higher intracellular concentrations of oncometabolites and a concurrent higher metastatic risk.

PHDs are involved in the inactivation of the HIF, a heterodimer that consists of two subunits, one α subunit and one β subunit. There are two different α-subunits (HIF1α and HIF2α) and two different β subunits (HIF1 β and aryl hydrocarbon receptor nuclear translocator ARNT2). The β subunits are constitutively expressed, whereas HIF1α and HIF2α are inactivated in the presence of oxygen through hydroxylation by PHDs and subsequent degradation by the VHL–ubiquitination complex (pVHL). The hydroxylation reaction performed by the PHDs requires oxygen and α-ketoglutarate as substrates as well as iron and ascorbate as cofactors [244].

Thus, PHD is inactive in the presence of hypoxia, resulting in stabilization of HIFα. The unmodified HIFα molecule translocates to the nucleus, where it forms a transcriptionally active heterodimer together with a HIFβ subunit, which is able to stimulate various target genes involved in angiogenesis, energy metabolism, and cell survival.

The epigenetic modifications are thought to play an important role in tumorigenesis by deregulating gene expression of key genes. Methylome analysis of a large PPGL cohort demonstrated a clear hypermethylator phenotype in the *SDHx*-related tumors [211].

Besides the *PNMT* gene, three other genes involved in the catecholamine pathway were also found to be hypermethylated, i.e., *DRD2*, *NPY*, and *SLC6A2* [211]. Transcription of *DRD2* results in the synthesis of the D2-dopamine receptor, and the *SLC6A2* gene or *solute carrier family 6, member 2* gene encodes the norepinephrine transporter (NET) responsible for reuptake of norepinephrine into presynaptic nerve terminals.

3.2.3. Relationship between Other Components of the Exocytotic Machinery and Metastatic Disease

The co-secreted neuropeptides neuropeptide Y, adrenomedullin, and PACAP are overexpressed in pheochromocytomas and stimulate catecholamine release [129]. These neuropeptides have also been implicated in influencing cell survival and tumor growth of PPGLs (Table 1) [119,120,129]. High expression levels of the adrenomedullin receptor RDC1 were demonstrated in a small series of metastatic PPGL. Overexpression of the adrenomedullin receptor RDC1 has been described in several cancers and has been found to be associated with invasiveness, survival, proliferation, and neo-angiogenesis [129]. These observations suggest a pathophysiological role of the adrenomedullin receptor RDC1 in metastatic PPGL.

Recently, overexpression of LAT-1, and to a lesser extent of LAT-2, has been demonstrated in pheochromocytoma. Moreover, LAT-1 overexpression was strongly correlated with higher levels of urinary catecholamine excretion. It seems plausible that this enhanced expression of LAT is required to ensure a sufficient supply of tyrosine as substrate for the increased catecholamine synthesis. Of interest, LAT-1 expression has been described as a poor prognostic marker in various malignancies, including lung, pancreas, breast, and hepatocellular cancer [245]. It is currently unknown whether LAT expression has any prognostic value in PPGL [246–249].

Connexins (Cx) are the specialized proteins of gap junctions, and these structures play an important role in cell proliferation and differentiation as well as in carcinogenesis. The connexion family consists of 21 different proteins, and it has been demonstrated that the expression pattern of connexins in pheochromocytomas is different from normal adrenal medulla tissue [170,250]. In addition, the expression of Cx50 was lower in metastatic as compared to benign pheochromocytomas [250]. However, data on the association between connexion expression pattern and biological behavior of pheochromocytomas are very limited.

In summary, our understanding of the intracellular molecular intricacies associated with metastatic PPGL has greatly improved in recent years. Although elucidation of these pathways is still incomplete, research of the genome–metabolome–phenotype relationship has already generated exciting and clinically important information of these rare neuro-endocrine tumors.

4. Conclusions and Future Perspectives

In conclusion, our increased knowledge of catecholamine synthesis, secretion, and regulation has improved our understanding of chromaffin cell tumorigenesis. Disregulation of these pathways is evident in pheochromocytomas and paragangliomas and varies between the different genomic backgrounds of the tumors. For example, the differences in PNMT, VMAT, RDC1, and LAT1 expression may signify a difference in cellular dedifferentiation, making certain tumors more aggressive. In addition, substances such as neuropeptide Y, PACAP, EM66, bombesin, and connexins might be differentially expressed by benign and metatstatic PPGL. These potential prognostic biomarkers will need to be examined in larger and more broad cohorts of PPGLs and in prospective studies to determine their true potential utility as prognostic markers. Moreover, further studies of chromaffin cell products with an unknown role in PPGL (Table 1) might also reveal clinically useful information.

Future research will continue to provide novel and relevant information that will enhance our current knowledge with respect to both the physiology and the pathophysiology of the chromaffin cell. To this end, an integrative and translational approach is required by combining clinical information with (epi)genomics, transcriptomics, and metabolomics. Such new information could, for example, elucidate the precise relationship between the net effect of the mixture of substances that are co-secreted with catecholamines and the clinical picture. In addition, it would allow better discrimination between benign and potentially metastatic PPGL at the time of initial diagnosis. Moreover, improved insight into the molecular pathways that drive the transformation of the normal chromaffin cell into the malignant chromaffin cell will also offer novel targets for treatment that hopefully will provide a definitive cure for these rare metastatic neuroendocrine tumors in the future.

Author Contributions: Conceptualization: A.M.A.B., M.N.K., G.E., J.W.M.L.; Writing—original draft preparation: A.M.A.B., M.N.K., G.E.; Writing—review and editing: A.M.A.B., G.E., L.F., A.N.A.v.d.H.-S., T.P.L., I.P.K., J.W.M.L., M.N.K.; Visualization: A.M.A.B., M.N.K., A.N.A.v.d.H.-S.

Funding: This research received no external funding.

Acknowledgments: We are grateful to Anna Siebers for the artwork.

Conflicts of Interest: The authors declare no conflict of interest.

References

1. Melmed, S.; Polonsky, K.S.; Larsen, P.R.; Kronenberg, H.M. *Williams Textbook Endocrinology*, 13th ed.; Elsevier: Amsterdam, The Netherlands, 2017; ISBN 978-0-323-29738-7.
2. Eisenhofer, G.; Ehrhart-Bornstein, M.; Bornstein, S. The Adrenal Medulla. Physiology and Pathophysiology. In *Handbook of the Autonomic Nervous System in Health and Disease*; Bolis, C.L., Govoni, S., Eds.; Marcel Dekker Inc.: New York, NY, USA; Basel, Switzerland, 2003; pp. 185–224.
3. Lenders, J.W.M.; Eisenhofer, G. Pathophysiology and diagnosis of disorder of the adrenal medulla: Focus on pheochromocytoma. *Compr. Physiol.* **2014**, *4*, 691–713. [PubMed]
4. Pihlajoki, M.; Dörmer, J.; Cochran, R.S.; Heikinheimo, M.; Wilson, D.B. Adrenocortical zonation, renewal and remodeling. *Front. Endocrinol. (Lausanne)* **2015**, *6*. [CrossRef] [PubMed]
5. Lumb, R.; Schwartz, Q. Sympathoadrenal neural crest cells: The known, unknown and forgotten? *Dev. Growth Differ.* **2015**, *57*, 146–157. [CrossRef] [PubMed]
6. Wong, D.L. Why is the adrenal adrenergic (review). *Endocr. Pathol.* **2003**, *14*, 25–36. [CrossRef]
7. Schinner, S.; Bornstein, S.R. Cortical-chromaffin cell interactions in the adrenal gland. *Endocr. Pathol.* **2005**, *16*, 91–98. [CrossRef]
8. Merke, D.P.; Chrousos, G.P.; Eisenhofer, G.; Weise, M.; Keil, M.F.; Rogol, A.D.; van Wyk, J.J.; Bornstein, S.R. Adrenomedullary dysplasia and hypofunction in patients with classic 21-hydroxylase deficiency. *N. Engl. J. Med.* **2000**, *343*, 1362–1368. [CrossRef]
9. Haase, M.; Willenberg, H.S.; Bornstein, S.R. Update on the corticomedullary interaction in the adrenal gland. *Endocr. Dev.* **2011**, *20*, 28–37.
10. Bornstein, S.R.; Gonzalez-Hernandez, J.A.; Ehrhart-Bornstein, M.; Adler, G.; Scherbaum, W.A. Intimate contact of chromaffin and cortical cells within the human adrenal gland forms the cellular basis for important intraadrenal interactions. *J. Clin. Endocrinol. Metab.* **1994**, *78*, 225–232.
11. Eisenhofer, G.; Huynh, T.T.; Hiroi, M.; Pacak, K. Understanding catecholamine metabolism as a guide to the biochemical diagnosis of pheochromocytoma. *Rev. Endocr. Metab. Disord.* **2001**, *2*, 297–311. [CrossRef]
12. Tank, A.W.; Lee Wong, D. Peripheral and central effects of circulating catecholamines. *Compr. Physiol.* **2015**. [CrossRef]
13. McCarty, R. Learning about stress: Neuronal, endocrine and behavioural adaptations. *Stress* **2016**, *19*, 449–475. [CrossRef] [PubMed]
14. Lenders, J.W.; Eisenhofer, G.; Mannelli, M.; Pacak, K. Phaeochromocytoma. *Lancet* **2005**, *366*, 665–675. [CrossRef]
15. McNicol, A.M. Update on tumours of the adrenal cortex, pheochromocytoma and extra-adrenal paraganglioma. *Histopathology* **2011**, *58*, 155–168. [CrossRef] [PubMed]

16. Lam, A.K. Update on adrenal tumours in 2017 World Health Organization (WHO) of endocrine tumours. *Endocr. Pathol.* **2017**, *28*, 213–227. [CrossRef] [PubMed]
17. Liao, W.B.; Liu, C.F.; Chiang, C.W.; Kung, C.T.; Lee, C.W. Cardiovascular manifestations of pheochromocytoma. *Am. J. Emerg. Med.* **2000**, *18*, 622–625. [CrossRef] [PubMed]
18. Brouwers, F.M.; Lenders, J.W.; Eisenhofer, G.; Pacak, K. Pheochromocytoma as an endocrine emergency. *Rev. Endocr. Metab. Disord.* **2003**, *4*, 121–128. [CrossRef] [PubMed]
19. Prejbisz, A.; Lenders, J.W.; Eisenhofer, G.; Januszewicz, A. Mortality associated with phaeochromocytoma. *Horm. Metab. Res.* **2013**, *45*, 154–158. [CrossRef] [PubMed]
20. Stolk, R.F.; Bakx, C.; Mulder, J.; Timmers, H.J.; Lenders, J.W. Is the excess cardiovascular morbidity in pheochromocytoma related to blood pressure or to catecholamines? *J. Clin. Endocrinol. Metab.* **2013**, *98*, 1100–1106. [CrossRef] [PubMed]
21. Berends, A.M.A.; Buitenwerf, E.; de Krijger, R.R.; Veeger, N.J.G.M.; van der Horst-Schrivers, A.N.A.; Links, T.P.; Kerstens, M.N. Incidence of pheochromocytoma and sympathetic paraganglioma in the Netherlands: A nationwide study and systematic review. *Eur. J. Intern. Med.* **2018**, *51*, 68–73. [CrossRef]
22. Eisenhofer, G.; Prejbisz, A.; Peitzsch, M.; Pamporaki, C.; Masjkur, J.; Rogowski-Lehmann, N.; Langton, K.; Tsourdi, E.; Peczkowska, M.; Fliedner, S.; et al. Biochemical diagnosis of chromaffin cell tumours in patients at high and low risk of disease: Plasma versus urinary free or deconjugated O-methylated catecholamine metabolites. *Clin. Chem.* **2018**, *64*, 1646–1656. [CrossRef]
23. Bozkurt, M.F.; Virgolini, I.; Balogova, S.; Beheshti, M.; Rubello, D.; Decristoforo, C.; Ambrosini, V.; Kjaer, A.; Delgado-Bolton, R.; Kunikowska, J.; et al. Guideline for PET/CT imaging of neuroendocrine neoplasms with ^{68}Ga-DOTA-conjugated somatostatin receptor targeting peptides and ^{18}F-DOPA. *Eur. J. Nucl. Med. Mol. Imaging* **2017**, *44*, 1588–1601. [CrossRef] [PubMed]
24. Pacak, K. Pheochromocytoma: A catecholamine and oxidative stress disorder. *Endocr. Regul.* **2011**, *45*, 65–90. [CrossRef] [PubMed]
25. Eisenhofer, G.; Klink, B.; Richter, S.; Lenders, J.W.M.; Robledo, M. Metabologenomics of pheochromocytoma and paraganglioma: An integrated approach for personalised biochemical and genetic testing. *Clin. Biochem. Rev.* **2017**, *38*, 69–100. [PubMed]
26. Gupta, G.; Pacak, K.; AACE Adrenal Scientific Committee. Precision medicine: An update on genotype/biochemical phenotype relationships in pheochromocytoma/paraganglioma patients. *Endocr. Pract.* **2017**, *23*, 690–704. [CrossRef]
27. Lehnert, H. Regulation of catecholamine synthesizing enzyme gene expression in human pheochromocytoma. *Eur. J. Endocrinol.* **1998**, *138*, 363–367. [CrossRef] [PubMed]
28. Garibotto, G.; Tessari, P.; Verzola, D.; Dertenois, L. The metabolic conversion of phenylalanine into tyrosine in the human kidney: Does it have nutritional implications in renal patients? *J. Ren. Nutr.* **2002**, *12*, 8–16. [CrossRef] [PubMed]
29. Koopmans, K.P.; Neels, O.N.; Kema, I.P.; Elsinga, P.H.; Links, T.P.; de Vries, E.G.E.; Jager, P.L. Molecular imaging in neuroendocrine tumours: Molecular uptake mechanisms and clinical results. *Crit. Rev. Oncol. Hematol.* **2009**, *71*, 199–213. [CrossRef]
30. Salisbury, T.B.; Arthur, S. The regulation and function of the L-type amino acid transporter 1 (LAT1) in cancer. *Int. J. Mol. Sci.* **2018**, *19*, 2373. [CrossRef]
31. Eisenhofer, G.; Rundquist, B.; Aneman, A.; Friberg, P.; Dakak, N.; Kopin, I.J.; Jacobs, M.C.; Lenders, J.W. Regional release and removal of catecholamines and extraneuronal metabolism to metanephrines. *J. Clin. Endocrinol. Metab.* **1995**, *80*, 3009–3017.
32. Nagatsu, T.; Levitt, M.; Udenfriend, S. Tyrosine hydroxylase: The initial step in norepinephrine biosynthesis. *J. Biol. Chem.* **1964**, *239*, 2910–2917.
33. Wolf, M.E.; LeWitt, P.A.; Bannon, M.J.; Dragovic, L.J.; Kapatos, G. Effect of ageing on tyrosine hydroxylase protein content and the relative number of dopamine nerve terminals in human caudate. *J. Neurochem.* **1991**, *56*, 1191–1200. [CrossRef] [PubMed]
34. Nagatsu, T. Tyrosine hydroxylase: Human isoforms, structure and regulation in physiology and pathology. *Essays Biochem.* **1995**, *30*, 15–35. [PubMed]
35. Rao, F.; Zhang, K.; Zhang, L.; Rana, B.K.; Wessel, J.; Fung, M.M.; Rodriquez-Flores, J.L.; Taupenot, L.; Ziegler, M.G.; O'Connor, D.T. Human tyrosine hydroxylase natural allelic variation: Influcence on autonomic function and hypertension. *Cell. Mol. Neurobiol.* **2010**, *30*, 1391–1394. [CrossRef]

36. Daubner, S.C.; Le, T.; Wang, S. Tyrosine hydroxylase and regulation of dopamine synthesis. *Arch. Biochem. Biophys.* **2011**, *508*, 1–12. [CrossRef] [PubMed]
37. Doskeland, A.P.; Flatmark, T. Ubiquitination of soluble and membrane bound tyrosine hydroxylase and degradation of the soluble form. *Eur. J. Biochem.* **2002**, *269*, 1561–1569. [CrossRef] [PubMed]
38. Chen, Y.; Best, J.A.; Nagamoto, K.; Tank, A.W. Regulation of tyrosine hydroxylase gene expression by the m1 muscarinic acetylcholine receptor in rat pheochromocytoma cells. *Mol. Brain Res.* **1996**, *40*, 42–54. [CrossRef]
39. Sabban, E.L.; Kvetnansky, R. Stress-triggered activation of gene expression in catecholaminergic systems: Dynamics of transcriptional events. *Trends Neurosci.* **2001**, *24*, 91–98. [CrossRef]
40. Eiden, L.E.; Jiang, S.Z. What's new in endocrinology: The chromaffin cell. *Front. Endocrinol. (Lausanne)* **2018**, *9*, 711. [CrossRef]
41. Lee, Y.H.; Gyun, Y.; Moon, J.Y.; Kim, J.S.; Jeong, K.H.; Lee, T.W.; Ihm, C.G.; Lee, S.H. Genetic variations of tyrosine hydroxylase in the pathogenesis of hypertension. *Electrolyte Blood Press* **2016**, *14*, 21–26. [CrossRef]
42. Zhu, M.Y.; Juorio, A.V. Aromatic L-amino acid decarboxylase: Biological characterization and functional role. *Gen. Pharmacol.* **1995**, *26*, 681–696. [CrossRef]
43. Barth, M.; Serre, V.; Hubert, L.; Chaabouni, Y.; Bahi-Buisson, N.; Cadoudal, M.; Rabier, D.; Tich, S.N.; Ribeiro, M.; Ricquier, D.; et al. Kinetic analyses guide the therapeutic decision in a novel form of moderate aromatic acid decarboxylase deficiency. *JIMD Rep.* **2012**, *3*, 25–32. [PubMed]
44. Berends, A.M.A.; Kerstens, M.N.; Bolt, J.W.; Links, T.P.; Korpershoek, E.; de Krijger, R.R.; Walenkamp, A.M.E.; Noordzij, W.; van Etten, B.; Kats-Ugurlu, G.; et al. False-positive findings on 6-[18F]fluor-L-3,4-dihydroxyphenylalanine PET (18F-FDOPA-PET) performed for imaging of neuroendocrine tumors. *Eur. J. Endocrinol.* **2018**, *179*, 127–135. [CrossRef] [PubMed]
45. Waymire, J.C.; Haycock, J.W. Lack of regulation of aromatic L-amino acid decarboxylase in intact bovine chromaffin cells. *J. Neurochem.* **2002**, *81*, 589–593. [CrossRef] [PubMed]
46. Li, X.M.; Juorio, A.V.; Boulton, A.A. NSD-1015 alters the gene expression of aromatic L-amino acid decarboxylase in rat PC12 pheochromocytoma cells. *Neurochem. Res.* **1993**, *18*, 915–919. [CrossRef]
47. Lee, J.J.; Jin, C.M.; Kim, Y.K.; Ryu, S.Y.; Lim, S.C.; Lee, M.K. Effects of anonaine on dopamine biosynthesis and L-dopa induced cytotoxicity in PC12 cells. *Molecules* **2008**, *13*, 475–487. [CrossRef]
48. Friedman, S.; Kaufman, S. 3,4-Dihydroxyphenylethylamine β-hydroxylase. Physical properties, copper content, and role of copper in the catalytic activity. *J. Biol. Chem.* **1965**, *240*, 4763–4773.
49. Weinshilboum, R.; Axelrod, J. Serum dopamine-beta-hydroxylase activity. *Circ. Res.* **1971**, *28*, 307–315. [CrossRef]
50. Palatini, P. Fumarate is the cause of the apparent ping-pong kinetics of dopamine beta-hydroxylase. *Biochem. Int.* **1985**, *11*, 565–572.
51. Wimalasena, K.; Dharmasena, S.; Wimalasena, D.S.; Hughbanks-Wheaton, D.K. Reduction of dopamine beta-monooxygenase. A unified model for apparent negative cooperativity and fumarate activation. *J. Biol. Chem.* **1996**, *271*, 26032–26043. [CrossRef]
52. Patak, P.; Willenberg, H.S.; Bornstein, S.R. Vitamin C is an important cofactor for both adrenal cortex and adrenal medulla. *Endocr. Res.* **2004**, *30*, 871–875. [CrossRef]
53. Trifaro, J. Molecular biology of the chromaffin cell. *Ann. N. Y. Acad. Sci.* **2002**, *971*, 11–18. [CrossRef] [PubMed]
54. Yu, P.H. Phenylethanolamine N-methyltransferase from the brain and adrenal medulla of the rat: A comparison of their properties. *Neurochem. Res.* **1978**, *3*, 755–762. [CrossRef] [PubMed]
55. Livett, B.G. Adrenal medullary chromaffin cells in vitro. *Physiol. Rev.* **1984**, *64*, 1103–1161. [CrossRef] [PubMed]
56. Wong, D.L.; Lesage, A.; Siddall, B.; Funder, J.W. Glucocorticoid regulation of phenylethanolamine N-methyltransferase in vivo. *FASEB J.* **1992**, *6*, 3310–3315. [CrossRef] [PubMed]
57. Wong, D.L.; Siddall, B.J.; Ebert, S.N.; Bell, R.A.; Her, S. Phenylethanolamine N-methyltransferase gene expression: Synergistic activation by Egr-1, AP-2 and the glucocorticoid receptor. *Brain Res. Mol. Brain Res.* **1998**, *61*, 154–161. [CrossRef]
58. Ceccatelli, S.; Dagerlind, A.; Schalling, M.; Wikström, A.C.; Okret, S.; Gustafsson, J.A.; Goldstein, M.; Hökfelt, T. The glucocorticoid receptor in the adrenal gland is localized in the cytoplasm of adrenaline cells. *Acta Physiol. Scand.* **1989**, *137*, 559–560. [CrossRef] [PubMed]

59. Zuckerman-Levin, N.; Tiosano, D.; Eisenhofer, G.; Bornstein, S.; Hochberg, Z. The importance of adrenocortical glucocorticoids for adrenomedullary and physiological response to stress: A study in isolated glucocorticoid deficiency. *J. Clin. Endocrinol. Metab.* **2001**, *86*, 5920–5924. [CrossRef]
60. Kennedy, B.; Bigby, T.D.; Ziegler, M.G. Nonadrenal epinephrine-forming enzymes in humans. Characteristics, distribution, regulation, and relationship to epinephrine levels. *J. Clin. Investig.* **1995**, *95*, 2896–2902. [CrossRef] [PubMed]
61. Osuala, K.; Telusma, K.; Khan, S.M.; Wu, S.; Shah, M.; Baker, C.; Alam, S.; Abukenda, I.; Fuentes, A.; Seifein, H.B.; et al. Distinctive left-sided distribution of adrenergic derived cells in the adult mouse heart. *PLoS ONE* **2011**, *6*, e22811. [CrossRef]
62. Winkler, H.; Apps, D.K.; Fischer-Colbrie, R. The molecular function of adrenal chromaffin granules: Established facts and unresolved topics. *Neuroscience* **1986**, *18*, 261–290. [CrossRef]
63. Crivellato, E.; Nico, B.; Ribatti, D. The chromaffin vesicle: Advances in understanding the composition of a versatile, multifunctional secretory organelle. *Anat. Rec. (Hoboken)* **2008**, *291*, 1587–1602. [CrossRef] [PubMed]
64. Estévez-Herrera, J.; González-Santana, A.; Baz-Dávila, R.; Machado, J.D.; Borges, R. The intravesicular cocktail and its role in the regulation of exocytosis. *J. Neurochem.* **2016**, *137*, 897–903. [CrossRef] [PubMed]
65. Estevez-Herrera, J.; Pardo, M.R.; Dominguez, N.; Pereda, D.; Machado, J.D.; Borges, R. The role of chromogranins in the secretory pathway. *Biomol. Concepts* **2013**, *4*, 605–609. [CrossRef] [PubMed]
66. Kim, T.; Tao-Cheng, J.H.; Eiden, L.E.; Loh, Y.P. Chromogranin A, an "on/off" switch controlling dense-core secretory granule biogenesis. *Cell* **2001**, *106*, 499–509. [CrossRef]
67. Stenman, A.; Svahn, F.; Hoijat-Farsangi, M.; Zedenius, J.; Söderkvist, P.; Gimm, O.; Larsson, C.; Juhlin, C.C. Molecular profiling of pheochromocytoma and abdominal paraganglioma stratified by the PASS algorithm reveals chromogranin B as associated with histologic prediction of malignant behavior. *Am. J. Surg. Pathol.* **2019**, *43*, 409–421. [CrossRef]
68. Zuber, S.; Wesley, R.; Prodanov, T.; Eisenhofer, G.; Pacak, K.; Kantorovich, V. Clinical utility of chromogranin A in SDHx-related paragangliomas. *Eur. J. Clin. Investig.* **2014**, *44*, 365–371. [CrossRef] [PubMed]
69. O'Connor, D.; Deftos, L. Secretion of chromogranin A by peptide producing endocrine neoplasms. *N. Engl. J. Med.* **1986**, *314*, 1145–1151. [CrossRef]
70. Hsiao, R.J.; Parmer, R.J.; Takiyyuddin, M.A.; O'Connor, D.T. Chromogranin A storage and secretion: Sensitivity and specificity for the diagnosis of pheochromocytoma. *Medicine (Baltimore)* **1991**, *70*, 33–45. [CrossRef]
71. Stridsberg, M.; Husebye, E.S. Chromogranin A and chromogranin B are sensitive circulating markers for pheochromocytoma. *Eur. J. Endocrinol.* **1997**, *136*, 67–73. [CrossRef]
72. Brouwers, F.M.; Gläsker, S.; Nave, A.F.; Vortmeyer, A.O.; Lubensky, I.; Huang, S.; Abu-Asab, M.S.; Eisenhofer, G.; Weil, R.J.; Park, D.M.; et al. Proteomic profiling of von Hippel-Lindau syndrome and multiple endocrine neoplasia type 2 pheochromocytomas reveals different expression of chromogranin B. *Endocr. Relat. Cancer* **2007**, *14*, 463–471. [CrossRef]
73. Guillemot, J.; Thouënnon, E.; Guérin, M.; Vallet-Erdtmann, V.; Ravni, A.; Montéro-Hadjadje, M.; Lefebvre, H.; Klein, M.; Muresan, M.; Seidah, N.G.; et al. Differential expression and processing of secretogranin II in relation to the status of pheochromocytoma: Implications for the production of the tumoral marker EM66. *J. Mol. Endocrinol.* **2012**, *48*, 115–127. [CrossRef] [PubMed]
74. Huh, Y.H.; Jeon, S.H.; Yoo, S.H. Chromogranin B-induced secretory granule biogenesis: Comparison with the similar role of chromogranin A. *J. Biol. Chem.* **2003**, *278*, 40581–40589. [CrossRef] [PubMed]
75. Guillemot, J.; Guerin, M.; Thouënnon, E.; Montero-Hadjadje, M.; Leprince, J.; Lefebvre, H.; Klein, M.; Muresan, M.; Anouar, Y.; Yon, L. Characterization and plasma measurement of the WE-14 peptide in patients with pheochromocytoma. *PLoS ONE* **2014**, *9*, e88698. [CrossRef] [PubMed]
76. Cleary, S.; Phillips, J.K.; Huynh, T.T.; Pacak, K.; Elkahloun, A.G.; Barb, J.; Worrell, R.A.; Goldstein, D.S.; Eisenhofer, G. Neuropeptide Y expression in phaeochromocytomas: Relative absence in tumours from patients with von Hippel-Lindau syndrome. *J. Endocrinol.* **2007**, *193*, 225–233. [CrossRef] [PubMed]
77. Guillemot, J.; Barbier, L.; Thouënnon, E.; Vallet-Erdtmann, V.; Montero-Hadjadje, M.; Lefebvre, H.; Klein, M.; Muresan, M.; Plouin, P.F.; Sei dah, N.; et al. Expression and processing of the neuroendocrine protein secretogranin II in benign and malignant pheochromocytomas. *Ann. N. Y. Acad. Sci.* **2006**, *107*, 527–532. [CrossRef] [PubMed]

78. Stridsberg, M.; Eriksson, B.; Janson, E.T. Measurement of secretogranins II, III, V and proconvertases 1/3 and 2 in plasma from patients with neuroendocrine tumours. *Regul. Pept.* **2008**, *148*, 95–98. [CrossRef] [PubMed]
79. Shimizu, K.; Namimatsu, S.; Kitagawa, W.; Akasu, H.; Takatsu, K.; Sugisaki, Y.; Tanaka, S. Immunohistochemical, biochemical and immunoelectron microscopic analysis of antigenic proteins on neuroendocrine cell tumors using monoclonal antibody HISL-19. *J. Nippon. Med. Sch.* **2002**, *69*, 365–372. [CrossRef]
80. Marcinkiewicz, M.; Benjannet, S.; Falgueyret, J.P.; Seidah, N.G.; Schurch, W.; Verdy, M.; Cantin, M.; Chretien, M. Identification and localization of 7B2 protein in human, porcine, and rat thyroid gland and in human medullary carcinoma. *Endocrinology* **1988**, *123*, 866–873. [CrossRef]
81. Hacker, G.W.; Bishop, A.E.; Terenghi, G.; Varndell, I.M.; Aghahowa, J.; Pollard, K.; Thurner, J.; Polak, J.M. Multiple peptide production and presence of general markers detected in 12 cases of human pheochromocytoma and in mammalian adrenal glands. *Virchows Arch. A Pathol. Anat. Histopathol.* **1988**, *412*, 399–411. [CrossRef]
82. Natori, S.; Iguchi, H.; Ohashi, M.; Nawata, H. Plasma 7B2 (a novel pituitary protein) immunoreactivity concentrations in patients with various endocrine disorders. *Endocrinol. Jpn.* **1988**, *35*, 651–654. [CrossRef]
83. Srivastava, A.; Padilla, O.; Fischer-Colbrie, R.; Tischler, A.S.; Dayal, Y. Neuroendocrine secretory protein-55 (NESP-55) expression discriminates pancreatic endocrine tumors and pheochromocytomas from gastrointestinal and pulmonary carcinoids. *Am. J. Surg. Pathol.* **2004**, *28*, 1371–1378. [CrossRef] [PubMed]
84. Jakobsen, A.M.; Ahlman, H.; Kolby, L.; Abrahamsson, J.; Fischer-Colbrie, R.; Nilsson, O. NESP55, a novel chromogranin-like peptide, is expressed in endocrine tumours of the pancreas and adrenal medulla but not in ileal carcinoids. *Br. J. Cancer* **2003**, *88*, 1746–1754. [CrossRef] [PubMed]
85. Rindi, G.; Licini, L.; Necchi, V.; Bottarelli, L.; Campanini, N.; Azzoni, C.; Favret, M.; Giordano, G.; D'Amato, F.; Brancia, C.; et al. Peptide products of the neurotrophin-inducible gene vgf are produced in human neuroendocrine cells from early development and increase in hyperplasia and neoplasia. *J. Clin. Endocrinol. Metab.* **2007**, *92*, 2811–2815. [CrossRef] [PubMed]
86. Salton, S.R. Neurotrophins, growth-factor-regulated genes and the control of energy balance. *Mt. Sinai J. Med.* **2003**, *70*, 93–100. [PubMed]
87. Salton, S.R.; Ferri, G.L.; Hahm, S.; Snyder, S.E.; Wilson, A.J.; Possenti, R.; Levi, A. VGF: A novel role for this neuronal and neuroendocrine polypeptide in the regulation of energy balance. *Front. Neuroendocr.* **2000**, *21*, 199–219. [CrossRef] [PubMed]
88. Isobe, K.; Nakai, T.; Yukimasa, N.; Nanmoku, T.; Takekoshi, K.; Nomura, F. Expression of mRNA coding for four catecholaminesynthesizing enzymes in human adrenal pheochromocytomas. *Eur. J. Endocrinol.* **1998**, *138*, 383–387. [CrossRef] [PubMed]
89. Jarrot, B.; Louis, W.J. Abnormalities in enzymes involved in catecholamine synthesis and catabolism in phaeochromocytoma. *Clin. Sci. Mol. Med.* **1977**, *53*, 529–535. [CrossRef]
90. Supek, F.; Supekova, L.; Mandiyan, S.; Pan, Y.C.E.; Nelson, H.; Nelson, N. A novel accessory subunit for vacuolar H1-ATPase from chromaffin granules. *J. Biol. Chem.* **1994**, *269*, 24102–24106.
91. Balogh, A.; Cadel, S.; Foulon, T.; Picart, R.; der Garabedian, A.; Rousselet, A.; Tougard, C.; Cohen, P. Aminopeptidase B: A processing enzyme secreted and associated with the plasma membrane of rat pheochromocytoma (PC12) cells. *J. Cell Sci.* **1998**, *111*, 161–169.
92. Azaryan, A.V.; Schiller, M.R.; Hook, V.Y. Chromaffin granule aspartic proteinase processes recombinant proopiomelanocortin (POMC). *Biochem. Biophys. Res. Commun.* **1995**, *215*, 937–944. [CrossRef]
93. Murthy, S.R.; Pacak, K.; Loh, Y.P. Carboxypeptidase E: Elevated expression correlated with tumor growth and metastasis in pheochromocytomas and other cancers. *Cell. Mol. Neurobiol.* **2010**, *30*, 1377–1381. [CrossRef] [PubMed]
94. Murthy, S.R.K.; Dupart, E.; Al-Sweel, N.; Chen, A.; Cawley, N.X.; Loh, Y.P. Carboxypeptidase E promotes cancer cell survival, but inhibits migration and invasion. *Cancer Lett.* **2013**, *341*, 204–213. [CrossRef] [PubMed]
95. Yasothornsrikul, S.; Greenbaum, D.; Medzihradszky, K.F.; Toneff, T.; Bundey, R.; Miller, R.; Schilling, B.; Petermann, I.; Dehnert, J.; Logvinova, A.; et al. Cathepsin L in secretory vesicles functions as a prohormone-processing enzyme for production of the enkephalin peptide neurotransmitter. *Proc. Natl. Acad. Sci. USA* **2003**, *100*, 9590–9595. [CrossRef] [PubMed]

96. Funkelstein, L.; Beinfeld, M.; Minokadeh, A.; Zadina, J.; Hook, V. Unique biological function of cathepsin L in secretory vesicles for biosynthesis of neuropeptides. *Neuropeptides* **2010**, *44*, 457–466. [CrossRef] [PubMed]
97. Laslop, A.; Weiss, C.; Savaria, D.; Eiter, C.; Tooze, S.A.; Seidah, N.G.; Winkler, H. Proteolytic processing of chromogranin B and secretogranin II by prohormone convertases. *J. Neurochem.* **1998**, *70*, 374–383. [CrossRef] [PubMed]
98. Parmer, R.J.; Mahata, M.; Mahata, S.; Sebald, M.T.; O'Connor, D.T.; Miles, L.A. Tissue plasminogen activator (t-PA) is targeted to the regulated secretory pathway. Catecholamine storage vesicles as a reservoir for the rapid release of t-PA. *J. Biol. Chem.* **1997**, *272*, 1976–1982. [CrossRef] [PubMed]
99. Parmer, R.J.; Mahata, M.; Gong, Y.; Mahata, S.K.; Jiang, Q.; O'Connor, D.T.; Xi, X.P.; Miles, L.A. Processing of chromogranin A by plasmin provides a novel mechanism for regulating catecholamine secretion. *J. Clin. Investig.* **2000**, *106*, 907–915. [CrossRef] [PubMed]
100. Hwang, S.R.; Bundey, R.; Toneff, T.; Hook, V. Endopin serpin protease inhibitors localize with neuropeptides in secretory vesicles and neuroendocrine tissues. *Neuroendocrinology* **2009**, *89*, 210–216. [CrossRef]
101. Thouënnon, E.; Piere, A.; Yon, L.; Anouar, Y. Expression of trophic peptides and their receptors in chromaffin cells and pheochromocytoma. *Cell. Mol. Neurobiol.* **2010**, *30*, 1383–1389. [CrossRef]
102. Hu, W.; Shi, L.; Zhou, P.H.; Zhang, X.B. Plasma concentrations of adrenomedullin and atrial and brain natriuretic peptides in patients with adrenal pheochromocytoma. *Oncol. Lett.* **2015**, *10*, 3163–3170. [CrossRef]
103. Shimosawa, T.; Fujita, T. Adrenomedullin and its related peptide. *Endocr. J.* **2005**, *52*, 1–10. [CrossRef] [PubMed]
104. Zudaire, E.; Martinez, A.; Cuttitta, F. Adrenomedullin and cancer. *Regul. Pept.* **2003**, *112*, 175–183. [CrossRef]
105. Morimoto, R.; Satoh, F.; Murakami, O.; Hirose, T.; Totsune, K.; Imai, Y.; Arai, Y.; Suzuki, T.; Sasano, H.; Ito, S.; et al. Expression of adrenomedullin 2/intermedin in human adrenal tumors and attached non-neoplastic adrenal tissues. *J. Endocrinol.* **2008**, *198*, 175–183. [CrossRef] [PubMed]
106. Chejfec, G.; Lee, I.; Warren, W.H.; Gould, V.E. Bombesin in human neuroendocrine (NE) neoplasms. *Peptides* **1985**, *6*, 107–112. [CrossRef]
107. Bostwick, D.G.; Bensch, K.G. Gastrin releasing peptide in human neuroendocrine tumours. *J. Pathol.* **1985**, *147*, 237–244. [CrossRef] [PubMed]
108. Linnoila, R.I.; Lack, E.E.; Steinberg, S.M.; Keiser, H.R. Decreased expression of neuropeptides in malignant paragangliomas: An immunohistochemical study. *Hum. Pathol.* **1988**, *19*, 41–50. [CrossRef]
109. Fedorak, I.; Prinz, R.A.; Fiscus, R.R.; Wang, X.; Chaumont, J.; Chejfec, G.; Glisson, S. Plasma calcitonin gene-related peptide and atrial natriuretic peptide levels during resection of pheochromocytoma. *Surgery* **1991**, *110*, 1094–1098. [PubMed]
110. Mazzocchi, G.; Musajo, F.G.; Neri, G.; Gottardo, G.; Nussdorfer, G.G. Adrenomedullin stimulates steroid secretion by the isolated perfused rat adrenal gland in situ: Comparison with calcitonin gene-related peptide effects. *Peptides* **1996**, *17*, 853–857. [CrossRef]
111. Mahata, S.K.; Mahata, M.; Fung, M.; O'Connor, D.T. Catestatin: A multifunctional peptide from chromogranin A. *Regul. Pept.* **2010**, *162*, 33–43. [CrossRef] [PubMed]
112. Mahata, S.K.; O'Connor, D.T.; Mahata, M.; Yoo, S.H.; Taupenot, L.; Wu, H.; Gill, B.M.; Parmer, R.J. Novel autocrine feedback control of catecholamine release. A discrete chromogranin a fragment is a noncompetitive nicotinic cholinergic antagonist. *J. Clin. Investig.* **1997**, *100*, 123–133. [CrossRef] [PubMed]
113. Guillemot, J.; Ait-Ali, D.; Turquier, V.; Montero-Hadjadje, M.; Fournier, A.; Vaudry, H.; Anouar, Y.; Yon, L. Involvement of multiple signalling pathways in PACAP induced EM66 secretion from chromaffin cells. *Regul. Pept.* **2006**, *137*, 79–88. [CrossRef] [PubMed]
114. Yon, L.; Guillemot, J.; Montero-Hadjadje, M.; Grumolato, L.; Leprince, J.; Lefebvre, H.; Contesse, V.; Plouin, P.F.; Vaudry, H.; Anouar, Y. Identification of the secretogranin II-derived peptide EM66 in pheochromocytomas as a potential marker for discriminating benign versus malignant tumors. *J. Clin. Endocrinol. Metab.* **2003**, *88*, 2579–2585. [CrossRef] [PubMed]
115. Babinski, K.; Haddad, P.; Vallerand, D.; McNicoll, N.; De Lean, A.; Ong, H. Natriuretic peptides inhibit nicotine-induced whole-cell currents and catecholamine secretion in bovine chromaffin cells: Evidence for the involvement of the atrial natriuretic factor R2 receptors. *J. Neurochem.* **1995**, *64*, 1080–1087. [CrossRef] [PubMed]
116. Suga, S.; Nakao, K.; Mukoyama, M.; Arai, H.; Hosoda, K.; Ogawa, Y.; Imura, H. Characterization of natriuretic peptide receptors in cultured cells. *Hypertension* **1992**, *19*, 762–765. [CrossRef] [PubMed]

117. Lymperopoulos, A.; Brill, A.; McCrink, K.A. GPCRs of adrenal chromaffin cells and catecholamines: The plot thickens. *Int. J. Biochem. Cell Biol.* **2016**, *77*, 213–219. [CrossRef]
118. Spinazzi, R.; Andreis, P.G.; Nussdorfer, G. Neuropeptide Y and Y receptors in the autocrine-paracrine regulation of adrenal gland under physiological and pathophysiological conditions (review). *Int. J. Mol. Med.* **2005**, *15*, 3–13. [CrossRef]
119. Cavadas, C.; Cefai, D.; Rosmaninho-Salgado, J.; Vieira-Coelho, M.A.; Moura, E.; Busso, N.; Pedrazzini, T.; Grand, D.; Rotman, S.; Waeber, B.; et al. Deletion of the neuropeptide Y (NPY) Y1 receptor gene reveals a regulatory role of NPY on catecholamine synthesis and secretion. *Proc. Natl. Acad. Sci. USA* **2006**, *103*, 10497–10502. [CrossRef]
120. Kitlinska, J.; Abe, K.; Kuo, L.; Pons, J.; Yu, M.; Li, L.; Tilan, J.; Everhart, L.; Lee, E.W.; Zukowska, Z.; et al. Differential effects of neuropeptide Y on the growth and vascularizaton of neural crest-derived tumors. *Cancer Res.* **2005**, *65*, 1719–1728. [CrossRef]
121. Helman, L.J.; Cohen, P.S.; Averbuch, S.D.; Cooper, M.J.; Keiser, H.R.; Isreal, M.A. Neuropeptide Y expression distinguishes malignant from benign pheochromocytoma. *J. Clin. Oncol.* **1989**, *7*, 1720–1725. [CrossRef]
122. Grouzmann, E.; Comoy, E.; Bohuon, C. Plasma neuropeptide Y concentration in patients with neuroendocrine tumors. *J. Clin. Endocrinol. Metab.* **1989**, *68*, 808–813. [CrossRef]
123. Tischler, A.S.; Lee, Y.C.; Perlman, R.L.; Costopoulos, D.; Slayton, V.W.; Bloom, S.R. Production of "ectopic" vasoactive intestinal peptide-like and Neurotensin-like immunoreactivity in human pheochromocytoma cell cultures. *J. Neurosci.* **1984**, *4*, 1398–1404. [CrossRef] [PubMed]
124. Tischler, A.S.; Lee, Y.C.; Slayton, V.W.; Bloom, S.R. Content and release of neurotensin in PC12 pheochromocytoma cell cultures: Modulation by dexamethasone and nerve growth factor. *Regul. Pept.* **1982**, *3*, 415–421. [CrossRef]
125. Pellizzari, E.H.; Barontini, M.; Figuerola, M.; Cigorraga, S.B.; Levin, G. Possible autocrine enkephalin regulation of catecholamine release in human pheochromocytoma cells. *Life Sci.* **2008**, *83*, 413–420. [CrossRef] [PubMed]
126. Gupta, N.; Bark, S.J.; Lu, W.D.; Taupenot, L.; O'Connor, D.T.; Pevzner, P.; Hook, V. Mass spectrometry based neuropeptidomics of secretory vesicles form human adrenal medullary pheochromocytoma reveals novel peptide products of prohormone processing. *J. Proteome Res.* **2010**, *9*, 5065–5075. [CrossRef] [PubMed]
127. Yoshimasa, T.; Nakao, K.; Li, S.; Ikeda, Y.; Suda, M.; Sakamoto, M.; Imura, H. Plasma methionine-enkephalin and leucine-enkephalin in normal subjects and patients with pheochromocytoma. *J. Clin. Endocrinol. Metab.* **1983**, *57*, 706–712. [CrossRef] [PubMed]
128. Albillos, A.; Gandia, L.; Michelena, P.; Gilabert, J.A.; del Valle, M.; Carbone, E.; Garcia, A.G. The mechanism of calcium channel facilitation in bovine chromaffin cells. *J. Physiol.* **1996**, *494*, 687–695. [CrossRef] [PubMed]
129. Thouënnon, E.; Piere, A.; Tanguy, Y.; Guillemot, J.; Manecka, D.L.; Guérin, M.; Ouafik, L.; Muresan, M.; Klein, M.; Bertherat, J.; et al. Expression of trophic amidated peptides and their receptors in benign and malignant pheochromocytomas: High expression of adrenomedullin RDC1 receptor and implication in tumoral cell survival. *Endocr. Relat. Cancer* **2010**, *17*, 637–651. [CrossRef] [PubMed]
130. Smith, C.B.; Eiden, L. Is PACAP the major neurotransmitter for stress transduction at the adrenomedullary synapse? *J. Mol. Neurosci.* **2012**, *48*, 403–412. [CrossRef]
131. Turquier, V.; Yon, L.; Grumolato, L.; Alexandre, D.; Fournier, A.; Vaudry, H.; Anouar, Y. Pituitary adenylate cyclase-activating polypeptide stimulates secretoneurin release and secretogranin II gene transcription in bovine adrenochromaffin cells through multiple signalling pathways and increased binding of pre-existing activator protein-1-like transcription factors. *Mol. Pharm.* **2001**, *60*, 42–52.
132. Fischer-Colbrie, R.; Kirchmair, R.; Kahler, C.M.; Wiedermann, C.J.; Saria, A. Secretoneurin: A new player in angiogenesis and chemotaxis linking nerves, blood vessels and the immune system. *Curr. Protein Pept. Sci.* **2005**, *6*, 373–385. [CrossRef] [PubMed]
133. Wiedermann, C.J. Secretoneurin: A functional neuropeptide in health and disease. *Peptides* **2000**, *21*, 1289–1298. [CrossRef]
134. Unsicker, K.; Krieglstein, K. Growth factors in chromaffin cells. *Prog. Neurobiol.* **1996**, *48*, 307–324. [CrossRef]
135. Combs, S.E.; Ernsberger, U.; Krieglstein, K.; Unsicker, K. Reduction of endogenous TGF-B does not affect phenotypic development of sympathoadrenal progenitors into adrenal chromaffin cells. *Mech. Dev.* **2001**, *109*, 295–302. [CrossRef]

136. Flanders, K.C.; Lüdecke, G.; Engels, S.; Cissel, D.S.; Roberts, A.B.; Kondaiah, P.; Lafyatis, R.; Sporn, M.B.; Unsicker, K. Localization and actions of transforming growth factor-Bs in the embryonic nervous system. *Development* **1991**, *113*, 183–191. [PubMed]

137. Lugardon, K.; Raffner, R.; Goumon, Y.; Corti, A.; Delmas, A.; Bulet, P.; Aunis, D.; Metz-Boutigue, M.H. Antibacterial and antifungal activities of vasostatin-1, the N-terminal fragment of chromogranin A. *J. Biol. Chem.* **2000**, *275*, 10745–10753. [CrossRef] [PubMed]

138. Russell, J.; Gee, P.; Liu, S.M.; Angeletti, R.H. Inhibition of parathyroid hormone secretion by amino-terminal chromogranin peptides. *Endocrinology* **1994**, *135*, 227–342. [CrossRef]

139. Aardal, S.; Helle, K.B. The vasoinhibitory activity of bovine chromogranin A fragment (vasostatin) and its independence of extracellular calcium in isolated segments of human blood vessels. *Regul. Pept.* **1992**, *41*, 9–18. [CrossRef]

140. Strub, J.M.; Goumon, Y.; Lugardon, K.; Capon, C.; Lopez, M.; Moniatte, M.; van Dorsselaer, A.; Aunis, D.; Metz-Boutigue, M.H. Antibacterial activity of glycosylated and phosphorylated chromogranin-A derived peptide 173–184 from bovine adrenal medullary chromaffin granules. *J. Biol. Chem.* **1996**, *271*, 28533–28540. [CrossRef]

141. Strub, J.M.; Garcia-Sablone, P.; Lonning, K.; Taupenot, L.; Hubert, P.; Van Dorsselaer, A.; Aunis, D.; Metz-Boutigue, M.H. Processing of chromogranin B in bovine adrenal medulla. Identification of secretolytin, the endogenous C-terminal fragment of residues 614–626 with antibacterial activity. *Eur. J. Biochem.* **1995**, *229*, 356–368. [CrossRef]

142. Metz-Boutigue, M.H.; Kieffer, A.E.; Goumon, Y.; Aunis, D. Innate immunity: Involvement of new neuropeptides. *Trends Microbiol.* **2003**, *11*, 585–592. [CrossRef]

143. Levine, E.Y.; Levenberg, B.; Kaufman, S. The enzymatic conversion of 3,4-dihydroxyphenylethylamine to norepinephrine. *J. Biol. Chem.* **1960**, *235*, 2080–2086.

144. Schlüter, H.; Meissner, M.; van der Giet, M.; Tepel, M.; Bachmann, J.; Gross, I.; Nordhoff, E.; Karas, M.; Spieker, C.; Witzel, H.; et al. Coenzyme A glutathione disulfide. A potent vasoconstrictor derived from the adrenal gland. *Circ. Res.* **1995**, *76*, 675–680. [CrossRef]

145. Burgoyne, R.D.; Morgan, A. Secretory granule exocytosis. *Physiol. Rev.* **2003**, *83*, 581–632. [CrossRef] [PubMed]

146. Tadros, T.S.; Strauss, R.M.; Cohen, C.; Gal, A.A. Galanin immunoreactivity in paragangliomas but not in carcinoid tumors. *Appl. Immunohistochem. Mol. Morphol.* **2003**, *11*, 250–252. [CrossRef]

147. Bauer, F.E.; Hacker, G.W.; Terenghi, G.; Adrian, T.E.; Polak, J.M.; Bloom, S.R. Localization and molecular forms of galanin in human adrenals: Elevated levels in pheochromocytomas. *J. Clin. Endocrinol. Metab.* **1986**, *63*, 1372–1378. [CrossRef] [PubMed]

148. Painter, G.R.; Diliberto, E.J.; Knoth, J. 31P nuclear magnetic resonance study of the metabolic pools of adenosine triphosphate in cultured bovine adrenal medullary chromaffin cells. *Proc. Natl. Acad. Sci. USA* **1989**, *86*, 2239–2242. [CrossRef] [PubMed]

149. Sala, F.; Nistri, A.; Criado, M. Nicotinic acetylcholine receptors of adrenal chromaffin cells. *Acta Physiol.* **2008**, *192*, 203–212. [CrossRef]

150. Simasko, S.M.; Durkin, J.A.; Weiland, G.A. Effects of substance P on nicotinic acetylcholine receptor function in PC12 cells. *J. Neurochem.* **1987**, *49*, 253–260. [CrossRef]

151. Zhou, X.F.; Livett, B.G. Substance P has biphasic effects on catecholamine secretion evoked by electrical stimulation of perfused rat adrenal glands in vitro. *J. Auton. Nerv. Syst.* **1990**, *31*, 31–39. [CrossRef]

152. Oehme, P.; Hecht, H.D.; Faulhaber, K.; Nieber, I.; Roske, I.; Rathsack, R. Relationship of substance P to catecholamines, stress and hypertension. *J. Cardiovasc. Pharmacol.* **1987**, *10*, 109–111. [CrossRef]

153. Vinik, A.I.; Shapiro, B.; Thompson, N.W. Plasma gut hormone levels in 37 patients with pheochromocytomas. *World J. Surg.* **1986**, *10*, 593–604. [CrossRef] [PubMed]

154. Hu, X.; Cao, W.; Zhao, M. Octreotide reverses shock due to vasoactive intestinal peptide-secreting adrenal pheochromocytoma: A case report and review of literature. *World J. Clin. Cases* **2018**, *6*, 862–868. [CrossRef] [PubMed]

155. Jiang, J.; Zhang, L.; Wu, Z.; Ai, Z.; Hou, Y.; Lu, Z.; Gao, X. A rare case of watery diarrhea, hypokalemia and achlorhydria syndrome caused by pheochromocytoma. *BMC Cancer* **2014**, *14*, 533. [CrossRef] [PubMed]

156. Leibowitz-Amit, R.; Mete, O.; Asa, S.L.; Ezzat, S.; Joshua, A.M. Malignant pheochromocytoma secreting vasoactive intestinal peptide and response to Sunitinib: A case report and literature review. *Endocr. Pr.* **2014**, *20*, e145–e150. [CrossRef] [PubMed]
157. Ghzili, H.; Grumolato, L.; Thouennon, E.; Tanguy, Y.; Turquier, V.; Vaudry, H.; Anouar, Y. Role of PACAP in the physiology and pathology of the sympathoadrenal system. *Front. Neuroendocrinol.* **2008**, *29*, 128–141. [CrossRef] [PubMed]
158. Henry, J.P.; Sagne, C.; Bedet, C.; Gasnier, B. The vesicular monoamine transporter: From chromaffin granule to brain. *Neurochem. Int.* **1998**, *32*, 227–246. [CrossRef]
159. Wimalasena, K. Vesicular monoamine transporters: Structure-function, pharmacology, and medicinal chemistry. *Med. Res. Rev.* **2011**, *31*, 483–519. [CrossRef]
160. Schuldiner, S.; Shirvan, A.; Linial, M. Vesicular neurotransmitter transporters: From bacteria to humans. *Physiol. Rev.* **1995**, *75*, 369–392. [CrossRef]
161. Hillarp, N.A.; Hokfelt, B. Evidence of adrenaline and noradrenaline in separate adrenal medullary cells. *Acta Physiol. Scand* **1953**, *30*, 55–68. [CrossRef]
162. Carmichael, S.W. The adrenal chromaffin vesicle: An historical perspective. *J. Auton. Nerv. Syst.* **1983**, *7*, 7–12. [CrossRef]
163. Eisenhofer, G. The role of neuronal and extraneuronal plasma membrane transporters. *Pharmacol. Ther.* **2001**, *91*, 35–62. [CrossRef]
164. Huynh, T.T.; Pacak, K.; Brouwers, F.M.; Abu-Asab, M.S.; Worrel, R.A.; Walther, M.M.; Elkahloun, A.G.; Goldstein, D.S.; Cleary, S.; Eisenhofer, G. Different expression of catecholamine transporters in phaeochromocytomas from patients with von Hippel-Lindau syndrome and multiple endocrine neoplasia type 2. *Eur. J. Endocrinol.* **2005**, *153*, 551–563. [CrossRef] [PubMed]
165. Motulsky, H.J.; Insel, P.A. Adrenergic receptors in man: Direct identification, physiologic regulation, and clinical alterations. *N. Engl. J. Med.* **1982**, *307*, 18–29. [CrossRef] [PubMed]
166. Guimaraes, S.; Moura, D. Vascular Adrenoceptors: An update. *Pharm. Rev.* **2001**, *53*, 319–356. [PubMed]
167. Aunis, D.; Langley, K. Physiological aspects of exocytosis in chromaffin cells of the adrenal medulla. *Acta Physiol. Scand* **1999**, *167*, 89–97. [CrossRef] [PubMed]
168. Wong, D.L.; Anderson, L.J.; Tai, T.C. Cholinergic and peptidergic regulation of phenylethanolamine N-methyltransferase gene expression. *Ann. N. Y. Acad. Sci.* **2002**, *971*, 19–26. [CrossRef] [PubMed]
169. Eisenhofer, G.; Huynh, T.T.; Elkahloun, A.; Morris, J.C.; Bratslavsky, G.; Linehan, W.M.; Zhuang, Z.; Balgley, B.M.; Lee, C.S.; Manelli, M.; et al. Differential expression of the regulated catecholamine secretory pathway in different hereditary forms of pheochromocytoma. *Am. J. Physiol. Endocrinol. Metab.* **2008**, *295*, E1223–E1233. [CrossRef] [PubMed]
170. Colomer, C.; Desarmenien, M.G.; Guerineau, N.C. Revisiting the stimulus-secretion coupling in the adrenal medulla: Role of gap junction-mediated intercellular communication. *Mol. Neurobiol.* **2009**, *40*, 87–100. [CrossRef] [PubMed]
171. García, A.G.; Garciá-de Diego, A.M.; Gandía, L.; Borges, R.; García-Sancho, J. Calcium signalling and exocytosis in adrenal chromaffin cells. *Physiol. Rev.* **2006**, *86*, 1093–1131. [CrossRef] [PubMed]
172. Marengo, F.D.; Cardenas, A.M. How does the stimulus define exocytosis in adrenal chromaffin cells (review). *Pflug. Arch.* **2018**, *470*, 155–167. [CrossRef] [PubMed]
173. Trifaro, J.M.; Gasman, S.; Gutierrez, L.M. Cytoskeletal control of vesicle transport and exocytosis in chromaffin cells. *Acta Physiol. (Oxf.)* **2008**, *192*, 165–172. [CrossRef] [PubMed]
174. Burgoyne, R.; Morgan, A. Analysis of regulated exocytosis in adrenal chromaffin cells: Insights into NSF/SNAP/SNARE function. *BioEssays* **1998**, *20*, 328–335. [CrossRef]
175. Holz, R.W.; Brondyk, W.H.; Senter, R.A.; Kuizon, L.; Macara, I.G. Evidence for the involvement of Rab3A in Ca(2+)-dependent exocytosis from adrenal chromaffin cells. *J. Biol. Chem.* **1994**, *269*, 10229–10234. [CrossRef] [PubMed]
176. Burgoyne, R.D.; Morgan, A.; Robinson, I.; Pender, N.; Cheek, T.R. Exocytosis in adrenal chromaffin cells. *J. Anat.* **1993**, *183*, 309–314.
177. Umbrecht-Jenck, E.; Demais, V.; Calco, V.; Bailly, Y.; Bader, M.F.; Chasserot-Golaz, S. S100A10 mediated translocation of annexin A2 to SNARE proteins in adrenergic chromaffin cells undergoing exocytosis. *Traffic* **2010**, *11*, 958–971. [CrossRef] [PubMed]

178. Gabel, A.G.; Chasserot-Golaz, S. Annexin A2, an essential partner of the exocytotic process in chromaffin cells. *J. Neurochem.* **2016**, *137*, 890–896. [CrossRef] [PubMed]
179. Cavadas, C.; Silva, A.L.P.; Mosimann, F.; Cotrim, M.D.; Ribeiro, C.A.; Brunner, H.R.; Grouzmann, E. NPY regulates catecholamine secretion from human adrenal chromaffin cells. *J. Clin. Endocrinol. Metab.* **2001**, *86*, 5956–5963. [CrossRef]
180. Fishbein, L.; Merrill, S.; Fraker, D.L.; Cohen, D.L.; Nathanson, K.L. Inherited mutations in pheochromocytoma and paraganglioma: Why all patients should be offered genetic testing. *Ann. Surg. Oncol.* **2013**, *20*, 1440–1450. [CrossRef]
181. Dahia, P.L. Pheochromocytoma and paraganglioma pathogenesis: Learning from genetic heterogeneity. *Nat. Rev. Cancer* **2014**, *14*, 108–119. [CrossRef]
182. Crona, J.; Nordling, M.; Maharjan, R.; Granberg, D.; Stålberg, P.; Hellman, P.; Björklund, P. Integrative genetic characterization and phenotype correlations in pheochromocytoma and paraganglioma tumours. *PLoS ONE* **2014**, *9*, e86756. [CrossRef]
183. Burnichon, N.; Buffet, A.; Gimenez-Roqueplo, A.P. Pheochromocytoma and paraganglioma: Molecular testing and personalized medicine. *Curr. Opin. Oncol.* **2016**, *28*, 5–10. [CrossRef] [PubMed]
184. NGS in PPGL (NGSnPPGL) Study Group; Toledo, R.A.; Burnichon, N.; Cascon, N.; Cascon, A.; Benn, D.E.; Bayley, J.P.; Welander, J.; Tops, C.M.; Firth, H.; et al. Consensus statement on next-generation-sequencing-based diagnostic testing of hereditary phaeochromocytomas and paragangliomas. *Nat. Rev. Endocrinol.* **2017**, *13*, 233–247. [CrossRef] [PubMed]
185. Dahia, P.L.; Ross, K.N.; Wright, M.E.; Hayashida, C.Y.; Santagata, S.; Barontini, M.; Kung, A.L.; Sanso, G.; Powers, J.F.; Tischler, A.S.; et al. A HIF1alpha regulatory loop links hypoxia and mitochondrial signals in pheochromocytomas. *PLoS Genet.* **2005**, *1*, 72–80. [CrossRef] [PubMed]
186. Eisenhofer, G.; Huynh, T.T.; Pacak, K.; Brouwers, F.M.; Walther, M.M.; Linehan, W.M.; Munson, P.J.; Mannelli, M.; Goldstein, D.S.; Elkahloun, A.G. Distinct gene expression profiles in norepinephrine- and epinephrine- producing hereditary and sporadic pheochromocytomas: Activation of hypoxia-driven angiogenic pathways in von Hippel-Lindau syndrome. *Endocr. Relat. Cancer* **2004**, *11*, 897–911. [CrossRef] [PubMed]
187. Fishbein, L.; Leshchiner, I.; Walter, V.; Danilova, L.; Robertson, A.G.; Johnson, A.R.; Lichtenberg, T.M.; Murray, B.A.; Ghayee, H.K.; Else, T.; et al. Comprehensive Molecular Characterization of Pheochromocytoma and Paraganglioma. *Cancer Cell* **2017**, *31*, 181–193. [CrossRef] [PubMed]
188. Crona, J.; Taïeb, D.; Pacak, K. New perspectives on pheochromocytoma and paraganglioma: Toward a molecular classification. *Endocr. Rev.* **2017**, *38*, 489–515. [CrossRef] [PubMed]
189. Fishbein, L.; Wilkerson, M.D. Chromaffin cell biology: Interferences from the Cancer Genome Atlas. *Cell Tissue Res.* **2018**, *372*, 339–346. [CrossRef] [PubMed]
190. Calsina, B.; Curras-Freixes, M.; Buffet, A.; Pons, T.; Contreras, L.; Leton, R.; Comino-Mendez, I.; Remacha, L.; Calatayud, M.; Obispo, B.; et al. Role of MDH2 pathogenic variant in pheochromocytoma and paraganglioma patients. *Genet. Med.* **2018**, *20*, 1652–1662. [CrossRef] [PubMed]
191. Richter, S.; Gieldon, L.; Pang, Y.; Peitzsch, M.; Huynh, T.; Leton, R.; Viana, B.; Ercolino, T.; Mangelis, A.; Rapizzi, E.; et al. Metabolome-guided genomics to identify pathogenic variants in isocitrate dehydrogenase, fumarate hydratase, and succinate dehydrogenase genes in pheochromocytoma and paraganglioma. *Genet. Med.* **2019**, *21*, 705–717. [CrossRef]
192. Yang, C.; Zhuang, Z.; Fliedner, S.M.; Shankavaram, U.; Sun, M.G.; Bullova, P.; Zhu, R.; Elkahloun, A.G.; Kourlas, P.J.; Merino, M. Germ-line PHD1 and PHD2 mutations detected in patients with pheochromocytoma/paraganglioma-polycythemia. *J. Mol. Med.* **2015**, *93*, 93–104. [CrossRef]
193. Alrezk, R.; Suarez, A.; Tena, I.; Pacak, K. Update of pheochromocytoma syndromes: Genetics, biochemical evaluation and imaging. *Front. Endocrinol. (Lausanne)* **2018**, *9*, 515. [CrossRef] [PubMed]
194. Crona, J.; Delgado Verdugo, A.; Maharjan, R.; Stålberg, P.; Granberg, D.; Hellman, P.; Björklund, P. Somatic mutations in H-RAS in sporadic pheochromocytoma and paraganglioma identified by exome sequencing. *J. Clin. Endocrinol. Metab.* **2013**, *98*, E1266–E1271. [CrossRef] [PubMed]
195. Nakada, T.; Furuta, H.; Katayama, T. Catecholamine metabolism in pheochromocytoma and normal adrenal medullae. *J. Urol.* **1988**, *140*, 1348–1351. [CrossRef]

196. Kimura, N.; Miura, Y.; Nagatsu, I.; Nagura, H. Catecholamine synthesizing enzymes in 70 cases of functioning and non-functioning phaeochromocytoma and extra-adrenal paraganglioma. *Virchows Arch. A Pathol. Anat. Histopathol.* **1992**, *421*, 25–32. [CrossRef] [PubMed]
197. Funahashi, H.; Imai, T.; Tanaka, Y.; Tobinaga, J.; Wada, M.; Matsuyama, T.; Tsukamura, K.; Yamada, F.; Takagi, H.; Narita, T.; et al. Discrepancy between PNMT presence and relative lack of adrenaline production in extra-adrenal pheochromocytoma. *J. Surg. Oncol.* **1994**, *57*, 196–200. [CrossRef] [PubMed]
198. Meijer, W.G.; Copray, S.C.; Hollema, H.; Kema, I.P.; Zwart, N.; Mantingh-Otter, I.; Links, T.P.; Willemse, P.H.; de Vries, E.G. Catecholamine-synthesizing enzymes in carcinoid tumors and pheochromocytomas. *Clin. Chem.* **2003**, *49*, 586–593. [CrossRef]
199. Grouzmann, E.; Tschopp, O.; Triponez, F.; Matter, M.; Bilz, S.; Brändle, M.; Drechser, T.; Sigrist, S.; Zulewski, H.; Henzen, C.; et al. Catecholamine metabolism in paraganglioma and pheochromocytoma: Similar tumors in different sites? *PLoS ONE* **2015**, *10*, e0125426. [CrossRef] [PubMed]
200. Konosu-Fukaya, S.; Omata, K.; Tezuka, Y.; Ono, Y.; Aoyama, Y.; Satoh, F.; Fujishima, F.; Sasano, H.; Nakamura, Y. Catecholamine-synthesizing enzymes in pheochromocytoma and extra adrenal paraganglioma. *Endocr. Pathol.* **2018**, *29*, 302–309. [CrossRef] [PubMed]
201. Iwase, K.; Nagasaka, A.; Nagatsu, I.; Kikuchi, K.; Nagatsu, T.; Funahashi, H.; Tsujimura, T.; Inagaki, A.; Nakai, A.; Kishikawa, T.; et al. Tyrosine hydroxylase induces cell differentiation of catecholamine biosynthesis in neuroendocrine tumors. *J. Endocrinol. Investig.* **1994**, *17*, 235–239. [CrossRef]
202. Feldman, J.M. Phenylethanolamine-N-methyltransferase activity determines the epinephrine concentration of pheochromocytomas. *Res. Commun. Chem. Pathol. Pharm.* **1981**, *34*, 389–398. [CrossRef]
203. Fliedner, S.M.; Breza, J.; Kvetnansky, R.; Powers, J.F.; Tischler, A.S.; Wesley, R.; Merino, M.; Lehnert, H.; Pacak, K. Tyrosine hydroxylase, chromogranin A, and steroidogenic acute regulator as markers for successful separation of human adrenal medulla. *Cell Tissue Res.* **2010**, *340*, 607–612. [CrossRef] [PubMed]
204. Feldman, J.M.; Blalock, J.A.; Zern, R.T.; Wells, S.A., Jr. The relationship between enzyme activity and the catecholamine content and secretion of pheochromocytomas. *J. Clin. Endocrinol. Metab.* **1979**, *49*, 445–451. [CrossRef] [PubMed]
205. Dubois, L.A.; Gray, D.K. Dopamine-secreting pheochromocytomas: In search of a syndrome. *World J. Surg.* **2005**, *29*, 909–913. [CrossRef] [PubMed]
206. Eisenhofer, G.; Lenders, J.W.; Timmers, H.; Mannelli, M.; Grebe, S.K.; Hofbauer, L.C.; Bornstein, S.R.; Tiebel, O.; Adams, K.; Bratslavsky, G.; et al. Measurements of plasma Methoxytyramine, normetanephrine, and metanephrine as discriminators of different hereditary forms of pheochromocytoma. *Clin. Chem.* **2011**, *57*, 411–420. [CrossRef] [PubMed]
207. Eisenhofer, G.; Pacak, K.; Huynh, T.T.; Qin, N.; Bratslavsky, G.; Linehan, W.M.; Mannelli, M.; Friberg, P.; Timmers, H.J.; Bornstein, S.R.; et al. Catecholamine metabolomics and secretory phenotypes in phaeochromocytoma. *Endocr. Relat. Cancer* **2011**, *18*, 97–111. [CrossRef] [PubMed]
208. Timmers, H.J.; Pacak, K.; Huynh, T.T.; Abu-Asab, M.; Tsokos, M.; Merino, M.J.; Baysal, B.E.; Adams, K.T.; Eisenhofer, G. Biochemically silent abdominal paragangliomas in patients with mutations in the succinate dehydrogenase subunit B gene. *J. Clin. Endocrinol. Metab.* **2008**, *93*, 4826–4832. [CrossRef]
209. Dreijerink, K.M.A.; Rijken, J.A.; Compaijen, C.J.A.C.; Timmers, H.J.L.M.; van der Horst-Schrivers, A.N.A.; van Leeuwaarde, R.S.; van Dam, S.; Leemans, C.R.; van Dam, E.W.C.M.; Dickhoff, C.; et al. Biochemically silent sympathetic paraganglioma, pheochromocytoma or metastatic disease in SDHD mutation carriers. *J. Clin. Endocrinol. Metab.* **2019**. [CrossRef]
210. Eisenhofer, G.; Walther, M.; Huynh, T.T.; Li, S.T.; Bornstein, S.R.; Vortmeyer, A.; Mannelli, M.; Goldstein, D.S.; Linehan, W.M.; Lenders, J.W.; et al. Pheochromocytomas in von Hippel-Lindau Syndrome and multiple endocrine neoplasia type 2 display distinct biochemical and clinical phenotypes. *J. Clin. Endocrinol. Metab.* **2001**, *86*, 1999–2008. [CrossRef]
211. Letouzé, E.; Martinelli, C.; Loriot, C.; Burnichon, N.; Abermil, N.; Ottolenghi, C.; Janin, M.; Menara, M.; Nguyen, A.T.; Benit, P.; et al. SDH mutations establish a hypermethylator phenotype in paraganglioma. *Cancer Cell* **2013**, *23*, 739–752. [CrossRef]
212. Favier, J.; Briere, J.J.; Burnichon, N.; Riviere, J.; Vescovo, L.; Benit, P.; Giscos-Douriez, I.; De Reynies, A.; Bertherat, J.; Badoual, C.; et al. The Warburg effect is genetically determined in inherited pheochromocytomas. *PLoS ONE* **2009**, *4*, e7094. [CrossRef]

213. Lopez-Jimenez, E.; Gomez-Lopez, G.; Leandro-Garcia, L.J.; Munoz, I.; Schiavi, F.; Montero-Conde, C.; de Cubas, A.A.; Ramires, R.; Landa, I.; Leskelä, S.; et al. Research resource: Transcriptional profiling reveals different pseudohypoxic signatures in SDHB and VHL-related pheochromocytomas. *Mol. Endocrinol.* **2010**, *24*, 2382–2391. [CrossRef] [PubMed]
214. Burnichon, N.; Vescovo, L.; Amar, L.; Libé, R.; de Reynies, A.; Venisse, A.; Jouanno, E.; Laurendeau, I.; Parfait, B.; Bertherat, J.; et al. Integrative genomic analysis reveals somatic mutations in pheochromocytoma and paraganglioma. *Hum. Mol. Genet.* **2011**, *20*, 3974–3985. [CrossRef] [PubMed]
215. Qin, N.; de Cubas, A.A.; Garcia-Martin, R.; Richter, S.; Peitzsch, M.; Menschikowski, M.; Lenders, J.W.; Timmers, H.J.; Mannelli, M.; Opocher, G.; et al. Opposing effects of HIF1a and HIF2a on chromaffin cell phenotypic features and tumor cell proliferation: Insights from MYC associated factor X. *Int. J. Cancer* **2014**, *135*, 2054–2064. [CrossRef] [PubMed]
216. Tian, H.; Hammer, R.E.; Matsumoto, A.M.; Russell, D.W.; McKnight, S.L. The hypoxia-responsive transcription factor EPAS1 is essential for catecholamine homeostasis and protection against heart failure during embryonic development. *Genes Dev.* **1998**, *12*, 3320–3324. [CrossRef] [PubMed]
217. Favier, J.; Kempf, H.; Corvol, P.; Casc, J.M. Cloning and expression pattern of EPAS1 in the chicken embryo. Colocalization with tyrosine hydroxylase. *FEBS Lett.* **1999**, *462*, 19–24. [CrossRef]
218. Nilsson, H.; Jögi, A.; Beckman, S.; Harris, A.L.; Poellinger, L.; Pahlman, S. HIF-2alpha expression in human fetal paraganglia and neuroblastoma: Relation to sympathetic differentiation, glucose deficiency, and hypoxia. *Exp. Cell Res.* **2005**, *303*, 447–456. [CrossRef]
219. Wang, H.; Cui, J.; Yang, C.; Rosenblum, R.S.; Zhang, Q.; Song, Q.; Pang, Y.; Fang, F.; Sun, M.; Dmitriev, P. A transgenic mouse model of Pacak-Zhuang syndrome with an EPAS1 gain of function mutation. *Cancers* **2019**, *11*, 667. [CrossRef] [PubMed]
220. Burnichon, N.; Cascon, A.; Schiavi, F.; Morales, N.P.; Comino-Mendez, I.; Abermil, N.; Inglada-Perez, L.; de Cubas, A.A.; Amar, L.; Barontini, M.; et al. MAX mutations cause hereditary and sporadic pheochromocytoma and paraganglioma. *Clin. Cancer Res.* **2012**, *18*, 2828–2837. [CrossRef] [PubMed]
221. Lloyd, R.V.; Osamura, R.Y.; Kloppel, G.; Rosai, J. *WHO Classification of Tumours: Pathology and Genetics of Tumours of Endocrine Organs*, 4th ed.; IARC: Lyon, France, 2017.
222. Tischler, A.S.; de Krijger, R.R. Pathology of pheochromocytoma and paraganglioma. *Endocr. Relat. Cancer* **2015**, *22*, 123–133. [CrossRef]
223. Thompson, L.D. Pheochromocytoma of the adrenal gland scaled score (PASS) to separate benign from malignant neoplasms: A clinicopathological and immunophenotypic study of 100 cases. *Am. J. Surg. Pathol.* **2002**, *26*, 551–566. [CrossRef]
224. Wu, D.; Tischler, A.S.; Lloyd, R.V.; DeLellis, R.A.; de Krijger, R.; van Nederveen, F.; Nosé, V. Obserer variation in the application of the pheochromocytoma of the adrenal gland scaled score. *Am. J. Surg. Pathol.* **2009**, *33*, 599–608. [CrossRef] [PubMed]
225. Kimura, N.; Takayanagi, R.; Takizawa, N.; Itagaki, E.; Katabami, T.; Kakoi, N.; Rakugi, H.; Ikeda, Y.; Tanabe, A.; Nigawara, T.; et al. Pathological grading for predicting metastasis in phaeochromocytoma and paraganglioma. *Endocr. Relat. Cancer* **2014**, *21*, 405–414. [CrossRef] [PubMed]
226. Szalat, A.; Fraenkel, M.; Doviner, V.; Salmon, A.; Gross, D.J. Malignant pheochromocytoma: Predictive factors of malignancy and clinical course in 16 patients at a single tertiary medical center. *Endocrine* **2010**, *39*, 160–166. [CrossRef] [PubMed]
227. Ayala-Ramirez, M.; Feng, L.; Johnson, M.M.; Ejaz, S.; Habra, M.A.; Rich, T.; Busaidy, N.; Cote, G.J.; Perrier, N.; Phan, A.; et al. Clinical risk factors for malignancy and overall survival in patients with pheochromocytomas and sympathetic paragangliomas: Primary tumor size and primary tumor location as prognostic indicators. *J. Clin. Endocrinol. Metab.* **2011**, *96*, 717–725. [CrossRef] [PubMed]
228. Goffredo, P.; Sosa, J.A.; Roman, S.A. Malignant pheochromocytoma and paraganglioma; a population level analysis of long-term survival over two decades. *J. Surg. Oncol.* **2013**, *107*, 659–664. [CrossRef] [PubMed]
229. Hamidi, O.; Young, W.F., Jr.; Iniguez-Ariza, N.M.; Kittah, N.E.; Gruber, L.; Bancos, C.; Tamhane, S.; Bancos, I. Malignant pheochromocytoma and paraganglioma: 272 patients over 55 years. *J. Clin. Endocrinol. Metab.* **2017**, *102*, 3296–3305. [CrossRef] [PubMed]

230. Hescot, S.; Curras-Freixes, M.; Deutschbein, T.; van Berkel, A.; Vezzosi, D.; Amar, L.; de la Fouchardiere, C.; Valdes, N.; Riccardi, F.; Do Cao, C.; et al. Prognosis of malignant pheochromocytoma and paraganglioma (MAPP Prono Study): A European Network for the Study of Adrenal Tumors Retrospective Study. *J. Clin. Endocrinol. Metab.* **2019**, *104*, 2367–2374. [CrossRef]
231. Amar, L.; Bertherat, J.; Baudin, E.; Ajzenberg, C.; Bressac-de Paillerets, B.; Chabre, O.; Chamontin, B.; Delemer, B.; Giraud, S.; Murat, A. Genetic testing in pheochromocytoma or functional paraganglioma. *J. Clin. Oncol.* **2005**, *23*, 8812–8818. [CrossRef]
232. Amar, L.; Baudin, E.; Burnichon, N.; Peyrard, S.; Silvera, S.; Bertherat, J.; Bertagna, X.; Schlumberger, M.; Jeunemaitre, X.; Gimenez-Roqueplo, A.P.; et al. Succinate dehydrogenase B gene mutations predict survival in patients with malignant pheochromocytomas or paragangliomas. *J. Clin. Endocrinol. Metab.* **2007**, *92*, 3822–3828. [CrossRef]
233. Burnichon, N.; Rohmer, V.; Amar, L.; Herman, P.; Leboulleux, S.; Darrouzet, V.; Niccoli, P.; Gaillard, D.; Chabrier, G.; Chabolle, F.; et al. The succinate dehydrogenase genetic testing in a large prospective series of patients with paragangliomas. *J. Clin. Endocrinol. Metab.* **2009**, *94*, 2817–2827. [CrossRef]
234. Castro-Vega, L.J.; Buffet, A.; De Cubas, A.A.; Cascon, A.; Menara, M.; Khalifa, E.; Amar, L.; Azriel, S.; Bourdeau, I.; Chabre, O.; et al. Germline mutations in FH confer predisposition to malignant pheochromocytomas and paragangliomas. *Hum. Mol. Genet.* **2014**, *23*, 2440–2446. [CrossRef] [PubMed]
235. Buffet, A.; Morin, A.; Castro-Vega, L.J.; Habarou, F.; Lussey-Lepoutre, C.; Letouzé, E.; Lefebvre, H.; Guilhem, I.; Haissaguerre, M.; Raingeard, I.; et al. Germline mutations in the mitochrondrial 2-oxoglutarate/malate carrier SLC25A11 gene confer a predisposition to metastatic paragangliomas. *Cancer Res.* **2018**, *78*, 1914–1922. [CrossRef] [PubMed]
236. Bausch, B.; Schiavi, F.; Ni, Y.; Welander, J.; Patocs, A.; Ngeow, J.; Wellner, U.; Malinoc, A.; Taschin, E.; Barbon, G.; et al. Clinical characterization of the pheochromocytoma and paraganglioma susceptibility genes SDHA, TMEM127, MAX, and SDHAF2 for gene-informed prevention. *JAMA Oncol.* **2017**, *3*, 1204–1212. [CrossRef] [PubMed]
237. Eisenhofer, G.; Lenders, J.W.; Siegert, G.; Bornstein, S.R.; Friberg, P.; Milosevic, D.; Mannelli, M.; Linehan, W.M.; Adams, K.; Timmers, H.J.; et al. Plasma methoxytyramine; a novel biomarker of metastatic pheochromocytoma and paraganglioma in relation to established risk factors of tumor size, location and SDHB mutation status. *Eur. J. Cancer* **2012**, *48*, 1739–1749. [CrossRef] [PubMed]
238. Peitzsch, M.; Prejbisz, A.; Kroiβ, M.; Beuschlein, F.; Arlt, W.; Januszewicz, A.; Siegert, G.; Eisenhofer, G. Analysis of plasma 3-methoxytyramine, normetanephrine and metanephrine by ultraperformance liquid chromatography tandem mass spectrometry: Utility for diagnosis of dopamineproducing metastatic phaeochromocytoma. *Ann. Clin. Biochem.* **2013**, *50*, 147–155. [CrossRef]
239. Van der Harst, E.; de Herder, W.W.; de Krijger, R.R.; Bruining, H.A.; Bonjer, H.J.; Lamberts, S.W.; van den Meiracker, A.H.; Stijnen, T.H.; Boomsma, F. The value of plasma markers for the clinical behaviour of phaeochromocytomas. *Eur. J. Endocrinol.* **2002**, *147*, 85–94. [CrossRef] [PubMed]
240. Sue, M.; Martucci, V.; Frey, F.; Lenders, J.M.; Timmers, H.J.; Peczkowska, M.; Prejbisz, A.; Swantje, B.; Bornstein, S.R.; Arlt, W.; et al. Lack of utility of SDHB mutation testing in adrenergic metastatic phaeochromocytoma. *Eur. J. Endocrinol.* **2015**, *172*, 89–95. [CrossRef]
241. Selak, M.A.; Armour, S.M.; MacKenzie, E.D.; Boulahbel, H.; Watson, D.G.; Mansfield, K.D.; Pan, Y.; Simon, M.C.; Thompson, C.B.; Gottlieb, E. Succinate links TCA cycle dysfunction to oncogenesis by inhibiting HIF-alpha prolyl hydroxylase. *Cancer Cell* **2005**, *7*, 77–85. [CrossRef]
242. Xiao, M.; Yang, H.; Xu, W.; Ma, S.; Lin, H.; Zhu, H.; Liu, L.; Liu, Y.; Yang, C.; Xu, Y.; et al. Inhibition of alpha-KG-dependent histone and DNA demethylases by fumarate and succinate that are accumulated in mutations of FH and SDH tumor suppressors. *Genes Dev.* **2012**, *26*, 1326–1338. [CrossRef]
243. Richter, S.; Peitzsch, M.; Rapizzi, E.; Lenders, J.W.; Qin, N.; de Cubas, A.A.; Schiavi, F.; Rao, J.U.; Beuschlein, F.; Quinkler, M.; et al. Krebs cycle metabolite profiling for identification and stratification of pheochromocytoma/paragangliomas due to succinate dehydrogenase deficiency. *J. Clin. Endocrinol. Metab.* **2014**, *99*, 3903–3911. [CrossRef]
244. Ploumakis, A.; Coleman, M.L. OH, the places you'll go! Hydroxylation, gene expression and cancer. *Mol. Cell* **2015**, *58*, 729–741. [CrossRef] [PubMed]

245. Barollo, S.; Bertazza, L.; Watutantrige-Fernando, S.; Censi, S.; Cavedon, E.; Galuppini, F.; Pennelli, G.; Fassina, A.; Citton, M.; Rubin, B.; et al. Overexpression of L-type amino acid transporter 1 (LAT1) and 2 (LAT2): Novel markers of neuroendocrine tumors. *PLoS ONE* **2016**, *11*, e0156044. [CrossRef] [PubMed]
246. Yanagida, O.; Kanai, Y.; Chairoungdua, A.; Kim, D.K.; Segawa, H.; Nii, T.; Cha, S.H.; Matsuo, H.; Fukushima, J.; Fukasawa, Y.; et al. Human L-type amino acid transporter 1 (LAT1): Characterization of function and expression in tumour cell lines. *Biochem. Biophys. Acta* **2001**, *1*, 291–302. [CrossRef]
247. Zhao, Y.; Wang, L.; Pan, J. The role of L-type amino acid transporter 1 in human tumours. *Intractable Rare Dis. Res.* **2015**, *4*, 165–169. [CrossRef] [PubMed]
248. Kongpracha, P.; Nagamori, S.; Wiriyasermkul, P.; Tanaka, Y.; Kaneda, K.; Okuda, S.; Ohgaki, R.; Kanai, Y. Structure-activity relationship of novel series of inhibitors for cancer type transporter L-type amino acid transporter 1 (LAT1). *J. Pharmacol. Sci.* **2017**, *133*, 96–102. [CrossRef] [PubMed]
249. Lamberti, G.; Brighi, N.; Maggio, I.; Manuzzi, L.; Peterle, C.; Ambrosini, V.; Ricci, C.; Casadei, R.; Campana, D. The role of the mTOR in neuroendocrine tumors: Future cornerstone of a winning strategy? *Int. J. Mol. Sci.* **2018**, *19*, 747. [CrossRef]
250. Willenberg, H.S.; Schott, M.; Saeger, W.; Tries, A.; Scherbaum, W.A.; Bornstein, S.R. Expression of connexins in chromaffin cells of normal human adrenals and in benign and malignant pheochromocytomas. *Ann. N. Y. Acad. Sci.* **2006**, *1073*, 578–583. [CrossRef] [PubMed]

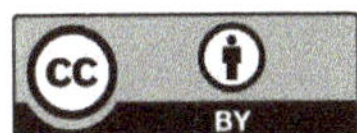

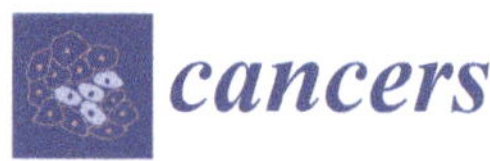

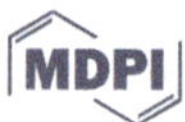

Review

Pheochromocytomas and Paragangliomas: Bypassing Cellular Respiration

Alberto Cascón [1,2,*], Laura Remacha [1], Bruna Calsina [1] and Mercedes Robledo [1,2,*]

1 Hereditary Endocrine Cancer Group, Spanish National Cancer Research Centre (CNIO), 28029 Madrid, Spain; l.remacha.m@gmail.com (L.R.); bcalsina@cnio.es (B.C.)

2 Centro de Investigación Biomédica en Red de Enfermedades Raras (CIBERER), 28029 Madrid, Spain

* Correspondence: acascon@cnio.es (A.C.); mrobledo@cnio.es (M.R.); Tel.: +34-91-224-69-47; Fax: +34-91-224-69-23

Received: 8 April 2019; Accepted: 13 May 2019; Published: 16 May 2019

Abstract: Pheochromocytomas and paragangliomas (PPGL) are rare neuroendocrine tumors that show the highest heritability of all human neoplasms and represent a paradoxical example of genetic heterogeneity. Amongst the elevated number of genes involved in the hereditary predisposition to the disease (at least nineteen) there are eleven tricarboxylic acid (TCA) cycle-related genes, some of which are also involved in the development of congenital recessive neurological disorders and other cancers such as cutaneous and uterine leiomyomas, gastrointestinal tumors and renal cancer. Somatic or germline mutation of genes encoding enzymes catalyzing pivotal steps of the TCA cycle not only disrupts cellular respiration, but also causes severe alterations in mitochondrial metabolite pools. These latter alterations lead to aberrant accumulation of "oncometabolites" that, in the end, may lead to deregulation of the metabolic adaptation of cells to hypoxia, inhibition of the DNA repair processes and overall pathological changes in gene expression. In this review, we will address the TCA cycle mutations leading to the development of PPGL, and we will discuss the relevance of these mutations for the transformation of neural crest-derived cells and potential therapeutic approaches based on the emerging knowledge of underlying molecular alterations.

Keywords: pheochromocytoma; paraganglioma; TCA cycle; germline mutation

---

1. Metabolism and Cancer

Almost a century ago, Nobel Prize winner Otto Warburg described how cancer cells can reprogram glucose metabolism by dramatically increasing the rate of glucose uptake, which is fermented to produce lactate even in the presence of oxygen and fully functioning mitochondria [1]. This observation suggested that defects in mitochondrial respiration could be the underlying cause of cancer. Although this aerobic glycolytic mechanism, known as the Warburg effect, has been studied extensively, its benefits for cell growth and survival are not well understood. In fact, nowadays it is more accepted that genetic events occurring in cancer cells are the cause of the alterations in metabolism observed by Warburg in the 1920s. At the beginning of the 21st century, the first mutations in the *SDHD* gene were reported, providing for the first time a link between germline alterations in a metabolic gene and the development of cancer, and demonstrating how disruption of mitochondrial respiration may lead to tumor development [2]. Moreover, the description of the first germline mutations in the *SDHD* gene in patients with hereditary pheochromocytoma (PCC) and paraganglioma (PGL) (together referred to as PPGL) marked a milestone in the study of this rare disease.

2. Germline or Somatic Disruption of the Tricarboxylic Acid (TCA) Cycle Leads to PPGL Development

For a long time it was thought that the tricarboxylic acid (TCA) cycle was so crucial to the metabolism of living cells that any significant defect, including mutations affecting the pivotal enzymatic activities, would be highly unlikely and probably incompatible with life. To date, thirteen TCA cycle-related genes have been described to be involved in the development of different cancers such as cutaneous and uterine leiomyomas, gastrointestinal tumors, gliomas, renal cancer, and especially PPGL. Thus, ~23% of PPGLs are found carrying mutations in genes encoding energy metabolism enzymes such as the succinate dehydrogenase (SDH) subunits (SDHx genes), fumarate hydratase or fumarase (*FH*), malate dehydrogenase 2 (*MDH2*), isocitrate dehydrogenases 1 (cytosolic), 2 and 3 (*IDH1/2/3*), glutamic-oxaloacetic transaminase 2 (*GOT2*) and solute carrier family 25 member 11 (*SLC25A11*) (Figure 1).

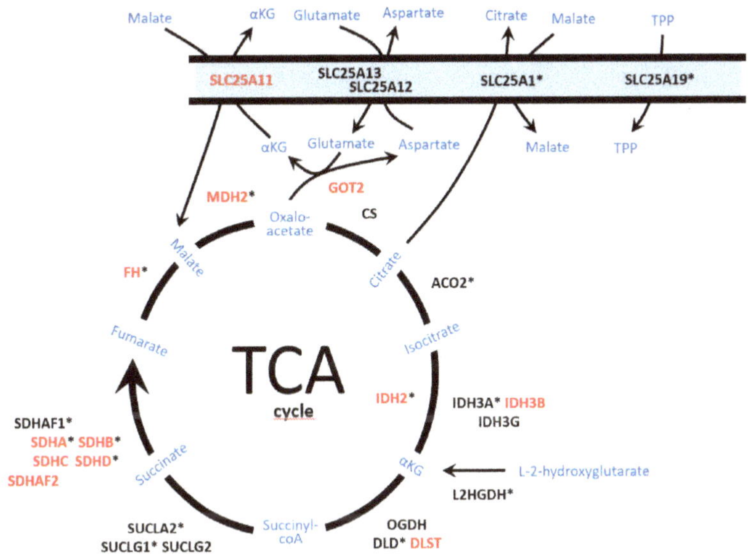

Figure 1. Schematic representation of the enzymes and mitochondrial metabolic pathways, tricarboxylic acid (TCA) cycle, malate/aspartate shuttle, nicotinamide adenine dinucleotide (NADH) exchange and metabolite efflux from the mitochondria, involved in pheochromocytoma and paraganglioma (PPGL) development and/or neurodegenerative disorders. Enzymes reported as altered in PPGL are denoted in red capital letters. Enzymes involved in neurodegenerative disorders are denoted with an asterisk. SLC25A11: solute carrier family 25 member 11; SLC25A12/SLC25A13: carriers solute carrier family 25 members 12/13; SLC25A1: solute carrier family 25 member 1; SLC25A19: solute carrier family 25 member 19; GOT2: mitochondrial glutamic-oxaloacetic transaminase 2; FH: fumarate hydratase; MDH2: mitochondrial malate dehydrogenase; CS: citrate synthase; ACO2: mitochondrial aconitase; IDH2: isocitrate dehydrogenase 2; IDH3A/IDH3B/IDH3G: subunits of isocitrate dehydrogenase 3; L2HGDH: L-2-hydroxyglutarate dehydrogenase; OGDH/DLD/DLST: subunits of the αKG (alpha-ketoglutarate) dehydrogenase complex; SUCLA2/SUCLG1/SUCLG2: subunits of succinyl-CoA synthetase; SDHA/B/C/D: subunits of the succinate dehydrogenase complex; SDHAF1/SDHAF2: succinate dehydrogenase assembly factors; αKG: α-ketoglutarate; TPP: thiamine pyrophosphate.

PPGLs are neuroendocrine tumors derived from chromaffin cells of the adrenal medulla and from neural crest progenitors of extra-adrenal paraganglia. Sympathetic PPGLs, including PCC and thoracic-abdominal-pelvic (TAP) PGLs, are mostly catecholamine-producing tumors, whereas those derived from parasympathetic paraganglia, mainly located in the head and neck (H&N) region, are non-secreting tumors. Although PPGLs are predominantly benign and patients can be cured by surgical removal of these tumors, they present a significant morbidity and mortality due to the clinical aggressiveness of metastatic tumors (especially those carrying mutations in TCA cycle-related genes), for which therapeutic options remain scarce. To note, PPGL is considered a very rare disease with an incidence of 2–8 patients per million per year (1000–2000 new cases diagnosed worldwide every year). Therefore, the discovery of new susceptibility genes involved in hereditary predisposition to develop metastatic PPGLs, which is crucial for genetic counseling, guiding follow-up and developing targeted therapies, has only been possible through the joint efforts of many groups studying this extremely rare disease.

3. SDH Genes and PPGL

Germline loss-of-function mutations in *SDHA, SDHB, SDHC, SDHD* and *SDHAF2* (together accounting for 20% of all PPGLs) cause the well-characterized familial PGL syndromes known as PGL5 [3], PGL4 [4], PGL3 [5], PGL1 [2] and PGL2 [6], respectively (Table 1). Additional solid tumors such as gastrointestinal stromal tumors (GISTs) [7], clear cell renal cell carcinomas (ccRCCs) [8] and pituitary adenomas (PAs) [9] have been associated, albeit rarely, with these familial PGL syndromes [10].

The SDH enzyme complex is a hetero-oligomer that comprises four structural subunits: two hydrophilic catalytic subunits, SDHA and SDHB, and two hydrophobic subunits that anchor the catalytic ones to the inner mitochondrial membrane, SDHC and SDHD. The fifth SDH gene associated with PPGL development, *SDHAF2*, encodes a cofactor responsible for flavination of SDHA. The SDH complex catalyzes the oxidative dehydrogenation of succinate to fumarate in the TCA cycle [11], and it is also functionally involved in the electron transport chain forming the mitochondrial complex II. Germline or somatic mutations in any of the SDH genes (SDHx) cause disassembly of the mitochondrial complex, with loss of SDH enzymatic activity and thus triggering the accumulation of its substrate, succinate. When succinate accumulates pathologically, it acts as a competitor of alpha-ketoglutarate (αKG) to broadly inhibit the activity of αKG-dependent dioxygenases, such as ten-eleven translocation (TET) DNA hydroxylases and Jumonji (JMJ) histone lysine demethylases (KDM) [12,13]. This causes a global hypermethylation with a characteristic CpG island methylation phenotype (CIMP) profile in the tumors, which leads to altered gene expression and contributes to tumorigenesis; this same mechanism was earlier observed in glioblastomas [14] and ccRCCs [15] carrying metabolic alterations such as *IDH1/2* and *FH/SDHB* mutations, respectively. Apart from the aforementioned CIMP profile, the accumulation of succinate competitively inhibits the family of prolyl hydroxylase domain-containing proteins (PHD1-3), leading to hypoxia-inducible factor 1 α (HIF-1α) stabilization under normoxic conditions, and contributing to activation of the pseudohypoxic pathway [16,17]. More recently, it was reported that the succinate-mediated inhibition of two αKG-dependent dioxygenases, histone lysine demethylases KDM4A and KDM4B, leads to suppression of homologous recombination [18]. Moreover, the accumulation of succinate also causes downregulation of the enzyme responsible for the conversion of norepinephrine to epinephrine, thus inducing the characteristic noradrenergic phenotype of SDHx tumors [13]. All these processes orchestrated by succinate (and fumarate) accumulation (both referred to as oncometabolites) have been proposed to be involved in tumorigenesis (Figure 2) and/or in the particular phenotype of PPGLs carrying TCA cycle-related mutations. This will be discussed in more detail below.

Table 1. Summary of phenotypic and genetic features associated with the TCA cycle-related PPGL genes.

TCA Cycle Gene	Chr. Location	Mean Age	% of Germline Mutations (Penetrance by Age) ¥	Risk of Malignancy (%)	Predominant Tumor Location	Number of Tumors (% Multiple)	BC	Related Syndromes; Associated Tumors
SDHD	11q23.1	35y	9–10 (43%, 60y)	Low (3–10%)	H&N > TAP > PCC	M (56%)	NA, DA	PGL1, Carney-Stratakis syndrome, encephalomyopathy *; ccRCC, GIST, PA
SDHB	1p36.13	30y	10 (13–21%, 50y)	High (30–50%)	TAP > H&N > PCC	S>M (20–25%)	NA, DA	PGL4, Carney-Stratakis syndrome, hypotonia and leukodystrophy *; ccRCC, GIST, PA
SDHC	1q23.3	40–50y	1–5 (25%, 60y)	Low (<3%)	H&N > TAP > PCC	S>M (15–20%)	NA, DA	PGL3, Carney-Stratakis syndrome; GIST, PA
SDHA	5p15.33	40y	3 (10%, 70y)	Moderate (12%)	H&N > TAP >> PCC	S>M (10–15%)	NA	PGL5, Leigh syndrome *, cardiomyopathy *, leukodystrophy *; ccRCC, GIST, PA
SDHAF2	11q12.2	30–40y	0.1–1	Low	H&N >> PCC	M (74%)	NA	PGL2; infantile leukoencephalopathy *
FH	1q42.1	-	1	High (60%)	PCC + TAP> H&N	M (60%)	NA	HLRCC, progressive encephalopathy in early childhood *; multiple cutaneous and uterine leiomyomatosis; cutaneous and uterine leiomyomas, type 2 papillary renal carcinoma
MDH2	7q11.23	45y	<1	High (50%)	TA	S > M (33%)	NA	Early-onset severe encephalopathy *
IDH1	2q34	>60y	NA	Low	TAP, H&N	S	NA	
SLC25A11	17p13.3	59y	1	High (70%)	TAP >> H&N	S	NA	
DLST	14q24.3	29y	<1	Low	TAP >> PCC	M (100%)	NA	

Chr: chromosome; ¥: penetrance data was included for genes with prevalence >1%; TCA: tricarboxylic acid; PGL: paraganglioma; NA: not applicable; H&N: head and neck paraganglioma; TAP: thoracic-abdominal-pelvic paraganglioma; PCC: pheochromocytoma; S: single; M: multiple BC: Biochemical predominant secretion; NA: noradrenergic (predominant secretion of noradrenaline/normetanephrine); A: adrenergic (predominant secretion of adrenaline/metanephrine); DA: dopaminergic (secretion of dopamine/3-methoxytyramine); GIST: gastrointestinal stromal tumor; ccRCC: clear cell renal cell carcinoma; PA: pituitary adenoma; HLRCC: hereditary leiomyomatosis and renal cell cancer. Other genes found mutated in single cases, such as *GOT2*, *IDH2* or *IDH3B*, are not included in the table. *: caused by autosomal-recessive mutations.

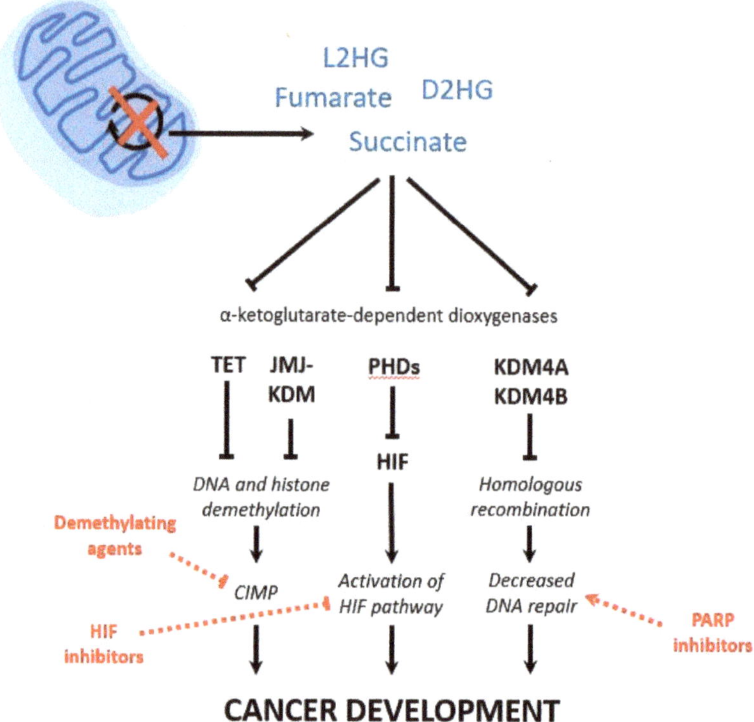

Figure 2. Schematic representation of the consequences of tricarboxylic acid (TCA) cycle disruption in pheochromocytomas and paragangliomas (PPGL). Upon disruption of the activity of pivotal TCA cycle enzymes, there is an accumulation of metabolites (i.e., succinate, fumarate, D2HG and L2HG). Their efflux from the mitochondria to the cytosol and their subsequent competition with α-ketoglutarate lead to the inhibition of α-ketoglutarate-dependent dioxygenases involved in DNA and histone demethylation, regulation of HIF, and homologous recombination. As a result, different mechanisms are proposed as the cause of tumorigenesis in PPGL: aberrant global hypermethylation (CIMP), activation of the HIF pathway and decreased DNA repair. Finally, different therapeutic options may target each altered pathway: demethylating agents, HIF inhibitors, and poly-(ADP-ribose)-polymerase (PARP) inhibitors, respectively. D2HG: D-2-hydroxyglutarate; L2HG: L-2-hydroxyglutarate; TET: ten-eleven translocation DNA hydroxylase; JMJ: Jumonji; KDM: histone lysine demethylase; PHDs: prolyl hydroxylase domain-containing proteins; HIF: hypoxia-inducible factor; CIMP: CpG island methylation phenotype.

3.1. *SDHD*

Baysal and colleagues described in 2000 the first gene responsible for hereditary PGL [2]. *SDHD*, referred to at that time as *PGL1* (the gene responsible for hereditary PGL type 1), had been mapped before to chromosome band 11q23, and was identified by direct sequencing of the best candidate gene contained in a subsequently narrowed critical interval [19]. The initial link with head and neck (H&N) PGLs, highly vascular tumors mainly arising in the main sensor of blood oxygenation (the carotid body), was rapidly extended to PCCs and TAP PGLs [20–22]. Although the original reports proposed that maternal imprinting accounted for the inheritance pattern observed in *SDHD*-related pedigrees, recent studies found that the "almost exclusive" paternal transmission of the disease can be explained by a somatic genetic mechanism targeting both the *SDHD* locus and a paternally imprinted gene on

11p15.5 [23]. Regardless the mechanism involved, the preferential paternal transmission of the disease may lead to generation skipping, making genetic counselling challenging. Moreover, though it can be considered as a rare scenario, development of PPGL may occur after maternal transmission of an *SDHD* mutation [24–26]. The estimated risk of PPGL in *SDHD* mutation carriers (excluding probands) at age 60 years is 43.2% [11]. Regarding the clinical presentation of *SDHD* mutations carriers, they primarily develop (multiple) H&N PGLs (84% of cases), although up to 22% also develop TAP PGLs and 12–24% develop PCCs (mainly unilateral); 3–10% of carriers develop metastases [27–29]. GISTs, PAs and, more rarely, ccRCCs can develop in *SDHD* mutation carriers [30]. It seems that the type of mutation, either impairing or not SDHD stability, influences the mutation-associated phenotype [27].

3.2. *SDHB*

One year after the finding of the first *SDHD* germline mutations in patients with PGL, mutations in *SDHB*, the gene encoding the SDH iron-sulfur subunit, were described as the genetic cause of hereditary PGL type 4 [4]. Soon, the presence of either point mutations or gross deletions affecting *SDHB* far surpassed the prevalence of *SDHD* mutations in patients with PPGL. Overall, mutations in *SDHB* and *SDHD* account for the great majority (over 60%) of all SDHx-related PGL patients, and *SDHB* itself accounts for approximately 10% of all PPGLs [31]. Unlike *SDHD*-associated clinical manifestations (i.e., multiple H&N PGLs), *SDHB* mutation carriers are usually diagnosed with single tumors that can arise in different locations (i.e., PCC, TAP PGL and H&N PGL) [32]. Paradoxically, mutations in *SDHB* show one of the lowest penetrances amongst the SDHx genes (13–21% at the age of 50 years) [11,31,33–35], but patients carrying germline *SDHB* mutations present a higher risk of malignancy (~50%) than other SDHx mutation carriers [11,32,36,37]. This latter observation favors the recommendation of prioritizing genetic testing of this gene in patients affected with PPGL [38]. In fact, the presence of mutations in *SDHB* is the best biomarker of poor prognosis and malignancy in PGL syndromes [36,39]. In addition, the absence of SDHB immunostaining in tumor cells, probably caused by altered assembly or SDH complex stability, is a reliable identifier of PPGLs caused not only by *SDHB* mutations, but also by any other SDHx mutation [40]. Although there is no explanation yet, it has been reported that male *SDHB* mutation carriers are at higher risk of disease than females [31]. Amongst the five SDHx genes, *SDHB* is the one with the most hereditary extra-paraganglial manifestations, such as ccRCCs [8,41], oncocytomas [42,43], GISTs [7], and PAs [44].

3.3. *SDHC*

The SDHC subunit anchors, along with SDHD, the SDH complex to the mitochondrial inner membrane. Though *SDHC* was the second SDHx gene identified as a cause of hereditary PGL (PGL type 3) [5], the frequency of patients carrying mutations in this gene is much lower than *SDHB*- and *SDHD*-related PPGLs, accounting for less than 1% of the patients. *SDHC* mutations result primarily in benign and non-functional H&N PGLs, but they have also been identified in patients with sympathetic PGLs [45,46]. Although no somatic point mutation affecting *SDHC* has been reported to date in PPGL, postzygotic epimutations in the gene promoter region have been identified in patients with PGLs [47], Carney triad (GIST, pulmonary chondroma and PGLs) [48], and Carney-Stratakis syndrome (PGL and GIST) [49]. This specific molecular mechanism of inactivation of the *SDHC* gene was first described in GISTs [50], and has been found in patients developing more than one PGL and/or having syndromic features resembling a hereditary case, as occurs with endothelial PAS domain protein 1 (*EPAS1*, also known as *HIF2A*) and *H3F3A* postzygotic somatic mutations. To identify these "genetically hidden" SDHx cases, a negative immunohistochemistry for SDHB appears to be essential. Although until now there are few patients reported, it seems that in general *SDHC* mutation carriers have low risk of developing GISTs and PAs [11].

3.4. SDHA

Paradoxically, mutations affecting the gene encoding one of the two major catalytic subunits of the SDH complex were described subsequently to mutations affecting the other members of the complex. Homozygous germline mutations of *SDHA* in patients with Leigh syndrome have been known since 1995 [51], but the involvement of this gene in the development of PPGL was elusive until 2010 [3]. This can be explained because, although *SDHA* variants are significantly enriched in PPGL cases, several *SDHA* alleles show a high prevalence amongst the normal population (i.e., 0.1–1% in gnomAD), and were therefore not considered as causative mutations in PPGL patients [52]. Mutations in *SDHA* have the lowest penetrance of all major PGL predisposition genes (10% at age 70 years) [53], and therefore most *SDHA* mutation carriers will not manifest the disease. Familial PPGL related to mutations in *SDHA* shows a prevalence of 3%, especially in patients with PGL, although it is not rare to find mutations in cases developing PCC [54]. The presence of metastasis in *SDHA* mutation carriers is 12%, and extraparaganglial manifestations such as PAs, GIST and ccRCC have also been described [53–55].

3.5. SDHAF2

Only two different mutations in *SDHAF2*, encoding one of the known SDH complex assembly factors, have been described to date in families with H&N PGLs [6,56,57], and one of them (i.e., p.Gly78Arg) exhibits a founder effect in the Dutch population [58]. As occurs with *SDHD* mutation carriers, carriers of *SDHAF2* mutations show an exclusively paternal transmission of the disease, maybe because both genes are located on the same chromosome and may follow the same route to tumorigenesis [59]. Patients carrying mutations in *SDHAF2* develop PGLs only in the H&N region, and frequently (74% of mutation carriers) in multiple locations [60,61]. Though the *SDHAF1* gene has been found mutated in SDH-defective infantile leukoencephalopathy, no mutations have been reported in PPGL to date [62].

4. Other TCA Cycle-Related Genes

4.1. FH

Fumarate hydratase (FH) catalyzes the reversible hydration of fumarate to malate in the TCA cycle. Deficiency in FH activity leads to the accumulation of the oncometabolite fumarate and to the subsequent inhibition of multiple αKG-dependent enzymes, which drives critical epigenetic changes and signaling pathway activation. Thus, overabundance of fumarate, as occurs with succinate, leads to stabilization of HIF-1α, deregulation of DNA/histone methylation, increase of glutaminolysis and glycolysis, and production of reactive oxygen species (something not found in SDH-mutant PPGLs) [63]. All these altered phenomena could promote carcinogenesis by stimulating proliferation and cell survival. Inactivating germline mutations affecting the *FH* gene are the cause of hereditary leiomyomatosis and renal cell carcinoma (HLRCC) [64], but, as far as we know, no PPGL has been reported in families with HLRCC. In 2013, a germline mutation in *FH* was found in a patient with PCC by whole exome sequencing (WES) applied to a tumor displaying transcriptional and methylation (CIMP profile) similarities to SDH-mutant tumors [13]. Subsequently, the study of two large series of patients allowed the identification of additional patients carrying inactivating germline *FH* mutations [65,66]. The prevalence of alterations in the gene is about 1% in PPGL patients, and a metastatic phenotype and presence of multiple tumors located in the adrenal gland or in TAP paraganglia are the clinical characteristics of PPGLs associated with *FH* mutations. In addition, fumarate causes a non-enzymatic covalent modification of cysteine residues in proteins, S-(2-succinyl) cysteine (2SC) [67], that can be detected by immunohistochemistry and has been proposed as a biomarker for *FH*-associated neoplasia. This protein modification, called succination, is different from succinylation, another post-translational modification that will be discussed later in this review. The extent of succination and the implications it may have for the function of targeted proteins is poorly studied, but it seems that this process is more likely to lead to inactivation of critical enzymes [68,69].

4.2. *MDH2*

MDH2 encodes the enzyme malate dehydrogenase 2, which is essential for the reversible oxidation of malate to oxaloacetate in the TCA cycle. This tumor suppressor gene was first reported mutated, with an incomplete penetrance, in a single family with multiple malignant PGLs [70]. Very recently, additional variants have been reported, accounting for <1% of the patients, and their involvement in noradrenergic PPGLs with malignant behavior has been suggested [71]. Tumors carrying *MDH2* mutations showed no accumulation of malate, and though knockdown of *MDH2* in HeLa cells triggered the accumulation of both malate and fumarate, the connection between mutations in this gene and tumorigenesis is not clear. Subsequent to the finding of *MDH2* mutations in PPGL, biallelic mutations of the gene were found as the cause of severe encephalopathy in pediatric patients [72], reinforcing the pathological role of alterations in this particular gene.

4.3. *IDH Genes*

Isocitrate dehydrogenases IDH1 (cytoplasmic) and IDH2 (mitochondrial) catalyze the oxidative decarboxylation of isocitrate to αKG. Recurrent, and mutually exclusive, mutations in the genes *IDH1* (involving R132) and *IDH2* (involving R172), result in neomorphic production of the oncometabolite D-2-hydroxyglutarate (D2HG) that ultimately causes the characteristic CIMP profile previously mentioned for succinate and fumarate accumulation [73]. Somatic mutations in the *IDH1* gene (p.R132C), frequently found in central nervous system tumors [74], have been rarely identified in PGLs (i.e., three benign tumors in TAP or H&N locations) [49,75,76]. On the other hand, only one somatic *IDH2* mutation has been found in a patient with a single H&N PGL by metabolome-guided genomic analysis [77]. Moreover, we recently found a germline truncating mutation affecting *IDH3B* in a patient with a single H&N PGL showing an altered αKG/isocitrate ratio and a CIMP-like profile [49]. Homozygous loss-of-function mutations in *IDH3B* have been found in families with retinitis pigmentosa, a hereditary neurodegeneration of rod and cone photoreceptors in the retina [78]. IDH3 is a heterotetramer, with two catalytic subunits encoded by *IDH3A* and two regulatory subunits encoded by *IDH3B* and *IDH3G*, which catalyzes the irreversible conversion of isocitrate to αKG in the TCA cycle. Although the finding of an *IDH3B* loss-of-function variant in a neuroendocrine tumor such as PGL suggests a causative role for this gene in the disease, and also for the other two genes encoding the remaining subunits of the tetramer, further studies are needed to definitively confirm this association.

4.4. *SLC25A11 and GOT2*

Another WES study applied to a tumor exhibiting an SDHx-like molecular phenotype (i.e., pseudohypoxic and CIMP profiles) in the absence of SDHx or *FH* mutations, identified a germline mutation in the *SLC25A11* gene, which encodes the mitochondrial α-KG/malate carrier [79]. Five additional patients, most of them developing metastatic TAP PGLs, were found in this study carrying *SLC25A11* mutations. This gene is not directly involved in the TCA cycle, but it participates in the exchange between two major intermediates of the cycle, which suggests that inactivation of other genes causing alterations in mitochondrial homeostasis can be responsible for PPGL development as well. Moreover, a single gain-of-function mutation in the *GOT2* gene, encoding the mitochondrial glutamic-oxaloacetic transaminase and also involved in stimulating the malate/aspartate shuttle, was recently reported in a patient with multiple metastatic PGL [49], further reinforcing the link between dysfunction of proteins involved in the exchange of metabolites between the mitochondria and the cytoplasm and PPGL.

4.5. New TCA Cycle-Related Genes Involved in PPGL Development

Recently, a recurrent germline variant affecting *DLST* was found in PPGL patients with multiple tumors [80]. DLST (dihydrolipoamide *S*-succinyltransferase) is one of the three components (the E2 component) of the 2-oxoglutarate dehydrogenase (OGDH) complex that catalyzes the overall conversion of αKG to succinyl-CoA and CO_2. Accumulation of L-2-hydroxyglutarate (L2HG) was found both in *DLST*-mutated tumors and in DLST-knockout (KO) cells transfected with the mutated protein. Surprisingly, and despite the mentioned accumulation, *DLST*-mutated tumors did not exhibit a CIMP profile, but they showed methylation and expression profiles similar to those observed for *EPAS1*-mutated PPGLs, suggesting a link between DLST disruption and pseudohypoxia. Moreover, a high *HIF3A* expression and a positive DLST immunostaining exclusively found in tumors carrying TCA cycle mutations or *EPAS1* mutations further supported this pseudohypoxic link.

5. Metabolic Remodeling not Associated with TCA-Cycle Alterations

Apart from the mentioned TCA cycle alterations, metabolic reprograming of cancer cells can be achieved in PPGLs by other molecular mechanisms. Mutations in *EPAS1*, as well as the stabilization of HIF-1α occurring in *VHL*- and PHD-mutated PPGLs, trigger a pseudohypoxic switch of metabolism from mitochondrial respiration to glycolysis irrespective of oxygen levels. On the other hand, MYC deregulation caused by mutations in *MAX* may increase, in cooperation with HIF-2α, glucose uptake and glycolysis. Moreover, activating alterations of the phosphatidylinositol 3-kinase (PI3K)/AKT serine-threonine kinase (Akt)/mammalian target of rapamycin (mTOR) pathway (by loss-of-function mutations in *NF1* and *TMEM127*, or gain-of-function mutations in *RET*, *FGFR1* and *HRAS*) can also increase glycolysis through the transcription of glycolytic enzymes [63].

6. Inborn TCA Cycle Alterations: Neurodegenerative Disorders versus Cancer

The relevance of hereditary alterations in TCA cycle-related genes to the etiology of severe mitochondrial disorders is well known. Thus, autosomal-recessive mutations in almost any of the genes encoding the main enzymes of the TCA cycle lead to different forms of encephalopathies (Figure 1). This is the case for recessive germline mutations in *SUCLG1* [81] and *SUCLA2* [82]. Moreover, *ACO2* alterations cause infantile cerebellar-retinal degeneration [83] and severe optic atrophy and spastic paraplegia [84]; *IDH3A* mutations lead to severe encephalopathy in infancy [85]; mutations in *DLD* cause severe encephalopathy and hyperlactatemia with neonatal onset [86]; homozygous *IDH2* mutations provoke developmental delay, epilepsy, hypotonia, cardiomyopathy, and dysmorphic features [87]; *SDHAF1* mutations lead to infantile leukoencephalopathy [62]; *SDHA* alteration is a well-known cause of Leigh syndrome, cardiomyopathy and leukodystrophy [51]; recessive *SDHB* mutations lead to hypotonia and leukodystrophy [88] and *SDHD* mutations cause encephalomyopathy [89]; *FH* alterations cause progressive encephalopathy in early childhood [90]; and *MDH2* mutations provoke early-onset severe encephalopathy [72]. In addition, homozygous mutations in *SLC25A1*, encoding a mitochondrial citrate carrier, cause combined D-2- and L-2-hydroxyglutaric aciduria, severe neonatal epileptic encephalopathy, absence of developmental progress, and often early death [91], and mutations in *SLC25A19*, encoding a mitochondrial transporter of a TCA cycle cofactor (thiamine pyrophosphate), cause encephalopathy and progressive polyneuropathy [92]. Finally, *L2HGDH* alterations cause macrocephaly, developmental delay, epilepsy, and cerebellar ataxia [93].

Considering that complete abrogation of the TCA cycle in cells is highly unlikely to be compatible with cell viability, how is it possible that homozygous germline mutations in TCA cycle-related genes exist? The first mammalian model lacking a protein of the TCA cycle was obtained in 1997. Johnson et al. generated viable $DLD^{+/-}$ mice, while the homozygous knockout animals ($DLD^{-/-}$) died at early embryonic stages [94]. This also occurred with *SDHD* [95], *FH* [96], *DLST* [97], *SDHB* [13] and *SUCLA2*/*SUCLG2* [98] knockout mice. Overall, these data suggest that complete lack of activity of TCA cycle enzymes appears to be deleterious during embryonic development. These observations imply that homozygous or compound heterozygous variants in TCA cycle-related genes associated with neurological disorders do not completely abolish the corresponding enzymatic activity and retain part of their functionality. However, the presence of homozygous or compound heterozygous SDHx mutations in patients with neurological disorders gives rise to a controversial situation, which is the absence of tumors in mutation carriers. In heterozygous mutation carriers, this can be either accounted for by the low penetrance of TCA cycle-related mutations (especially in the case of *SDHA* and *SDHB* variants) or by the aforementioned modest effect of the alterations found in these patients. In addition, though clinical presentation and survival may be variable [99], patients carrying homozygous or compound heterozygous germline mutations in TCA cycle genes are usually diagnosed at a young age and die within a few years of diagnosis before reaching adulthood [100], so tumor diagnosis is unlikely to occur in these patients. However, taking into account that patients with L-2-hydroxyglutaric aciduria show increased risk of brain tumors [101], the tumorigenic potential of recessive mutations in TCA cycle-related genes cannot be ruled out. Both PPGL patients carrying TCA cycle-related mutations and patients with encephalopathies associated with the presence of recessive mutations in the aforementioned genes may benefit from therapeutic approaches targeting the aberrant DNA/histone methylation and the DNA-repair pathway, such as the use of demethylating agents (5-aza-2′-deoxycytidine or decitabine, for instance) or PARP inhibitors, respectively.

7. TCA Cycle-Related Omics Profiling in PPGLs

7.1. Pseudohypoxic Transcriptional Profile

The major regulator of cellular response to limited levels of oxygen (hypoxia) is the heterodimeric (composed of alpha and beta subunits) basic helix-loop-helix transcription factor HIF-1α. Under low oxygen conditions, HIF-1α (and also HIF-2α) activates the transcription of many genes involved in the metabolic adaptation to hypoxia, including transporters for increased glucose import (favoring anaerobic growth by glycolysis) and genes encoding angiogenesis factors [102]. The regulation of HIF-1α activity involves oxygen-limited hydroxylation of prolyl residues carried out by PHD1-3 prolyl hydroxylases. This prolyl hydroxylation induces the binding of HIF-1α to the von Hippel–Lindau (VHL) protein-associated complex, which is in charge of targeting HIF-1α by ubiquitination for proteosomal degradation [103,104]. Prolyl hydroxylation of HIF-1α requires oxygen, iron, and αKG, and the reaction produces succinate. Under hypoxia, prolyl hydroxylation is inhibited, HIF-1α is not ubiquitinated and this leads to the transcription of HIF-responsive genes. However, cancer cells may reproduce the hypoxic gene expression signature regardless of the oxygen condition in a process known as pseudohypoxia. This process is the hallmark of the VHL syndrome, in which mutations of *VHL* lead to HIF-1α stabilization in normoxia, leading to the development of tumors (e.g., ccRCCs and PPGLs). The pseudohypoxic transcriptional profile associated with the presence of mutations in TCA cycle-related genes in PPGL was first described by Patricia L Dahia in 2005. In this pioneering study, it was shown that SDH mutations, and the subsequent accumulation of succinate, caused a pseudohypoxic transcription profile similar to the one originated by VHL dysfunction [16,63,105]. Chronic pseudohypoxic signaling could be a mitogenic tumor initiator in neuroendocrine cells, and therefore inappropriate HIF-1α or HIF-2α persistence due to loss of SDH function in PPGL could drive tumorigenesis [106,107]. To note, the only environmental risk factor described in PPGL is chronic hypoxia which, in populations living at high altitude, leads to an increased incidence of H&N PGLs [108–111]. However, though the accumulation of oncometabolites is undoubtedly linked to tumor development in PPGLs, the subsequent pseudohypoxic response is not the only downstream mechanism proposed to explain tumorigenesis caused by TCA cycle dysfunction. The identification and validation of HIF-2α as one of the main oncogenic drivers in PPGLs [112–114] provides a rationale for exploring direct inhibition of HIF-2α as a therapeutic target in metastatic patients [115]. Preclinical studies have shown that HIF-2α antagonists are capable of inhibiting tumor growth in several models of renal cancer, and clinical trials of the first-in-class HIF-2α antagonist PT2385

[(S)-3-((2,2-difluoro-1-hydroxy-7-(methylsulfonyl)-2,3-dihydro-1H-inden-4-yl)oxy)-5-fluorobenzonitrile] have achieved promising results in ccRCC [116]. These findings set the stage for future trials focused on metastatic PPGL, a tumor type that, similar to ccRCC, harbors the pseudo-hypoxia molecular signature as its main molecular hallmark [117,118].

7.2. TCA-Cycle Mutations and CpG Island Methylator Phenotype (CIMP)

The association between the presence of SDHx mutations and CIMP in PPGL has been known since 2008 [119]. Geli et al. performed a quantitative evaluation of promoter methylation of a set of tumor suppressor genes (i.e., *RASSF1A*, *RASSF5*, *CDKN2A*, *RARB*, *TNFRSF10D*, *CDH1*, and *APC*), and found that five of seven tumors exhibiting a targeted CIMP profile were mutated in *SDHB*. Moreover, this particular CIMP profile (defined by the presence of methylation in at least three of the genes included in the analysis) was associated with metastatic behavior and extra-adrenal location (both clinical characteristics related to SDHx mutations). Later, it was published that the accumulation of fumarate and succinate, upon *FH* or SDHx mutations respectively, led to enzymatic inhibition of multiple α-KG-dependent dioxygenases and consequent alterations of genome-wide histone and DNA methylation, linking the TCA cycle mutations to tumorigenesis by their effect on the epigenome [12]. Interestingly, and like a snake that bites its tail, the methylation of the promoter of *SDHC* is a very well-known mechanism leading to CIMP in GIST [50] and PPGLs [47,49]. In 2013, two separate studies based on DNA methylation profiling of samples carrying SDHx mutations further explored the connection between metabolic disruption and altered epigenetic modifications [13,120]. These studies uncovered that SDH deficiency, and the subsequent accumulation of succinate, led to DNA hypermethylation in multiple tumor lineages (e.g., PPGLs and GISTs). These epigenomic changes were particularly severe in *SDHB*-mutated tumors, potentially explaining their malignancy. To note, one of these methylation-based studies also uncovered mutations in *FH* as a cause of hereditary PPGL [13], expanding the CIMP to another TCA cycle-related gene beyond the SDHx genes. In addition, a sporadic PPGL has been also described showing CIMP associated with the presence of a *IDH1* mutation [49] but, as previously mentioned, tumors carrying *DLST* mutations do not exhibit the characteristic CIMP profile despite their accumulation of TCA metabolites [80]. To date, the presence of mutations in other genes involved in the epigenetic machinery in PPGLs exhibiting hypermethylation [121,122], and the finding of tumors with a CIMP profile not associated with mutations in any TCA cycle-related gene [49], further suggest that other genes and pathways may be involved in this particular phenotype. Additional studies are required to elucidate whether the accumulation of metabolites, and the subsequent CIMP, is the cause or a consequence of the tumorigenic process and the adverse outcome associated with some TCA cycle mutations in PPGL.

7.3. Metabolome-Guided Genetic Characterization of the TCA Cycle

Since a link between pathological accumulation of TCA cycle metabolites and tumorigenesis was established, the study of the PPGL-associated metabolome has been used in the characterization of tumors carrying common genetic alterations, and additionally, in the identification of new candidate genes [49], the interpretation of genetic variants, and the improvement of diagnostics [77,123,124]. Mass spectrometry-based measurements of succinate:fumarate ratios allow to distinguish between SDH-deficient PPGLs and tumors without dysfunction of the SDH complex [123]. This is true, except in the case of some H&N PGLs, which may exhibit higher fumarate levels and therefore lower succinate:fumarate ratios compared to those at adrenal or TAP locations. The absence of this particular metabolic signature in some H&N PGLs is probably due to their higher content of stromal cells that dilute the signal from the tumor cells. In addition, alterations in the metabolites' ratios can be used to identify hidden alterations in other TCA cycle-related genes. Thus, a tumor with a gain-of-function *GOT2* mutation exhibited a high succinate:fumarate ratio, probably due to the accumulation of αKG and its subsequent conversion to succinate [49]. Moreover, high fumarate:malate ratios have been observed in PPGLs carrying *FH* mutations, high absolute values of D2HG can be detected in PPGLs carrying *IDH1/2* mutations [49,77], and accumulation of L2HG was found both in *DLST*-mutated PPGLs and in DLST-KO cells transfected with the mutated protein [80].

In addition, hypermethylation (and the subsequent downregulation) of genes involved in the biosynthesis (*PNMT*, *DRD2* and *SULT1A1*), transport (*SLC6A2*), and secretion (*NPY*) of catecholamines found in SDH- and FH-mutant PPGLs [13], may contribute to the immature catecholamine phenotypic features of PGLs carrying mutations in TCA cycle-related genes [124]. Thus, the reduced *PNMT* expression reported in SDH-mutant tumors has been proposed to cause the predominant secretion of noradrenaline or dopamine observed in these tumors.

8. Link Between Defective TCA Cycle and DNA Repair

On the whole, mutations affecting TCA cycle-related genes are associated with metastatic PPGLs for which curative chances, if any, are very limited. For that reason, the recently reported link between accumulation of TCA cycle oncometabolites and homologous recombination paves the way for new therapeutic approaches to the treatment of metastatic PPGL. Moreover, FH enzymatic activity is required for the cellular DNA damage response to double-strand breaks, and it is known that it is involved in the non-homologous end joining repair pathway [125,126]. Thus, in this unexpected connection between metabolism and DNA repair, the excess of fumarate and succinate not only would inhibit αKG-dependent dioxygenase activities, specifically the lysine demethylases KDM4A and KDM4B, but also would suppress the homologous recombination pathway [18]. This blockage would avoid the maintenance of genomic integrity and would make cells vulnerable to synthetic-lethal targeting with poly [adenosine diphosphate (ADP)]-ribose polymerase (PARP) inhibitors. Recent findings have revealed that the expression of mitochondrial complex I core subunits were upregulated in PPGLs with a pseudohypoxic profile. This augmented complex I activity increases intracellular nicotinamide adenine dinucleotide (NAD^+) levels, which serves as an important cofactor to support the PARP DNA repair pathway. Thus, pseudohypoxic PPGLs would present more efficient DNA repair, resulting in potential chemoresistance.Interestingly, a combined treatment with a PARP inhibitor and temozolomide improved cytotoxicity in vitro, reducing tumor proliferation and metastatic lesions with prolonged overall survival in mice with SDHB-KO allografts [127].

9. Defective TCA Cycle Metabolism, Succinylation of Histones and Transcriptional Responses

In addition to the mentioned effects that the accumulation of TCA cycle metabolites has on overall DNA methylation, there are other less known implications of disruption of the cycle. Lysine succinylation is a known post-translational protein modification [128] that when occurring in histones may affect chromosome structure and function [129]. It was recently demonstrated that a fraction of the OGDH complex localizes in the nucleus and binds to lysine acetyltransferase 2A (KAT2A) in the promoter regions of genes [130], and this nuclear translocation of the complex depends on a nuclear localization sequence in DLST. Preventing the OGDH complex from entering the nucleus avoids nuclear generation of succinyl-CoA and the subsequent KAT2A-dependent H3 succinylation, reducing gene expression and inhibiting tumor cell proliferation and tumor growth. These results are consistent with previous observations linking nucleosome succinylation with enhanced in vitro transcription. These interesting findings not only might explain the tumorigenic potential of DLST, as part of the OGDH complex, but also open a new avenue of research into the connection of metabolism and cancer. A subsequent study also demonstrated a potential role of chromatin succinylation in modulating gene expression using an inducible cell culture model of SDH loss, which results in accumulation of succinyl-CoA [131]. This study also demonstrated that defective TCA cycle metabolism results in a DNA repair defect. Chromatin succinylation may thus represent a mechanism by which metabolism modulates both genome-wide transcription and DNA repair activities.

Apart from the aforementioned effect on the succinylation of histones, inhibition of the OGDH complex also reduces lysine succinylation of cytosolic and mitochondrial proteins altering rates of enzymes and pathways, especially mitochondrial metabolic pathways [132,133]. Moreover, ablation of specific enzymes of the TCA cycle affects the availability of succinyl CoA and global enzymatic and non-enzymatic succinylation patterns [134], providing a novel mechanism in which mitochondrial intermediates act as sensors to regulate metabolism.

10. Can We Open New Therapeutic Avenues for TCA Cycle-Altered PPGLs?

Apart from the known approaches to treating malignant PPGLs [135,136], we will discuss here novel therapeutic strategies that should be pursued for tumors carrying alterations in the TCA cycle. Though overall PPGLs present a low degree of chromosome instability, about 2–3% of tumors show chromothripsis involving chromosome arm 1p, where SDHB is located [129]. Chromothripsis phenomenon is a form of genome instability, associated with poor prognosis [137,138], in which one or a few chromosomes are affected by an alternating copy number profile with both loss and retention of heterozygosity [139,140]. One of the mechanisms involved in the initiation of chromothripsis is telomere dysfunction that leads to attrition of chromosome ends [141]. Subsequently, cancer cells showing this phenomenon become stabilized in order to avoid additional chromosomal aberrations that would be incompatible with cell survival. A well-known telomere stabilization mechanism involves the presence of high levels of *TERT* mRNA, mainly through amplification, promoter point mutations, methylation or rearrangements. Interestingly, increased *TERT* expression and telomere length has been observed in chromothripsis-positive ependymomas and glioblastomas [142], and in high-stage neuroblastomas [143] among other cancers, suggesting that telomere maintenance pathways may represent therapeutic targets in chromothripsis-positive tumors. With regard to PPGL, high to moderate *TERT* expression has been observed in 18–51% of patients, which are often metastatic cases [75,144,145], and in an important proportion of patients associated with deficiency of SDHx [146]. Moreover, the presence of somatic *ATRX* mutations, found preferentially in *SDHB/FH*-mutated tumors, and the associated alternative lengthening of telomeres have been described as an independent risk factor for metastatic PPGL [75,146,147]. It is tempting to speculate that metastatic PPGLs related to mutations in other TCA cycle genes that also exhibit telomere dysfunction, could benefit from the multiple telomerase-targeting therapeutic strategies that have been pursued in the past two decades (reviewed in [148]).

Another important avenue of potential treatments for metastatic PPGLs focuses on investigating whether a specific driver mutation could be associated with the tumor's immune profile, and therefore with the potential efficacy of immunotherapy. In this regard, one of the main problems related to the potential lack of response is immune evasion, in which the tumor microenvironment (TME) plays a pivotal role [149]. The TME can be influenced by different conditions, but there are two in particular that gain importance when considering PPGLs with TCA-mutated genes: the hypoxic state, and an aberrant production of metabolites. Whether the PPGL immune subtypes are genotype-specific, or if there is an enrichment of any immune subtype among *SDHB*-mutated tumors or among those related to TCA genes with a higher metastatic risk is still to be addressed. Regardless these upcoming knowledge, it seems clear that a highly heterogeneous disease such as PPGL will benefit from a personalize treatment based on the specific genetic background, as well as from a deep characterization of the tumor microenvironment.

11. Conclusions

More than 20% of PPGLs are found carrying mutations in genes encoding TCA cycle metabolic enzymes. These mutations cause the disruption of the cycle, and the subsequent accumulation of "oncometabolites" lead to overall pathological changes in gene expression (i.e., by DNA methylation and post-translational protein modification), metabolic adaptation of cells to hypoxia, and DNA repair processes. Unraveling the pathological mechanisms associated with the presence of different PPGL mutations could pave the way to new personalized therapeutic approaches.

Author Contributions: Conceptualisation, A.C. and M.R.; Original draft preparation, A.C., L.R., B.C. and M.R.; Writing—review and editing, A.C., L.R., B.C. and M.R.; Supervision, A.C. and M.R.

Funding: This work was supported by the Instituto de Salud Carlos III (ISCIII), through the "Acción Estratégica en Salud" (AES) (projects PI18/00454 and PI17/01796, to A.C. and M.R., respectively, cofounded by the European Regional Development Fund (ERDF)), and the Paradifference Foundation.

Conflicts of Interest: The authors declare no conflict of interest.

References

1. Warburg, O. The metabolism of carcinoma cells 1. *J. Cancer Res.* **1925**, *9*, 148–163. [CrossRef]
2. Baysal, B.E.; Ferrell, R.E.; Willett-Brozick, J.E.; Lawrence, E.C.; Myssiorek, D.; Bosch, A.; Van Der Mey, A.; Taschner, P.E.M.; Rubinstein, W.S.; Myers, E.N.; et al. Mutations in SDHD, a mitochondrial complex II gene, in hereditary paraganglioma. *Science* **2000**, *287*, 848–851. [CrossRef] [PubMed]
3. Burnichon, N.; Brière, J.J.; Libé, R.; Vescovo, L.; Rivière, J.; Tissier, F.; Jouanno, E.; Jeunemaitre, X.; Bénit, P.; Tzagoloff, A.; et al. SDHA is a tumor suppressor gene causing paraganglioma. *Hum. Mol. Genet.* **2010**, *19*, 3011–3020. [CrossRef]
4. Astuti, D.; Latif, F.; Dallol, A.; Dahia, P.L.M.; Douglas, F.; George, E.; Sköldberg, F.; Husebye, E.S.; Eng, C.; Maher, E.R. Gene Mutations in the Succinate Dehydrogenase Subunit SDHB Cause Susceptibility to Familial Pheochromocytoma and to Familial Paraganglioma. *Am. J. Hum. Genet.* **2001**, *69*, 49–54. [CrossRef] [PubMed]
5. Niemann, S.; Muller, U. Mutations in SDHC cause autosomal dominant paraganglioma, type 3. *Nat. Genet.* **2000**, *26*, 268–270.
6. Hao, H.X.; Khalimonchuk, O.; Schraders, M.; Dephoure, N.; Bayley, J.P.; Kunst, H.; Devilee, P.; Cremers, C.W.R.J.; Schiffman, J.D.; Bentz, B.G.; et al. SDH5, a gene required for flavination of succinate dehydrogenase, is mutated in paraganglioma. *Science* **2009**, *325*, 1139–1142. [CrossRef] [PubMed]
7. McWhinney, S.R.; Pasini, B.; Stratakis, C.A. Familial Gastrointestinal Stromal Tumors and Germ-Line Mutations. *N. Engl. J. Med.* **2007**, *357*, 1054–1056. [CrossRef] [PubMed]
8. Vanharanta, S.; Buchta, M.; McWhinney, S.R.; Virta, S.K.; Peçzkowska, M.; Morrison, C.D.; Lehtonen, R.; Januszewicz, A.; Järvinen, H.; Juhola, M.; et al. Early-Onset Renal Cell Carcinoma as a Novel Extraparaganglial Component of SDHB-Associated Heritable Paraganglioma. *Am. J. Hum. Genet.* **2004**, *74*, 153–159. [CrossRef] [PubMed]
9. Xekouki, P.; Pacak, K.; Almeida, M.; Wassif, C.A.; Rustin, P.; Nesterova, M.; De La Luz Sierra, M.; Matro, J.; Ball, E.; Azevedo, M.; et al. Succinate dehydrogenase (SDH) D subunit (SDHD) inactivation in a growth-hormone-producing pituitary tumor: A new association for SDH? *J. Clin. Endocrinol. Metab.* **2012**, *97*, 357–366. [CrossRef]
10. Mannelli, M.; Canu, L.; Ercolino, T.; Rapizzi, E.; Martinelli, S.; Parenti, G.; De Filpo, G.; Nesi, G. DIAGNOSIS of ENDOCRINE DISEASE: SDHx mutations: Beyond pheochromocytomas and paragangliomas. *Eur. J. Endocrinol.* **2018**, *178*, R11–R17. [CrossRef]
11. Andrews, K.A.; Ascher, D.B.; Pires, D.E.V.; Barnes, D.R.; Vialard, L.; Casey, R.T.; Bradshaw, N.; Adlard, J.; Aylwin, S.; Brennan, P.; et al. Tumour risks and genotype–phenotype correlations associated with germline variants in succinate dehydrogenase subunit genes *SDHB*, *SDHC* and *SDHD*. *J. Med. Genet.* **2018**, *55*, 384–394.
12. Xiao, M.; Yang, H.; Xu, W.; Ma, S.; Lin, H.; Zhu, H.; Liu, L.; Liu, Y.; Yang, C.; Xu, Y.; et al. Inhibition of α-KG-dependent histone and DNA demethylases by fumarate and succinate that are accumulated in mutations of FH and SDH tumor suppressors. *Genes Dev.* **2012**, *26*, 1326–1338. [CrossRef]
13. Letouzé, E.; Martinelli, C.; Loriot, C.; Burnichon, N.; Abermil, N.; Ottolenghi, C.; Janin, M.; Menara, M.; Nguyen, A.T.; Benit, P.; et al. SDH Mutations Establish a Hypermethylator Phenotype in Paraganglioma. *Cancer Cell* **2013**, *23*, 739–752. [CrossRef]
14. Turcan, S.; Rohle, D.; Goenka, A.; Walsh, L.A.; Fang, F.; Yilmaz, E.; Campos, C.; Fabius, A.W.M.; Lu, C.; Ward, P.S.; et al. IDH1 mutation is sufficient to establish the glioma hypermethylator phenotype. *Nature* **2012**, *483*, 479–483. [CrossRef]
15. Ricketts, C.; Killian, J.K.; Vocke, C.D.; Sourbier, C.; Yang, Y.; Merino, M.J.; Meltzer, P.S.; Linehan, W.M. Abstract 2660: A renal CpG island methylator phenotype (R-CIMP) in kidney tumors associated with germline mutations of *FH* and *SDHB*. *Cancer Res.* **2016**, *76*, 2660. [CrossRef]
16. Selak, M.A.; Armour, S.M.; MacKenzie, E.D.; Boulahbel, H.; Watson, D.G.; Mansfield, K.D.; Pan, Y.; Simon, M.C.; Thompson, C.B.; Gottlieb, E. Succinate links TCA cycle dysfunction to oncogenesis by inhibiting HIF-α prolyl hydroxylase. *Cancer Cell* **2005**, *7*, 77–85. [CrossRef]

17. Pollard, P.J.; Brière, J.J.; Alam, N.A.; Barwell, J.; Barclay, E.; Wortham, N.C.; Hunt, T.; Mitchell, M.; Olpin, S.; Moat, S.J.; et al. Accumulation of Krebs cycle intermediates and over-expression of HIF1α in tumours which result from germline FH and SDH mutations. *Hum. Mol. Genet.* **2005**, *14*, 2231–2239. [CrossRef]
18. Sulkowski, P.L.; Sundaram, R.K.; Oeck, S.; Corso, C.D.; Liu, Y.; Noorbakhsh, S.; Niger, M.; Boeke, M.; Ueno, D.; Kalathil, A.N.; et al. Krebs-cycle-deficient hereditary cancer syndromes are defined by defects in homologous-recombination DNA repair. *Nat. Genet.* **2018**, *50*, 1086–1092. [CrossRef]
19. Baysal, B.E.; Van Schothorst, E.M.; Farr, J.E.; Grashof, P.; Myssiorek, D.; Rubinstein, W.S.; Taschner, P.; Cornelisse, C.J.; Devlin, B.; Devilee, P.; et al. Repositioning the hereditary paraganglioma critical region on chromosome band 11q23. *Hum. Genet.* **1999**, *104*, 219–225. [CrossRef]
20. Astuti, D.; Douglas, F.; Lennard, T.W.J.; Aligianis, I.A.; Woodward, E.R.; Evans, D.G.R.; Eng, C.; Latif, F.; Maher, E.R. Germline SDHD mutation in familial phaeochromocytoma. *Lancet* **2001**, *357*, 1181–1182. [CrossRef]
21. Neumann, H.P.H.; Bausch, B.; McWhinney, S.R.; Bender, B.U.; Gimm, O.; Franke, G.; Schipper, J.; Klisch, J.; Altehoefer, C.; Zerres, K.; et al. Germ-Line Mutations in Nonsyndromic Pheochromocytoma. *N. Engl. J. Med.* **2002**, *346*, 1459–1466. [CrossRef]
22. Cascon, A.; Ruiz-Llorente, S.; Cebrian, A.; Telleria, D.; Rivero, J.C.; Diez, J.J.; Lopez-Ibarra, P.J.; Jaunsolo, M.A.; Benitez, J.; Robledo, M. Identification of novel SDHD mutations in patients with phaeochromocytoma and/or paraganglioma. *Eur. J. Hum. Genet.* **2002**, *10*, 457–461. [CrossRef]
23. Hensen, E.F.; Jordanova, E.S.; Van Minderhout, I.J.H.M.; Hogendoorn, P.C.W.; Taschner, P.E.M.; Van Der Mey, A.G.L.; Devilee, P.; Cornelisse, C.J. Somatic loss of maternal chromosome 11 causes parent-of-origin-dependent inheritance in SDHD-linked paraganglioma and phaeochromocytoma families. *Oncogene* **2004**, *23*, 4076–4083. [CrossRef] [PubMed]
24. Burnichon, N.; Mazzella, J.M.; Drui, D.; Amar, L.; Bertherat, J.; Coupier, I.; Delemer, B.; Guilhem, I.; Herman, P.; Kerlan, V.; et al. Risk assessment of maternally inherited SDHD paraganglioma and phaeochromocytoma. *J. Med. Genet.* **2017**, *54*, 100–103. [CrossRef]
25. Pigny, P.; Vincent, A.; Bauters, C.C.; Bertrand, M.; De Montpreville, V.T.; Crepin, M.; Porchet, N.; Caron, P. Paraganglioma after maternal transmission of a succinate dehydrogenase gene mutation. *J. Clin. Endocrinol. Metab.* **2008**, *93*, 1609–1615. [CrossRef] [PubMed]
26. Yeap, P.M.; Tobias, E.S.; Mavraki, E.; Fletcher, A.; Bradshaw, N.; Freel, E.M.; Cooke, A.; Murday, V.A.; Davidson, H.R.; Perry, C.G.; et al. Molecular analysis of pheochromocytoma after maternal transmission of SDHD mutation elucidates mechanism of parent-of-origin effect. *J. Clin. Endocrinol. Metab.* **2011**, *96*, E2009–E2013. [CrossRef] [PubMed]
27. Ricketts, C.J.; Forman, J.R.; Rattenberry, E.; Bradshaw, N.; Lalloo, F.; Izatt, L.; Cole, T.R.; Armstrong, R.; Ajith Kumar, V.K.; Morrison, P.J.; et al. Tumor risks and genotype-phenotype-proteotype analysis in 358 patients with germline mutations in SDHB and SDHD. *Hum. Mutat.* **2010**, *31*, 41–51. [CrossRef]
28. Mannelli, M.; Castellano, M.; Schiavi, F.; Filetti, S.; Giacchè, M.; Mori, L.; Pignataro, V.; Bernini, G.; Giachè, V.; Bacca, A.; et al. Clinically guided genetic screening in a large cohort of Italian patients with pheochromocytomas and/or functional or nonfunctional paragangliomas. *J. Clin. Endocrinol. Metab.* **2009**, *94*, 1541–1547. [CrossRef]
29. Cascón, A.; Pita, G.; Burnichon, N.; Landa, I.; López-Jiménez, E.; Montero-Conde, C.; Leskelä, S.; Leandro-García, L.J.; Letón, R.; Rodríguez-Antona, C.; et al. Genetics of pheochromocytoma and paraganglioma in Spanish patients. *J. Clin. Endocrinol. Metab.* **2009**, *94*, 1701–1705. [CrossRef]
30. Evenepoel, L.; Papathomas, T.G.; Krol, N.; Korpershoek, E.; De Krijger, R.R.; Persu, A.; Dinjens, W.N.M. Toward an improved definition of the genetic and tumor spectrum associated with SDH germ-line mutations. *Genet. Med.* **2015**, *17*, 610–620. [CrossRef]
31. Jochmanova, I.; Wolf, K.I.; King, K.S.; Nambuba, J.; Wesley, R.; Martucci, V.; Raygada, M.; Adams, K.T.; Prodanov, T.; Fojo, A.T.; et al. SDHB-related pheochromocytoma and paraganglioma penetrance and genotype–phenotype correlations. *J. Cancer Res. Clin. Oncol.* **2017**, *143*, 1421–1435. [CrossRef]
32. Niemeijer, N.D.; Rijken, J.A.; Eijkelenkamp, K.; Van Der Horst-Schrivers, A.N.A.; Kerstens, M.N.; Tops, C.M.J.; Van Berkel, A.; Timmers, H.J.L.M.; Kunst, H.P.M.; Leemans, C.R.; et al. The phenotype of SDHB germline mutation carriers: A nationwide study. *Eur. J. Endocrinol.* **2017**, *177*, 115–125. [CrossRef]

33. Rijken, J.A.; Niemeijer, N.D.; Jonker, M.A.; Eijkelenkamp, K.; Jansen, J.C.; van Berkel, A.; Timmers, H.J.L.M.; Kunst, H.P.M.; Bisschop, P.H.L.T.; Kerstens, M.N.; et al. The penetrance of paraganglioma and pheochromocytoma in SDHB germline mutation carriers. *Clin. Genet.* **2018**, *93*, 60–66. [CrossRef]
34. Schiavi, F.; Milne, R.L.; Anda, E.; Blay, P.; Castellano, M.; Opocher, G.; Robledo, M.; Cascón, A. Are we overestimating the penetrance of mutations in SDHB? *Hum. Mutat.* **2010**, *31*, 761–762. [CrossRef]
35. Jafri, M.; Whitworth, J.; Rattenberry, E.; Vialard, L.; Kilby, G.; Kumar, A.V.; Izatt, L.; Lalloo, F.; Brennan, P.; Cook, J.; et al. Evaluation of SDHB, SDHD and VHL gene susceptibility testing in the assessment of individuals with non-syndromic phaeochromocytoma, paraganglioma and head and neck paraganglioma. *Clin. Endocrinol.* **2013**, *78*, 898–906. [CrossRef]
36. Gimenez-Roqueplo, A.-P.; Favier, J.; Rustin, P.; Rieubland, C.; Crespin, M.; Nau, V.; Khau Van Kien, P.; Corvol, P.; Plouin, P.-F.; Jeunemaitre, X.; et al. Mutations in the SDHB gene are associated with extra-adrenal and/or malignant phaeochromocytomas. *Cancer Res.* **2003**, *63*, 5615–5621.
37. Dhir, M.; Li, W.; Hogg, M.E.; Bartlett, D.L.; Carty, S.E.; McCoy, K.L.; Challinor, S.M.; Yip, L. Clinical Predictors of Malignancy in Patients with Pheochromocytoma and Paraganglioma. *Ann. Surg. Oncol.* **2017**, *24*, 3624–3630. [CrossRef]
38. Cascón, A.; López-Jiménez, E.; Landa, I.; Leskelä, S.; Leandro-García, L.J.; Maliszewska, A.; Letón, R.; Vega, L.D.L.; García-Barcina, M.J.; Sanabria, C.; et al. Rationalization of genetic testing in patients with apparently sporadic pheochromocytoma/paraganglioma. *Horm. Metab. Res.* **2009**, *41*, 672–675. [CrossRef]
39. Amar, L.; Baudin, E.; Burnichon, N.; Peyrard, S.; Silvera, S.; Bertherat, J.; Bertagna, X.; Schlumberger, M.; Jeunemaitre, X.; Gimenez-Roqueplo, A.P.; et al. Succinate dehydrogenase B gene mutations predict survival in patients with malignant pheochromocytomas or paragangliomas. *J. Clin. Endocrinol. Metab.* **2007**, *92*, 3822–3828. [CrossRef]
40. Van Nederveen, F.H.; Gaal, J.; Favier, J.; Korpershoek, E.; Oldenburg, R.A.; de Bruyn, E.M.; Sleddens, H.F.; Derkx, P.; Rivière, J.; Dannenberg, H.; et al. An immunohistochemical procedure to detect patients with paraganglioma and phaeochromocytoma with germline SDHB, SDHC, or SDHD gene mutations: A retrospective and prospective analysis. *Lancet Oncol.* **2009**, *10*, 764–771. [CrossRef]
41. Ricketts, C.; Woodward, E.R.; Killick, P.; Morris, M.R.; Astuti, D.; Latif, F.; Maher, E.R. Germline SDHB mutations and familial renal cell carcinoma. *J. Natl. Cancer Inst.* **2008**, *100*, 1260–1262. [CrossRef] [PubMed]
42. Cascón, A.; Landa, Í.; López-Jiménez, E.; Díez-Hernández, A.; Buchta, M.; Montero-Conde, C.; Leskelä, S.; Leandro-García, L.J.; Letón, R.; Rodríguez-Antona, C.; et al. Molecular characterisation of a common SDHB deletion in paraganglioma patients. *J. Med. Genet.* **2008**, *45*, 233–238. [CrossRef] [PubMed]
43. Henderson, A.; Douglas, F.; Perros, P.; Morgan, C.; Maher, E.R. SDHB-associated renal oncocytoma suggests a broadening of the renal phenotype in hereditary paragangliomatosis. *Fam. Cancer* **2009**, *8*, 257–260. [CrossRef]
44. Dénes, J.; Swords, F.; Rattenberry, E.; Stals, K.; Owens, M.; Cranston, T.; Xekouki, P.; Moran, L.; Kumar, A.; Wassif, C.; et al. Heterogeneous genetic background of the association of pheochromocytoma/paraganglioma and pituitary adenoma: Results from a large patient cohort. *J. Clin. Endocrinol. Metab.* **2015**, *100*, E531–E541. [CrossRef] [PubMed]
45. Mannelli, M.; Ercolino, T.; Giachè, V.; Simi, L.; Cirami, C.; Parenti, G. Genetic screening for pheochromocytoma: Should SDHC gene analysis be included? *J. Med. Genet.* **2007**, *44*, 586–587. [CrossRef]
46. Else, T.; Marvin, M.L.; Everett, J.N.; Gruber, S.B.; Arts, H.A.; Stoffel, E.M.; Auchus, R.J.; Raymond, V.M. The clinical phenotype of SDHC-associated hereditary paraganglioma syndrome (PGL3). *J. Clin. Endocrinol. Metab.* **2014**, *99*, E1482–E1486. [CrossRef]
47. Richter, S.; Klink, B.; Nacke, B.; De Cubas, A.A.; Mangelis, A.; Rapizzi, E.; Meinhardt, M.; Skondra, C.; Mannelli, M.; Robledo, M.; et al. Epigenetic mutation of the succinate dehydrogenase c promoter in a patient with two paragangliomas. *J. Clin. Endocrinol. Metab.* **2016**, *101*, 359–363. [CrossRef] [PubMed]
48. Haller, F.; Moskalev, E.A.; Faucz, F.R.; Barthelmeß, S.; Wiemann, S.; Bieg, M.; Assie, G.; Bertherat, J.; Schaefer, I.M.; Otto, C.; et al. Aberrant DNA hypermethylation of SDHC: A novel mechanism of tumor development in Carney triad. *Endocr. Relat. Cancer* **2014**, *21*, 567–577. [CrossRef]
49. Remacha, L.; Comino-Mendez, I.; Richter, S.; Contreras, L.; Curras-Freixes, M.; Pita, G.; Leton, R.; Galarreta, A.; Torres-Perez, R.; Honrado, E.; et al. Targeted exome sequencing of Krebs cycle genes reveals candidate cancer–predisposing mutations in pheochromocytomas and paragangliomas. *Clin. Cancer Res.* **2017**, *23*, 6315–6325. [CrossRef]

50. Killian, J.K.; Miettinen, M.; Walker, R.L.; Wang, Y.; Zhu, Y.J.; Waterfall, J.J.; Noyes, N.; Retnakumar, P.; Yang, Z.; Smith, W.I.; et al. Recurrent epimutation of SDHC in gastrointestinal stromal tumors. *Sci. Transl. Med.* **2014**, *6*, 268ra177. [CrossRef]
51. Bourgeron, T.; Rustin, P.; Chretien, D.; Birch-Machin, M.; Bourgeois, M.; Viegas-Péquignot, E.; Munnich, A.; Rötig, A. Mutation of a nuclear succinate dehydrogenase gene results in mitochondrial respiratory chain deficiency. *Nat. Genet.* **1995**, *11*, 144–149. [CrossRef]
52. Maniam, P.; Zhou, K.; Lonergan, M.; Berg, J.N.; Goudie, D.R.; Newey, P.J. Pathogenicity and penetrance of germline SDHA variants in pheochromocytoma and paraganglioma (PPGL). *J. Endocr. Soc.* **2018**, *2*, 806–816. [CrossRef]
53. Van Der Tuin, K.; Mensenkamp, A.R.; Tops, C.M.J.; Corssmit, E.P.M.; Dinjens, W.N.; Van De Horst-Schrivers, A.N.; Jansen, J.C.; De Jong, M.M.; Kunst, H.P.M.; Kusters, B.; et al. Clinical aspects of SDHA-related pheochromocytoma and paraganglioma: A nationwide study. *J. Clin. Endocrinol. Metab.* **2018**, *103*, 438–445. [CrossRef]
54. Bausch, B.; Schiavi, F.; Ni, Y.; Welander, J.; Patocs, A.; Ngeow, J.; Wellner, U.; Malinoc, A.; Taschin, E.; Barbon, G.; et al. Clinical characterization of the pheochromocytoma and paraganglioma susceptibility genes SDHA, TMEM127, MAX, and SDHAF2 for gene-informed prevention. *JAMA Oncol.* **2017**, *3*, 1204–1212. [CrossRef]
55. Jha, A.; de Luna, K.; Balili, C.A.; Millo, C.; Paraiso, C.A.; Ling, A.; Gonzales, M.K.; Viana, B.; Alrezk, R.; Adams, K.T.; et al. Clinical, Diagnostic, and Treatment Characteristics of SDHA-Related Metastatic Pheochromocytoma and Paraganglioma. *Front. Oncol.* **2019**, *9*, 53. [CrossRef]
56. Bayley, J.P.; Kunst, H.P.M.; Cascon, A.; Sampietro, M.L.; Gaal, J.; Korpershoek, E.; Hinojar-Gutierrez, A.; Timmers, H.J.L.M.; Hoefsloot, L.H.; Hermsen, M.A.; et al. SDHAF2 mutations in familial and sporadic paraganglioma and phaeochromocytoma. *Lancet Oncol.* **2010**, *11*, 366–372. [CrossRef]
57. Piccini, V.; Rapizzi, E.; Bacca, A.; Di Trapani, G.; Pulli, R.; Giachè, V.; Zampetti, B.; Lucci-Cordisco, E.; Canu, L.; Corsini, E.; et al. Head and neck paragangliomas: Genetic spectrum and clinical variability in 79 consecutive patients. *Endocr. Relat. Cancer* **2012**, *19*, 149–155. [CrossRef]
58. Hensen, E.F.; van Duinen, N.; Jansen, J.C.; Corssmit, E.P.M.; Tops, C.M.J.; Romijn, J.A.; Vriends, A.H.J.T.; van der Mey, A.G.L.; Cornelisse, C.J.; Devilee, P.; et al. High prevalence of founder mutations of the succinate dehydrogenase genes in The Netherlands. *Clin. Genet.* **2012**, *81*, 284–288. [CrossRef]
59. Hensen, E.F.; Siemers, M.D.; Jansen, J.C.; Corssmit, E.P.M.; Romijn, J.A.; Tops, C.M.J.; Van Der Mey, A.G.L.; Devilee, P.; Cornelisse, C.J.; Bayley, J.P.; et al. Mutations in SDHD are the major determinants of the clinical characteristics of Dutch head and neck paraganglioma patients. *Clin. Endocrinol.* **2011**, *75*, 650–655. [CrossRef]
60. Favier, J.; Amar, L.; Gimenez-Roqueplo, A.P. Paraganglioma and phaeochromocytoma: From genetics to personalized medicine. *Nat. Rev. Endocrinol.* **2015**, *11*, 101–111. [CrossRef]
61. Kunst, H.P.M.; Rutten, M.H.; De Mönnink, J.P.; Hoefsloot, L.H.; Timmers, H.J.L.M.; Marres, H.A.M.; Jansen, J.C.; Kremer, H.; Bayley, J.P.; Cremers, C.W.R.J. SDHAF2 (PGL2-SDH5) and hereditary head and neck paraganglioma. *Clin. Cancer Res.* **2011**, *17*, 247–254. [CrossRef]
62. Ghezzi, D.; Goffrini, P.; Uziel, G.; Horvath, R.; Klopstock, T.; Lochmüller, H.; D'Adamo, P.; Gasparini, P.; Strom, T.M.; Prokisch, H.; et al. SDHAF1, encoding a LYR complex-II specific assembly factor, is mutated in SDH-defective infantile leukoencephalopathy. *Nat. Genet.* **2009**, *41*, 654–656. [CrossRef]
63. Dahia, P.L.M. Pheochromocytoma and paraganglioma pathogenesis: Learning from genetic heterogeneity. *Nat. Rev. Cancer* **2014**, *14*, 108–119. [CrossRef]
64. Tomlinson, I.P.M.; Alam, N.A.; Rowan, A.J.; Barclay, E.; Jaeger, E.E.M.; Kelsell, D.; Leigh, I.; Gorman, P.; Lamlum, H.; Rahman, S.; et al. Germline mutations in FH predispose to dominantly inherited uterine fibroids, skin leiomyomata and papillary renal cell cancer the multiple leiomyoma consortium. *Nat. Genet.* **2002**, *30*, 406–410.
65. Castro-Vega, L.J.; Buffet, A.; De Cubas, A.A.; Cascón, A.; Menara, M.; Khalifa, E.; Amar, L.; Azriel, S.; Bourdeau, I.; Chabre, O.; et al. Germline mutations in FH confer predisposition to malignant pheochromocytomas and paragangliomas. *Hum. Mol. Genet.* **2014**, *23*, 2440–2446. [CrossRef]
66. Clark, G.R.; Sciacovelli, M.; Gaude, E.; Walsh, D.M.; Kirby, G.; Simpson, M.A.; Trembath, R.C.; Berg, J.N.; Woodward, E.R.; Kinning, E.; et al. Germline FH mutations presenting with pheochromocytoma. *J. Clin. Endocrinol. Metab.* **2014**, *99*, E2046–E2050. [CrossRef]

67. Bardella, C.; El-Bahrawy, M.; Frizzell, N.; Adam, J.; Ternette, N.; Hatipoglu, E.; Howarth, K.; O'Flaherty, L.; Roberts, I.; Turner, G.; et al. Aberrant succination of proteins in fumarate hydratase-deficient mice and HLRCC patients is a robust biomarker of mutation status. *J. Pathol.* **2011**, *225*, 4–11. [CrossRef]
68. Ternette, N.; Yang, M.; Laroyia, M.; Kitagawa, M.; O'Flaherty, L.; Wolhulter, K.; Igarashi, K.; Saito, K.; Kato, K.; Fischer, R.; et al. Inhibition of Mitochondrial Aconitase by Succination in Fumarate Hydratase Deficiency. *Cell Rep.* **2013**, *3*, 689–700. [CrossRef]
69. Frizzell, N.; Lima, M.; Baynes, J.W. Succination of proteins in diabetes. *Free Radic. Res.* **2011**, *45*, 101–109. [CrossRef]
70. Cascon, A.; Comino-Mendez, I.; Curras-Freixes, M.; de Cubas, A.A.; Contreras, L.; Richter, S.; Peitzsch, M.; Mancikova, V.; Inglada-Perez, L.; Perez-Barrios, A.; et al. Whole-Exome Sequencing Identifies MDH2 as a New Familial Paraganglioma Gene. *JNCI J. Natl. Cancer Inst.* **2015**, *107*, djv053. [CrossRef]
71. Calsina, B.; Currás-Freixes, M.; Buffet, A.; Pons, T.; Contreras, L.; Letón, R.; Comino-Méndez, I.; Remacha, L.; Calatayud, M.; Obispo, B.; et al. Role of MDH2 pathogenic variant in pheochromocytoma and paraganglioma patients. *Genet. Med.* **2018**, *20*, 1652–1662. [CrossRef]
72. Ait-El-Mkadem, S.; Dayem-Quere, M.; Gusic, M.; Chaussenot, A.; Bannwarth, S.; François, B.; Genin, E.C.; Fragaki, K.; Volker-Touw, C.L.M.; Vasnier, C.; et al. Mutations in MDH2, Encoding a Krebs Cycle Enzyme, Cause Early-Onset Severe Encephalopathy. *Am. J. Hum. Genet.* **2017**, *100*, 151–159. [CrossRef] [PubMed]
73. Lu, C.; Ward, P.S.; Kapoor, G.S.; Rohle, D.; Turcan, S.; Abdel-Wahab, O.; Edwards, C.R.; Khanin, R.; Figueroa, M.E.; Melnick, A.; et al. IDH mutation impairs histone demethylation and results in a block to cell differentiation. *Nature* **2012**, *483*, 474–478. [CrossRef]
74. Yan, H.; Parsons, D.W.; Jin, G.; McLendon, R.; Rasheed, B.A.; Yuan, W.; Kos, I.; Batinic-Haberle, I.; Jones, S.; Riggins, G.J.; et al. *IDH1* and *IDH2* Mutations in Gliomas. *N. Engl. J. Med.* **2009**, *360*, 765–773. [CrossRef]
75. Fishbein, L.; Leshchiner, I.; Walter, V.; Danilova, L.; Robertson, A.G.; Johnson, A.R.; Lichtenberg, T.M.; Murray, B.A.; Ghayee, H.K.; Else, T.; et al. Comprehensive Molecular Characterization of Pheochromocytoma and Paraganglioma. *Cancer Cell* **2017**, *31*, 181–193. [CrossRef]
76. Gaal, J.; Burnichon, N.; Korpershoek, E.; Roncelin, I.; Bertherat, J.; Plouin, P.F.; De Krijger, R.R.; Gimenez-Roqueplo, A.P.; Dinjens, W.N.M. Isocitrate dehydrogenase mutations are rare in pheochromocytomas and paragangliomas. *J. Clin. Endocrinol. Metab.* **2010**, *95*, 1274–1278. [CrossRef] [PubMed]
77. Richter, S.; Gieldon, L.; Pang, Y.; Peitzsch, M.; Huynh, T.; Leton, R.; Viana, B.; Ercolino, T.; Mangelis, A.; Rapizzi, E.; et al. Metabolome-guided genomics to identify pathogenic variants in isocitrate dehydrogenase, fumarate hydratase, and succinate dehydrogenase genes in pheochromocytoma and paraganglioma. *Genet. Med.* **2018**, *21*, 705–717. [CrossRef] [PubMed]
78. Hartong, D.T.; Dange, M.; McGee, T.L.; Berson, E.L.; Dryja, T.P.; Colman, R.F. Insights from retinitis pigmentosa into the roles of isocitrate dehydrogenases in the Krebs cycle. *Nat. Genet.* **2008**, *40*, 1230–1234. [CrossRef]
79. Buffet, A.; Morin, A.; Castro-Vega, L.J.; Habarou, F.; Lussey-Lepoutre, C.; Letouze, E.; Lefebvre, H.; Guilhem, I.; Haissaguerre, M.; Raingeard, I.; et al. Germline mutations in the mitochondrial 2-oxoglutarate/malate carrier SLC25A11 gene confer a predisposition to metastatic paragangliomas. *Cancer Res.* **2018**, *78*, 1914–1922. [CrossRef]
80. Remacha, L.; Pirman, D.; Mahoney, C.E.; Coloma, J.; Calsina, B.; Currás-Freixes, M.; Letón, R.; Torres-Pérez, R.; Richter, S.; Pita, G.; et al. Recurrent Germline DLST Mutations in Individuals with Multiple Pheochromocytomas and Paragangliomas. *Am. J. Hum. Genet.* **2019**, *104*, 651–664. [CrossRef]
81. Carrozzo, R.; Verrigni, D.; Rasmussen, M.; de Coo, R.; Amartino, H.; Bianchi, M.; Buhas, D.; Mesli, S.; Naess, K.; Born, A.P.; et al. Succinate-CoA ligase deficiency due to mutations in SUCLA2 and SUCLG1: Phenotype and genotype correlations in 71 patients. *J. Inherit. Metab. Dis.* **2016**, *39*, 243–252. [CrossRef]
82. Carrozzo, R.; Dionisi-Vici, C.; Steuerwald, U.; Lucioli, S.; Deodato, F.; Di Giandomenico, S.; Bertini, E.; Franke, B.; Kluijtmans, L.A.J.; Meschini, M.C.; et al. SUCLA2 mutations are associated with mild methylmalonic aciduria, Leigh-like encephalomyopathy, dystonia and deafness. *Brain* **2007**, *130*, 862–874. [CrossRef]
83. Spiegel, R.; Pines, O.; Ta-Shma, A.; Burak, E.; Shaag, A.; Halvardson, J.; Edvardson, S.; Mahajna, M.; Zenvirt, S.; Saada, A.; et al. Infantile cerebellar-retinal degeneration associated with a mutation in mitochondrial aconitase, ACO2. *Am. J. Hum. Genet.* **2012**, *90*, 518–523. [CrossRef]

84. Bouwkamp, C.G.; Afawi, Z.; Fattal-Valevski, A.; Krabbendam, I.E.; Rivetti, S.; Masalha, R.; Quadri, M.; Breedveld, G.J.; Mandel, H.; Tailakh, M.A.; et al. ACO2 homozygous missense mutation associated with complicated hereditary spastic paraplegia. *Neurol. Genet.* **2018**, *4*, e223. [CrossRef]
85. Fattal-Valevski, A.; Eliyahu, H.; Fraenkel, N.I.D.; Elmaliach, G.; Hausman-Kedem, M.; Shaag, A.; Mandel, D.; Pines, O.; Elpeleg, O. Homozygous mutation, p. Pro304His, in IDH3A, encoding isocitrate dehydrogenase subunit is associated with severe encephalopathy in infancy. *Neurogenetics* **2017**, *18*, 57–61. [CrossRef]
86. Odièvre, M.-H.; Chretien, D.; Munnich, A.; Robinson, B.H.; Dumoulin, R.; Masmoudi, S.; Kadhom, N.; Rötig, A.; Rustin, P.; Bonnefont, J.-P. A novel mutation in the dihydrolipoamide dehydrogenase E3 subunit gene (DLD) resulting in an atypical form of α-ketoglutarate dehydrogenase deficiency. *Hum. Mutat.* **2005**, *25*, 323–324. [CrossRef]
87. Kranendijk, M.; Struys, E.A.; Van Schaftingen, E.; Gibson, K.M.; Kanhai, W.A.; Van Der Knaap, M.S.; Amiel, J.; Buist, N.R.; Das, A.M.; De Klerk, J.B.; et al. IDH2 mutations in patients with D-2-hydroxyglutaric aciduria. *Science* **2010**, *330*, 336. [CrossRef]
88. Alston, C.L.; Davison, J.E.; Meloni, F.; van der Westhuizen, F.H.; He, L.; Hornig-Do, H.T.; Peet, A.C.; Gissen, P.; Goffrini, P.; Ferrero, I.; et al. Recessive germline SDHA and SDHB mutations causing leukodystrophy and isolated mitochondrial complex II deficiency. *J. Med. Genet.* **2012**, *49*, 569–577. [CrossRef]
89. Jackson, C.B.; Nuoffer, J.M.; Hahn, D.; Prokisch, H.; Haberberger, B.; Gautschi, M.; Häberli, A.; Gallati, S.; Schaller, A. Mutations in SDHD lead to autosomal recessive encephalomyopathy and isolated mitochondrial complex II deficiency. *J. Med. Genet.* **2014**, *51*, 170–175. [CrossRef]
90. Bourgeron, T.; Chretien, D.; Poggi-Bach, J.; Doonan, S.; Rabier, D.; Letouzé, P.; Munnich, A.; Rötig, A.; Landrieu, P.; Rustin, P. Mutation of the fumarase gene in two siblings with progressive encephalopathy and fumarase deficiency. *J. Clin. Investig.* **1994**, *93*, 2514–2518. [CrossRef]
91. Nota, B.; Struys, E.A.; Pop, A.; Jansen, E.E.; Fernandez Ojeda, M.R.; Kanhai, W.A.; Kranendijk, M.; Van Dooren, S.J.M.; Bevova, M.R.; Sistermans, E.A.; et al. Deficiency in SLC25A1, encoding the mitochondrial citrate carrier, causes combined D-2- and L-2-hydroxyglutaric aciduria. *Am. J. Hum. Genet.* **2013**, *92*, 627–631. [CrossRef] [PubMed]
92. Spiegel, R.; Shaag, A.; Edvardson, S.; Mandel, H.; Stepensky, P.; Shalev, S.A.; Horovitz, Y.; Pines, O.; Elpeleg, O. SLC25A19 mutation as a cause of neuropathy and bilateral striatal necrosis. *Ann. Neurol.* **2009**, *66*, 419–424. [CrossRef]
93. Rzem, R.; Veiga-da-Cunha, M.; Noel, G.; Goffette, S.; Nassogne, M.-C.; Tabarki, B.; Scholler, C.; Marquardt, T.; Vikkula, M.; Van Schaftingen, E. A gene encoding a putative FAD-dependent L-2-hydroxyglutarate dehydrogenase is mutated in L-2-hydroxyglutaric aciduria. *Proc. Natl. Acad. Sci. USA* **2004**, *101*, 16849–16854. [CrossRef]
94. Johnson, M.T.; Yang, H.-S.; Magnuson, T.; Patel, M.S. Targeted disruption of the murine dihydrolipoamide dehydrogenase gene (Dld) results in perigastrulation lethality (gene targeting embryonic lethal mutation embryonic metabolism). *Dev. Boil.* **1997**, *94*, 14512–14517.
95. Piruat, J.I.; Pintado, C.O.; Ortega-Saenz, P.; Roche, M.; Lopez-Barneo, J. The Mitochondrial SDHD Gene Is Required for Early Embryogenesis, and Its Partial Deficiency Results in Persistent Carotid Body Glomus Cell Activation with Full Responsiveness to Hypoxia. *Mol. Cell. Biol.* **2004**, *24*, 10933–10940. [CrossRef]
96. Pollard, P.J.; Spencer-Dene, B.; Shukla, D.; Howarth, K.; Nye, E.; El-Bahrawy, M.; Deheragoda, M.; Joannou, M.; McDonald, S.; Martin, A.; et al. Targeted Inactivation of Fh1 Causes Proliferative Renal Cyst Development and Activation of the Hypoxia Pathway. *Cancer Cell* **2007**, *11*, 311–319. [CrossRef] [PubMed]
97. Yang, L.; Shi, Q.; Ho, D.J.; Starkov, A.A.; Wille, E.J.; Xu, H.; Chen, H.L.; Zhang, S.; Stack, C.M.; Calingasan, N.Y.; et al. Mice deficient in dihydrolipoyl succinyl transferase show increased vulnerability to mitochondrial toxins. *Neurobiol. Dis.* **2009**, *36*, 320–330. [CrossRef] [PubMed]
98. Kacso, G.; Ravasz, D.; Doczi, J.; Nemeth, B.; Madgar, O.; Saada, A.; Ilin, P.; Miller, C.; Ostergaard, E.; Iordanov, I.; et al. Two transgenic mouse models for-subunit components of succinate-CoA ligase yielding pleiotropic metabolic alterations. *Biochem. J.* **2016**, *473*, 3463–3485. [CrossRef] [PubMed]
99. Pagnamenta, A.T.; Hargreaves, I.P.; Duncan, A.J.; Taanman, J.W.; Heales, S.J.; Land, J.M.; Bitner-Glindzicz, M.; Leonard, J.V.; Rahman, S. Phenotypic variability of mitochondrial disease caused by a nuclear mutation in complex II. *Mol. Genet. Metab.* **2006**, *89*, 214–221. [CrossRef] [PubMed]

100. Levitas, A.; Muhammad, E.; Harel, G.; Saada, A.; Caspi, V.C.; Manor, E.; Beck, J.C.; Sheffield, V.; Parvari, R. Familial neonatal isolated cardiomyopathy caused by a mutation in the flavoprotein subunit of succinate dehydrogenase. *Eur. J. Hum. Genet.* **2010**, *18*, 1160–1165. [CrossRef]
101. Aghili, M.; Zahedi, F.; Rafiee, E. Hydroxyglutaric aciduria and malignant brain tumor: A case report and literature review. *J. Neurooncol.* **2009**, *91*, 233–236. [CrossRef]
102. Maher, L.J., III; Smith, E.H.; Rueter, E.M.; Becker, N.A.; Bida, J.P.; Nelson-Holte, M.; Palomo, J.I.P.; García-Flores, P.; López-Barneo, J.; van Deursen, J. Mouse Models of Human Familial Paraganglioma. In *Pheochromocytoma-A New View of the Old Problem*; Intech: London, UK, 2011.
103. Semenza, G.L. Targeting HIF-1 for cancer therapy. *Nat. Rev. Cancer* **2003**, *3*, 721–732. [CrossRef]
104. Schofield, C.J.; Ratcliffe, P.J. Oxygen sensing by HIF hydroxylases. *Nat. Rev. Mol. Cell Biol.* **2004**, *5*, 343–354. [CrossRef] [PubMed]
105. Dahia, P.L.M.; Ross, K.N.; Wright, M.E.; Hayashida, C.Y.; Santagata, S.; Barontini, M.; Kung, A.L.; Sanso, G.; Powers, J.F.; Tischler, A.S.; et al. A HIf1α regulatory loop links hypoxia and mitochondrial signals in pheochromocytomas. *PLoS Genet.* **2005**, *1*, 72–80. [CrossRef] [PubMed]
106. Her, Y.F.; Maher, L.J. Succinate dehydrogenase loss in familial paraganglioma: Biochemistry, genetics, and epigenetics. *Int. J. Endocrinol.* **2015**, *2015*, 296167. [CrossRef] [PubMed]
107. Jochmanová, I.; Yang, C.; Zhuang, Z.; Pacak, K. Hypoxia-inducible factor signaling in pheochromocytoma: Turning the rudder in the right direction. *J. Natl. Cancer Inst.* **2013**, *105*, 1270–1283. [CrossRef]
108. Waguespack, S.G.; Rich, T.; Grubbs, E.; Ying, A.K.; Perrier, N.D.; Ayala-Ramirez, M.; Jimenez, C. A current review of the etiology, diagnosis, and treatment of pediatric pheochromocytoma and paraganglioma. *J. Clin. Endocrinol. Metab.* **2010**, *95*, 2023–2037. [CrossRef]
109. Astrom, K.; Cohen, J.E.; Willett-Brozick, J.E.; Aston, C.E.; Baysal, B.E. Altitude is a phenotypic modifier in hereditary paraganglioma type 1: Evidence for an oxygen-sensing defect. *Hum. Genet.* **2003**, *113*, 228–237. [CrossRef] [PubMed]
110. Cerecer-Gil, N.Y.; Figuera, L.E.; Llamas, F.J.; Lara, M.; Escamilla, J.G.; Ramos, R.; Estrada, G.; Hussain, A.K.; Gaal, J.; Korpershoek, E.; et al. Mutation of SDHB is a cause of hypoxia-related high-altitude paraganglioma. *Clin. Cancer Res.* **2010**, *16*, 4148–4154. [CrossRef]
111. Opotowsky, A.R.; Moko, L.E.; Ginns, J.; Rosenbaum, M.; Greutmann, M.; Aboulhosn, J.; Hageman, A.; Kim, Y.; Deng, L.X.; Grewal, J.; et al. Pheochromocytoma and paraganglioma in cyanotic congenital heart disease. *J. Clin. Endocrinol. Metab.* **2015**, *100*, 1325–1334. [CrossRef] [PubMed]
112. Zhuang, Z.; Yang, C.; Lorenzo, F.; Merino, M.; Fojo, T.; Kebebew, E.; Popovic, V.; Stratakis, C.A.; Prchal, J.T.; Pacak, K. Somatic *HIF2A* Gain-of-Function Mutations in Paraganglioma with Polycythemia. *N. Engl. J. Med.* **2012**, *367*, 922–930. [CrossRef]
113. Comino-Méndez, I.; de Cubas, A.A.; Bernal, C.; Álvarez-Escolá, C.; Sánchez-Malo, C.; Ramírez-Tortosa, C.L.; Pedrinaci, S.; Rapizzi, E.; Ercolino, T.; Bernini, G.; et al. Tumoral EPAS1 (HIF2A) mutations explain sporadic pheochromocytoma and paraganglioma in the absence of erythrocytosis. *Hum. Mol. Genet.* **2013**, *22*, 2169–2176. [CrossRef] [PubMed]
114. Toledo, R.A.; Qin, Y.; Srikantan, S.; Morales, N.P.; Li, Q.; Deng, Y.; Kim, S.W.; Pereira, M.A.A.; Toledo, S.P.A.; Su, X.; et al. In vivo and in vitro oncogenic effects of HIF2A mutations in pheochromocytomas and paragangliomas. *Endocr. Relat. Cancer* **2013**, *20*, 349–359. [CrossRef] [PubMed]
115. Toledo, R.; Jimenez, C. Recent advances in the management of malignant pheochromocytoma and paraganglioma: Focus on tyrosine kinase and hypoxia-inducible factor inhibitors. *F1000Research* **2018**, *7*, 1148. [CrossRef]
116. Courtney, K.D.; Infante, J.R.; Lam, E.T.; Figlin, R.A.; Rini, B.I.; Brugarolas, J.; Zojwalla, N.J.; Lowe, A.M.; Wang, K.; Wallace, E.M.; et al. Phase I dose-escalation trial of PT2385, a first-in-class hypoxia-inducible factor-2a antagonist in patients with previously treated advanced clear cell renal cell carcinoma. *J. Clin. Oncol.* **2018**, *36*, 867–874. [CrossRef]
117. Chen, W.; Hill, H.; Christie, A.; Kim, M.S.; Holloman, E.; Pavia-Jimenez, A.; Homayoun, F.; Ma, Y.; Patel, N.; Yell, P.; et al. Targeting renal cell carcinoma with a HIF-2 antagonist. *Nature* **2016**, *539*, 112–117. [CrossRef] [PubMed]
118. Cho, H.; Kaelin, W.G. Targeting HIF2 in Clear Cell Renal Cell Carcinoma. *Cold Spring Harb. Symp. Quant. Biol.* **2016**, *81*, 113–121. [CrossRef]

119. Geli, J.; Kiss, N.; Karimi, M.; Lee, J.J.; Bäckdahl, M.; Ekström, T.J.; Larsson, C. Global and regional CpG methylation in pheochromocytomas and abdominal paragangliomas: Association to malignant behavior. *Clin. Cancer Res.* **2008**, *14*, 2551–2559. [CrossRef]
120. Killian, J.K.; Kim, S.Y.; Miettinen, M.; Smith, C.; Merino, M.; Tsokos, M.; Quezado, M.; Smith, W.I.; Jahromi, M.S.; Xekouki, P.; et al. Succinate dehydrogenase mutation underlies global epigenomic divergence in gastrointestinal stromal tumor. *Cancer Discov.* **2013**, *3*, 648–657. [CrossRef] [PubMed]
121. Remacha, L.; Currás-Freixes, M.; Torres-Ruiz, R.; Schiavi, F.; Torres-Pérez, R.; Calsina, B.; Letón, R.; Comino-Méndez, I.; Roldán-Romero, J.M.; Montero-Conde, C.; et al. Gain-of-function mutations in DNMT3A in patients with paraganglioma. *Genet. Med.* **2018**, *20*, 1644–1651. [CrossRef]
122. Toledo, R.A.; Qin, Y.; Cheng, Z.M.; Gao, Q.; Iwata, S.; Silva, G.M.; Prasad, M.L.; Ocal, I.T.; Rao, S.; Aronin, N.; et al. Recurrent Mutations of Chromatin-Remodeling Genes and Kinase Receptors in Pheochromocytomas and Paragangliomas. *Clin. Cancer Res.* **2016**, *22*, 2301–2310. [CrossRef] [PubMed]
123. Richter, S.; Peitzsch, M.; Rapizzi, E.; Lenders, J.W.; Qin, N.; De Cubas, A.A.; Schiavi, F.; Rao, J.U.; Beuschlein, F.; Quinkler, M.; et al. Krebs cycle metabolite profiling for identification and stratification of pheochromocytomas/paragangliomas due to succinate dehydrogenase deficiency. *J. Clin. Endocrinol. Metab.* **2014**, *99*, 3903–3911. [CrossRef]
124. Eisenhofer, G.; Klink, B.; Richter, S.; Lenders, J.W.M.; Robledo, M. Metabologenomics of phaeochromocytoma and paraganglioma: An integrated approach for personalised biochemical and genetic testing. *Clin. Biochem. Rev.* **2017**, *38*, 69–100. [PubMed]
125. Leshets, M.; Silas, Y.B.H.; Lehming, N.; Pines, O. Fumarase: From the TCA Cycle to DNA Damage Response and Tumor Suppression. *Front. Mol. Biosci.* **2018**, *5*, 68. [CrossRef] [PubMed]
126. Yogev, O.; Yogev, O.; Singer, E.; Shaulian, E.; Goldberg, M.; Fox, T.D.; Pines, O. Fumarase: A mitochondrial metabolic enzyme and a cytosolic/nuclear component of the dna damage response. *PLoS Biol.* **2010**, *8*, e1000328. [CrossRef]
127. Pang, Y.; Lu, Y.; Caisova, V.; Liu, Y.; Bullova, P.; Huynh, T.T.; Zhou, Y.; Yu, D.; Frysak, Z.; Hartmann, I.; et al. Targeting NADþ/PARP DNA repair pathway as a novel therapeutic approach to SDHB-mutated cluster I pheochromocytoma and paraganglioma. *Clin. Cancer Res.* **2018**, *24*, 3423–3432. [CrossRef]
128. Zhang, Z.; Tan, M.; Xie, Z.; Dai, L.; Chen, Y.; Zhao, Y. Identification of lysine succinylation as a new post-translational modification. *Nat. Chem. Biol.* **2011**, *7*, 58–63. [CrossRef]
129. Sabari, B.R.; Zhang, D.; Allis, C.D.; Zhao, Y. Metabolic regulation of gene expression through histone acylations. *Nat. Rev. Mol. Cell Biol.* **2017**, *18*, 90–101. [CrossRef]
130. Wang, Y.; Guo, Y.R.; Liu, K.; Yin, Z.; Liu, R.; Xia, Y.; Tan, L.; Yang, P.; Lee, J.H.; Li, X.J.; et al. KAT2A coupled with the α-KGDH complex acts as a histone H3 succinyltransferase. *Nature* **2017**, *552*, 273–277. [CrossRef]
131. Smestad, J.; Erber, L.; Chen, Y.; Maher, L.J., III. Chromatin Succinylation Correlates with Active Gene Expression and Is Perturbed by Defective TCA Cycle Metabolism. *iScience* **2018**, *2*, 63–75. [CrossRef] [PubMed]
132. Yang, Y.; Gibson, G.E. Succinylation Links Metabolism to Protein Functions. *Neurochem. Res.* **2019**, 1–14. [CrossRef] [PubMed]
133. Park, J.; Chen, Y.; Tishkoff, D.X.; Peng, C.; Tan, M.; Dai, L.; Xie, Z.; Zhang, Y.; Zwaans, B.M.M.; Skinner, M.E.; et al. SIRT5-Mediated Lysine Desuccinylation Impacts Diverse Metabolic Pathways. *Mol. Cell* **2013**, *50*, 919–930. [CrossRef]
134. Weinert, B.T.; Schölz, C.; Wagner, S.A.; Iesmantavicius, V.; Su, D.; Daniel, J.A.; Choudhary, C. Lysine succinylation is a frequently occurring modification in prokaryotes and eukaryotes and extensively overlaps with acetylation. *Cell Rep.* **2013**, *4*, 842–851. [CrossRef] [PubMed]
135. Lowery, A.J.; Walsh, S.; McDermott, E.W.; Prichard, R.S. Molecular and therapeutic advances in the diagnosis and management of malignant pheochromocytomas and paragangliomas. *Oncologist* **2013**, *18*, 391–407. [CrossRef]
136. Jimenez, C. Treatment for patients with malignant pheochromocytomas and paragangliomas: A perspective from the hallmarks of cancer. *Front. Endocrinol.* **2018**, *9*, 227. [CrossRef]
137. Molenaar, J.J.; Koster, J.; Zwijnenburg, D.A.; Van Sluis, P.; Valentijn, L.J.; Van Der Ploeg, I.; Hamdi, M.; Van Nes, J.; Westerman, B.A.; Van Arkel, J.; et al. Sequencing of neuroblastoma identifies chromothripsis and defects in neuritogenesis genes. *Nature* **2012**, *483*, 589–593. [CrossRef] [PubMed]

138. Rausch, T.; Jones, D.T.W.; Zapatka, M.; Stütz, A.M.; Zichner, T.; Weischenfeldt, J.; Jäger, N.; Remke, M.; Shih, D.; Northcott, P.A.; et al. Genome sequencing of pediatric medulloblastoma links catastrophic DNA rearrangements with TP53 mutations. *Cell* **2012**, *148*, 59–71. [CrossRef]
139. Stephens, P.J.; Greenman, C.D.; Fu, B.; Yang, F.; Bignell, G.R.; Mudie, L.J.; Pleasance, E.D.; Lau, K.W.; Beare, D.; Stebbings, L.A.; et al. Massive genomic rearrangement acquired in a single catastrophic event during cancer development. *Cell* **2011**, *144*, 27–40. [CrossRef]
140. Zhang, C.Z.; Leibowitz, M.L.; Pellman, D. Chromothripsis and beyond: Rapid genome evolution from complex chromosomal rearrangements. *Genes Dev.* **2013**, *27*, 2513–2530. [CrossRef] [PubMed]
141. Maher, C.A.; Wilson, R.K. Chromothripsis and human disease: Piecing together the shattering process. *Cell* **2012**, *148*, 29–32. [CrossRef]
142. Ernst, A.; Jones, D.T.W.; Maass, K.K.; Rode, A.; Deeg, K.I.; Jebaraj, B.M.C.; Korshunov, A.; Hovestadt, V.; Tainsky, M.A.; Pajtler, K.W.; et al. Telomere dysfunction and chromothripsis. *Int. J. Cancer* **2016**, *138*, 2905–2914. [CrossRef]
143. Valentijn, L.J.; Koster, J.; Zwijnenburg, D.A.; Hasselt, N.E.; Van Sluis, P.; Volckmann, R.; Van Noesel, M.M.; George, R.E.; Tytgat, G.A.M.; Molenaar, J.J.; et al. TERT rearrangements are frequent in neuroblastoma and identify aggressive tumors. *Nat. Genet.* **2015**, *47*, 1411–1414. [CrossRef] [PubMed]
144. Dwight, T.; Flynn, A.; Amarasinghe, K.; Benn, D.E.; Lupat, R.; Li, J.; Cameron, D.L.; Hogg, A.; Balachander, S.; Candiloro, I.L.M.; et al. TERT structural rearrangements in metastatic pheochromocytomas. *Endocr. Relat. Cancer* **2018**, *25*, 1–9. [CrossRef]
145. Liu, T.; Brown, T.C.; Juhlin, C.C.; Andreasson, A.; Wang, N.; Bäckdahl, M.; Healy, J.M.; Prasad, M.L.; Korah, R.; Carling, T.; et al. The activating TERT promoter mutation C228T is recurrent in subsets of adrenal tumors. *Endocr. Relat. Cancer* **2014**, *21*, 427–434. [CrossRef] [PubMed]
146. Job, S.; Draskovic, I.; Burnichon, N.; Buffet, A.; Cros, J.; Lépine, C.; Venisse, A.; Robidel, E.; Verkarre, V.; Meatchi, T.; et al. Telomerase Activation and ATRX Mutations Are Independent Risk Factors for Metastatic Pheochromocytoma and Paraganglioma. *Clin. Cancer Res.* **2019**, *25*, 760–770. [CrossRef] [PubMed]
147. Fishbein, L.; Khare, S.; Wubbenhorst, B.; Desloover, D.; D'Andrea, K.; Merrill, S.; Cho, N.W.; Greenberg, R.A.; Else, T.; Montone, K.; et al. Whole exome sequencing identifies somatic ATRX mutations in pheochromocytomas and paragangliomas. *Nat. Commun.* **2015**, *6*, 6140. [CrossRef] [PubMed]
148. Xu, Y.; Goldkorn, A. Telomere and telomerase therapeutics in cancer. *Genes* **2016**, *7*, 22. [CrossRef]
149. Joyce, J.A.; Fearon, D.T. T cell exclusion, immune privilege, and the tumor microenvironment. *Science* **2015**, *348*, 74–80. [CrossRef]

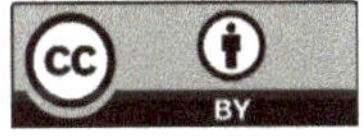

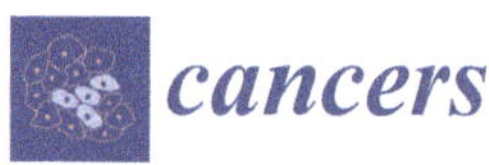

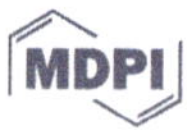

Article

Optimizing Genetic Workup in Pheochromocytoma and Paraganglioma by Integrating Diagnostic and Research Approaches

Laura Gieldon [1,2,3,4,†], Doreen William [2,3,4,†], Karl Hackmann [1,2,3,4], Winnie Jahn [2,3,4], Arne Jahn [1,2,3,4], Johannes Wagner [1,2,3,4], Andreas Rump [1,2,3,4], Nicole Bechmann [5], Svenja Nölting [6], Thomas Knösel [7], Volker Gudziol [8], Georgiana Constantinescu [9], Jimmy Masjkur [9], Felix Beuschlein [10], Henri JLM Timmers [11], Letizia Canu [12], Karel Pacak [13], Mercedes Robledo [14], Daniela Aust [15], Evelin Schröck [1,2,3,4], Graeme Eisenhofer [5,9], Susan Richter [5] and Barbara Klink [1,2,3,4,16,*]

1 Institute for Clinical Genetics, Medical Faculty Carl Gustav Carus, Technische Universität Dresden, 01307 Dresden, Germany; Laura.Gieldon@tu-dresden.de (L.G.); Karl.Hackmann@uniklinikum-dresden.de (K.H.); Arne.Jahn@uniklinikum-dresden.de (A.J.); Johannes.Wagner@uniklinikum-dresden.de (J.W.); Andreas.Rump@uniklinikum-dresden.de (A.R.); Evelin.Schroeck@uniklinikum-dresden.de (E.S.)

2 Core Unit for Molecular Tumor Diagnostics (CMTD), National Center for Tumor Diseases (NCT), 01307 Dresden, Germany; doreen.william@nct-dresden.de (D.W.); w.jahn@dkfz-heidelberg.de (W.J.)

3 German Cancer Consortium (DKTK), 01307 Dresden, Germany

4 German Cancer Research Center (DKFZ), 69120 Heidelberg, Germany

5 Institute of Clinical Chemistry and Laboratory Medicine, University Hospital Carl Gustav Carus, Medical Faculty Carl Gustav Carus, Technische Universität Dresden, 01307 Dresden, Germany; Nicole.Bechmann@uniklinikum-dresden.de (N.B.); Graeme.Eisenhofer@uniklinikum-dresden.de (G.E.); Susan.Richter@uniklinikum-dresden.de (S.R.)

6 Medizinische Klinik und Poliklinik IV, Klinikum der Universität, LMU München, 80336 Munich, Germany; Svenja.Noelting@med.uni-muenchen.de

7 Institute of Pathology, Ludwig-Maximilians-University, 80337 Munich, Germany; Thomas.Knoesel@med.uni-muenchen.de

8 Department of Otorhinolaryngology Head and Neck Surgery, Municipal Hospital Dresden, 01067 Dresden, Germany; Volker.Gudziol@uniklinikum-dresden.de (V.G.)

9 Department of Internal Medicine III, University Hospital Carl Gustav Carus at Technische Universität Dresden, 01307 Dresden, Germany; Georgiana.Constantinescu@uniklinikum-dresden.de (G.C.), Jimmy.Masjkur@med.uni-heidelberg.de (J.M.)

10 Klinik für Endokrinologie, Diabetologie und Klinische Ernährung, Universitätsspital Zürich, 8091 Zürich, Switzerland; felix.beuschlein@usz.ch

11 Department of Internal Medicine, Radboud University Medical Centre, 6525 Nijmegen, The Netherlands; henri.timmers@radboudumc.nl

12 Department of Experimental and Clinical Biomedical Sciences, University of Florence, 50149 Florence, Italy; letizia.canu@unifi.it

13 Eunice Kennedy Shriver National Institute of Child Health and Human Development, National Institutes of Health, Bethesda, MD 20892, USA; karel@mail.nih.gov

14 Hereditary Endocrine Cancer Group, CNIO, Madrid, Spain and Centro de Investigación Biomédica en Red de Enfermedades Raras (CIBERER), 28029 Madrid, Spain; mrobledo@cnio.es

15 Institute of Pathology, Tumor and Normal Tissue Bank of the UCC/NCT Dresden, University Hospital Carl Gustav Carus, Technische Universität Dresden, 01307 Dresden, Germany; Daniela.Aust@uniklinikum-dresden.de

16 National Center for Genetics (NCG), Laboratoire national de santé (LNS), 1, rue Louis Rech, 3555 Dudelange, Luxembourg

* Correspondence: Barbara.Klink@lns.etat.lu; Tel.: +352-28100-429

† These authors contributed equally.

Received: 30 April 2019; Accepted: 5 June 2019; Published: 11 June 2019

Abstract: Pheochromocytomas and paragangliomas (PPGL) are rare neuroendocrine tumors with a strong hereditary background and a large genetic heterogeneity. Identification of the underlying genetic cause is crucial for the management of patients and their families as it aids differentiation between hereditary and sporadic cases. To improve diagnostics and clinical management we tailored an enrichment based comprehensive multi-gene next generation sequencing panel applicable to both analyses of tumor tissue and blood samples. We applied this panel to tumor samples and compared its performance to our current routine diagnostic approach. Routine diagnostic sequencing of 11 PPGL susceptibility genes was applied to blood samples of 65 unselected PPGL patients at a single center in Dresden, Germany. Predisposing germline mutations were identified in 19 (29.2%) patients. Analyses of 28 PPGL tumor tissues using the dedicated PPGL panel revealed pathogenic or likely pathogenic variants in known PPGL susceptibility genes in 21 (75%) cases, including mutations in *IDH2*, *ATRX* and *HRAS*. These mutations suggest sporadic tumor development. Our results imply a diagnostic benefit from extended molecular tumor testing of PPGLs and consequent improvement of patient management. The approach is promising for determination of prognostic biomarkers that support therapeutic decision-making.

Keywords: pheochromocytoma; paraganglioma; next-generation sequencing; sporadic; hereditary; CNV detection

---

1. Introduction

Pheochromocytomas and paragangliomas (PPGL) are rare neuroendocrine tumors that originate from neural crest-derived chromaffin cells and develop either in the adrenal medulla or in extra-adrenal sympathetic and parasympathetic ganglia. PPGLs show the highest heritability of all cancers with almost 40% of patients carrying pathogenic germline mutations in one of the known PPGL susceptibility genes. [1–5] For this reason, current guidelines recommend that germline genetic testing should be considered in all patients with PPGLs, regardless of family history and age at diagnosis [6]. Identification of a predisposing germline variant enables predictive testing in PPGL families, clinical surveillance of healthy mutation carriers and risk stratification for malignant disease and for development of synchronous and metachronous tumors.

The majority of hereditary PPGLs are caused by mutations affecting *NF1, RET, VHL, SDHA, SDHB, SDHC* and *SDHD*. Rare underlying germline mutations have been described in *FH, MAX, SDHAF2* and *TMEM127*. [2,7–11]. Genetic testing of these genes in PPGL patients in routine diagnostics has previously been conducted according to a step-wise diagnostic algorithm [2]. With next generation sequencing techniques becoming cheaper and more commonly available, multi-gene panel sequencing is increasingly replacing targeted approaches. Recently, several additional susceptibility and candidate genes accounting for a small proportion of cases have been identified. These are, however, not yet commonly included in routine diagnostic analyses of affected patients. These include germline mutations in genes encoding components of metabolic pathways, e.g. *MDH2*, *GOT2* and *DLST* [12–14] and in hypoxia pathway related genes *EGLN2* (*PHD1*), *EGLN1* (*PHD2*), and *EPAS1* (*HIF2α*) [15,16]. Mutations in the latter usually occur somatically but can be associated with a syndromic presentation when they occur in mosaic forms [17]. Similarly, a case with a postzygotic mosaic mutation in *H3F3A* presenting with PPGLs and a giant cell tumor of the bone has recently been described [18].

Recent efforts in genomic analyses of PPGLs revealed that about 30% of tumors carry somatic mutations in known susceptibility and driver genes [19]. Furthermore, somatic mutations in known cancer associated genes have been identified as driver-alterations in a subset of PPGLs due to recent efforts in genome sequencing projects, such as somatic activating hot-spot cases, and somatic hot-spot mutations in *IDH1* or *IDH2*, recognized as drivers of tumorigenesis in PPGL, were identified [20,21].

In addition, somatic alterations in other cancer-associated genes, such as *SETD2, EZH2, FGFR1, BRAF, MET,* and *TP53,* have been reported [18,19,22].

Supporting analyses of tumor tissue by immunohistochemistry and metabolite measurements provide further information, aiding in identification and interpretation of genetic variants [21]. We previously demonstrated that quantification of Krebs cycle metabolites in tumor tissue can classify PPGLs and identify tumors with underlying alteration in *SDH*-genes (*SDHx*), *FH*, and *IDH*-genes *(IDHx)* and can furthermore aid in classification of variants of unknown significance in *SDHx* [21,23].

To improve PPGL diagnostics and patient management we developed a comprehensive customized PPGL multi-gene panel for the analysis of PPGL tumor tissue, comprising 84 PPGL associated and candidate genes. We applied this to a cohort of 28 PPGL tumor samples and compared the results to our in-house PPGL cohort of patients who, over the course of several years, have undergone germline sequencing within a routine diagnostic setting.

2. Results

2.1. Routine Germline Testing in PPGL Patients Solves 30% of Cases

Between 2008 and 2017, 65 patients with PPGLs were referred to the Institute of Clinical Genetics in Dresden for genetic counselling and/or genetic testing. Thirty-one patients primarily presented with pheochromocytoma (PHEO) and 34 patients with paraganglioma (PGL), of which 25 were head and neck paragangliomas (HNP). The median age at diagnosis was 46.5 years (ranging from 13 to 77 years) and did not differ between those patients diagnosed with pheochromocytoma and those with paraganglioma. Eleven patients (17.2%) had developed PPGL until 30 years of age (y), while 27 patients had an age of onset over 50y (41.5%). Forty-two patients (64.6%) were female (18 PHEOs, 24 PGLs) and 23 patients (35.4%) were male (13 PHEOs, 10 PGLs).

Five of these patients (7.7%) had multiple PPGL tumors and 8 patients (12.3%) had additional tumors including adrenocortical adenoma/carcinoma, thyroid carcinoma, renal cell carcinoma, a testicular tumor, mamma carcinoma, Hodgkin's lymphoma and cervical carcinoma. Pedigree information was available in 53 of the patients and inconspicuous regarding relatives with tumors in 34 of them (64.2%). Three patients had relatives affected by paraganglioma, pheochromocytoma or gastrointestinal stromal tumor (GIST), indicating hereditary disease in these families, which was molecularly confirmed in all three cases. One family was known to carry a pathogenic *BRCA2* germline mutation causing hereditary breast and ovarian cancer. In addition, pedigree analysis of 3 further families was suspicious of hereditary breast and ovarian cancer, hereditary gastric cancer and hereditary colon cancer, respectively. Another 15 families were affected by additional cancers unrelated to PPGL and without fulfillment of criteria for a specific hereditary tumor predisposing syndrome. Clinical data are summarized in Supplementary Table S1.

Germline testing of 11 PPGL susceptibility genes associated with known hereditary tumor predisposition syndromes associated with PPGLs (*SDHA, SDHB, SDHC, SDHD, SDHAF2, MAX, FH, NF1, RET, TMEM127* and *VHL*) was done in all of these patients, in the majority of cases using a combination of targeted multi-gene sequencing with the TruSight Cancer panel (Illumina, Inc., San Diego, CA, USA) in combination with customized array-based Comparative Genomic Hybridization (array-CGH) for copy number variation (CNV) calling [24] and Sanger Sequencing of *SDHA* (for details see Supplementary Table S1)

In 19 of 65 cases (29.2%) we identified pathogenic or likely pathogenic germline mutations in a PPGL susceptibility gene, confirming a PPGL related hereditary tumor predisposition syndrome in these cases (Table 1). The majority (14) of these patients had germline mutations in an *SDHx* gene, which is associated with an aberrant succinate to fumarate ratio (S:F ratio) in the tumor tissue. In eight cases with pathogenic germline *SDHx* variants, succinate and fumarate concentrations in the tumors were analyzed and aberrant S:F ratios were evident in six of these cases (Table 1).

Table 1. Overview of (likely) pathogenic germline variants (ACMG classes 4/5) identified during routine testing.

ID	Diagnosis	Solitary/Multiple	AD/Gender	Family History	Gene	Nucleotide Change	Amino Acid Change	S:F Ratio in Tumor Tissue
ID45	PHEO	unknown	30/f	unknown	FH	c.434C > G	p.(Ser145*)	0.14
ID11	PHEO	solitary	59/m	unknown	FH	c.1431_1433dupAAA	p.(Lys477dup)	n.a.
ID32	PHEO	multiple	39/f	1 melanoma (AO 35)	NF1	c.6084+1G > A	p.?	n.a.
ID52	PHEO	multiple	47/f	inconspicuous	RET	c.1901G > T	p.(Cys634Phe)	5.5
ID56	HNP	unknown	23/m	unknown	SDHA	c.553_554insA	p.(Ala186fs)	n.a.
ID62	PGL	solitary	37/f	inconspicuous	SDHA	c.1338delA	p.(His447fs)	n.a.
ID35	PGL/HNP	multiple	52/f	1 melanoma (AO 48)	SDHAF2	c.232G > A	p.(Gly78Arg)	217.3
ID3	HNP	solitary	17/m	inconspicuous	SDHB CHEK2	c.649C > T c.1100delC	p.(Arg217Cys) p.(Thr367fs)	24.1
ID42	PGL	solitary	51/m	cancers (AO > 50)	SDHB	c.287-3 C > G	p.?	1472.7
ID4	PGL/HNP	multiple	23/f	cancers (AO > 50)	SDHB	deletion exon 3		n.a.
ID55	HNP	unknown	26/f	unknown	SDHB	c.806delT	p.(Met269fs)	n.a.
ID86	PGL	solitary	33/m	unknown	SDHB	c.649C > T	p.(Arg217Cys)	n.a.
ID19	HNP	solitary	36/f	cancers (AO > 50)	SDHB	c.725G > A	p.(Arg242His)	5908.3
ID63	PGL	solitary	48/m	cancers (AO > 50)	SDHC	c.397C > T	p.(Arg133*)	45.4
ID48	HNP	solitary	69/f	inconspicuous	SDHC	c.43C > T	p.(Arg15*)	n.a.
ID43	PHEO	solitary	50/m	cancers (AO > 50)	SDHC	c.379C > T	p.(His127Tyr)	795.5
ID34	HNP	solitary	34/m	2 PGLs	SDHD	c.53-2A > G	p.?	278.3
ID38	HNP	solitary	47/f	1 PGL	SDHD	c.49C > T	p.(Arg17*)	920.6
ID59	HNP	unknown	68/f	unknown	TMEM127	c.465_466insACTTG	p.(Ala156fs)	n.a.

AD: age at diagnosis, AO: age of onset, PHEO: pheochromocytoma, PGL: paraganglioma, HNP: head & neck paraganglioma, S:F ratio: succinate to fumarate ratio.

In one patient (ID3) with a pathogenic *SDHB* variant, we found an additional pathogenic germline variant in *CHEK2* (c.1100delC, p.(Thr367fs)) that is known to be associated with hereditary breast and ovarian cancer (Table 1). In this case, an aberrant S:F ratio was not observed in the tumor although a pathogenic *SDHB* variant was identified, which might be explained by reported inconsistencies between *SDHx* mutations and aberrant S:F ratios in head and neck paragangliomas (HNPs) [21].

2.2. Development of a Dedicated PPGL Custom Panel for Germline and Tumor Testing

We designed a custom PPGL panel comprising a total of 84 genes, including 20 well-defined PPGL susceptibility genes (*EGLN1, EGLN2, MDH2, FH, SDHA, SDHB, SDHC, SDHD, SDHAF2, MAX, RET, TMEM127, VHL, EPAS1, NF1, H3F3A, IDH1, IDH2, ATRX,* and *HRAS*) that have been described to occur as germline, somatic or mosaic mutations in PPGL [2,4]. Additionally, we included further common known tumor genes such as *TP53, PTEN, FGFR1,* and *BRAF* that have been described to be mutated in PPGL tumors and might be secondary mutations [18,19,22]. Furthermore, we included candidate genes for PPGLs based on their gene function or gene family, e.g., genes encoding for metabolic enzymes or genes involved in epigenetic regulation (such as *TET1* and *TET2*) (Figure 1, Supplementary Table S2). Some of these candidate genes have already been implicated to play a role in PPGL development, such as *KIF1B, GOT2,* and *IDH3B* [13,25].

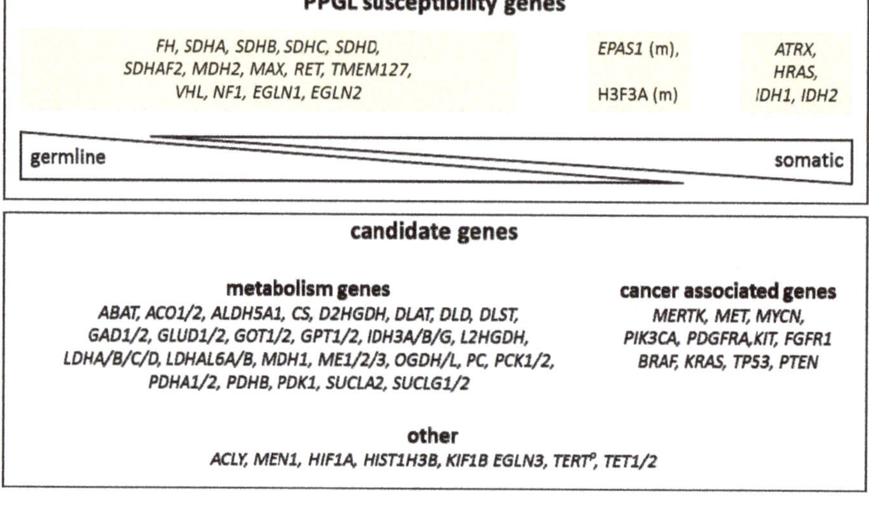

Figure 1. Schematic overview of the custom pheochromocytoma and paraganglioma (PPGL) panel. Known PPGL susceptibility genes and expected occurrences (germline, somatic) are depicted in the upper panel. Candidate gene categories are depicted in the lower panel. (m): mosaic, *TERT*^{P}: *TERT promoter region.*

Importantly, we chose an enrichment-based protocol to enable even nucleotide coverages across target regions and to limit coverage fluctuations as best as possible. Even overall coverage enables robust CNV detection using next generation sequencing (NGS) data. Furthermore, the enrichment-based design can be adapted to be used, not only for high-quality DNA, but also for low-quality and fragmented DNA from paraffin-embedded (FFPE) tumor tissues. [26]

2.3. Comprehensive Tumor Testing Improves Detection Rate of Underlying Mutations in PPGL-Patients

We first applied our novel customized PPGL panel to available tumor tissues of ten cases from our Dresden cohort that had undergone routine diagnostic germline testing. Four of the analyzed tumors were FFPE samples and six were freshly cryo-conserved tissue samples. Two of the cases (ID42 and ID43) had pathogenic germline variants in known PPGL susceptibility genes (*SDHB, SDHC*), whereas in eight cases, no pathogenic variants had been identified during routine germline testing (Table 2). Sequencing of tumor tissue from the aforementioned ten patients led to the identification of pathogenic variants in known PPGL susceptibility genes in nine cases (Table 2). In the two cases with pathogenic germline mutations, we could confirm both mutations in tumor tissue. In one of these cases (ID42), we observed increased allele frequency (85.4%) of the pathogenic *SDHB* variant, suggesting a loss of heterozygosity in this tumor (Table 2). In the other case (ID43) with a pathogenic germline variant in *SDHC*, we found an additional pathogenic somatic variant in *ATRX* (Table 2). In seven out of eight cases with inconspicuous germline analysis results, we identified pathogenic somatic variants in tumor tissue of the patients (Table 2). Four of these cases (ID69, ID66, ID67 and ID24) had a somatic variant in a known PPGL susceptibility gene (*SDHB*, *SDHD*, and 2x *VHL*) that was not present in the matched blood sample, indicating a sporadic tumor development in these cases. The tumor ID69 with a pathogenic *SDHD* variant additionally harbored a somatic missense variant of unknown significance in *FH* (p.(Ala198Val)) with a low allele frequency (7.3%), indicating a potential secondary event. Pathogenic hot-spot variants in *HRAS* were identified in two cases (ID1 and ID68). In the seventh tumor (ID72), we found pathogenic variants in *TP53* and in *ATRX*. In all of these cases, the family history was inconspicuous and, to our knowledge, no other tumors were diagnosed in those patients. All cases with pathogenic variants in *SDHx* also had aberrant S:F ratios in tumor tissue, whereas cases with pathogenic variants in non-*SDHx* genes did not show elevated S:F ratios, demonstrating correlation between genomic and metabolomic analyses (Table 2). Altogether, combined tumor and germline testing revealed causative mutations in 90% of the cases (9/10), confirming a sporadic tumor in seven cases.

Table 2. (Likely) pathogenic variants (ACMG classes 4/ 5) identified in tumor samples.

	Diagnosis	AD/Gender	Gene	Nucleotide Change	Amino Acid Change	VAF (Tumor)	LOH	Somatic Status	Germline Testing *	S:F Ratio
ID80	PHEO	65/m	*ATRX*	c.1441G > T	p.(Glu481*)	5.4%	no	likely somatic	no	46.2
ID82	PHEO	31/f	*FH*	c.700A > G	p.(Thr234Ala)	82.0%	yes	germline	yes (targeted)	0.4
ID41	PHEO	37/m	*FH*	c.816_836del	p.(Ala273_Val279del)	92.3%	yes	germline	yes (targeted)	0.3
ID68	PHEO	66/f	*HRAS*	c.182A > G	p.(Gln61Arg)	56.8%	no	somatic	yes	66.3
ID1	PHEO	52/f	*HRAS*	c.182A > G	p.(Gln61Arg)	72.0%		somatic	yes	17.7
ID60	PHEO	27/f	*HRAS*	c.37G > C	p.Gly13Arg	26.0%	no	somatic	no	12.8
ID75	HNP	53/f	*IDH2*	c.514A > G	p.Arg172Gly	24.5%	no	somatic	yes (targeted)	5.3
ID73	PHEO	56/f	*NF1*	c.1540C > T	p.(Gln514*)	62.1%		unknown	no	16.6
ID79	PHEO	58/f	*NF1*	c.7798_7799insA	p.(Ser2601fs)	83.2%	yes	unknown	no	47.5
ID91	PHEO	50/m	*NF1*	c.205-1G > T	p.?	39.9%	no	unknown	no	unknown
ID92	PHEO	73/f	*NF1*	c.1318C > T	p.(Arg440*)	15.9%	no	likely somatic	no	unknown
			NF1	c.7549C > T	p.(Arg2517*)	33.2%	no	unknown		unknown
ID51	PGL	56/m	*SDHB*	c.183T > G	p.(Tyr61*)	80.0%	yes	somatic	yes (targeted)	5178.2
ID42	PGL	51/m	*SDHB*	c.287-3C > G	p.?	85.4%	yes	germline	yes	1472.7
ID71	HNP	49/m	*SDHB*	c.724C > T	p.(Arg242Cys)	16.4%	no	likely somatic	no	24.7
ID43	PHEO	50/m	*SDHC*	c.379C > T	p.(His127Tyr)	46.6%	no	germline	yes	795.5
			ATRX	c.2817del	p.(Ala940fs)	65.8%		likely somatic		
ID69	HNP	27/f	*SDHD*	c.3G > T	p.(Met1Ile)	18.2%	no	somatic	yes	405.9
ID24	PGL	21/m	*SDHD*	c.337_340del	p.(Asp113fs)	41.5%		somatic	yes	1756.8
ID72	PHEO	66/f	*TP53*	c.817C > T	p.(Arg273Cys)	74.1%		somatic	yes	5.7
			ATRX	c.4744_4745insA	p.(Thr1582fs)	61.2%		unknown		
ID67	PGL	31/f	*VHL*	c.193T > G	p.(Ser65Ala)	8.5%	no	somatic	yes	24.1
ID66	PHEO	13/m	*VHL*	c.193T > G	p.(Ser65Ala)	17.4%	no	somatic	yes	21.4
ID78	PHEO	47/f	*VHL*	c.500G > A	p.(Arg167Gln)	49.6%	no	unknown	no	17.4

* Information about germline status was either available from routine germline testing in the patients included from our clinical cohort (indicated with "Germline testing yes") or due to targeted Sanger sequencing of blood samples ("yes (targeted)"). ACMG: American College of Medical Genetics, AD: age at diagnosis, LOH: loss of heterozygosity PHEO: pheochromocytoma, PGL: paraganglioma, HNP: head and neck paraganglioma, S:F ratio: succinate to fumarate ratio, VAF: variant allele frequency.

Next, we applied our PPGL custom panel to 18 PPGL tumor samples (twelve freshly cryo-conserved and six FFPE samples) within the scope of a multi-center research project. This cohort consisted of twelve pheochromocytomas and six paragangliomas, two of which were head and neck paragangliomas.

In twelve of these 18 tumors, pathogenic variants in a known PPGL susceptibility gene were identified by PPGL custom panel sequencing (Table 2). In four cases, germline status of pathogenic variants could be evaluated by targeted Sanger sequencing. In two cases (ID51, ID71), we found pathogenic variants in *SDHB*. The pathogenic nonsense mutation p.(Tyr61*) in *SDHB* in case ID51 was confirmed to be a somatic variant [21]. Furthermore, metabolome analysis of tumor tissue of case ID51 showed an elevated S:F ratio of 5178.2, which is concurrent with the pathogenic *SDHB* variant [21]. The *SDHB* missense variant p.(Arg242Cys) in case ID71 showed a low allele frequency of 16.4%, indicating that this variant is likely somatic as well. However, in this case no elevated S:F ratio was detected in tumor tissue, which is likely attributable to known deviations between pathogenic *SDHx* variants and S:F ratio in head and neck paragangliomas [21]. Pathogenic variants in *FH* were identified in tumor tissue of two cases (ID41 and ID82) and showed elevated fumarate to malate ratios, demonstrating correlation between genomic and metabolomic analyses [21]. Both pathogenic *FH* variants were also identified in the germline of the patients by targeted analysis (Table 2) [21].

In four cases, we identified pathogenic variants in *NF1* (ID73, ID79, ID91 and ID92). One of these cases (ID92) had two different nonsense mutations in *NF1* (p.(Arg440*) and p.(Arg2517*)) at allele frequencies of 15.9% and 33.2%, respectively, which could also indicate somatic origin. Case ID73 had a *NF1* nonsense variant (p.(Gln514*) at an allele frequency of 62.1%, case ID79 showed a pathogenic frameshift variant (p.(Ser2601fs)) in *NF1* with an allele frequency of 83.2% and ID91 had a pathogenic splice variant in *NF1* with an allele frequency of 39.9%. A pathogenic missense variant in *VHL* (p.(Arg167Gln) was identified in ID78 at an allele frequency of 49.6%. No blood samples were available for analysis in these five cases and thus, presence of the respective *NF1* or *VHL* variants in the germline of these patients could not be determined.

One tumor (ID75) harbored a somatic *IDH2* hot-spot mutation, in line with elevated D-2-hydroxyglutarate [21]. Tumor ID60 presented with a known hot-spot mutation in *HRAS*. Although no germline sequencing data were available, it can be assumed that this hot-spot mutation was somatic based on the gene involved and the low allele frequency of the variant. In one tumor (ID80) we identified a nonsense mutation in ATRX (p.Glu481*), however, only at a frequency of 5.4%. This might imply the alteration was a secondary event contributing to tumor maintenance, although no other pathogenic variants were found in this tumor using the PPGL custom panel.

Taken together, by sequencing analyses of altogether 28 tumor tissues using our PPGL panel, we identified 24 (likely) pathogenic variants in 21 tumor samples (Table 2, Figure 2). The spectrum of genes involved in these 21 samples differs from the spectrum of mutated genes identified by routine germline testing in our clinical cohort of 65 patients (Figure 2b). For example, the majority of variants identified by germline testing involved *SDHx* genes, while *SDHx* mutations only account for about 30% of mutations found by tumor testing (14/19 germline variants in the clinical cohort compared to 7/24 variants in tumor tissues). In contrast, variants in *IDH2*, *TP53*, *ATRX*, *HRAS*, and *VHL* were exclusively found by tumor sequencing, and variants in *NF1* were more frequently found in tumor tissues (5/24 variants in 21 tumor cases) compared to germline testing (1/19 variants identified in our clinical cohort of 65 patients (Figure 2b).

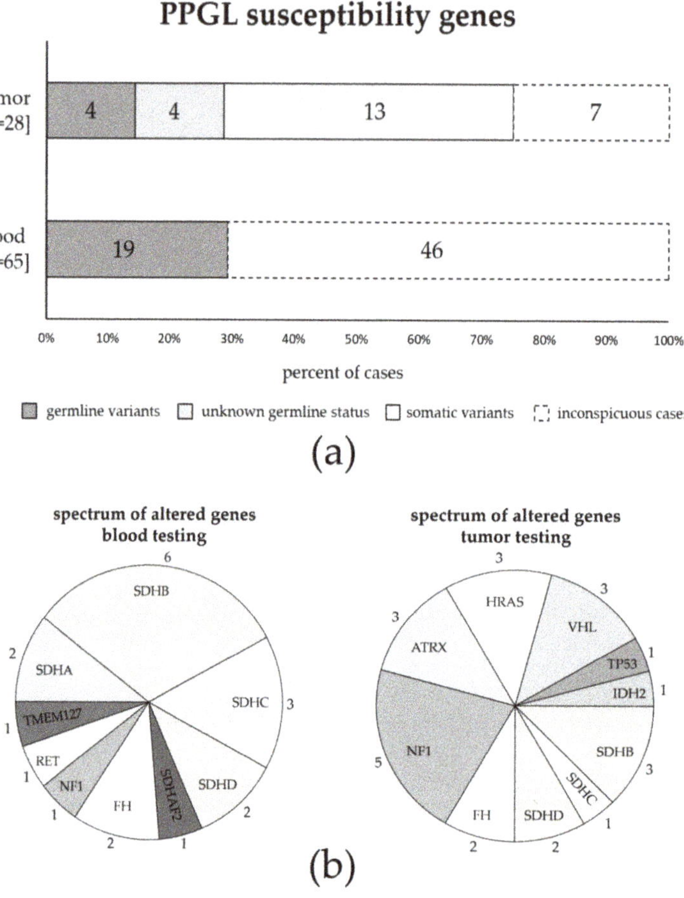

Figure 2. Summarized outcome of sequencing analysis of pheochromocytoma and paraganglioma (PPGL) susceptibility genes by diagnostic sequencing of blood samples in a clinical cohort of 65 patients and next generation sequencing analysis of 28 tumor tissues using our PPGL panel. Ten patients received both, diagnostic blood sequencing and tumor analysis, and are included in both cohorts. (**a**) We found (likely) pathogenic mutations in 21 of 28 tumors (75%), including three samples with more than one mutation (see Table 2); four of those patients had confirmed germline variants (dark grey); in four patients, germline status of the variant is unknown (grey); 13 cases had either confirmed somatic mutations or presumably somatic mutations based on the genes involved and/or the allele frequencies of the variants (light grey). Routine clinical blood testing in the clinical cohort of 65 patients identified 19 cases with germline mutations (29.2%). (**b**) Different spectrum of genes found to be mutated when performing blood testing (19 (likely) pathogenic variants identified in 19 of 65 blood samples) or tumor testing (24 (likely) pathogenic variants identified in 21 of 28 tumor samples). Numbers indicate how many variants were identified per gene.

In seven of 28 analyzed PPGL tumor samples, we found no underlying pathogenic variants in any of the 20 known PPGL susceptibility genes. In two of these seven cases, we identified potentially disease relevant variants. One tumor (ID61) had a missense variant in *ATRX* (p.(Asn53His)) at an allele frequency of 25%. This variant was not listed in databases such as gnomAD, ClinVar or dbSNP and has, to the best of our knowledge, not described in the literature [27–29]. In the tumor of patient ID90 we identified a missense variant in the candidate gene *TET1* (p.(Val128Leu)) with an allele frequency of 26.1%. The variant was found two times in heterozygous state in the general population (gnomAD database) and is listed in dbSNP (rs142008363), but not in ClinVar. Based on current knowledge, we classified both variants as variants of unknown significance. Unfortunately, blood samples to confirm the somatic status were unavailable in both cases, although the allele frequencies indicate that these variants might be somatic.

2.4. Tumor Testing with Our PPGL Custom Panel Can Provide Additional Information about Secondary Somatic Changes

To gain additional information about further potentially pathogenic alterations, we performed NGS-based copy number variant (CNV) detection in all samples that were sequenced with the PPGL custom panel. A blood sample with a confirmed deletion of one *NF1* allele served as positive control for CNV detection and the *NF1* loss was reliably detected by the applied algorithms (Figure 3F).

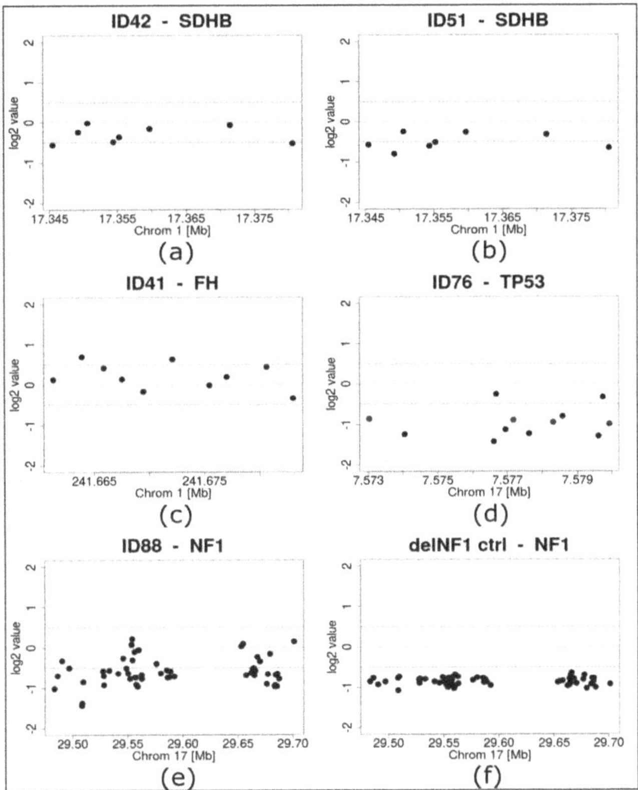

Figure 3. Results of next generation sequencing based copy number variant detection. (**a**) *SDHB* of case ID42, (**b**) *SDHB* of case ID51, (**c**) *FH* of case ID41, (**d**) *TP53* of case ID76, (**e**) *NF1* of case ID88, (**f**) *NF1* of a control sample with an experimentally proven *NF1* deletion; dots represent single targets of the respective genes, green lines highlight a log2 value of 0, dotted red lines mark log2 values of +0.5 and −0.5.

Within our cohort of 28 PPGL tumors that were analyzed by custom panel sequencing, several pathogenic variants were found at high allele frequencies indicating a loss of heterozygosity (Table 2). In two cases with pathogenic *SDHB* variants (ID42: frequency of 85.4% and ID51: frequency of 80%)

loss of one *SDHB* allele was identified by CNV detection analysis (Figure 3a,b). Similarly, pathogenic variants at high allele frequencies in *FH* were found in ID41 (92.3%) and ID82 (82%). Neither of these cases showed an *FH* deletion, supporting a copy number neutral mechanism of loss of heterozygosity (LOH) (Figure 3C, Supplementary Table S3).

Two tumors with inconspicuous sequencing results (ID76 and ID88) had high frequencies of CNVs compared to the other samples (Supplementary Table S3, Supplementary Figure S1), including heterozygous loss of *TP53* in one tumor (ID76) and of *NF1* in the other tumor (ID88) (Figure 3D,E).

2.5. Identification of Variants in Candidate Genes

Sequencing of PPGL tumor tissue with the custom panel revealed rare variants in candidate genes in nine cases (Table 3). All of these variants were missense variants and the significance of these variants is currently unknown. Two of these variants were found at low allele frequencies (ID61: *ATRX* p.(Asn53His) 25.2% and ID88: *TET1* p.(Val128Leu) 26.1%) in tumors that otherwise did not harbor a clear pathogenic or likely pathogenic mutation in a known PPGL susceptibility gene (see Section 2.3).

Table 3. Overview of variants of unknown significance in candidate genes.

ID	Gene	Nucleotide Change	Amino Acid Change	VAF (Tumor)	gnomAD het/hom	SIFT	PolyPhen	COSMIC	dbSNP	Pathogenic Variants
ID61	*ATRX*	c.157A > C	p.(Asn53His)	25.2%	0/0	tolerated	probably damaging	-	-	no
ID78	*FGFR1*	c.2104C > A	p.(Pro702Thr)	49.6%	0/0	damaging	probably damaging	1 × lung	-	yes (*VHL*)
ID69	*FH*	c.593C > T	p.(Ala198Val)	7.3%	0/0	damaging	probably damaging	-	-	yes (*SDHD*)
ID68	*GPT*	c.628G > A	p.(Glu210Lys)	46.0%	0/0	damaging	probably damaging	1 × large intestine	rs1366336459	yes (*HRAS*)
ID79	*HIST1H3B*	c.131C > A	p.(Pro44Gln)	52.3%	0/0	damaging	n.a.	-	-	yes (*NF1*)
ID41	*OGDHL*	c.1340A > G	p.(Tyr447Cys)	51.1%	32/0	damaging	probably damaging	-	rs148307090	yes (*FH*)
ID82	*PCK2*	c.463C > T	p.(Arg155Cys)	50.9%	30/0	damaging	probably damaging	-	rs141787425	yes (*FH*)
ID71	*PDHB*	c.520G > A	p.(Val174Met)	47.7%	1/0	damaging	probably damaging	-	rs760966357	yes (*SDHB*)
ID88	*TET1*	c.382G > C	p.(Val128Leu)	26.1%	2/0	tolerated	benign	-	rs142008363	no

VAF: variant allele frequency, het: heterozygous, hom: homozygous, SIFT: Sorting Intolerant From Tolerant (*in silico* variant effect prediction), COSMIC: the Catalogue Of Somatic Mutations In Cancer.

The other seven variants were identified in cases that also carried a pathogenic variant in a PPGL susceptibility gene and occurred at allele frequencies between 46% and 52.3% with the exception of *FH* p.(Ala198Val) with a frequency of 7.3% (Table 3).

All seven variants were predicted to be pathogenic by several *in silico* prediction programs (ID41: *OGDHL* p.(Tyr447Cys), ID68: *GPT* p.(Glu210Cys), ID69: *FH* p.(Ala198Val), ID71: *PDHB* p.(Val174Met), ID78: *FGFR1* p.(Pro702Tyr), ID79: *HIST1H3B* p.(Pro44Gln) and ID82: *PCK2* p.(Arg155Cys), Table 3). None of the selected variants was listed in ClinVar or occurred at a significant frequency in the general population (gnomAD) [27,28]. Five of these variants were listed in dbSNP and two variants were identified as somatic variants in lung cancer (*FGFR1* p.(Pro702Tyr)) or in a colon carcinoma ((*GPT* p.(Glu210Cys), COSMIC database; (Table 3)) [29,30].

Since these variants occurred together with clearly pathogenic variants and (with the exception of the *FH* variant) with an allele frequency of about 50%, they might be rare/private germline variants that are coincidental findings. Unfortunately, blood samples of these nine cases were not available to confirm or exclude the somatic status of these variants.

3. Discussion

PPGLs are rare but known to be the tumor type with the highest heritability, with 30–40% of patients carrying a predisposing germline mutation. A steadily growing number of 20 PPGL susceptibility genes has been identified to date, and several candidate genes are being investigated [2,5]. Some of these genes have been found to be mutated both in the germline and somatically, while others only occur as somatic mutations [7,8,13,16–19,22,31,32].

Analyses of both tumor and blood-derived DNA therefore aid in discrimination of sporadic from hereditary tumor forms [31]. This information is crucial for stratifying the risk of synchronous or metachronous tumor development in PPGL patients both regarding additional PPGLs and regarding other tumor types that, respectively, are associated with some of the PPGL susceptibility genes such as gastrointestinal stromal tumors (GIST) with *SDH*x mutations [33].

In some patients, occurrence of PPGL is the first manifestation of a heritable syndrome such as Neurofibromatosis type 1 (NF1) that besides a tumor predisposition is usually accompanied by additional symptoms [34,35]. Patients with hereditary conditions need to undergo genetic counselling and predictive testing can be offered to healthy family members. Healthy mutation carriers should then be included in tailored clinical surveillance programs for early detection of tumor development or other manifestations of disease. Depending on the gene affected, predictive testing can even be indicated in children and prenatal testing needs to be considered for severe conditions with highly variable phenotypic expression.

On the other hand, knowledge of somatic mutations can also be crucial for patient treatment and follow-up. Patients with pathogenic mutations in *SDHB* and *FH*, for example, have an elevated risk for malignant tumor development, regardless of whether the mutation was inherited or whether it occurred somatically [10,36]. Diagnosis of malignancy of PPGLs can, with certainty, only be made based on detection of metastases and not histology [37]. Therefore, patients with mutations associated with malignancy of tumors need to be followed up closely for metastatic disease. Moreover, knowledge of mutations, both somatic and germline, increasingly opens up the possibility for targeted therapeutic approaches [38].

Taking these implications on clinical management into account, it is evident that patients can substantially benefit from combined genetic analysis of both blood and tumor-derived DNA. We found that in our cohort germline testing identified pathogenic mutations in PPGL core genes in 19 out of 65 patients (29.2%). This number complies with reported germline mutational rates of 30–40% in PPGL patients in the literature [1–4,31]. Tumor analysis of 28 samples using the custom tailored PPGL panel revealed pathogenic mutations in 21 tumors (75%) of which 13 were available for germline testing (9 were from our routine clinical cohort who had received routine diagnostic testing, and 4 cases from our research cohort received targeted blood sequencing of variants after tumor testing, see Table 2).

About one third of these 13 mutations found in tumor tissue were also present in blood and therefore presumed to be germline, while two third of these pathogenic mutations had developed somatically. Aim et al. recently published similar results with a mutation detection rate of 74% for combined germline and somatic mutation testing with a custom panel comprising 17 genes. This study, however, identified half of the mutations to be of germline and half of somatic origin [31]. This discrepancy could be explained by a high percentage of patients with seemingly sporadic tumors in our cohort. Average age of tumor onset for those 13 patients who received both germline and tumor analysis was 42 years and only one patient had proven malignant disease. None of these patients had a positive family history for PPGL-associated tumors.

While patients can benefit from combined tumor and germline analysis, this approach is generally hindered by both financial issues and organizational obstacles. We did observe such obstacles in our cohort for those patients of whom, due to anonymous inclusion in a multi-center trial, we could only analyze tumor tissue without having access to germline information. Interdisciplinary approaches, especially between pathologists and clinical geneticists, could aid in bringing together both germline and tumor sequencing results in order to provide attending physicians with comprehensive genetic data.

Commonly used commercial sequencing panels for cancers are usually designed to either be used in clinical genetics in search for predisposing germline variants (such as the TruSight Cancer panel used in our routine diagnostic approach) or for application in molecular pathology for identification of somatic (hot-spot) variants in tumor tissues with focus on FFPE samples. Our custom panel covers both, i.e., genes that are typically mutated in the germline in context of hereditary tumor diseases (such as *SDHx* or *FH*) and genes that are almost exclusively somatically mutated in PPGLs (such as *HRAS*, *ATRX*, *IDHx*, etc.). It is moreover suitable for testing of high-quality DNA from blood samples as well as low-quality DNA from FFPE tissue samples. Therefore, our PPGL panel can be applied to combined germline and tumor analysis, leading to a significant increase in detected mutations.

The mutational spectrum we observed was generally compliant with previously reported results [3,4,31]. We did find a total of 3/28 (10.7%) somatically *ATRX* mutated tumors, which is presumed to be associated with aggressive disease [22,39,40]. One of these patients had not developed any metastases at the time of investigation, one patient had recurrence of disease and for one patient, follow-up information was unavailable. The first patient additionally carried a pathogenic *SDHC* germline mutation, which is in line with the reported enrichment of *ATRX* mutations in *SDHx* mutated tumors [32]. The second tumor showed a somatic pathogenic *TP53* mutation in addition to the *ATRX* truncating mutation. *TP53* mutations are rare in PPGLs compared to most other tumor types. However, it has been proposed they could have a synergistic effect on other driver mutations, and it seems plausible that both the *ATRX* and *TP53* mutations affected tumor development in this patient. Different from *ATRX* mutations, however, *TP53* mutations in PPGL have not been associated with more aggressive disease. [3,22] The third patient in our cohort with an *ATRX* mutation was not identified to carry any other driver alterations and did only show a read frequency of 5.4% for the *ATRX* mutation. While sole *ATRX* mutations have been described to drive sporadic PPGL development, it could also be considered that in this patient a relevant second mutation might have escaped the analysis [32,39].

Copy number variants (CNVs), for instance, are typically not detected by NGS-based variant calling [26]. We therefore applied a CNV detection approach based on the sequencing data generated by our custom panel in order to complement single nucleotide variant (SNV) detection from both cryo-conserved tumor samples and paraffin embedded tissues. This approach detected both loss-of-heterozygosity and possibly disease-related mutations in several tumors. However, further improvements and validations would be needed in order to reliably apply this technique in a diagnostic setting. This might be of value, since array-CGH can be unreliable for highly degraded DNA from FFPE tumor samples. CNV-detection based on our NGS custom-panel data could therefore provide a feasible alternative for CNV detection in these cases.

Apart from possible CNV detection and combined tumor and germline analysis, our broad customized PPGL panel did show further advantages over limited diagnostic panels, such as possible detection of rare or unexpected genetic events. For example, we identified a somatic *IDH2* hot spot mutation (Arg172Gly) in a paraganglioma sample, as reported previously [21]. In addition, several variants of unknown significance were identified in PPGL candidate genes, allowing for further investigation of these potentially relevant genes. Considering steady research advances in underlying genetic mechanisms of PPGLs, the panel can easily be extended to further target regions.

However, one limitation of common sequencing approaches, which also applies to our panel, is the identification of epigenetic events leading to PPGL development. In one patient in our cohort, who developed multiple tumors, no pathogenic mutation was identified by common sequencing approaches, since the underlying epigenetic event was hypermethylation of the *SDHC* promoter region, as was reported earlier [41]. This example emphasizes that even with broad diagnostic sequencing panels, unsolved cases with suspicion of hereditary disease should be directed to research approaches. Metabolic data can substantially aid diagnostics by guiding the search for genetic alterations that escape routine genetic testing [21,23,41].

Taking these results together, we propose an interdisciplinary approach for genetic analysis of PPGL that encompasses both tumor and germline sequencing and conclude that our custom designed PPGL panel provides a valid tool for the identification of SNVs from fresh frozen and paraffin-embedded tumor tissues. CNV detection can further be performed based on the data generated by our panel. Combined diagnostic and research approaches yield optimal results for comprehensive genetic characterization of PPGL patients.

4. Materials and Methods

4.1. Patient Cohort and Genetic Testing Strategy

Sequencing of blood or tumor samples was conducted either within a diagnostic or a research setting after informed written consent was given by all patients at their respective centers of study inclusion. In a diagnostic setting, patients were initially seen by endocrinologists and referred to the Institute for Clinical Genetics for genetic counselling. Pedigrees were analyzed and germline analysis was initiated, covering PPGL core genes *SDHB, SDHC, SDHD, SDHAF2, MAX, FH, NF1, RET, TMEM127* and *VHL* either via Sanger-Sequencing and/or next generation sequencing using a commercially available gene panel (TruSight Cancer Panel, Illumina) [34,42]. This was complemented by custom array-CGH analysis for detection of copy number variations and multiplex ligation-dependent probe amplification (MLPA) (*SDHA*). If a causative mutation was identified, genetic counselling and predictive testing in families as well as appropriate clinical management and/or study inclusion were initiated. If tumor samples were available, cases with no identified causative germline mutations were analyzed using our dedicated PPGL multi gene panel comprising 84 genes. Additionally, blood or tumor tissue samples were provided in anonymized fashion by several centers from Madrid, Nijmegen, Munich and Bethesda under the clinical protocol of the Prospective Monoamine-producing Tumor Study (coordinator Graeme Eisenhofer). A number of samples reported here have already been published in a study with a different research focus [21]. Patients from the research cohort were either part of the Prospective Monoamine-producing Tumor Study (PMT study; https://pmt-study.pressor.org/) and/or Registry and Repository of biological samples of the European Network for the Study of Adrenal Tumours (ENS@T) with ethic approval given at each participating institution (ethic codes: EK 189062010 (Dresden), 2011-334 (Nijmegen), 173-11 and 379-10 (Munich), 15/024 (Madrid), 2011/0020149 Ref. n. 59/11 (Florence)), or enrolled under the IRB Protocol 00-CH-0093 (NIH/Bethesda/USA). Patients from the diagnostic cohort signed informed consent for genetic testing in accordance with the German Genetic Diagnostics Act (GenDG).

4.2. Next Generation Sequencing Analysis

DNA was isolated either from blood or from tumor tissue samples provided fresh or formalin fixed paraffin embedded. NGS analysis was conducted on a NextSeq or MiSeq sequencing instrument

(Illumina Inc., San Diego, CA, USA) using the TruSight Cancer sequencing panel (Illumina Inc., San Diego, CA, USA) in the case of diagnostic analysis or the custom designed PPGL Panel (Illumina Inc., San Diego, CA, USA Supplementary Table S1) for research analysis.

Resulting fastq sequence files were aligned to the human reference genome hg19 (GRCh37) using the Biomedical Genomics Workbench 5.0 (Qiagen, Hilden, Germany). In the case of diagnostic analysis, variants were called with a fixed ploidy algorithm with a required minimum frequency of 10 %, 3 reads supporting the variant and a required minimum coverage of 10 reads. For research analysis of tumor tissue or blood, variants were called using a low frequency variant detection algorithm (no assumption of known sample ploidy) with a required minimum frequency of 5% and otherwise similar settings. Variant calling was restricted to target regions as defined by the bed files of the TruSight Cancer panel (Illumina Inc., San Diego, CA, USA) and the PPGL panel. Variant classification was performed in accordance with the standards and guidelines of the American College of Medical Genetics and Genomics and the Association for Molecular Pathology (ACMG-AMP) [43].

4.3. CNV Calling

NGS-based calling of copy number variations (CNVs) was performed with the R (https://www.r-project.org/, [44]) package panelcn.MOPS [45], a CNV detection tool for targeted panel NGS data, set to default parameters. DNA obtained from blood samples of ten healthy individuals was sequenced with the PPGL panel and served as normal controls for CNV detection. The absence of CNVs in known PPGL susceptibility genes (*SDHA, SDHB, SDHC, SDHD, SDHAF2, MAX, FH, NF1, RET, TMEM127* and *VHL)* in controls was confirmed by array-CGH. Additionally, a sample with a heterozygous deletion of *NF1* as previously identified by array-CGH was included as a positive control for CNV detection. For each sample, log2 values, statistical parameters and copy numbers (CNx; x = number of copies) were exported into a csv file (Supplementary Table S3). Furthermore, for each sample, median log2ratios per gene were plotted for visualization (Supplementary Figure S1).

4.4. Metabolite Analyses

Succinate and fumarate were extracted with methanol from fresh or FFPE tissue as previously reported [23] and analyzed by liquid chromatography tandem mass spectrometry (LC-MS/MS). Methodological details have previously been reported [21].

5. Conclusions

Comprehensive testing of tumor samples can improve diagnostics in PPGL patients. We propose parallel testing of blood and tumor tissue (fresh frozen or FFPE), accompanied by metabolite profiling, immunohistochemistry and additional analyses such as methylation detection to allow for better data interpretation. In the future, current NGS panel designs have to be updated to facilitate integration of newly discovered susceptibility genes or could even be replaced by exome sequencing. Patients can substantially benefit from integrating diagnostic and research approaches for molecular characterization of PPGLs.

Supplementary Materials: The following are available online at http://www.mdpi.com/2072-6694/11/6/809/s1, Supplementary Table S1: Cohort Overview and clinical information, Supplementary Table S2: PPGL custom panel design, Supplementary Table S3: CNV calling data, Supplementary Figure S1: CNV plots.

Author Contributions: Conceptualization, B.K., S.R.; methodology, B.K. software, D.W., L.G., A.R., B.K. and W.J.; formal analysis, K.H., D.W., L.G., A.R. and B.K.; investigation, B.K., L.G., D.W., K.H., A.J., J.W., N.B., S.N., T.K., V.G., G.C., J.M., F.B., H.J.T., L.C., K.P., M.R., D.A., S.R. and G.E.; resources, B.K., E.S., G.E., D.A.; data curation, D.W., L.G. and B.K.; writing—original draft preparation, D.W., L.G. and B.K.; writing—review and editing, D.W., L.G., B.K., A.J., A.R., S.R., G.E., K.P., S.N., N.B., M.R.; visualization, D.W., W.J.; supervision, B.K.; project administration, B.K.; funding acquisition, B.K., S.R.

Funding: This research was funded by the Deutsche Forschungsgemeinschaft (RI 2684/1-1; KL 2541/2-1 and CRC/Transregio 205/1, B10 for S.R., B12 for B.K., G.E.). M.R. receives funding support from Instituto de Salud

Carlos III (ISCIII), through the "Acción Estratégica en Salud" (AES) (projects PI17/01796), cofounded by the European Regional Development Fund (ERDF)), and the Paradifference Foundation.

Acknowledgments: We thank the patients and their families who have made this research possible. We want to thank Jacques W. Lenders for his support. We further thank Alexander Krüger, Lydia Rossow and Franziska Stübner for technical support as well as Katharina Langton and Uwe Siemon for their assistance in patient administration.

Conflicts of Interest: The authors declare no conflict of interest.

References

1. Dahia, P.L. Pheochromocytoma and paraganglioma pathogenesis: Learning from genetic heterogeneity. *Nat. Rev. Cancer* **2014**, *14*, 108–119. [CrossRef] [PubMed]
2. Eisenhofer, G.; Klink, B.; Richter, S.; Lenders, J.W.; Robledo, M. Metabologenomics of phaeochromocytoma and paraganglioma: An integrated approach for personalised biochemical and genetic testing. *Clin. Biochem. Rev.* **2017**, *38*, 69–100. [PubMed]
3. Fishbein, L.; Leshchiner, I.; Walter, V.; Danilova, L.; Robertson, A.G.; Johnson, A.R.; Lichtenberg, T.M.; Murray, B.A.; Ghayee, H.K.; Else, T.; et al. Comprehensive molecular characterization of pheochromocytoma and paraganglioma. *Cancer Cell* **2017**, *31*, 181–193. [CrossRef] [PubMed]
4. Jochmanova, I.; Pacak, K. Genomic landscape of pheochromocytoma and paraganglioma. *Trends Cancer* **2018**, *4*, 6–9. [CrossRef]
5. Huang, K.L.; Mashl, R.J.; Wu, Y.; Ritter, D.I.; Wang, J.; Oh, C.; Paczkowska, M.; Reynolds, S.; Wyczalkowski, M.A.; Oak, N.; et al. Pathogenic germline variants in 10,389 adult cancers. *Cell* **2018**, *173*, 355–370. [CrossRef]
6. Lenders, J.W.M.; Eisenhofer, G. Update on modern management of pheochromocytoma and paraganglioma. *Endocrinol. Metab.* **2017**, *32*, 152–161. [CrossRef]
7. Bayley, J.P.; Kunst, H.P.; Cascon, A.; Sampietro, M.L.; Gaal, J.; Korpershoek, E.; Hinojar-Gutierrez, A.; Timmers, H.J.; Hoefsloot, L.H.; Hermsen, M.A.; et al. Sdhaf2 mutations in familial and sporadic paraganglioma and phaeochromocytoma. *Lancet Oncol.* **2010**, *11*, 366–372. [CrossRef]
8. Qin, Y.; Yao, L.; King, E.E.; Buddavarapu, K.; Lenci, R.E.; Chocron, E.S.; Lechleiter, J.D.; Sass, M.; Aronin, N.; Schiavi, F.; et al. Germline mutations in tmem127 confer susceptibility to pheochromocytoma. *Nat. Genet.* **2010**, *42*, 229–233. [CrossRef]
9. Comino-Mendez, I.; Gracia-Aznarez, F.J.; Schiavi, F.; Landa, I.; Leandro-Garcia, L.J.; Leton, R.; Honrado, E.; Ramos-Medina, R.; Caronia, D.; Pita, G.; et al. Exome sequencing identifies max mutations as a cause of hereditary pheochromocytoma. *Nat. Genet.* **2011**, *43*, 663–667. [CrossRef]
10. Castro-Vega, L.J.; Buffet, A.; De Cubas, A.A.; Cascon, A.; Menara, M.; Khalifa, E.; Amar, L.; Azriel, S.; Bourdeau, I.; Chabre, O.; et al. Germline mutations in fh confer predisposition to malignant pheochromocytomas and paragangliomas. *Hum. Mol. Genet.* **2014**, *23*, 2440–2446. [CrossRef]
11. Clark, G.R.; Sciacovelli, M.; Gaude, E.; Walsh, D.M.; Kirby, G.; Simpson, M.A.; Trembath, R.C.; Berg, J.N.; Woodward, E.R.; Kinning, E.; et al. Germline fh mutations presenting with pheochromocytoma. *J. Clin. Endocrinol. Metab.* **2014**, *99*, E2046–E2050. [CrossRef] [PubMed]
12. Cascon, A.; Comino-Mendez, I.; Curras-Freixes, M.; de Cubas, A.A.; Contreras, L.; Richter, S.; Peitzsch, M.; Mancikova, V.; Inglada-Perez, L.; Perez-Barrios, A.; et al. Whole-exome sequencing identifies mdh2 as a new familial paraganglioma gene. *J. Natl. Cancer Inst.* **2015**, *107*. [CrossRef] [PubMed]
13. Remacha, L.; Comino-Mendez, I.; Richter, S.; Contreras, L.; Curras-Freixes, M.; Pita, G.; Leton, R.; Galarreta, A.; Torres-Perez, R.; Honrado, E.; et al. Targeted exome sequencing of krebs cycle genes reveals candidate cancer-predisposing mutations in pheochromocytomas and paragangliomas. *Clin. Cancer Res.* **2017**, *23*, 6315–6324. [CrossRef] [PubMed]
14. Remacha, L.; Pirman, D.; Mahoney, C.E.; Coloma, J.; Calsina, B.; Curras-Freixes, M.; Leton, R.; Torres-Perez, R.; Richter, S.; Pita, G.; et al. Recurrent germline dlst mutations in individuals with multiple pheochromocytomas and paragangliomas. *Am. J. Hum. Genet.* **2019**, *104*, 651–664. [CrossRef] [PubMed]
15. Zhuang, Z.; Yang, C.; Lorenzo, F.; Merino, M.; Fojo, T.; Kebebew, E.; Popovic, V.; Stratakis, C.A.; Prchal, J.T.; Pacak, K. Somatic hif2a gain-of-function mutations in paraganglioma with polycythemia. *N. Engl. J. Med.* **2012**, *367*, 922–930. [CrossRef]

16. Yang, C.; Zhuang, Z.; Fliedner, S.M.; Shankavaram, U.; Sun, M.G.; Bullova, P.; Zhu, R.; Elkahloun, A.G.; Kourlas, P.J.; Merino, M.; et al. Germ-line phd1 and phd2 mutations detected in patients with pheochromocytoma/paraganglioma-polycythemia. *J. Mol. Med.* **2015**, *93*, 93–104. [CrossRef]
17. Buffet, A.; Smati, S.; Mansuy, L.; Menara, M.; Lebras, M.; Heymann, M.F.; Simian, C.; Favier, J.; Murat, A.; Cariou, B.; et al. Mosaicism in hif2a-related polycythemia-paraganglioma syndrome. *J. Clin. Endocrinol. Metab.* **2014**, *99*, E369–E373. [CrossRef]
18. Toledo, R.A.; Qin, Y.; Cheng, Z.M.; Gao, Q.; Iwata, S.; Silva, G.M.; Prasad, M.L.; Ocal, I.T.; Rao, S.; Aronin, N.; et al. Recurrent mutations of chromatin-remodeling genes and kinase receptors in pheochromocytomas and paragangliomas. *Clin. Cancer Res.* **2016**, *22*, 2301–2310. [CrossRef]
19. Castro-Vega, L.J.; Letouze, E.; Burnichon, N.; Buffet, A.; Disderot, P.H.; Khalifa, E.; Loriot, C.; Elarouci, N.; Morin, A.; Menara, M.; et al. Multi-omics analysis defines core genomic alterations in pheochromocytomas and paragangliomas. *Nat. Commun.* **2015**, *6*, 6044. [CrossRef]
20. Gaal, J.; Burnichon, N.; Korpershoek, E.; Roncelin, I.; Bertherat, J.; Plouin, P.F.; de Krijger, R.R.; Gimenez-Roqueplo, A.P.; Dinjens, W.N. Isocitrate dehydrogenase mutations are rare in pheochromocytomas and paragangliomas. *J. Clin. Endocrinol. Metab.* **2010**, *95*, 1274–1278. [CrossRef]
21. Richter, S.; Gieldon, L.; Pang, Y.; Peitzsch, M.; Huynh, T.; Leton, R.; Viana, B.; Ercolino, T.; Mangelis, A.; Rapizzi, E.; et al. Metabolome-guided genomics to identify pathogenic variants in isocitrate dehydrogenase, fumarate hydratase, and succinate dehydrogenase genes in pheochromocytoma and paraganglioma. *Genet. Med.* **2019**, *21*, 705–717. [CrossRef] [PubMed]
22. Luchetti, A.; Walsh, D.; Rodger, F.; Clark, G.; Martin, T.; Irving, R.; Sanna, M.; Yao, M.; Robledo, M.; Neumann, H.P.; et al. Profiling of somatic mutations in phaeochromocytoma and paraganglioma by targeted next generation sequencing analysis. *Int. J. Endocrinol.* **2015**, *2015*, 138573. [CrossRef] [PubMed]
23. Richter, S.; Peitzsch, M.; Rapizzi, E.; Lenders, J.W.; Qin, N.; de Cubas, A.A.; Schiavi, F.; Rao, J.U.; Beuschlein, F.; Quinkler, M.; et al. Krebs cycle metabolite profiling for identification and stratification of pheochromocytomas/paragangliomas due to succinate dehydrogenase deficiency. *J. Clin. Endocrinol. Metab.* **2014**, *99*, 3903–3911. [CrossRef] [PubMed]
24. Hackmann, K.; Kuhlee, F.; Betcheva-Krajcir, E.; Kahlert, A.K.; Mackenroth, L.; Klink, B.; Di Donato, N.; Tzschach, A.; Kast, K.; Wimberger, P.; et al. Ready to clone: Cnv detection and breakpoint fine-mapping in breast and ovarian cancer susceptibility genes by high-resolution array cgh. *Breast Cancer Res. Treat.* **2016**, *159*, 585–590. [CrossRef] [PubMed]
25. Schlisio, S.; Kenchappa, R.S.; Vredeveld, L.C.; George, R.E.; Stewart, R.; Greulich, H.; Shahriari, K.; Nguyen, N.V.; Pigny, P.; Dahia, P.L.; et al. The kinesin kif1bbeta acts downstream from egln3 to induce apoptosis and is a potential 1p36 tumor suppressor. *Genes Dev.* **2008**, *22*, 884–893. [CrossRef] [PubMed]
26. Zakrzewski, F.; Gieldon, L.; Rump, A.; Seifert, M.; Grutzmann, K.; Kruger, A.; Loos, S.; Zeugner, S.; Hackmann, K.; Porrmann, J.; et al. Targeted capture-based ngs is superior to multiplex pcr-based ngs for hereditary brca1 and brca2 gene analysis in ffpe tumor samples. *BMC Cancer* **2019**, *19*, 396. [CrossRef]
27. Karczewski, K.J.; Francioli, L.C.; Tiao, G.; Cummings, B.B.; Alföldi, J.; Wang, Q.; Collins, R.L.; Laricchia, K.M.; Ganna, A.; Birnbaum, D.P.; et al. Variation across 141,456 human exomes and genomes reveals the spectrum of loss-of-function intolerance across human protein-coding genes. *bioRxiv* **2019**, 531210. [CrossRef]
28. Landrum, M.J.; Lee, J.M.; Benson, M.; Brown, G.R.; Chao, C.; Chitipiralla, S.; Gu, B.; Hart, J.; Hoffman, D.; Jang, W.; et al. Clinvar: Improving access to variant interpretations and supporting evidence. *Nucleic Acids Res.* **2018**, *46*, D1062–D1067. [CrossRef]
29. Sherry, S.T.; Ward, M.H.; Kholodov, M.; Baker, J.; Phan, L.; Smigielski, E.M.; Sirotkin, K. Dbsnp: The ncbi database of genetic variation. *Nucleic Acids Res.* **2001**, *29*, 308–311. [CrossRef]
30. Harsha, B.; Creatore, C.; Kok, C.Y.; Hathaway, C.; Cole, C.G.; Ramshaw, C.C.; Rye, C.E.; Beare, D.M.; Dawson, E.; Boutselakis, H.; et al. Cosmic: The catalogue of somatic mutations in cancer. *Nucleic Acids Res.* **2018**, *47*, D941–D947.
31. Ben Aim, L.; Pigny, P.; Castro-Vega, L.J.; Buffet, A.; Amar, L.; Bertherat, J.; Drui, D.; Guilhem, I.; Baudin, E.; Lussey-Lepoutre, C.; et al. Targeted next-generation sequencing detects rare genetic events in pheochromocytoma and paraganglioma. *J. Med Genet.* **2019**. [CrossRef] [PubMed]
32. Fishbein, L.; Khare, S.; Wubbenhorst, B.; DeSloover, D.; D'Andrea, K.; Merrill, S.; Cho, N.W.; Greenberg, R.A.; Else, T.; Montone, K.; et al. Whole-exome sequencing identifies somatic atrx mutations in pheochromocytomas and paragangliomas. *Nat. Commun.* **2015**, *6*, 6140. [CrossRef] [PubMed]

33. McWhinney, S.R.; Pasini, B.; Stratakis, C.A. Familial gastrointestinal stromal tumors and germ-line mutations. *N. Engl. J. Med.* **2007**, *357*, 1054–1056. [CrossRef] [PubMed]
34. Gieldon, L.; Masjkur, J.R.; Richter, S.; Darr, R.; Lahera, M.; Aust, D.; Zeugner, S.; Rump, A.; Hackmann, K.; Tzschach, A.; et al. Next-generation panel sequencing identifies nf1 germline mutations in three patients with pheochromocytoma but no clinical diagnosis of neurofibromatosis type 1. *Eur. J. Endocrinol.* **2018**, *178*, K1–K9. [CrossRef] [PubMed]
35. Welander, J.; Soderkvist, P.; Gimm, O. Genetics and clinical characteristics of hereditary pheochromocytomas and paragangliomas. *Endocr. Relat. Cancer* **2011**, *18*, R253–R276. [CrossRef]
36. Gimenez-Roqueplo, A.P.; Favier, J.; Rustin, P.; Rieubland, C.; Crespin, M.; Nau, V.; Khau Van Kien, P.; Corvol, P.; Plouin, P.F.; Jeunemaitre, X. Mutations in the sdhb gene are associated with extra-adrenal and/or malignant phaeochromocytomas. *Cancer Res.* **2003**, *63*, 5615–5621.
37. Ayala-Ramirez, M.; Feng, L.; Johnson, M.M.; Ejaz, S.; Habra, M.A.; Rich, T.; Busaidy, N.; Cote, G.J.; Perrier, N.; Phan, A.; et al. Clinical risk factors for malignancy and overall survival in patients with pheochromocytomas and sympathetic paragangliomas: Primary tumor size and primary tumor location as prognostic indicators. *J. Clin. Endocrinol. Metab.* **2011**, *96*, 717–725. [CrossRef]
38. Jimenez, C. Treatment for patients with malignant pheochromocytomas and paragangliomas: A perspective from the hallmarks of cancer. *Front. Endocrinol.* **2018**, *9*, 277. [CrossRef]
39. Job, S.; Draskovic, I.; Burnichon, N.; Buffet, A.; Cros, J.; Lepine, C.; Venisse, A.; Robidel, E.; Verkarre, V.; Meatchi, T.; et al. Telomerase activation and atrx mutations are independent risk factors for metastatic pheochromocytoma and paraganglioma. *Clin. Cancer Res.* **2019**, *25*, 760–770. [CrossRef]
40. Kantorovich, V.; Pacak, K. New insights on the pathogenesis of paraganglioma and pheochromocytoma. *F1000Research* **2018**, *7*. [CrossRef]
41. Richter, S.; Klink, B.; Nacke, B.; de Cubas, A.A.; Mangelis, A.; Rapizzi, E.; Meinhardt, M.; Skondra, C.; Mannelli, M.; Robledo, M.; et al. Epigenetic mutation of the succinate dehydrogenase c promoter in a patient with two paragangliomas. *J. Clin. Endocrinol. Metab.* **2016**, *101*, 359–363. [CrossRef] [PubMed]
42. Schroeder, C.; Faust, U.; Sturm, M.; Hackmann, K.; Grundmann, K.; Harmuth, F.; Bosse, K.; Kehrer, M.; Benkert, T.; Klink, B.; et al. Hboc multi-gene panel testing: Comparison of two sequencing centers. *Breast Cancer Res. Treat.* **2015**, *152*, 129–136. [CrossRef] [PubMed]
43. Richards, S.; Aziz, N.; Bale, S.; Blick, D.; Das, S.; Gastier-Foster, J.; Grody, W.W.; Hedge, M.; Lyon, E.; Spector, E.; et al. Standards and guidelines fot the interpretation of sequence variants: A joint consensus recommendation of the American College of Medical Genetics and Genomics and the Association for Molecular Pathology. *Genet. Med.* **2015**, *17*, 405–424. [CrossRef] [PubMed]
44. R Core Team. R: A Language and Environment for Statistical Computing. 2017. Available online: http://www.r-project.org/ (accessed on 11 March 2019).
45. Povysil, G.; Tzika, A.; Vogt, J.; Haunschmid, V.; Messiaen, L.; Zschocke, J.; Klambauer, G.; Hochreiter, S.; Wimmer, K. panelcn.MOPS: Copy-number detection in targeted NGS panel data for clinical diagnostics. *Hum. Mutat.* **2017**, *38*, 889–897. [CrossRef] [PubMed]

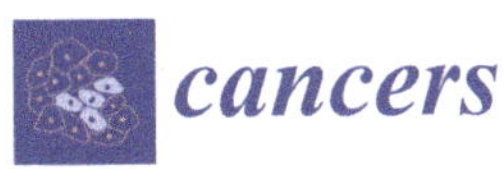

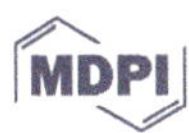

Article

Catecholamines Induce Left Ventricular Subclinical Systolic Dysfunction: A Speckle-Tracking Echocardiography Study

Jan Kvasnička [1], Tomáš Zelinka [1], Ondřej Petrák [1], Ján Rosa [1], Branislav Štrauch [1], Zuzana Krátká [1], Tomáš Indra [2], Alice Markvartová [1], Jiří Widimský Jr. [1] and Robert Holaj [1,*]

1 3rd Department of Medicine, Centre for Hypertension, General University Hospital and 1st Faculty of Medicine, Charles University in Prague, Ovocný trh 5, 116 36 Prague 1, Czech Republic; jan.kvasnicka3@vfn.cz (J.K.); tzeli@lf1.cuni.cz (T.Z.); ondrej.petrak@vfn.cz (O.P.); jan.rosa@vfn.cz (J.R.); branislav.strauch@vfn.cz (B.Š.); zuzana.kratka@vfn.cz (Z.K.); alice.vrankova@vfn.cz (A.M.); jwidi@lf1.cuni.cz (J.W.J.)

2 Department of Nephrology, General University Hospital and 1st Faculty of Medicine, Charles University in Prague, Ovocný trh 5, 116 36 Prague 1, Czech Republic; tomas.indra@vfn.cz

* Correspondence: robert.holaj@vfn.cz or rholaj@hotmail.com; Tel.: +420-224-963-509

Received: 9 January 2019; Accepted: 28 February 2019; Published: 6 March 2019

Abstract: *Background*: Pheochromocytomas (PHEO) are tumors arising from chromaffin cells from the adrenal medulla, having the ability to produce, metabolize and secrete catecholamines. The overproduction of catecholamines leads by many mechanisms to the impairment in the left ventricle (LV) function, however, endocardial measurement of systolic function did not find any differences between patients with PHEO and essential hypertension (EH). The aim of the study was to investigate whether global longitudinal strain (GLS) derived from speckle-tracking echocardiography can detect catecholamine-induced subclinical impairments in systolic function. *Methods*: We analyzed 17 patients (10 females and seven males) with PHEO and 18 patients (nine females and nine males) with EH. The groups did not differ in age or in 24-h blood pressure values. *Results*: The patients with PHEO did not differ in echocardiographic parameters including LV ejection fraction compared to the EH patients (0.69 ± 0.04 vs. 0.71 ± 0.05; NS), nevertheless, in spackle-tracking analysis, the patients with PHEO displayed significantly lower GLS than the EH patients (−14.8 ± 1.5 vs. −17.8 ± 1.7; $p < 0.001$). *Conclusions*: Patients with PHEO have a lower magnitude of GLS than the patients with EH, suggesting that catecholamines induce a subclinical decline in LV systolic function.

Keywords: pheochromocytoma; catecholamine; global longitudinal strain; speckle-tracking echocardiography; subclinical systolic dysfunction

1. Introduction

Pheochromocytomas (PHEO) and functional paragangliomas (PGLs) are rare and mostly non-metastatic tumors originating from chromaffin cells either from the adrenal medulla (PHEO) or from the sympathetic nervous system–associated chromaffin tissue (PGLs) [1]. The prevalence of PHEO and PGLs in non-selected population of patients with arterial hypertension is between 0.2 and 0.6% [2,3] and the prevalence of PHEO is higher than the prevalence of PGLs, when 80 to 85% of chromaffin-cell tumors are PHEO, whereas 15 to 20% are PGLs [4]. Due to the higher age of the population and smaller tumor sizes at diagnosis, the incidence has increased in recent years [5].

These tumors have the ability to produce, metabolize, and secrete catecholamines. Catecholamines produced by the tumor cells are responsible for a large variety of signs, in particular paroxysmal effects, such as headache, sweating, palpitations, and hypertension because of their effect on hemodynamics and metabolism [4,6]. In vitro [7] and in vivo studies [8] showed that catecholamines influence vascular wall growth and remodeling, independently of their hemodynamic impact. In general, patients with pheochromocytoma have a higher risk of cardiovascular complications (even life-threatening like arrhythmias, heart failure and myocardial infarction), than patients with essential hypertension (EH) [9]. The aforementioned heart failure may be manifested by a decrease in the ejection fraction (EF) or, in some patients, by a transient left ventricle (LV) dysfunction due to the so-called catecholamine-induced myocarditis, also called pheochromocytoma-associated catecholamine cardiomyopathy [10]. Adrenalectomy also leads to an improvement of LV mass in patients with PHEO in contrast to the impairment of this parameter in EH patients [11]. A reduction of LV EF or even heart failure are signs of already developed clinical impairment. We therefore focused on the detection of subclinical impairment before the onset of cardiac damage.

In recent years, global longitudinal strain (GLS) derived from two-dimensional speckle-tracking echocardiography seems to be a better parameter for evaluating LV systolic performance including myocardial motion and longitudinal deformation than LV EF [12]. GLS can also detect LV systolic impairment already in the preclinical stage, when EF remains in normal range [13]. Recently, GLS has been used for the assessments of LV subclinical systolic function in many indications. In clinical practice, it is most often the evaluation of various forms of LV hypertrophy such as hypertrophic cardiomyopathy, amyloidosis [14] or primary aldosteronism [15] and evaluation of cardiotoxicity in patients with oncological diseases undergoing chemotherapy [16]. Therefore, we designed a prospective study to detect catecholamines-induced myocardial impairment of LV systolic function in patients with PHEO already in the subclinical stage.

2. Results

2.1. Characteristic of Groups

The final group included seventeen patients with a diagnosis of PHEO (11 subjects with adrenergic phenotype and six subjects with noradrenergic phenotype), aged 28 to 67 years (10 females and seven males) and eighteen patients (nine females and nine males) with a diagnosis of EH. The patient subgroups do not significantly differ in age, body mass index, in presumptive duration of disease or in heart rate and blood pressure values measured casually or using 24-h ambulatory monitoring (ABPM).

Thirteen patients with PHEO (76%) had a history of sustained hypertension and used at least one antihypertensive drug. Four patients with PHEO (24%) had developed only paroxysmal symptoms in the history and displayed normal blood pressure levels during measurements in the hospital. On the contrary, two patients with PHEO (12%) showed repeatedly very high blood pressure levels. The other patients with PHEO showed only a mild form of hypertension. The average values of heart rate in patients with PHEO were only about +7 mmHg higher than those in patients with EH. Nevertheless, this slight difference did not achieve statistical significance. The patients with EH used a higher number of antihypertensive drugs before switching to the treatment with α-blockers and/or slow-release verapamil than the patients with PHEO ($p < 0.01$) (Table 1). Significantly higher proportion of EH patients were treated by β-blockers ($p < 0.01$), calcium channel blockers ($p < 0.01$), and diuretics ($p < 0.05$). Four patients with PHEO had diabetes (two of them were on insulin and three of them were on oral antidiabetic drugs) and seven patients in both groups were treated for dyslipidemia (Table 2).

Table 1. Clinical characteristic of the study population.

Clinical Characteristic	PHEO (n = 17)	EH (n = 18)	p-Value
Age (years)	50 ± 11	49 ± 6	NS
Gender: F/M (% female)	10/7 (58%)	9/9 (50%)	NS
Height (cm)	170 ± 8	173 ± 7	NS
Weight (kg)	82 ± 14	88 ± 11	NS
Body mass index (kg/m^2)	29 ± 5	30 ± 4	NS
Systolic office BP (mmHg)	141 ± 13	140 ± 8	NS
Diastolic office BP (mmHg)	88 ± 6	89 ± 5	NS
Heart Rate office (BPM)	81 ± 9	74 ± 8	NS
24 h ABPM systolic BP (mmHg)	127 ± 9	132 ± 8	NS
24 h ABPM diastolic BP (mmHg)	76 ± 7	80 ± 5	NS
24 h ABPM Heart Rate (BPM)	77 ± 10	71 ± 6	NS
Number of used antihypertensive drugs	1.5 ± 1.1	3.6 ± 1.4	<0.001
Manifestation of symptoms (years)	5.8 ± 3.4	6.7 ± 3.6	NS

Variables are shown as means ± SD, or absolute values and relative values in percent. PHEO, pheochromocytoma; EH, essential hypertension; BP, blood pressure; BPM, beats per minute; ABPM, ambulatory blood pressure monitoring; NS, non-significant.

Table 2. Use of antihypertensive, antidiabetic and lipid-lowering drugs in the study population.

Antihypertensive, Antidiabetic and Lipid-Lowering Drugs	PHEO (n = 17)	EH (n = 18)	p-Value
Diuretics [n (%)]	3 (18)	10 (56)	<0.05
β-blockers [n (%)]	3 (18)	11 (61)	<0.01
Calcium channel blockers [n (%)]	5 (29)	14 (78)	<0.01
Angiotensin-converting enzyme inhibitors [n (%)]	5 (29)	10 (56)	NS
Angiotensin receptor blockers [n (%)]	2 (12)	7 (39)	NS
α-blockers [n (%)]	4 (24)	2 (11)	NS
Central agonists [n (%)]	3 (18)	6 (33)	NS
Aldosterone antagonists [n (%)]	1 (6)	4 (22)	NS
Statins [n (%)]	7 (41)	7 (39)	NS
Insulin [n (%)]	2 (12)	0 (0)	NS
Oral antidiabetic drugs [n (%)]	3 (18)	0 (0)	NS

Values are presented in absolute numbers (in percents). PHEO, pheochromocytoma; EH, essential hypertension; NS, non-significant.

2.2. Laboratory Results

The patient subgroups did not differ in lipid parameters, in plasma creatinine or in creatinine clearance. As expected, all endocrine-related laboratory values in patients with PHEO (fasting plasma glucose, plasma metanephrines, normetanephrines) were higher than in patients with EH (Table 3).

Table 3. Laboratory data of the study population.

Laboratory Data	PHEO (n = 17)	EH (n = 18)	p-Value
Plasma creatinine (μmol/L)	69 ± 12	75 ± 12	NS
Creatinine clearance (mL/min)	135 ± 34	119 ± 25	NS
Plasma cholesterol (mmol/L)	4.4 ± 0.5	4.8 ± 0.5	NS
HDL cholesterol (mmol/L)	1.5 ± 0.3	1.5 ± 0.3	NS
LDL cholesterol (mmol/L)	2.4 ± 0.5	2.5 ± 0.5	NS
Triglycerides (mmol/L)	1.2 ± 0.5	1.4 ± 0.5	NS
Fasting plasma glucose (mmol/L)	6.0 ± 0.9	5.2 ± 0.5	<0.05
Plasma metanephrines (nmol/L)	4.87 ± 4.30	0.16 ± 0.09	<0.01
Plasma normetanephrines (nmol/L)	13.65 ± 13.80	0.27 ± 0.12	<0.05

Variables are shown as means ± S.D.; PHEO, pheochromocytoma; EH, essential hypertension; HDL, high-density lipoprotein; LDL, low-density lipoprotein; NS, non-significant.

2.3. Echocardiography Parameters

The patient subgroups did not differ in the LV and left atrial dimensions, LV mass indexes or Doppler-derived indexes characterizing diastolic function (Table 4).

Table 4. Echocardiographic parameters and Doppler-derived indexes of the study population.

Echocardiographic Parameters	PHEO (n = 17)	EH (n = 18)	p-Value
IVS (mm)	9.7 ± 1.6	9.6 ± 1.1	NS
LVED (mm)	49.6 ± 4.7	49.3 ± 3.1	NS
LVES (mm)	30.3 ± 2.6	29.1 ± 2.9	NS
PWT (mm)	9.6 ± 1.6	9.8 ± 1.1	NS
RWT	0.39 ± 0.05	0.40 ± 0.05	NS
LA (mm)	38.2 ± 5.1	37.0 ± 2.9	NS
LVMi/BSA (g/m^2)	91.2 ± 23.3	86.4 ± 16.2	NS
LVMi (g/m$^{2.7}$)	42.2 ± 12.1	40.3 ± 9.1	NS
LVEF	0.69 ± 0.04	0.71 ± 0.05	NS
E/A	1.04 ± 0.30	1.06 ± 0.25	NS
E/e′	8.5 ± 1.9	8.9 ± 1.6	NS

Variables are shown as means ± SD; LVEF, left ventricle ejection fraction; IVS, interventricular septum; LVED, left ventricle end-diastolic diameter; LVES, left ventricle end-systolic diameter; PWT, posterior wall thickness; RWT, relative wall thickness; LVMi/BSA, left ventricular mass index to the body surface area; LVMi, left ventricular mass index to the 2.7th power of height in meters; LA, left atrium; E/e′, Pulsed-Wave Doppler/Tissue Doppler Imaging ratio of E wave velocity, NS, non-significant.

When evaluating systolic function, the two groups did not differ in LV EF (0.69 ± 0.04 in the PHEO group vs. 0.71 ± 0.05 in the EH group, p = 0.25), nevertheless, in the speckle analysis, a significantly lower magnitude of GLS was found in patients with PHEO compared to those with EH.

The patients with PHEO displayed significantly lower strain than those with EH in all three views including: apical two-chamber view (−14.9 ± 1.6% in the PHEO group vs. −18.2 ± 2.1% in the EH group, $p < 0.001$), apical long axis view (−15.0 ± 1.7% in the PHEO group vs. −18.0 ± 1.9% in the EH group, $p < 0.001$), apical four-chamber view (−14.5 ± 1.4% in the PHEO group vs. −17.8 ± 1.7% in the EH group, $p < 0.001$), and GLS (−14.8 ± 1.5% in the PHEO group vs. −17.8 ± 1.7% in the EH group, $p < 0.001$, Figure 1). Comparing the individual LV segments, patients with PHEO showed a significantly reduced peak longitudinal strain in all segments (apical, mid-ventricular and basal, $p < 0.001$) compared to patients with EH (Table 5).

Table 5. Longitudinal strain parameters of the study population.

Longitudinal Strain Parameters	PHEO (n = 17)	EH (n = 18)	p-Value
Global LS (%)	−14.8 ± 1.5	−17.8 ± 1.7	<0.001
Basal LV LS (%)	−14.8 ± 2.1	−17.3 ± 2.3	<0.05
Mid-ventricular LV LS (%)	−15.7 ± 1.9	−18.9 ± 2.1	<0.001
Apical LV LS (%)	−16.1 ± 2.6	−19.9 ± 3.9	<0.05

Variables are shown as means ± SD; EF, ejection fraction; GLS, global longitudinal strain, LV LS, left ventricle longitudinal strain.

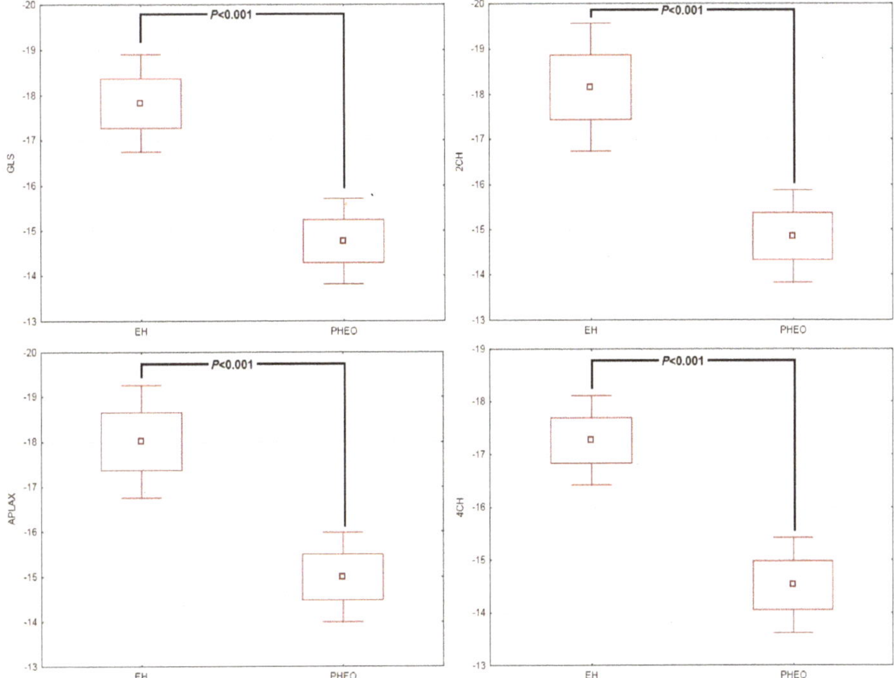

Figure 1. Speckle-tracking analysis in patients with pheochromocytoma and essential hypertension. The patients with pheochromocytoma showed significantly lower global longitudinal strain (GLS), strain in apical two-chamber view (2CH), strain in apical long axis view (APLAX), and strain in apical four-chamber view (4CH).

3. Discussion

Our results demonstrate that the patients with PHEO display a lower magnitude of GLS than patients with EH, although they display the same hemodynamic parameters and no difference in LVEF. Our study therefore indicates that the overproduction of catecholamines in patients with PHEO may cause subclinical LV systolic impairment.

A conventional approach to the assessment of LV systolic function usually involves measurement of LVEF and endocardial fractional shortening. Both of these methods are derived from endocardial movement without considering myocardium deformation [17]. However, an evaluation using the EF cannot detect LV affection in hypertrophic patients and thus distinguish these patients from healthy controls [18,19].

In contrast to the conventional methods of measuring LV from endocardial movement, methods taking myocardium deformation into consideration, such as mid-wall endocardial fractional shortening or speckle-tracking echocardiography, have the advantage of being able to detect systolic function impairments with a higher degree of sensitivity [12]. For example, in hypertensive patients, an impairment of LV longitudinal strain and geometric changes (such as concentric remodeling or hypertrophy) occur prior to a decrease in LVEF [20], and increased afterload-related cardiomyocyte hypertrophy and collagen deposition in the extracellular matrix may cause the deterioration in strain in hypertensive myocardium [21].

It is well known that catecholamine overproduction has an adverse effect on cardiac structure [22]. Catecholamine stimulates cell growth and cardiomyocyte hypertrophy, which may lead to cardiac wall thickening and LV mass increase. In addition, in animal studies, catecholamine infusion has been shown to induce cardiac hypertrophy and myocardial interstitial fibrosis and scarring in both left and right ventricles [23]. In our previous studies, we found that the patients with PHEO displayed higher LVMI than patients with essential hypertension in echocardiography and that adrenalectomy led to a reduction of cardiovascular remodeling [11]. Catecholamine-induced cardiomyocyte hypertrophy, elevated cardiac wall thickness and collagen deposition in the extracellular matrix may explain the decrease in GLS in patients with PHEO in the current study. With a more contemporary tool, cardiac magnetic resonance imaging, Ferreira at al. [24] demonstrated that patients with PHEO had broader extent of myocardial fibrosis and myocardial dysfunction than patients with EH and elevated LV mass, and cardiac fibrosis improved after the removal of catecholamine excess (after adrenalectomy). Taken together, these findings indicate that patients with PHEO had a more severe cardiac fibrosis. This reduction in GLS is well known from patients with hypertrophic cardiomyopathy in whom reductions in longitudinal strain may be found prior to the reduction in EF [12].

An important factor is the direct toxic effect of catecholamines on the myocardium. Long-term high levels of catecholamines lead to β-adrenergic receptor downregulation. This degrades the function of the myofibers and gradually leads to their necrosis [25]. A similar mechanism, where β-adrenergic receptors are stimulated, occurs in stress cardiomyopathy, also referred to as Takotsubo cardiomyopathy [26]. Also, patients with PHEO may develop Takotsubo-like cardiomyopathy [27] due to the overproduction of catecholamines or develop a different form of another cardiac dysfunction (inverted Takotsubo cardiomyopathy and diffuse hypokinesis of LV) [10,28], which may often be transient [29]. Known cardiotoxic effects have been also observed in different types of chemotherapeutics used in the treatment of oncological diseases (although not mediated through β-adrenergic receptors), and GLS is used for an early detection of this cardiotoxicity [30]. It is therefore suggested that the decrease in GLS is related to the direct toxic effect of catecholamines on the myocardial muscle fibers through β-adrenergic receptors.

Another mechanism that may also play a role in the acceleration of cardiovascular hypertrophy is the higher fasting plasma glucose concentration in subjects with PHEO [31]. Asymptomatic patients with type 2 diabetes mellitus have a significant reduction in GLS, which is associated with a worse prognosis in these groups of patients [32]. Similarly, patients with type 2 diabetes mellitus have lower GLS after ST-segment elevation myocardial infarction [33] than non-diabetic patients.

Finally, a chronic inflammatory process may also lead to vascular damage [34,35]. In our previous study, we showed that chronic catecholamine excess in subjects with PHEO was accompanied by an increase in inflammatory markers, which was reversed by the tumor removal [36]. The decline of GLS is well documented in patients with the systemic inflammatory response syndrome and the magnitude of decline of GLS is related to the prognosis of these patients [37], which can be also related to the results of our work.

There are several limitations to this study. First, the number of patients was relatively small, which prevented finding any association between GLS and catecholamine overproduction. However, this is the first study to demonstrate subclinical systolic functional changes in patients with PHEO using speckle-tracking echocardiography. Further large-scale studies are needed to confirm the link between the magnitude of GLS and the overproduction of catecholamines. Secondly, we tried to match the group of subjects with PHEO with the EH group as closely as possible. This is, however, an elusive goal, because the overproduction of catecholamines leads not only to hypertension and weight loss but also to abnormalities in glucose metabolism. This makes the exact matching of the two groups unachievable. Therefore, the possible impact of diabetes on the magnitude of GLS in subject with PHEO cannot be excluded. On the other hand, EH patients had definitely higher atherogenic risk profiles, namely longer duration of hypertension, higher 24 h ABPM systolic blood pressure and higher body weight which may counteract the GLS differences between the two groups. Thirdly, the frequency of various antihypertensive drugs was not identical in the two groups of patients. Intervention studies in EH patients found that a therapy with drugs affecting the renin–angiotensin aldosterone system and calcium channel blockers can have a superior effect on the regression of LV hypertrophy than a therapy with diuretics and β-blockers independently of BP lowering. In our study, the proportions of EH patients on angiotensin-converting enzyme inhibitors or calcium channel blockers therapy were higher than those of PHEO patients (56% vs. 29% and 78% vs. 29%, respectively). Fourthly, postoperative speckle-tracking data were not available at the time of the study. Therefore, we could not resolve whether the impaired subclinical systolic function was reversible or not. A follow-up study involving postoperative findings of speckle-tracking analysis is under way.

4. Materials and Methods

Patients were recruited from a cohort of almost 1100 patients investigated for severe or resistant hypertension and for suspected secondary hypertension at our tertiary hospital-based Centre for Hypertension at the 3rd Department of Medicine, General University Hospital and 1st Faculty of Medicine, Charles University in Prague between November 2015 and October 2018. Each participant provided his/her written informed consent, and the study protocol was approved by the local Ethics Committee which took place during the grant approval (on 21 May 2015, code 20/15).

The diagnosis of PHEO was newly confirmed in 35 patients during the aforementioned period, which is about 3% rate in this preselected population. The diagnosis of PHEO was based on elevated plasma metanephrines and normetanephrines above the upper reference limit, and positive finding of adrenal tumor on computed tomography or magnetic resonance imaging. After examination all subjects underwent surgical removal of the tumor, and the diagnosis was confirmed histo-pathologically.

Ten patients were not enrolled due to the poor quality of echocardiography images or impossibility of GLS determination and seven due to significant comorbidities, including coronary atherosclerosis, atrial fibrillation or cardiac dysfunction for reasons other than PHEO. One patient was excluded for persistent overproduction of catecholamines after surgical removal because of the generalization of metastatic PHEO.

The control group of patients with essential hypertension (EH) was composed of the same prospective cohort as for the PHEO patients, on the basis of matching age, gender, body mass index, office and 24 h systolic blood pressure (BP). The patients were selected, after exclusion of the main forms of secondary hypertension (primary aldosteronism, PHEO, Cushing syndrome, renal parenchymal disease, renovascular hypertension), non-compliance or drug-induced hypertension. The subjects were considered hypertensive or pre-hypertensive when their clinic BP, an average of 3 sphygmomanometric measurements performed on 3 separate days, was ≥140/90 mmHg or ≥130/80 mmHg, respectively [38]. Chronic antihypertensive therapy was discontinued at least 2 weeks before admission, and patients were switched to the treatment with α-blockers and/or slow-release verapamil. Diabetes mellitus was defined as medication with oral antidiabetic drugs or repeated fasting glucose levels of >7.0 mmol/L [39]. There were two insulin-dependent patients in the PHEO group and none in the control group. All subjects with dyslipidemia (total plasma cholesterol ≥5.0 mmol/L or low-density cholesterol ≥3.0 mmol/L or high-density lipoprotein cholesterol ≤1.0 mmol/L in men and ≤1.2 mmol/L in women or triglycerides ≥1.7 mmol/L) were on a diet and received lipid-lowering therapy [40]. All patients were examined during a short three-day hospitalization.

4.1. BP Measurement

Casual blood pressure was measured using an oscillometric device (Omron M6, Shimogyo-ku, Kyoto, Japan). The measurement was made in a silent, quiet room with the patient's arm situated at the heart level and on chronic antihypertensive treatment during the first ambulatory visit, prior to switching to the treatment with α-blockers and/or slow-release verapamil. Blood pressure was measured three times in sitting position after five minutes of rest. The resulting value of causal systolic and diastolic blood pressure was calculated as the average from the second and third measurements. The patient's 24-h blood pressure was measured during their stay in the hospital using an oscillometric device (SpaceLabs 90207, SpaceLabs Medical, Redmond, WA, USA) already on switched medication.

4.2. Laboratory

Plasma-fractioned metanephrines (metanephrine and normetanephrine) were quantified by liquid chromatography with electrochemical detection (Agilent 1100; Agilent Technologies, Wilmington, DE, USA) in the Laboratory for Endocrinology and Metabolism at the 3rd Department of Medicine, General University Hospital and 1st Faculty of Medicine, Charles University in Prague [41].

Blood biochemistry, including sodium, potassium, urea, creatinine, total cholesterol, low-density lipoprotein cholesterol, high-density lipoprotein cholesterol, triglycerides, and plasma glucose, was analyzed using a multianalyzer (Modular SWA; Roche Diagnostics, Basel, Switzerland) in the Institute of Medical Biochemistry and Laboratory Diagnostics of the General University Hospital and 1st Faculty of Medicine, Charles University in Prague. Creatinine clearance was calculated using the Cockcroft–Gault equation.

4.3. Echocardiography

M-mode, 2-dimensional, Doppler and speckle tracking echocardiography were performed according to a standard protocol on Vivid 9 ultrasound system (GE Healthcare, Chicago, IL, USA). The records were analyzed offline using the EchoPAC working station (v.113, Advanced Analysis Technologies; GE Healthcare) by one cardiologist (J.K.) blinded to participants final diagnoses due to at least a fourteen-day period for the analysis of plasmatic metanephrines. M-mode images of the left ventricle at the mitral valve tip were obtained, guided by 2-dimensional parasternal long-axis and short-axis view, with the subjects lying down in the left lateral decubitus position at end-expiration. The LV end-diastolic (LVED) diameter, interventricular septum (IVS) thickness and LV posterior wall (LVPW) thickness were measured at the end of diastole and relative wall thickness (RWT) was measured with the formula 2 × LVPW thickness/LVED according to the recommendations of the American Society of Echocardiography and the European Association of Cardiovascular Imaging [42].

The LVED index was calculated as the LVED diameter indexed to the body surface area in square meters (LVED diameter/body surface area). LV mass estimation using American Society of Echocardiography convention was used [43]: LV mass (grams) = $0.8 \times 1.04 \times [(\text{LVED diameter} + \text{IVS thickness} + \text{LVPW thickness})^3 - (\text{LVED diameter})^3] + 0.6$ (with diameters in centimeters). Two variants of LV mass indexing were used: to the body surface area in square meters and to the 2.7th power of height in meters. The LV EF was measured by the biplane method of disks (modified Simpson's rule) according to the last published recommendations [42]. Before the speckle-tracking analysis was performed, the image quality, frame rate and foreshortening were optimized. The speckle-tracking analysis was performed by automated detection of endocardial border after manually defining the basal and apical points of the LV myocardium. If necessary, a manual adjustment was applied. The seventeen ventricular segment model was obtained from three projections: apical four-chamber view, two-chamber view and apical long-axis view and then the GLS was computed as the mean of peak longitudinal strain values from each of these segments according to consensus of American Society of Echocardiography and European Association of Echocardiography endorsed by the Japanese Society of Echocardiography (Figure 2) [44]. As recommended, patients were excluded if tracking was insufficient in more than one segment because of not clear visualization or artefacts [45]. If tracking in only one segment was unsuccessful, this segment was discarded and not used when calculating the GLS. The mid-wall GLS and also peak longitudinal strain in individual segments were evaluated. Individual segments were unified like basal, mid-ventricular and apical for simplification. The normal range of GLS using GE Healthcare system was −18.0 to −21.5% ± 3.7% [45].

4.4. Statistical Analysis

Data were analyzed using the Stata 13.5 program (StataCorp LP, College Station, TX, USA). Differences between the two groups (PHEO and EH) were analyzed with the help of the χ^2 test for categoric data and with the help of non-paired t-test for normal distribution of variables for the two patient groups. Depending on the normality/nonnormality of the distributions of particular variables, the results were given as mean ± SD values or median values (interquartile range). A p-values of <0.05 were considered statistically significant.

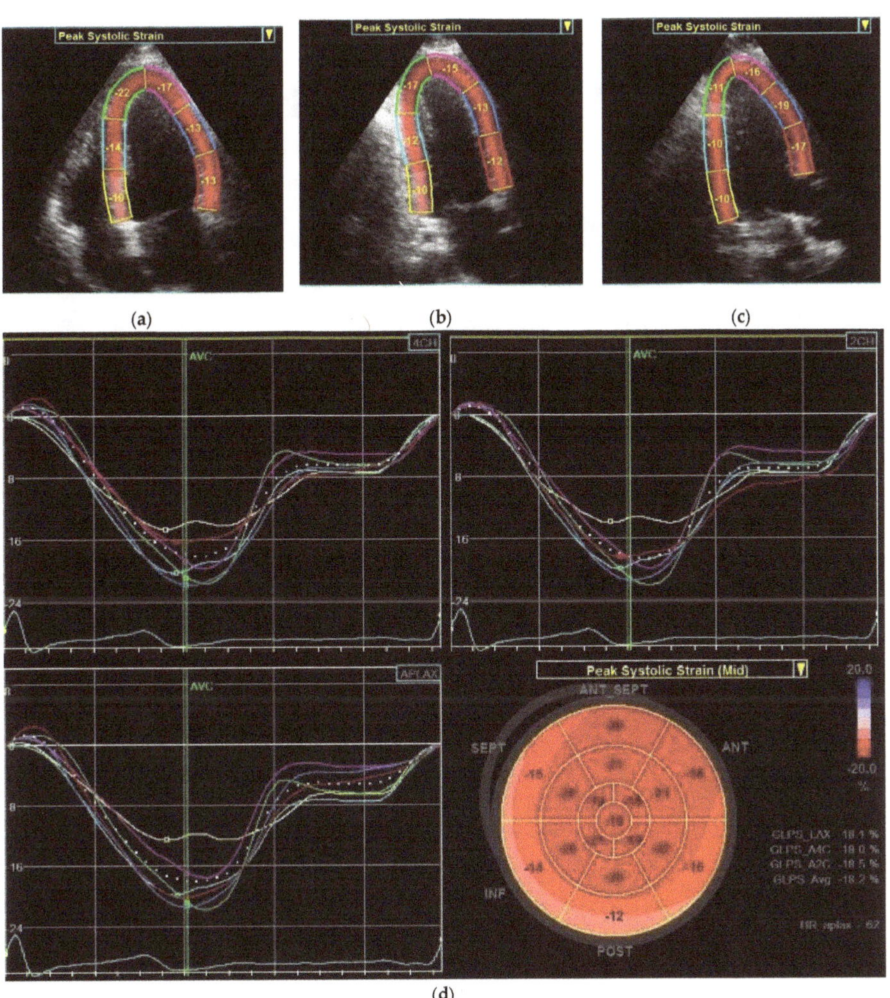

(a) (b) (c)

(d)

Figure 2. *Cont.*

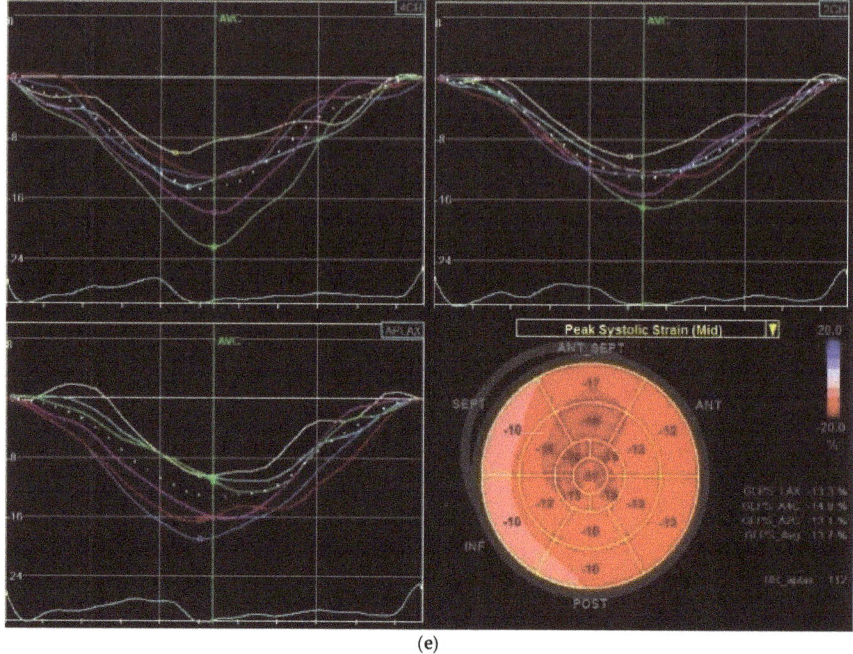

(e)

Figure 2. Distribution of individual left ventricular segments in which peak systolic strain is analyzed in apical four-chamber view (**a**), apical two-chamber view (**b**) and apical long-axis view (**c**). The resulting peak systolic strain-expressing curves in individual segments that correspond to the color designation of the segments in images a-c in a patient with essential hypertension (**d**) and in a patient with pheochromocytoma (**e**). The GLS (or GLPS) is calculated for the whole LV from each segment peak systolic strain and is expressed as the LV seventeen-segment model also called "bull eye" which is shown at the bottom right of images d-e. GLPS, global longitudinal peak strain; 4CH, apical four-chamber view, 2CH, apical two-chamber view; APLAX, apical long-axis view; MID, mid-wall; AVC, aortic valve closure; ANT-SEPT, anterior-septal; ANT, anterior; LAT, lateral; POST, posterior; INF, inferior; SEPT, septal; HR, heart rate

5. Conclusions

In conclusion, the patients with PHEO revealed lower magnitudes of GLS than the patients with EH. This finding is possibly caused by catecholamine-induced subclinical decline in LV systolic function, nevertheless, the link between the magnitude of GLS and the overproduction of catecholamines has not been proved in this study. At this stage, we can only express a suspicion of the diagnosis of PHEO in hypertensive patients based on measured lower magnitudes of GLS during routine echocardiographic examination.

Author Contributions: J.K., and R.H. designed the study and drafted the manuscript. J.K. performed and evaluated all echocardiographic examinations. T.Z., O.P., J.R., B.Š., T.I., Z.K. and J.W.J. collected clinical samples, patient information and provided statistical analysis. A.M. performed a laboratory analysis of plasma-fractioned metanephrines. R.H., as the corresponding author, made the final editing of the article. All authors were involved in the revision of the manuscript and approved the final version of the submitted manuscript.

Funding: This study was supported by grant projects AZV 16-30345A and AZV 15-27109A from the Ministry of Health of the Czech Republic and by research projects Progres Q25 and Q28 of Charles University in Prague.

Acknowledgments: The authors wish to express special thanks to nurses Terezie Holajová and Eva Straková of the echocardiography laboratory at the 3rd Department of Medicine for their assistance during the study.

Conflicts of Interest: The authors declare no conflict of interest. The funders had no role in the design of the study; in the collection, analysis, or interpretation of data; in the writing of the manuscript, or in the decision to publish the results.

References

1. Pacak, K.; Keiser, H.R.; Eisenhofer, G. Pheochromocytoma. In *Endocrinology*, 5th ed.; DeGroot, L.J., Jamenson, J.L., Eds.; Elsevier Saunders: Philadelphia, PA, USA, 2006; pp. 2501–2534.
2. Ariton, M.; Juan, C.S.; AvRuskin, T.W. Pheochromocytoma: Clinical observations from a Brooklyn tertiary hospital. *Endocr. Pract.* **2000**, *6*, 249–252. [CrossRef] [PubMed]
3. Omura, M.; Saito, J.; Yamaguchi, K.; Kakuta, Y.; Nishikawa, T. Prospective study on the prevalence of secondary hypertension among hypertensive patients visiting a general outpatient clinic in Japan. *Hypertens. Res.* **2004**, *27*, 193–202. [PubMed]
4. Lenders, J.W.; Eisenhofer, G.; Mannelli, M.; Pacak, K. Phaeochromocytoma. *Lancet* **2005**, *366*, 665–675. [CrossRef]
5. Berends, A.M.A.; Buitenwerf, E.; de Krijger, R.R.; Veeger, N.; van der Horst-Schrivers, A.N.A.; Links, T.P.; Kerstens, M.N. Incidence of pheochromocytoma and sympathetic paraganglioma in the Netherlands: A nationwide study and systematic review. *Eur. J. Intern. Med.* **2018**, *51*, 68–73. [CrossRef] [PubMed]
6. Zelinka, T.; Eisenhofer, G.; Pacak, K. Pheochromocytoma as a catecholamine producing tumor: Implications for clinical practice. *Stress* **2007**, *10*, 195–203. [PubMed]
7. Zhang, H.; Faber, J.E. Trophic effect of norepinephrine on arterial intima-media and adventitia is augmented by injury and mediated by different alpha1-adrenoceptor subtypes. *Circ. Res.* **2001**, *89*, 815–822. [PubMed]
8. Nakaki, T.; Nakayama, M.; Yamamoto, S.; Kato, R. Alpha 1-adrenergic stimulation and beta 2-adrenergic inhibition of DNA synthesis in vascular smooth muscle cells. *Mol. Pharm.* **1990**, *37*, 30–36.
9. Zelinka, T.; Petrák, O.; Turková, H.; Holaj, R.; Štrauch, B.; Kršek, M.; Vrankova, A.B.; Musil, Z.; Dušková, J.; Kubinyi, J.; et al. High incidence of cardiovascular complications in pheochromocytoma. *Horm. Metab. Res.* **2012**, *44*, 379–384. [CrossRef] [PubMed]
10. Park, J.H.; Kim, K.S.; Sul, J.Y.; Shin, S.K.; Kim, J.H.; Lee, J.H.; Choi, S.W.; Jeong, J.O.; Seong, I.W. Prevalence and patterns of left ventricular dysfunction in patients with pheochromocytoma. *J. Cardiovasc. Ultrasound* **2011**, *19*, 76–82. [CrossRef] [PubMed]
11. Majtan, B.; Zelinka, T.; Rosa, J.; Petrák, O.; Kratka, Z.; Štrauch, B.; Tuka, V.; Vránková, A.; Michalský, D.; Novák, K.; et al. Long-Term Effect of Adrenalectomy on Cardiovascular Remodeling in Patients With Pheochromocytoma. *J. Clin. Endocrinol. Metab.* **2017**, *102*, 1208–1217. [CrossRef] [PubMed]
12. Kalam, K.; Otahal, P.; Marwick, T.H. Prognostic implications of global LV dysfunction: A systematic review and meta-analysis of global longitudinal strain and ejection fraction. *Heart* **2014**, *100*, 1673–1680. [PubMed]
13. Smiseth, O.A.; Torp, H.; Opdahl, A.; Haugaa, K.H.; Urheim, S. Myocardial strain imaging: How useful is it in clinical decision making? *Eur. Heart J.* **2016**, *37*, 1196–1207. [CrossRef] [PubMed]
14. Sun, J.P.; Stewart, W.J.; Yang, X.S.; Donnell, R.O.; Leon, A.R.; Felner, J.M.; Thomas, J.D.; Merlino, J.D. Differentiation of hypertrophic cardiomyopathy and cardiac amyloidosis from other causes of ventricular wall thickening by two-dimensional strain imaging echocardiography. *Am. J. Cardiol.* **2009**, *103*, 411–415. [CrossRef] [PubMed]
15. Chen, Z.W.; Huang, K.C.; Lee, J.K.; Lin, L.C.; Chen, C.W.; Chang, Y.Y.; Liao, C.W.; Wu, V.C.; Hung, C.S.; Lin, Y.H. Aldosterone induces left ventricular subclinical systolic dysfunction: A strain imaging study. *J. Hypertens.* **2017**, *36*, 353–360.
16. Plana, J.C.; Galderisi, M.; Barac, A.; Ewer, M.S.; Ky, B.; Scherrer-Crosbie, M.; Ganame, J.; Sebag, I.A.; Agler, D.A.; Badano, L.P.; et al. Expert consensus for multimodality imaging evaluation of adult patients during and after cancer therapy: A report from the American Society of Echocardiography and the European Association of Cardiovascular Imaging. *J. Am. Soc. Echocardiogr.* **2014**, *27*, 911–939. [PubMed]
17. Park, K.; Chang, S.A.; Kim, H.K.; Park, H.E.; Na, S.H.; Kim, Y.J.; Sohn, D.W.; Oh, B.H.; Park, Y.B. Normal ranges and physiological changes of midwall fractional shortening in healthy korean population. *Korean Circ. J.* **2010**, *40*, 587–592. [PubMed]

18. Krzesinski, P.; Uzieblo-Zyczkowska, B.; Gielerak, G.; Stanczyk, A.; Kurpaska, M.; Piotrowicz, K. Global longitudinal two-dimensional systolic strain is associated with hemodynamic alterations in arterial hypertension. *J. Am. Soc. Hypertens. JASH* **2015**, *9*, 680–689. [CrossRef] [PubMed]
19. Mayet, J.; Ariff, B.; Wasan, B.; Chapman, N.; Shahi, M.; Senior, R.; Foale, R.A.; Thom, S.A. Midwall myocardial shortening in athletic left ventricular hypertrophy. *Int. J. Cardiol.* **2002**, *86*, 233–238. [PubMed]
20. Kouzu, H.; Yuda, S.; Muranaka, A.; Doi, T.; Yamamoto, H.; Shimoshige, S.; Hase, M.; Hashimoto, A.; Saitoh, S.; Tsuchihashi, K.; et al. Left ventricular hypertrophy causes different changes in longitudinal, radial, and circumferential mechanics in patients with hypertension: A two-dimensional speckle tracking study. *J. Am. Soc. Echocardiogr.* **2011**, *24*, 192–199. [CrossRef] [PubMed]
21. Ishizu, T.; Seo, Y.; Kameda, Y.; Kawamura, R.; Kimura, T.; Shimojo, N.; Xu, D.; Murakoshi, N.; Aonuma, K. Left ventricular strain and transmural distribution of structural remodeling in hypertensive heart disease. *Hypertension* **2014**, *63*, 500–506. [PubMed]
22. Galetta, F.; Franzoni, F.; Bernini, G.; Poupak, F.; Carpi, A.; Cini, G.; Tocchini, L.; Antonelli, A.; Santoro, G. Cardiovascular complications in patients with pheochromocytoma: A mini-review. *Biomed. Pharm.* **2010**, *64*, 505–509. [CrossRef] [PubMed]
23. Johnson, M.D.; Grignolo, A.; Kuhn, C.M.; Schanberg, S.M. Hypertension and cardiovascular hypertrophy during chronic catecholamine infusion in rats. *Life Sci.* **1983**, *33*, 169–180. [PubMed]
24. Ferreira, V.M.; Marcelino, M.; Piechnik, S.K.; Marini, C.; Karamitsos, T.D.; Ntusi, N.A.; Francis, J.M.; Robson, M.D.; Arnold, J.R.; Mihai, R.; et al. Pheochromocytoma Is Characterized by Catecholamine-Mediated Myocarditis, Focal and Diffuse Myocardial Fibrosis, and Myocardial Dysfunction. *J. Am. Coll. Cardiol.* **2016**, *67*, 2364–2374. [CrossRef] [PubMed]
25. De Miguel, V.; Arias, A.; Paissan, A.; de Arenaza, D.P.; Pietrani, M.; Jurado, A.; Jaén, A.; Day, P.F. Catecholamine-induced myocarditis in pheochromocytoma. *Circulation* **2014**, *129*, 1348–1349. [CrossRef] [PubMed]
26. Lyon, A.R.; Rees, P.S.; Prasad, S.; Poole-Wilson, P.A.; Harding, S.E. Stress (Takotsubo) cardiomyopathy—A novel pathophysiological hypothesis to explain catecholamine-induced acute myocardial stunning. *Nat. Clin. Pract. Cardiovasc. Med.* **2008**, *5*, 22–29. [CrossRef] [PubMed]
27. Chiang, Y.L.; Chen, P.C.; Lee, C.C.; Chua, S.K. Adrenal pheochromocytoma presenting with Takotsubo-pattern cardiomyopathy and acute heart failure: A case report and literature review. *Medicine* **2016**, *95*, e4846. [CrossRef] [PubMed]
28. Tafreshi, S.; Naqvi, S.Y.; Thomas, S. Extra-adrenal pheochromocytoma presenting as inverse takotsubo-pattern cardiomyopathy treated with surgical resection. *BMJ Case Rep.* **2018**, *11*, e226384. [PubMed]
29. Brilakis, E.S.; Young, W.F., Jr.; Wilson, J.W.; Thompson, G.B.; Munger, T.M. Reversible catecholamine-induced cardiomyopathy in a heart transplant candidate without persistent or paroxysmal hypertension. *J. Heart Lung Transplant.* **1999**, *18*, 376–380. [CrossRef]
30. Thavendiranathan, P.; Poulin, F.; Lim, K.D.; Plana, J.C.; Woo, A.; Marwick, T.H. Use of myocardial strain imaging by echocardiography for the early detection of cardiotoxicity in patients during and after cancer chemotherapy: A systematic review. *J. Am. Coll. Cardiol.* **2014**, *63*, 2751–2768. [PubMed]
31. Turnbull, D.M.; Johnston, D.G.; Alberti, K.G.; Hall, R. Hormonal and metabolic studies in a patient with a pheochromocytoma. *J. Clin. Endocrinol. Metab.* **1980**, *51*, 930–933. [PubMed]
32. Holland, D.J.; Marwick, T.H.; Haluska, B.A.; Leano, R.; Hordern, M.D.; Hare, J.L.; Fang, Z.Y.; Prins, J.B.; Stanton, T. Subclinical LV dysfunction and 10-year outcomes in type 2 diabetes mellitus. *Heart* **2015**, *101*, 1061–1066. [CrossRef] [PubMed]
33. Hoogslag, G.E.; Abou, R.; Joyce, E.; Boden, H.; Kamperidis, V.; Regeer, M.V.; van Rosendael, P.J.; Schalij, M.J.; Bax, J.J.; Marsan, N.A.; et al. Comparison of Changes in Global Longitudinal Peak Systolic Strain After ST-Segment Elevation Myocardial Infarction in Patients With Versus Without Diabetes Mellitus. *Am. J. Cardiol.* **2015**, *116*, 1334–1339. [CrossRef] [PubMed]
34. Wang, T.J.; Nam, B.H.; Wilson, P.W.; Wolf, P.A.; Levy, D.; Polak, J.F.; D'agostino, R.B.; O'donnell, C.J. Association of C-reactive protein with carotid atherosclerosis in men and women: The Framingham Heart Study. *Arterioscler. Thromb. Vasc. Biol.* **2002**, *22*, 1662–1667. [CrossRef] [PubMed]
35. Magyar, M.T.; Szikszai, Z.; Balla, J.; Valikovics, A.; Kappelmayer, J.; Imre, S.; Balla, G.; Jeney, V.; Csiba, L.; Bereczki, D. Early-onset carotid atherosclerosis is associated with increased intima-media thickness and elevated serum levels of inflammatory markers. *Stroke J. Cereb. Circ.* **2003**, *34*, 58–63. [CrossRef]

36. Zelinka, T.; Petrák, O.; Štrauch, B.; Holaj, R.; Kvasnička, J.; Mazoch, J.; Pacak, K.; Widimský, J., Jr. Elevated inflammation markers in pheochromocytoma compared to other forms of hypertension. *Neuroimmunomodulation* **2007**, *14*, 57–64. [CrossRef] [PubMed]
37. Sanfilippo, F.; Corredor, C.; Fletcher, N.; Tritapepe, L.; Lorini, F.L.; Arcadipane, A.; Vieillard-Baron, A.; Cecconi, M. Left ventricular systolic function evaluated by strain echocardiography and relationship with mortality in patients with severe sepsis or septic shock: A systematic review and meta-analysis. *Crit. Care* **2018**, *22*, 183. [CrossRef] [PubMed]
38. Mancia, G.; Fagard, R.; Narkiewicz, K.; Redon, J.; Zanchetti, A.; Boehm, M.; Christiaens, T.; Cifkova, R.; De Backer, G.; Dominiczak, A.; et al. 2013 ESH/ESC Guidelines for the management of arterial hypertension: The Task Force for the management of arterial hypertension of the European Society of Hypertension (ESH) and of the European Society of Cardiology (ESC). *J. Hypertens.* **2013**, *31*, 1281–1357. [CrossRef] [PubMed]
39. Force IDFCGT. Global Guideline for Type 2 Diabetes: Recommendations for standard, comprehensive, and minimal care. *Diabet. Med.* **2006**, *23*, 579–593.
40. Graham, I.; Atar, D.; Borch-Johnsen, K.; Boysen, G.; Burell, G.; Cifkova, R.; Dallongeville, J.; De Backer, G.; Ebrahim, S.; Gjelsvik, B.; et al. European guidelines on cardiovascular disease prevention in clinical practice: Executive summary: Fourth Joint Task Force of the European Society of Cardiology and Other Societies on Cardiovascular Disease Prevention in Clinical Practice (Constituted by representatives of nine societies and by invited experts). *Eur. Heart J.* **2007**, *28*, 2375–2414. [PubMed]
41. Lenders, J.W.; Eisenhofer, G.; Armando, I.; Keiser, H.R.; Goldstein, D.S.; Kopin, I.J. Determination of metanephrines in plasma by liquid chromatography with electrochemical detection. *Clin. Chem.* **1993**, *39*, 97–103. [PubMed]
42. Lang, R.M.; Badano, L.P.; Mor-Avi, V.; Afilalo, J.; Armstrong, A.; Ernande, L.; Flachskampf, F.A.; Foster, E.; Goldstein, S.A.; Kuznetsova, T.; et al. Recommendations for cardiac chamber quantification by echocardiography in adults: An update from the American Society of Echocardiography and the European Association of Cardiovascular Imaging. *Eur. Heart J. Cardiovasc. Imaging* **2015**, *16*, 233–270. [CrossRef] [PubMed]
43. Devereux, R.B.; Alonso, D.R.; Lutas, E.M.; Gottlieb, G.J.; Campo, E.; Sachs, I.; Reichek, N. Echocardiographic assessment of left ventricular hypertrophy: Comparison to necropsy findings. *Am. J. Cardiol.* **1986**, *57*, 450–458. [PubMed]
44. Mor-Avi, V.; Lang, R.M.; Badano, L.P.; Belohlavek, M.; Cardim, N.M.; Derumeaux, G.; Galderisi, M.; Marwick, T.; Nagueh, S.F.; Sengupta, P.P.; et al. Current and evolving echocardiographic techniques for the quantitative evaluation of cardiac mechanics: ASE/EAE consensus statement on methodology and indications endorsed by the Japanese Society of Echocardiography. *Eur. J. Echocardiogr.* **2011**, *12*, 167–205. [CrossRef] [PubMed]
45. Farsalinos, K.E.; Daraban, A.M.; Unlu, S.; Thomas, J.D.; Badano, L.P.; Voigt, J.U. Head-to-Head Comparison of Global Longitudinal Strain Measurements among Nine Different Vendors: The EACVI/ASE Inter-Vendor Comparison Study. *J. Am. Soc. Echocardiogr.* **2015**, *28*, 1171–1181.e2. [CrossRef] [PubMed]

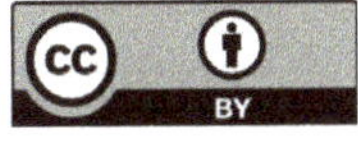

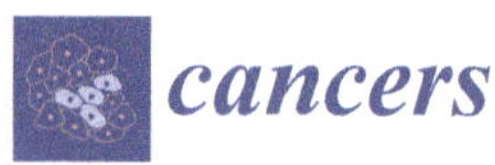

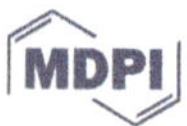

Article

The Significant Reduction or Complete Eradication of Subcutaneous and Metastatic Lesions in a Pheochromocytoma Mouse Model after Immunotherapy Using Mannan-BAM, TLR Ligands, and Anti-CD40

Veronika Caisova [1,2], Liping Li [1], Garima Gupta [1], Ivana Jochmanova [1], Abhishek Jha [1], Ondrej Uher [1,2], Thanh-Truc Huynh [1], Markku Miettinen [3], Ying Pang [1], Luma Abunimer [1], Gang Niu [4], Xiaoyuan Chen [4], Hans Kumar Ghayee [5], David Taïeb [6], Zhengping Zhuang [7], Jan Zenka [2] and Karel Pacak [1,*]

1 Section on Medical Neuroendocrinology, *Eunice Kennedy Shriver* National Institute of Child Health and Human Development, National Institutes of Health, Bethesda, MD 20814, USA; veronika.caisova@nih.gov (V.C.); bat.150@hotmail.com (L.L.); garima.gupta83@gmail.com (G.G.); ivana.jochmanova@gmail.com (I.J.); abhishek.jha@nih.gov (A.J.); ondrej.uher@nih.gov (O.U.); huynht@mail.nih.gov (T.-T.H.); ying.pang@nih.gov (Y.P.); luma.abunimer@nih.gov (L.A.)

2 Department of Medical Biology, Faculty of Science, University of South Bohemia, Ceske Budejovice 37005, Czech Republic; jzenka@gmail.com

3 Laboratory of Pathology, National Cancer Institute, National Institutes of Health, Bethesda, MD 20814, USA; markku.miettinen@nih.gov

4 Laboratory of Molecular Imaging and Nanomedicine, National Institute of Biomedical Imaging and Bioengineering, National Institutes of Health, Bethesda, MD 20814, USA; gang.niu@nih.gov (G.N.); shawn.chen@nih.gov (X.C.)

5 Biological Molecular Imaging Section, University of Florida College of Medicine, Gainesville, FL 32603, USA; Hans.Ghayee@medicine.ufl.edu

6 Department of Nuclear Medicine, La Timone University Hospital, CERIMED, Aix-Marseille University, 13385 Marseille, France; David.TAIEB@ap-hm.fr

7 Surgical Neurology Branch, National Institute of Neurological Disorders and Stroke, National Institutes of Health, Bethesda, MD 20814, USA; zhengping.zhuang@nih.gov

* Correspondence: karel@mail.nih.gov; Tel.: +1-301-402-4594

Received: 13 March 2019; Accepted: 6 May 2019; Published: 11 May 2019

Abstract: Therapeutic options for metastatic pheochromocytoma/paraganglioma (PHEO/PGL) are limited. Here, we tested an immunotherapeutic approach based on intratumoral injections of mannan-BAM with toll-like receptor ligands into subcutaneous PHEO in a mouse model. This therapy elicited a strong innate immunity-mediated antitumor response and resulted in a significantly lower PHEO volume compared to the phosphate buffered saline (PBS)-treated group and in a significant improvement in mice survival. The cytotoxic effect of neutrophils, as innate immune cells predominantly infiltrating treated tumors, was verified in vitro. Moreover, the combination of mannan-BAM and toll-like receptor ligands with agonistic anti-CD40 was associated with increased mice survival. Subsequent tumor re-challenge also supported adaptive immunity activation, reflected primarily by long-term tumor-specific memory. These results were further verified in metastatic PHEO, where the intratumoral injections of mannan-BAM, toll-like receptor ligands, and anti-CD40 into subcutaneous tumors resulted in significantly less intense bioluminescence signals of liver metastatic lesions induced by tail vein injection compared to the PBS-treated group. Subsequent experiments focusing on the depletion of T cell subpopulations confirmed the crucial role of $CD8^+$ T cells in inhibition of bioluminescence signal intensity of liver metastatic lesions. These data call for a new therapeutic approach in patients with metastatic PHEO/PGL using immunotherapy that initially activates innate immunity followed by an adaptive immune response.

Keywords: pheochromocytoma; paraganglioma; metastatic; immunotherapy; innate immunity; adaptive immunity; toll-like receptor; pathogen-associated molecular patterns; neutrophil; T cell

---

1. Introduction

Pheochromocytomas (PHEOs) and paragangliomas (PGLs) are rare catecholamine-producing neuroendocrine/neural crest cell tumors arising from the adrenal medulla and extra-adrenal paraganglia, respectively [1]. Approximately 10–30% of all PHEOs/PGLs become metastatic and therapeutic options for treating metastatic disease are limited [2]. Therefore, efforts to find new and more effective therapies are urgently needed for patients with either inoperable or metastatic PHEO/PGL.

Immunotherapy, in which immune cells of a patient are used to attack and subsequently eliminate tumor cells, is currently one of the most extensively studied therapeutic approaches in cancer research [3,4]. Not much is known about the interaction between PHEO/PGL and a patient's immune system. Overall, PHEO/PGL can be considered as immunologically "cold" compared to other cancer types because of their lack of leukocyte fraction, low amount of neoantigens, and low somatic sequence mutation rate [5–7]. To date, only one experimental study proposed the use of immunotherapy in PHEO/PGL, specifically chromogranin A, as a potential treatment target [8]. In this study, immunization with chromogranin A peptides induced the production of cytotoxic T cells with subsequent elimination of chromogranin A expressing PHEO cells. Moreover, chromogranin A peptides were suggested as a potential anti-tumor vaccine in PHEO patients with risk of metastatic disease [8]. Recently, two clinical trials focusing on the application of checkpoint inhibitors (specifically nivolumab, ipilimumab, and pembrolizumab) in rare tumors, including PHEO/PGL, were initiated and are in the stage of patient recruitment (ClinicalTrials.gov Identifier: NCT02834013 and NCT02721732).

Current immunotherapeutic approaches to cancer treatment are based either on the activation of innate or more frequently adaptive immunity [9–11]. The innate immune system is well conserved, and its response is uniform, robust, and short-lasting, but it can well contribute to cancer treatment and the elimination of metastatic lesions [12–14]. Recently, immunotherapy based on the activation of innate immunity via pathogen-associated molecular patterns (PAMPs) has been tested in melanoma, which is also a neural crest tumor. Intratumoral application of PAMPs, particularly ligands stimulating phagocytosis and toll-like receptor (TLR) ligands, resulted in the complete elimination of over 80% of subcutaneous tumors in the B16-F10 melanoma mouse model [15–17].

Ligands stimulating phagocytosis initiate ingestion of pathogens by phagocytic immune cells [18,19]. PAMP-based immunotherapy uses intratumoral administration of mannan, a simple polysaccharide from *Saccharomyces cerevisiae*, as a ligand stimulating phagocytosis [16]. Mannan recognized by mannan-binding lectin (MBL) activates the complement lectin pathway [20]. This activation results in iC3b molecule production, followed by iC3b tumor cell opsonization [21,22], and consequently their elimination by phagocytes, particularly neutrophils, macrophages, and dendritic cells. In this type of immunotherapy, mannan is bound to a tumor cell membrane by the biocompatible anchor for a membrane called BAM (Figure 1).

TLRs are expressed on the surface of various cells, mainly those belonging to the innate immune system. These receptors recognize their specific ligands and initiate immune system mobilization [23–25]. This process is well supported by previous reports showing that the intratumoral application of TLR ligands increased the number of tumor-infiltrating leukocytes in melanoma and renal cell carcinoma mouse models [15–17,26]. Resiquimod (R-848), polyinosinic-polycytidylic acid (poly(I:C)), and lipoteichoic acid (LTA) are TLR ligands used in the present study. R-848 is an imidazoquinoline compound with anti-viral effects that activates immune cells via TLR7/TLR8 in humans and TLR7 in mice [27]. Poly(I:C) is a synthetic analog of dsRNA that activates immune cells via TLR3 [28]. LTA is a constituent of the cell wall of Gram-positive bacteria that activates immune cells via TLR2 [29].

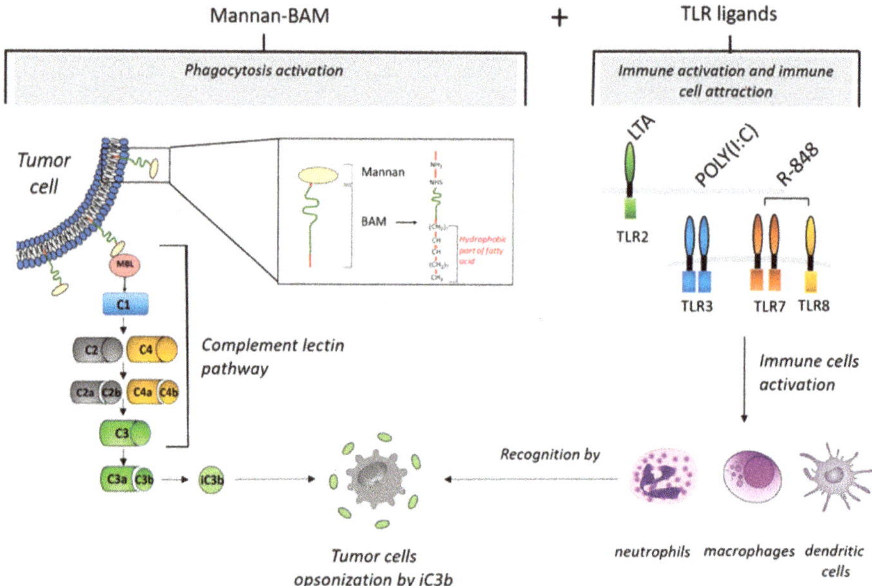

Figure 1. Mechanisms of tumor cell elimination during immunotherapy based on intratumoral application of mannan-BAM+TLR ligands (MBT). After intratumoral application of mannan with a biocompatible anchor for membrane-BAM, the hydrophobic part of BAM is incorporated into the lipid bilayer of tumor cells. Mannan attached to membranes activates innate immunity by the interaction of mannan with mannan binding lectin (MBL). This interaction initiates activation of the complement lectin pathway. This results in iC3b production and opsonization of tumor cells followed by migration of immune cells (macrophages, dendritic cells, or granulocytes) and phagocytosis activation. Further, simultaneous intratumoral application of TLR ligands (resiquimod (R-848), polyinosinic-polycytidylic acid (poly(I:C)), and lipoteichoic acid (LTA)) causes a strong attraction of immune cells (macrophages, dendritic cells, or granulocytes) to the tumor.

Thus, in the present study, we aimed to evaluate the therapeutic effects of intratumorally administered mannan-BAM and TLR ligands (MBT) in a subcutaneous and metastatic mouse PHEO. Specifically, we focused on the initial activation of innate immunity, an assessment of its role in the elimination of PHEO, and the detection of the potential role of subsequent engagement of adaptive immunity in elimination of distant metastatic PHEO organ lesions. This model was established using B6(Cg)-*Tyr*$^{c\text{-}2J}$/J mouse strains with subcutaneously and/or intravenously injected experimental PHEO cells called mouse tumor tissue (MTT)-luciferase cells [30,31]. Subsequently, the intratumoral application of MBT resulted in a significantly lower PHEO volume compared to the phosphate buffered saline (PBS)-treated group and in an improvement in mice survival. As neutrophils infiltrated the treated subcutaneous PHEOs, their role in this therapeutic model was established by measuring neutrophil cytotoxic activity and neutrophil-tumor cell interactions with MTT-luciferase and hPheo1 cell lines. An additional boost of MBT with anti-CD40 (this combination is henceforth referred to as MBTA) significantly improved the effect of the MBT application on the survival of experimental mice. Since re-challenge experiment suggested potential engagement of adaptive immunity, the therapy was tested in metastatic PHEO with a positive effect on the bioluminescence signal intensity of PHEO metastatic organ lesions compared to the PBS-treated group. Finally, the crucial role of $CD8^+$ cells in the inhibition of bioluminescence signal intensity of metastatic organ lesions was further supported by the antibody-dependent $CD4^+$/$CD8^+$ cell depletion experiment.

2. Results

2.1. A Syngeneic PHEO Mouse Model for Immunotherapy Evaluation

Since there is a very limited number of animal models for PHEO, we first decided to establish a PHEO mouse model that is appropriate for immunotherapy evaluation. Female B6(Cg)-*Tyr*$^{c\text{-}2J}$/J mice were subcutaneously injected with 3×10^6 MTT-luciferase cells in 0.2 mL of DMEM without additives in the right lower dorsal site or intravenously with 1.5×10^6 MTT-luciferase cells in 0.1 mL of PBS in a lateral tail vein. Subcutaneous PHEO tumors reached a mean volume of 118 mm^3 (range 8.5–407.2 mm^3) 45 days after tumor cell injection. Mice with intravenously injected tumor cells had detectable metastatic organ lesions 14 days after tumor cell transplantation. These metastatic organ lesions were located predominantly in the liver; small lesions were also detected in bones and lymph nodes (Figure 2A).

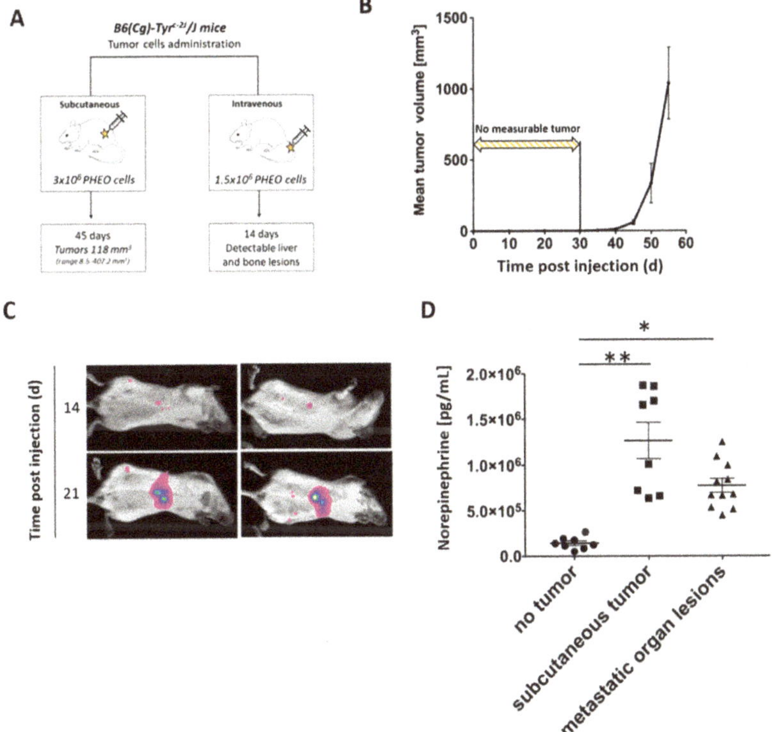

Figure 2. Subcutaneous and metastatic PHEO in mouse model suitable for immunotherapy testing established using MTT-luciferase cells. (**A**) B6(Cg)-Tyr$^{c\text{-}2J}$/J mice were subcutaneously (n = 24) or intravenously (n = 10) injected with MTT-luciferase cells. (**B**) Subcutaneous MTT-luciferase tumors reached a mean volume of 118 mm^3 45 days after tumor cell injection. No tumors were detected for 30 days after tumor cells injection. (**C**) Metastatic organ lesions were detectable 14 days after intravenous tumor cells injection using bioluminescence imaging. Metastatic organ lesions were predominantly located in the liver; small lesions were also detected in bones and lymph nodes. (**D**) Tumor-bearing mice, either with subcutaneous tumors or metastatic organ lesions, had significantly higher urine norepinephrine levels than those without tumors (* $p < 0.05$; ** $p < 0.01$ against no tumor).

Subcutaneous PHEO tumors were not measurable until 30 days after tumor cell injection. However, 40 days after tumor cell injection, the tumor volume increased significantly (Figure 2B). A diameter size of 2 cm was reached after 57 days (range 49–85 days) in most of the experimental mice. Subcutaneous tumors development was observed in 100% of mice. Metastatic organ lesions, after intravenous PHEO tumor cell injection, were detectable in 65% of mice 14 days after tumor cell injection using bioluminescence imaging. On the 21st day, 95% of mice had detectable metastatic liver lesions (Figure 2C).

To further characterize the established PHEO mouse model, urine catecholamine levels (norepinephrine, dopamine, and epinephrine) were measured in B6(Cg)-Tyr^{c-2J}/J tumor-bearing mice (subcutaneous tumor and metastatic organ lesions) after the injection of MTT-luciferase cells. Norepinephrine levels were significantly higher in tumor-bearing mice (subcutaneous tumor and metastatic organ lesions) compared to non-tumor-bearing mice (no tumor) (Figure 2D). Dopamine levels did not reveal any significant changes when comparing groups of tumor-bearing mice (subcutaneous tumor and metastatic organ lesions) to non-tumor-bearing mice (no tumor) (Figure S1A). Epinephrine levels were higher in mice with metastatic organ lesions compared to non-tumor-bearing mice (no tumor) and tumor-bearing mice (subcutaneous tumor) (Figure S1B).

2.2. MBT Immunotherapy Stabilize Tumor Volume and Improves Mice Survival

To evaluate the effect of MBT in PHEO, we applied MBT into subcutaneous PHEO tumors (on specific days as described in Materials and Methods). MBT application resulted in a significant stabilization of subcutaneous PHEO volume compared to the PBS-treated group (Figure 3A,B).

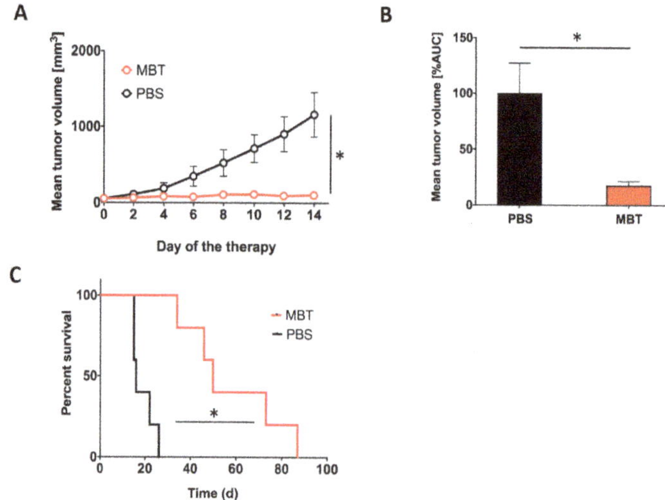

Figure 3. Intratumoral application of MBT in subcutaneous PHEO. B6(Cg)-Tyr^{c-2J}/J mice were subcutaneously injected with MTT-luciferase cells. After tumors grew to the desired size (about 100 mm^3), mice were randomized into two groups ($n = 5$/group): (i) the group treated with MBT; (ii) the group treated with PBS. MBT and PBS were given intratumorally on days 0, 1, 2, 8, 9, 10, 16, 17, 18, 24, 25, and 26. Tumor volume was measured with a caliper. (**A**) The tumor volume growth is presented as a growth curve (* $p < 0.05$ against PBS) and (**B**) as an area under the curve (AUC) (* $p < 0.05$ against PBS). (**C**) The survival analysis for the two groups are presented as a Kaplan–Meier curve (* $p < 0.05$ against PBS).

In addition, intratumoral application of MBT resulted in significantly longer survival of the treated mice. The median survival increased from 16 days (range 15–26 days) in the PBS-treated group to 50 days (range 34–87 days) in the MBT-treated group (Figure 3C).

2.3. Significant Participation of Innate Immunity in Subcutaneous PHEO Volume Stabilization

In the subsequent experiment, we used B6.CB17-*Prkdc*^{scid}/SzJ mice lacking functional T and B cells to verify the role of innate and adaptive immunity in the PHEO volume stabilization during MBT therapy. Subcutaneous PHEOs were treated intratumorally with MBT or PBS on specific days as described in Materials and Methods. Intratumoral application of MBT resulted in PHEO volume stabilization compared to the PBS-treated group (Figure 4A,B). Since we started this experiment with a lower tumor volume than in the previous experiment (about 50 mm^3), most of the experimental mice (five of six mice from both the MBT- and PBS-treated groups) survived during the whole course of the therapy (30 days). On the 30th day of therapy, mice from both groups were sacrificed, and subcutaneous tumors were harvested and then analyzed. The MBT-treated tumors were significantly smaller than the PBS-treated tumors (Figure 4C). Additional immunohistochemical analysis showed higher levels of tumor-infiltrating leukocytes (CD45$^+$ cells) in the MBT-treated group compared to the PBS-treated group (Figure 4D).

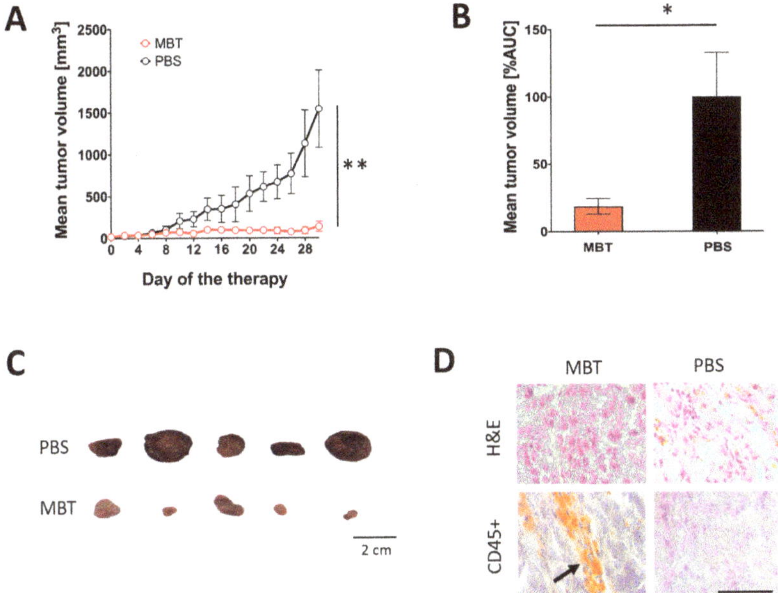

Figure 4. Significance of innate immunity in MBT immunotherapy in subcutaneous PHEO. B6.CB17-Prkdc^{scid}/SzJ mice were subcutaneously injected with MTT-luciferase cells. After tumors grew to the desired size (about 50 mm^3), mice were randomized into two groups (n = 6/group): (i) the group treated with MBT and (ii) the group treated with PBS. MBT and PBS were given intratumorally on days 0, 1, 2, 8, 9, 10, 16, 17, 18, 24, 25, and 26. Tumor volume was measured with a caliper. (**A**) The tumor volume growth is presented as a growth curve (** $p < 0.01$ against PBS) and (**B**) as an area under the curve (AUC) (* $p < 0.05$ against PBS). (**C**) Surviving mice were sacrificed on the 30th day of therapy (five mice from the MBT-treated group and five mice from the PBS-treated group), and tumors were documented. (**D**) Hematoxylin and eosin (H&E) staining and CD45$^+$ immunohistochemistry staining were performed on tumor cryosections (a thickness of 8 µm). Bar = 20 µm.

2.4. Characterization of Tumor-Infiltrating Leukocytes and Tumor Environment during MBT Immunotherapy

2.4.1. Flow Cytometry Analysis of Tumor-Infiltrating Leukocytes in the MBT-Treated Tumors

To identify immune cells infiltrating subcutaneous PHEO tumors during MBT therapy, we performed a flow cytometry analysis of tumor-infiltrating leukocytes. Since we limited the number of mice per group (n = 3/group), we decided to present tumor-infiltrating leukocytes data as individual values for each mouse, with a color legend based on the size of the analyzed tumors. The flow cytometry analysis of tumor-infiltrating leukocytes showed increased levels of CD45$^+$ cells in the MBT-treated group. This trend culminated on the 15th day of therapy (Figure 5A). T cells (CD3$^+$) were the most common leukocytes in the MBT-treated tumors (Figure 5A). The analysis of CD3$^+$ subpopulations revealed increased levels of Th cells (CD4$^+$) (Figure S2A) and Tc cells (CD8$^+$) (Figure S2B) in the MBT-treated group. Furthermore, a significant increase in granulocytes was observed on the 3rd and 19th days of therapy (Figure 5A). No significant changes were observed in B cells (CD19$^+$) (Figure S2C), monocytes/macrophages (F4/80$^+$) (Figure S2D), or natural killer (NK) cells (Figure S2E).

2.4.2. Histological Analysis of Tumor-Infiltrating Leukocytes in the MBT-Treated Tumors

To verify the flow cytometry results of tumor-infiltrating leukocytes, we performed hematoxylin and eosin (H&E) staining and immunohistochemistry staining on the same tumors, which were originally used for the flow cytometry analysis (Figure 5B). Tumors harvested on the 19th day of therapy are presented in Figure 5B as a representative example of infiltrating CD45$^+$ cells and their subpopulations. H&E staining showed extensive necrotic areas in tumor tissues in the MBT-treated group. In contrast, no or very small necrotic areas were detected in the PBS-treated group. CD45$^+$ immunostaining revealed higher levels of tumor-infiltrating leukocytes during the whole course of therapy in the MBT-treated group compared to the PBS-treated group (Figure 5B). CD45$^+$ cells were predominantly localized in necrotic areas of the tumor. Furthermore, CD3$^+$ immunohistochemistry staining revealed higher T cell infiltration in the MBT-treated group during the entire course of therapy compared to the PBS-treated group (Figure 5B). Ly6G/Ly6C immunostaining revealed increased infiltration of neutrophils on the 19th day of therapy in the MBT-treated group (Figure 5B).

2.4.3. Interferon Gamma (IFN-γ) and Interleukin 10 (IL-10) Levels Detection in the MBT-Treated Tumors

The high levels of IFN-γ (Figure 5C), low levels of IL-10 (Figure 5C), and high ratio of IFN-γ/IL-10 (Figure 5C) revealed a Th1 shift in the tumor microenvironment in the MBT-treated tumors.

2.5. *In Vitro Analysis of Neutrophil Cytotoxic Effects toward PHEO Cells and Neutrophil-PHEO Cell Interactions Based on Labeling of Tumor Cells with Mannan-BAM*

To verify the positive effect of mannan-BAM binding to PHEO cells on their recognition by innate immune cells, we measured (i) cytotoxic activity of neutrophils on PHEO cells with or without mannan-BAM and (ii) neutrophil-PHEO cell interactions. The cytotoxic experiments using PHEO cell lines (MTT-luciferase and hPheo1) revealed an increased cytotoxic effect of neutrophils toward PHEO cells labeled by mannan-BAM compared to the cells without mannan-BAM (Figure 6A,B). Microscopic evaluation of neutrophils and mannan-BAM-labeled PHEO cells showed enhanced frustrated phagocytosis and neutrophil rosette formation in the mannan-BAM group (Figure 6C).

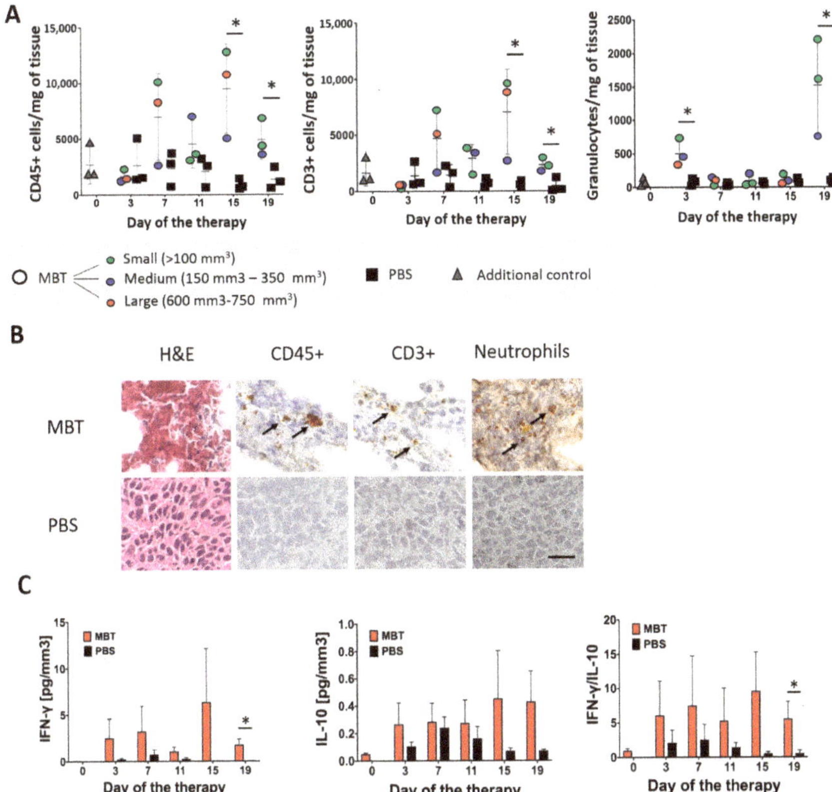

Figure 5. Flow cytometry and immunohistochemistry analysis of tumor-infiltrating leukocytes in the MBT-treated tumors. B6(Cg)-*Tyr*$^{c\text{-}2J}$/J mice were subcutaneously injected with MTT-luciferase cells. After tumors grew to the desired size (about 100 mm^3), mice were randomized into two groups (n = 24/group): (i) the group treated with MBT and (ii) the group treated with PBS. MBT and PBS were given intratumorally on days 0, 1, 2, 8, 9, 10, 16, 17, 18, 24, 25, and 26. Three mice from both groups were sacrificed on days 3, 7, 11, 15, and 19. One half of the harvested subcutaneous tumors was used for flow cytometry analysis of tumor-infiltrating leukocytes and the second half was used for immunohistochemistry analysis of tumor-infiltrating leukocytes. Three mice were sacrificed on day 0 and used as an additional control—gray triangles (no application of any compounds into the tumor). (**A**) The analysis of tumor-infiltrating CD45$^+$ and CD3$^+$ cells revealed their elevation on the 15th and 19th days of therapy in the MBT-treated group. Granulocytes (Ly6G$^+$ cells) were elevated on the 3rd and 19th days of therapy in the MBT-treated group. The results are presented as individual values for each mouse, with a color legend based on the size of the analyzed tumors. (* $p < 0.05$ against PBS). (**B**) Hematoxylin and eosin (H&E) staining and CD45$^+$, CD3$^+$, and Ly6G/Ly6C immunohistochemistry staining were performed on tumor cryosections (a thickness of 8 µm). Bar = 20 µm. (**C**) IFN-γ levels, measured by ELISA from tumor supernatants collected during tumor-infiltrating leukocyte analysis revealed significantly higher levels in the MBT-treated group compared to the PBS-treated group. The IL-10 analysis revealed low levels in both the MBT-treated group and the PBS-treated group. The IFN-γ/IL-10 ratio was significantly higher in the MBT-treated group compared to the PBS-treated group (* $p < 0.05$ against PBS).

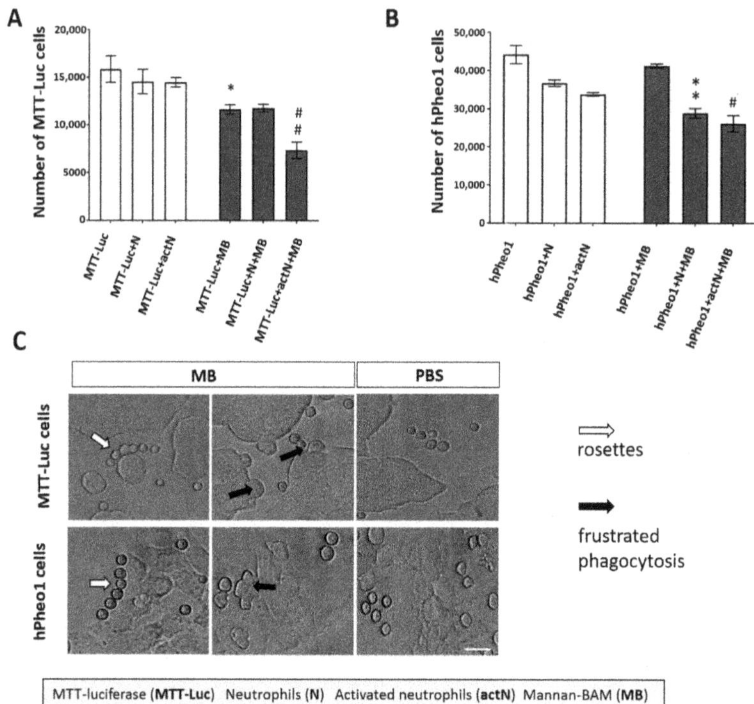

Figure 6. Neutrophil cytotoxicity against PHEO cells labeled with mannan-BAM and neutrophil-PHEO cell interactions. Mouse neutrophils (isolated from bone marrow of B6(Cg)-*Tyr*$^{c-2J}$/J non-tumor-bearing mice) and human neutrophils (isolated from whole blood of healthy donors) were activated by cytokines (granulocyte-macrophages colony-stimulatory factor (GM-CSF), tumor necrosis factor alpha (TNFα), and laminarin) and cultivated with MTT-luciferase and hPheo1 tumor cells with or without mannan-BAM attached to their surface. Mouse neutrophils were mixed with MTT-luciferase cells and human neutrophils were mixed with hPheo1 cells. After two hours of incubation, neutrophils were stained with anti-mouse or anti-human CD45 antibody. One microliter of DAPI was used for the staining of dead cells. Live tumor cells were measured using a BD FACSCanto II analyzer and evaluated using FlowJo software. (**A**) Analysis of mouse neutrophil cytotoxicity against MTT-luciferase cells revealed a statistically significant increase in neutrophil cytotoxicity toward MTT-luciferase cells with mannan-BAM attached to the tumor cell membrane (* $p < 0.05$ against MTT-luciferase (MTT-Luc) group, ## $p < 0.01$ against MTT-luciferase activated neutrophils group (MTT-Luc+actN)). (**B**) Analysis of human neutrophil cytotoxicity against hPheo1 cells revealed a statistically significant increase in neutrophil cytotoxicity toward hPheo1 cells with mannan-BAM attached to the tumor cell membrane (** $p < 0.01$ against hPheo1+neutrophils group (hPheo1+N), # $p < 0.05$ against hPheo1+activated neutrophils group (hPheo+actN)). (**C**) Frustrated phagocytosis (black arrows) and neutrophil rosettes (white arrows) were detected in the group with mannan-BAM attached to the tumor cell membrane. Bar = 100 μm.

2.6. Anti-CD40 Addition Improved Survival in the MBT-Treated Mice

In order to increase the therapeutic effect of MBT in the PHEO mouse model, we decided to combine MBT with an immunostimulatory monoclonal antibody: anti-CD40. Anti-CD40 is an agonist antibody binding to CD40 transmembrane protein expressed on a variety of cells such as macrophages, dendritic cells, and some tumor cells. The interaction of anti-CD40 with CD40 on the surface of immune cells supports their activation and enhances the immune response (Figure 7A).

Interestingly, the beneficial effect of anti-CD40 addition into the MBT therapeutic mixture was not evident during the first 14 days of the therapy (Figure 7B,C). However, the combination of MBT with anti-CD40 (MBTA), in the long term, increased mice survival when compared to the group treated only with MBT (Figure 7D). Moreover, five of eight mice from the MBTA-treated group manifested a complete elimination of subcutaneous tumor, compared to only two of eight mice from the MBT-treated group. A re-challenge experiment, performed with these mice manifested a complete elimination of tumors, revealed resistance against PHEO tumor cell re-injection in both groups, MBT and MBTA (Figure 7E). Interestingly, re-challenged mice initially developed small detectable tumors in the first 14 days; however, after that, all tumors were eradicated with the simultaneous development of skin lesions. These skin lesions were subsequently also eliminated and the whole re-challenged area healed completely.

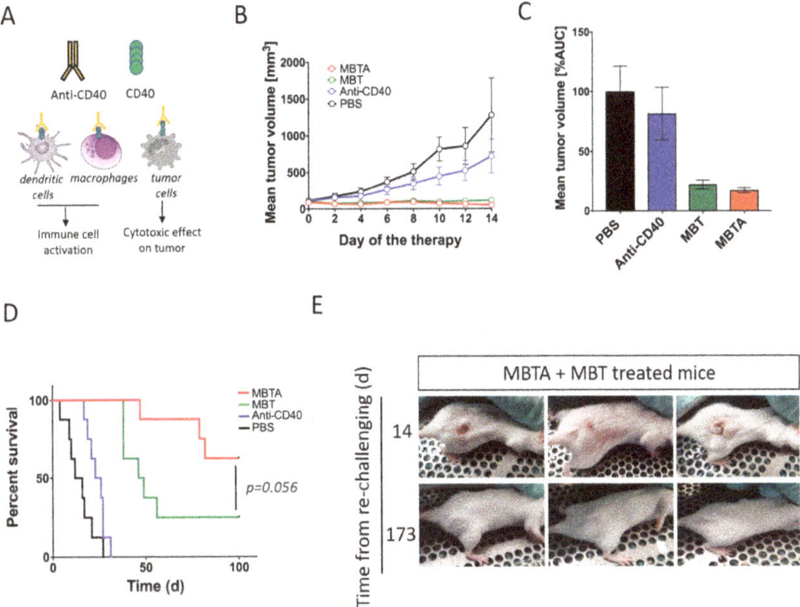

Figure 7. The effect of anti-CD40 addition into MBT therapeutic mixture and re-challenge experiment. B6(Cg)-*Tyr*$^{c-2J}$/J mice were subcutaneously injected with MTT-luciferase cells. After tumors grew to the desired size (about 100 mm^3), mice were randomized into four groups (n = 8/group): (i) the group treated with MBTA, (ii) the group treated with MBT, (iii) the group treated with anti-CD40, and (iv) the group treated with PBS. Therapy was given intratumorally on days 0, 1, 2, 8, 9, 10, 16, 17, 18, 24, 25, and 26. (**A**) Anti-CD40 is an agonist antibody binding to transmembrane protein CD40. CD40 is expressed on variety of cells, such as macrophages, dendritic cells, and some tumor cells. (**B**) The tumor volume growth is presented as a growth curve and (**C**) as an area under the curve (AUC). (**D**) The survival analysis is presented as a Kaplan–Meier curve (p = 0.056). (**E**) Mice with complete tumor elimination from the groups treated with MBTA (n = 5) and with MBT (n = 2) were re-challenged on day 120 (since the start of the therapy) by 3 × 10^6 MTT-luciferase cells. All animals rejected injected tumor cells.

2.7. MBTA Therapy in Metastatic PHEO

Our results from the re-challenge experiment suggested that MBTA therapy activate not only innate immunity but also adaptive immunity. Therefore, we decided to evaluate MBTA therapy in metastatic PHEO. Metastatic PHEO was established by prior subcutaneous injection of MTT cells into the right flank of experimental mice followed by intravenous injection of MTT-luciferase cells into the lateral tail vein (2 weeks after subcutaneous injection). These mice, which developed both subcutaneous tumors as well as metastatic organ lesions (predominantly in the liver), were selected for the subsequent experiment (Figure 8A).

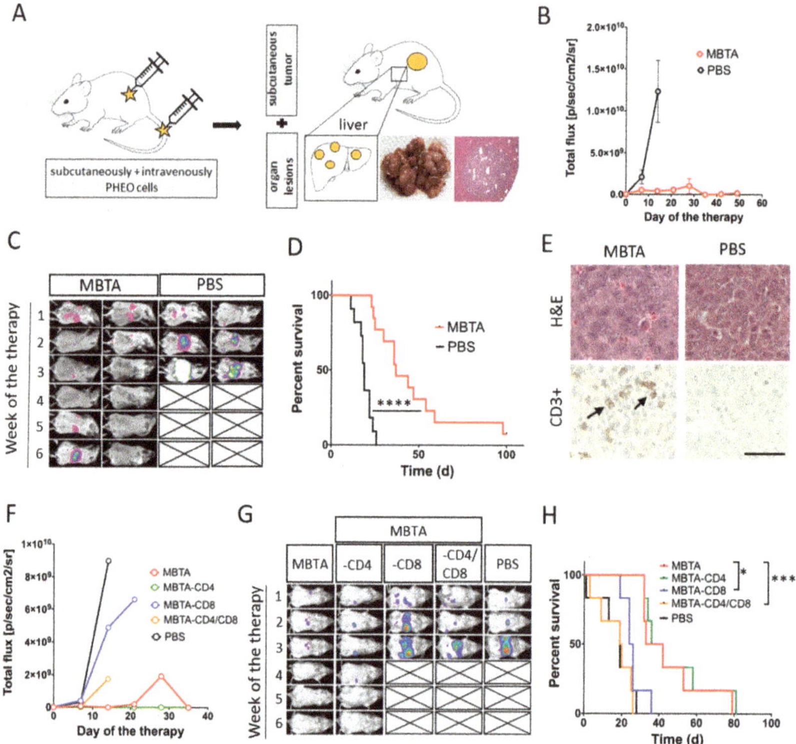

Figure 8. MBTA therapy in metastatic PHEO and the crucial role of $CD8^+$ T cells. (**A**) B6(Cg)-*Tyr*$^{c\text{-}2J}$/J mice were subcutaneously injected with MTT cells, with subsequent injection of MTT-luciferase cells into the lateral tail vein (2 weeks after subcutaneous injection). When mice developed subcutaneous tumors (around 250 mm^3) together with metastatic lesions (predominantly in the liver), they were randomized into two groups: (i) the group treated with MBTA (n = 13) and (ii) the group treated with PBS (n = 12). Therapy was given intratumorally on days 0, 1, 2, 8, 9, 10, 16, 17, 18, 24, 25, and 26. (**B**,**C**) An in vivo bioluminescence assay showed bioluminescence signal intensity inhibition of metastatic organ lesions in the MBTA-treated group compared to the PBS-treated group (p/sec/cm^2/sr = photons/second/cm^2/steradian). (**D**) The survival analysis is presented as a Kaplan–Meier curve (**** $p < 0.0001$ against PBS). (**E**) Immunohistochemistry analysis of $CD3^+$ cells in metastatic organ lesions in the MBTA- and the PBS-treated group revealed strong infiltration by $CD3^+$ cells in the MBTA-treated group. Bar = 20 µm. For the $CD4^+$ and $CD8^+$ T cell depletion experiment, mice with both subcutaneous PHEO tumor and metastatic organ lesions were randomized equally into five groups (n = 6/group): (a) the group treated with MBTA, (b) the group treated with MBTA with intraperitoneal application of anti-CD4, (c) the group treated with MBTA with intraperitoneal application of anti-CD8, (d) the group treated with MBTA with intraperitoneal application of anti-CD4 and anti-CD8, and (e) the group treated with PBS. (**F**,**G**) An in vivo bioluminescence assay showed the important role of $CD8^+$ cells in bioluminescence signal intensity inhibition of metastatic organ lesions during MBTA therapy. Part F is presented without SEM as a result of extensive overlap of SEM error bars. (**H**) The survival analysis is presented as a Kaplan–Meier curve (* $p < 0.05$, *** $p < 0.001$ against MBTA).

When MBTA therapy was tested in this metastatic PHEO (MBTA was applied intratumorally into subcutaneous tumors), we detected lower bioluminescence signal intensity of metastatic organ lesions in the MBTA-treated group compared to the PBS-treated group (Figure 8B,C). In addition, the survival in the MBTA-treated group increased significantly (median survival: 37 days) compared to the PBS-treated group (median survival: 19 days, $p < 0.0001$). Moreover, one mouse from the MBTA-treated group survived for more than 100 days since the beginning of the therapy and manifested a complete regression of metastatic organ lesions (Figure 8D). Histologic sections of metastatic liver lesions showed stronger T cell ($CD3^+$) infiltration in the MBTA-treated group compared to the PBS-treated group (Figure 8E).

We further evaluated the role of T cells, specifically $CD4^+$ and $CD8^+$ T cells, in MBTA therapy. The $CD4^+$ and $CD8^+$ T cell depletion in metastatic PHEO revealed the importance of $CD8^+$ T cells in inhibition of bioluminescence signal intensity of metastatic organ lesions (Figure 8F,G). When $CD8^+$ T cells, alone or simultaneously with CD4+ T cells, were depleted in the MBTA-treated group, the bioluminescence signal intensity of metastatic organ lesions was comparable to the PBS-treated group (Figure 8F,G). The same effect was reflected in survival analysis where the depletion of $CD8^+$ T cells alone (MBTA-CD8) or with $CD4^+$ T cells (MBTA-CD4/CD8) significantly decreased the survival of treated mice (Figure 8H).

3. Discussion

In the present study, we showed that the application of mannan anchored to a tumor cell membrane via BAM along with TLR ligands (R-848, poly(I:C), LTA) (a combination referred as MBT) resulted in the stabilization of subcutaneous PHEO volume and significantly improved mice survival. The crucial role of initial activation of innate immunity during MBT therapy was further verified using B6.CB17-*Prkdc*^{scid}/SzJ mice lacking functional T and B cells. Similar to B6(Cg)-*Tyr*$^{c\text{-}2J}$/J mice, in B6.CB17-*Prkdc*^{scid}/SzJ mice, the subcutaneous PHEO volume remained stable in the MBT-treated group compared to the PBS-treated group. Flow cytometry analysis of tumor-infiltrating leukocytes and in vitro experiments in this model showed the potential role of granulocytes (specifically neutrophils) in innate immunity-induced PHEO elimination. An additional combination of MBT with agonistic anti-CD40 antibody (MBTA) resulted in increased mice survival and increased incidence of complete subcutaneous PHEO elimination. Interestingly, a re-challenge experiment in animals with the complete elimination of subcutaneous PHEO showed a generation of an excellent memory immune response with subsequent rejection of MTT-luciferase cells. To verify the activation of specific immunity (which was suggested by the observed immune memory response), we performed an experiment in a metastatic PHEO mouse model, where MBTA therapy resulted in lower bioluminescence signal intensity of metastatic organ lesions compared to the PBS-treated group. The subsequent $CD4^+$ and $CD8^+$ T cell depletion experiment confirmed the role of $CD8^+$ T cells in this bioluminescence signal intensity inhibition of metastatic organ lesions.

As a first step, we developed a mouse model of PHEO for immunotherapy testing with an option to inject PHEO tumor cells subcutaneously or intravenously. We used the B6(Cg)-*Tyr*$^{c\text{-}2J}$/J mouse strain injected with MTT or MTT-luciferase cells. MTT cells were originally developed from liver metastases arising from MPC cells injected intravenously [31]. Moreover, this PHEO mouse model is known to release catecholamines from experimental tumors resembling PHEOs found in patients. However, there are two main limitations arising from the practical use of this PHEO mouse model: (i) a long waiting period from tumor cell injection to tumor formation and (ii) very inconsistent tumor growth, which caused difficulties with the randomization of mice into the groups, resulting in lower numbers of mice per group.

After establishing a subcutaneous PHEO mouse model, we initiated the evaluation of MBT immunotherapy in PHEO. The MBT immunotherapy was previously tested in a melanoma mouse model and a very challenging pancreatic adenocarcinoma mouse model. Specifically, in the melanoma mouse model, MBT immunotherapy resulted in an 83% survival rate of treated mice with a potential anti-metastatic effect [17]. In pancreatic adenocarcinoma, MBT immunotherapy resulted in the suppression of metastases growth, but no increase in the survival rate of treated mice was detected [17].

In a PHEO mouse model, MBT therapy resulted in a subcutaneous PHEO volume stabilization compared to the PBS-treated group. The strategy of promoting an anti-tumor immune response using TLR ligands is well known and was previously successfully tested in many types of tumors [32–34]. However, our concept is unique, because of the specific combination of TLR ligands (particularly TLR2, TLR3, and TLR7/8), which seems to have an extraordinary effect on innate immunity activation and tumor elimination, as previously presented in melanoma and pancreatic adenocarcinoma mouse models [15–17]. Moreover, an additional anti-tumor effect of TLR ligands in this novel concept is provided by a combination with phagocytosis-stimulating ligands, such as mannan, bound to the tumor cell surface [15–17].

To further investigate the role of innate and adaptive immunity in the stabilization of subcutaneous PHEO volume during MBT immunotherapy, we used mice lacking functional T and B cells (B6.CB17-Prkdc^{scid}/SzJ mice) and, therefore, lacking basic adaptive immunity function. The stabilization of PHEO volume in mice lacking adaptive immunity treated with MBT was comparable to the stabilization of PHEO volume in a mouse model with a fully functional immune system. These results clearly suggest that innate immunity is crucial for stabilization of subcutaneous PHEO volume during MBT immunotherapy.

In order to characterize the underlying innate immunity mechanisms and tumor environment during MBT therapy in subcutaneous PHEO, we analyzed tumor-infiltrating leukocytes in the MBT- and the PBS-treated groups. In the MBT-treated group, we observed a higher level of tumor-infiltrating leukocytes compared to the PBS-treated group. Tumor-infiltrating leukocytes were mainly represented by T cells and granulocytes. As demonstrated in previous experiments with mice lacking functional T and B cells, T cells do not seem to have an important role in the initial elimination of subcutaneous PHEO, so we decided to further focus on the role of granulocytes in this model.

The high ratio of IFN-γ and IL-10 in the MBT-treated tumors indicates that the Th1 polarization of the tumor environment. In general, the tumor environment can be characterized by Th1 or Th2 polarization. Th2 polarization is considered to favor tumor growth (e.g., promoting angiogenesis, inhibiting cell-mediated immunity and tumor cell killing), whereas Th1 polarization exerts antitumor effects [35]. It was also described previously that PHEO/PGL tumors present high levels of M2 macrophage fractions, leading to Th2 polarization and the promotion of tumor angiogenesis [6]. TLRs are known to play crucial roles in immune response polarization. The activation of TLR3 and TLR7 triggers Th1 polarization in a tumor through increased IL-12, IL-23, and type I IFN production [36].

In vitro cytotoxicity experiments confirmed the importance of mannan-BAM bound to the PHEO cell membrane. The decision to use neutrophils, as the most abundant granulocytes, for these in vitro experiments was based on our tumor-infiltrating leukocyte analysis results as described previously. The increase in neutrophil cytotoxicity was dependent on the presence of mannan-BAM attached to the PHEO cells. Moreover, the presence of complement proteins in the tumor-neutrophils reaction environment (ensured by non-heat inactivated fetal bovine serum (FBS) addition) was crucial for the recognition of tumor cells with mannan-BAM and subsequent neutrophil cytotoxicity toward them.

Moreover, the participation of frustrated phagocytosis in PHEO cell elimination was fully dependent on the presence of mannan-BAM. The same findings were observed in the melanoma model when mannan-BAM was used [37].

From the aforementioned results, we concluded that MBT immunotherapy is effective for the stabilization of subcutaneous PHEO volume and for improvement in survival in mouse models with a robust initial activation of innate immunity. However, the biggest challenge in PHEO is metastatic disease. Therefore, in the next part of our study, we focused on how to simultaneously boost activation of adaptive immunity in MBT immunotherapy to achieve a systematic anti-tumor response with subsequent metastatic organ lesion elimination.

In the first step, we chose the anti-CD40 antibody to boost activation of adaptive immunity. The Anti-CD40 agonistic antibody supports the activation of antigen presenting cells, such as B and T cells, dendritic cells, and macrophages, and so establishes an effective humoral and cellular immune response [38]. The combination of anti-CD40 with MBT applied in a pancreatic adenocarcinoma mouse model resulted in an 80% survival rate, which represented significant improvement compared to the MBT therapy without anti-CD40 [17]. In a PHEO mouse model, the combination of the anti-CD40 antibody with MBT increased the incidence of complete elimination of subcutaneous tumors and improved the overall survival of the treated mice. This effect can be explained by the support of tumor antigen presentation and the stronger participation of adaptive immunity via anti-CD40 [39]. A similar effect was previously reported, when the combination of TLR ligands with anti-CD40 significantly stimulated $CD8^+$ T cell responses and induced the migration of activated dendritic cells with a promotion in their capacity to present antigens [40,41]. The activation of adaptive immunity with the subsequent generation of a memory immune response was further verified by a re-challenge experiment in animals with a complete elimination of subcutaneous PHEO from the MBT- and MBTA-treated groups. All re-challenged mice rejected injected PHEO cells, which suggests that the MBT-treated mice also manifest partial activation of adaptive immunity. However, anti-CD40 beneficially boosted adaptive immunity, since 62.5% of mice in the MBTA-treated group completely eliminated subcutaneous PHEO compared to only 25% of mice in the MBT-treated group.

To further support our hypothesis of the adaptive immunity activation during MBTA immunotherapy, we tested MBTA immunotherapy in metastatic PHEO. MBTA immunotherapy resulted in a lower bioluminescence signal intensity of metastatic organ lesions compared to the PBS-treated group and in a significant prolongation of mice survival. Moreover, in this experiment, we observed an interesting phenomenon. Mice with fast initial elimination of subcutaneous tumors (complete elimination in the first week of MBTA therapy) manifested decreased bioluminescence signal intensity inhibition of metastatic organ lesions compared to those where subcutaneous tumors persisted during the first three weeks of MBTA therapy. This observation can be explained by insufficient activation of adaptive immunity caused by short-lasting tumor antigen stimulation since the main source of tumor antigens (the subcutaneous tumor) was eliminated very shortly after MBTA therapy initiation. This is also consistent with principles of tumor vaccines, where repeated applications of these vaccines are usually needed to develop a strong adaptive immune response [42,43]. Since we partially predicted this situation, we decided in advance to enroll mice with higher subcutaneous tumor volume (around 250 mm^3) compared to the previous experiments to provide enough tumor mass for tumor antigen release and adaptive immunity stimulation. The crucial role of T cells in the inhibition of bioluminescence signal intensity of metastatic organ lesions was further verified in the $CD4^+$ and $CD8^+$ T cell depletion experiment. The depletion of $CD8^+$ T cells, alone or both $CD4^+$ and $CD8^+$ T cells resulted in decreased survival and decreased bioluminescence signal intensity inhibition of metastatic organ lesions compared to the group treated by MTBA without depletion. These finding are consistent with several studies, where the importance of $CD8^+$ T cells on visceral disease was also highlighted [44,45].

Although the presented data may be important for future metastatic PHEO/PGL treatment, one important concern must be addressed. This therapy requires a direct application of MBT or MBTA into a tumor. Initially, this could be considered a limitation, particularly for metastatic PHEO/PGL, because metastases are exclusively found in deep organs, lymph nodes, or bones. However, current interventional radiology approaches are capable of treating metastases, even in those problematic locations [46]. Moreover, local therapy offers certain advantages over systemic therapies, such as a delivery of higher concentrations of the drug into the tumor, minimal systemic side effects, no required tumor antigen identification, in situ vaccination by tumor authentic antigens, no pretreatment biopsy, no major histocompatibility complex (MHC) restriction, polyclonal T and B cell stimulation, and low cost [4,47].

We also acknowledge that there are unanswered questions regarding the underlying immune mechanisms during the presented therapy. Therefore, our future directions involve a deeper understanding of adaptive immunity participation during MBTA therapy and its maximal boost for better control of metastatic organ lesion growth. Moreover, a possible combination of MBTA therapy with other therapies will be considered. There may be great potential in the combination of MBTA with checkpoint inhibitors, as MBTA can support the initial infiltration of leukocytes into the tumor or metastatic organ lesions. This can be especially beneficial, since PHEO/PGL are tumors with a low lymphocyte fraction [6] and the prediction for checkpoint inhibitor therapy, as a single treatment, is thus not favorable [48–50]. Interestingly, certain subsets of PHEO/PGL tumors showed programed cell death 1 (PD-L1) and programed cell death 2 (PD-L2) expression [51]. In these specific PHEO/PGL subsets, the combination of MBTA with checkpoint inhibitor therapy can potentially intensify the therapeutic response. The doors are also open to a possible combination of MBTA therapy with radiotherapy and/or chemotherapy [52].

4. Materials and Methods

4.1. Mannan-BAM Synthesis

Mannan-BAM synthesis was performed as previously reported [15–17]. Mannan was obtained from Sigma-Aldrich, Saint Louis, MO, USA. BAM was obtained from NOF Corporation, White Plains, NY, USA.

4.2. Cell Lines

MTT, MTT-luciferase, and human hPheo1 cell lines were used in this study [30,31]. MTT and MTT-luciferase cells are rapidly growing cells derived from liver metastases of MPC cells, and MTT-luciferase cells are transfected by a luciferase plasmid [30,31]. hPheo1 (obtained from University of Texas, Southwestern Medical Center, Dr. Hans Kumar Ghayee, D.O., MTA# 41611) is a progenitor cell line derived from human PHEO [53].

MTT and MTT-luciferase cells were maintained in Dulbecco's modified eagle media (DMEM) (Sigma-Aldrich) supplemented with 10% heat-inactivated fetal bovine serum (Gemini, West Sacramento, CA, USA) and penicillin/streptomycin (100 U/mL; Gemini). In MTT-luciferase cells, geneticin (750 μg/mL; Thermo Fisher Scientific, Waltham, MA, USA) was used for stable cell line selection. hPheo1 cells were maintained in RPMI (Sigma-Aldrich) supplemented with 10% heat-inactivated fetal bovine serum and penicillin/streptomycin (100 U/mL). Both cell lines were cultured at 37 °C in humidified air with 5% CO_2.

All cell lines used were routinely tested for mycoplasma using the MycoAlert^{TM} detection kit (Lonza, Walkersville, MD, USA). Cell authentication was performed per ATCC guidelines using morphology, growth curves, and mycoplasma testing. After thawing, cells were cultured for no longer than 3 weeks.

4.3. Establishment of a PHEO Mouse Model and Tumor Cell Injection

Female B6(Cg)-*Tyr*$^{c\text{-}2J}$/J and B6.CB17-*Prkdc*^{scid}/SzJ mice were purchased from the Jackson Laboratory, Bar Harbor, ME, USA. B6(Cg)-*Tyr*$^{c\text{-}2J}$/J mice were used for subcutaneous and metastatic PHEO and represent mouse models with fully functional immune systems. B6.CB17-*Prkdc*^{scid}/SzJ mice lacking functional T and B cells were used for subcutaneous PHEO and represent mouse models with dysfunctional adaptive immunity. Mice were housed in specific pathogen-free conditions and all experiments were approved by the *Eunice Kennedy Shriver* National Institute of Child Health and Human Development animal protocol (ASP: 15 028).

For subcutaneous PHEO, B6(Cg)-*Tyr*$^{c\text{-}2J}$/J and B6.CB17-*Prkdc*^{scid}/SzJ mice were subcutaneously injected in the right lower dorsal site with 3×10^6 and 1.5×10^6 MTT-luciferase cells in 0.2 mL of DMEM without additives, respectively. For metastatic PHEO, B6(Cg)-*Tyr*$^{c\text{-}2J}$/J mice were also subcutaneously injected in the right lower dorsal site with 3×10^6 MTT cells in 0.2 mL of DMEM without additives and were simultaneously injected intravenously with 1.5×10^6 MTT-luciferase cells in 0.1 mL of PBS. MTT cells without luciferase where used for the establishment of subcutaneous PHEO to prevent the possibility that the signal from MTT-luciferase cells in large subcutaneous tumors will cover the signal from small metastatic organ lesions during bioluminescence imaging.

For a re-challenge experiment, 3×10^6 MTT-luciferase cells in 0.2 mL of DMEM without additives were injected subcutaneously on day 120 since the beginning of therapy in the animals manifested a complete elimination of tumors due to used immunotherapy.

4.4. Treatment

Treatment in subcutaneous PHEO was initiated when subcutaneous tumors reached an average volume of 100 mm^3 in B6(Cg)-*Tyr*$^{c\text{-}2J}$/J mice. In B6.CB17-*Prkdc*^{scid}/SzJ mice, lacking functional T and B cells, the treatment was initiated with a lower tumor volume (average volume of 50 mm^3) to prevent the potential early reach of a tumor endpoint size as a result of the rapid growth of subcutaneous PHEO in mice with a specific immunity disfunction. Treatment in metastatic PHEO was initiated when subcutaneous tumors reached an average volume of 250 mm^3 with a simultaneous presence of detectable signal in organs using bioluminescence imaging. This greater starting tumor volume was purposely chosen to ensure enough tumor mass for tumor antigen gradual release during the whole course of the therapy. Mice, with both subcutaneous PHEO and metastatic PHEO, were treated intratumorally (into the subcutaneous tumor) on days 0, 1, 2, 8, 9, 10, 16, 17, 18, 24, 25, and 26 with 50 μL of the following mixtures: (a) 0.5 mg of R-848 hydrogen chloride (HCl) (Tocris, Minneapolis, MN, USA), 0.5 mg of poly(I:C) (Sigma-Aldrich), 0.5 mg of LTA/mL (Sigma-Aldrich), and 0.2 mM mannan-BAM (MBT), and later on in combination with anti-CD40, clone FGK4.5/FGK45 (BioXCell, West Lebanon, NH, USA) (MBTA), in PBS; and (b) PBS.

4.5. Tumor Size Evaluation

Subcutaneous tumor volume was measured every other day with a caliper and calculated as $V = (\pi/6)\ AB^2$ (A and B = the largest and the smallest dimension of the tumor, respectively) [54]. Survival curves are based on the time of death caused by tumor growth or on the time of sacrifice of mice reaching the maximally allowed tumor size of 2 cm in diameter.

In metastatic PHEO, mice were imaged by an IVIS system (Bruker, Billerica, MA, USA) once a week to detect a bioluminescence signal intensity of metastatic organ lesions, and the signal was evaluated using Bruker MI SE software.

4.6. Urine Catecholamine Determination

Urine specimens from B6(Cg)-*Tyr*$^{c\text{-}2J}$/J tumor-bearing mice were collected after subcutaneous or intravenous injection of MTT-luciferase cells. B6(Cg)-*Tyr*$^{c\text{-}2J}$/J mice without tumors were used as controls. All specimens were collected at the same time of the day to prevent any variance in catecholamine levels caused by circadian rhythms. Urine catecholamines (norepinephrine, epinephrine, and dopamine) were analyzed by liquid chromatography with electrochemical detection as described previously [55].

4.7. Analysis of Tumor Infiltrating Leukocytes and Spleen Leukocytes

B6(Cg)-*Tyr*$^{c\text{-}2J}$/J tumor-bearing mice were euthanized by cervical dislocation. Tumors were harvested from the body. Tumors were washed in cold DMEM and cut into small pieces. For tumor cell dissociation, a tumor dissociation kit (Miltenyi Biotech, Auburn, CA, USA) was used. One hour after incubation in 37 °C with constant agitation, samples were centrifuged. Supernatant was collected and used for the detection of cytokines (interferon gamma (IFN-γ) and interleukin 10 (IL-10)) by an enzyme-linked immunosorbent assay (ELISA). The tumor cell pellet was passed through a 70 μm strainer. The red blood cells were removed using ammonium-chloride-potassium (ACK) lysing buffer (Thermo Fisher Scientific). Leukocytes ($CD45^+$ cells) and their subpopulations were stained using the following antibodies: APC anti-mouse CD45, clone: 30-F11 (BioLegend, Dedham, MA, USA); Brilliant Violet 650 anti-mouse CD19, clone: 6D5 (BioLegend); FITC anti-mouse CD3, clone: 17A2

(BioLegend); Brilliant Violet 605 anti-mouse CD4, clone: RM4-5 (BioLegend); APC/Cy7 anti-mouse CD8a, clone: 53-6.7 (BioLegend); PE/Cy7 anti-mouse Ly-6G/Ly-6C (GR-1), clone: RB6-8C5 (BioLegend); PE anti-mouse NK-1.1, clone: PK136 (BioLegend); and Brilliant Violet 421 anti-mouse F4/80, clone: BM8 (BioLegend). LIVE/DEAD® fixable yellow dead cell stain (Invitrogen, Carlsbad, CA, USA) was used to eliminate dead cells. Samples were measured using a BD Fortessa analyzer (San Jose, CA, USA) and evaluated with FlowJo software (Ashland, OR, USA). CountBright absolute counting beads (Invitrogen) were used to count absolute numbers of individual $CD45^+$ cells.

4.8. Cytokine Assay

Supernatant collected during the analysis of tumor infiltrating leukocytes was used to measure INF-γ and IL-10 levels in the tumors during the therapy. The following ELISA kits were used for the detection: IFN-γ Mouse ELISA Kit, Extra Sensitive (Thermo Fisher), and Mouse IL-10 ELISA Kit (LSBio, Seattle, WA, USA).

4.9. Immunohistochemistry

Tumor tissue samples embedded in Tissue-Tek optimum cutting temperature (OCT) were sectioned by a microtome-cryostat (8 µm). Formalin fixed, paraffin-embedded tissue specimen was prepared for 5 µm sections. Frozen sections were fixed in HistoChoice MB tissue Fixative solution (Ambresco, Cleveland, OH, USA). Subsequently in both frozen and paraffin-embedded sections, peroxidase activity was inhibited by 3% hydrogen peroxide. Additionally, samples were blocked using SuperBlock blocking buffer (Thermo Fisher Scientific). Anti-mouse CD45 antibody, anti-mouse Ly6G/Ly6C antibody, and anti-mouse CD3 antibody (Abcam, Cambridge, MA, USA) were used for immunohistochemistry staining. The signal was developed by diaminobenzidine (DAB) substrate (Dako, Santa Clara, CA, USA).

4.10. Neutrophil Cytotoxicity toward PHEO Cells

Bone marrow from B6(Cg)-$Tyr^{c\text{-}2J}$/J non-tumor-bearing mice was used as a source of mouse neutrophils. Bone marrow isolation was performed according to Stassen et al. [56]. Untouched mouse neutrophils were isolated by magnetic-activated cell sorting using a neutrophil isolation kit (Miltenyi Biotec). Human neutrophils were isolated from whole blood of healthy donors received from the National Institutes of Health (NIH) Blood Bank using an EasySep Direct Human Neutrophils Isolation kit (Stemcell Technologies, Cambridge, MA, USA). Both human and mouse neutrophils were activated for 20 min by a mixture of GM-CSF (12 ng/mL) (Sigma-Aldrich), TNFα (2.5 ng/mL) (Sigma-Aldrich), and 2 µM laminarin (Sigma) as previously described [57].

MTT-luciferase or hPheo1 cells were incubated with 0.02 mM mannan-BAM in culture medium for 30 min in 37 °C. After incubation and washing by centrifugation, mouse MTT-luciferase cells were co-cultured with activated or non-activated murine neutrophils and human hPheo1 cells with activated or non-inactivated human neutrophils for 2 h in 37 °C. The tumor cell/neutrophil ratio was 1:5 (50,000 tumor cells to 250,000 neutrophils). Dead cells were stained with DAPI (1 µM) (Invitrogen). APC anti-mouse CD45 antibody, clone 30-F11 (BioLegend), and APC anti-human CD45 antibody, clone H130 (BioLegend), were used to stain leukocytes (in this specific case neutrophils). CountBright absolute counting beads (Invitrogen) were used to count absolute numbers of live tumor cells in the samples. Samples were measured by FACSCantoII. FlowJo software was used for analysis.

4.11. Imaging of PHEO Cell–Neutrophil Interactions

Adhered hPheo1 or MTT-luciferase cells were incubated with 0.02 mM mannan-BAM in culture medium for 30 min in 37 °C. Following incubation, unbound mannan-BAM was washed by centrifugation and human neutrophils were added to the hPheo1 cells and mouse neutrophils to the MTT-luciferase cells (the ratio of tumor cells to neutrophils was 1:2 (50,000 tumor cells:100,000 neutrophils). Neutrophils and hPheo1/MTT-luciferase cell interactions were documented after 2 h of co-culturing in 37 °C. A Leica DMRB microscope and Leica LAS AF software were used for analysis.

4.12. Depletions

Cellular subsets were depleted by administering 300 μg of depleting antibody intraperitoneally twice weekly starting one day prior to immunotherapy: $CD8^+$ T-cells with anti-CD8α, clone 2.43 (BioXCell), and $CD4^+$ T-cells with anti-CD4, clone GK1.5 (BioXCell). Cellular depletion of $CD8^+$ and $CD4^+$ T-cells were confirmed by flow cytometry of PBMC blood levels (Figure S3). Samples were measured by FACSCantoII. FlowJo software was used for analysis.

4.13. Statistical Analysis

Data were analyzed using STATISTICA 12 (StatSoft, Tulsa, OK, USA) or Prism 7 (GraphPad Software, San Diego, CA, USA). Individual data sets were compared using a dependent/independent Student's t-test. Analyses across multiple groups and times were performed using repeated measures ANOVA (for data with normal distribution) with individual groups assessed using Tukey's multiple comparison. For data without normal distribution, non-parametric ANOVA was used with individual groups were assessed by Kruskal–Wallis test. Kaplan–Meier survival curves were compared using a log-rank test. Error bars indicate the standard error of the mean (SEM). * $p < 0.05$; ** $p < 0.01$; *** $p < 0.001$; **** $p < 0.0001$. # $p < 0.05$; ## $p < 0.01$.

5. Conclusions

We demonstrate here promising therapeutic effects of enhanced innate immunity with subsequent activation of adaptive immunity using intratumoral application of ligands stimulating phagocytosis combined with TLR ligands in subcutaneous and metastatic PHEO in mouse models. This effect was verified in vitro in mouse PHEO and human PHEO cell lines. We suggest that this immunotherapeutic approach could potentially become a novel treatment option in patients with metastatic PHEO/PGL.

Supplementary Materials: The following are available online at http://www.mdpi.com/2072-6694/11/5/654/s1. Figure S1: Urine dopamine and epinephrine levels in the subcutaneous and metastatic PHEO, Figure S2: Tumor CD4+, CD8+, CD19+, F4/80+, and NK cells levels in the course of MBT therapy, Figure S3: Depletion of CD4+ and CD8+ T cells during MBTA therapy.

Author Contributions: Conceptualization: V.C., J.Z., and K.P.; methodology: V.C., J.Z., and K.P.; validation: V.C.; formal analysis: V.C.; investigation: V.C., L.L., G.G., I.J., TT.H., L.A. and M.M.; resources: G.N., X.C., H.K.G., and K.P.; writing—original draft preparation: V.C.; writing—review and editing: V.C., L.L., G.G., A.J., O.U., Y.P., H.K.G., D.T., Z.Z., J.Z., and K.P.; visualization: V.C.; supervision: J.Z. and K.P.; project administration: V.C. and K.P.; funding acquisition: K.P.

Funding: This research was supported by the Intratumoral Research Program of the National Institutes of Health, *Eunice Kennedy Shiver* National Institutes of Child Health and Human Development (grant number ZIAHD008735).

Acknowledgments: The authors would like to thank Pradeep K. Dagur, and Ankit Saxena, for their technical assistance during flow cytometry analyses, as well as the staff of the Flow Cytometry Core, National Heart, Lung, and Blood Institute, NIH, MD 20892. The authors would also like to thank Dale Kiesewetter, Laboratory of Molecular Imaging and Nanomedicine, National Institute of Biomedical Imaging and Bioengineering, National Institutes of Health, Bethesda, Maryland, MD, USA, for his assistance during the bioluminescence imaging of experimental mice.

Conflicts of Interest: The authors declare no conflict of interest.

References

1. Lenders, J.W.; Eisenhofer, G.; Mannelli, M.; Pacak, K. Phaeochromocytoma. *Lancet* **2005**, *366*, 665–675. [CrossRef]
2. Crona, J.; Taieb, D.; Pacak, K. New Perspectives on Pheochromocytoma and Paraganglioma: Toward a Molecular Classification. *Endocr. Rev.* **2017**, *38*, 489–515. [CrossRef]

3. Mellman, I.; Coukos, G.; Dranoff, G. Cancer immunotherapy comes of age. *Nature* **2011**, *480*, 480–489. [CrossRef]
4. Marabelle, A.; Tselikas, L.; de Baere, T.; Houot, R. Intratumoral immunotherapy: Using the tumor as the remedy. *Ann. Oncol.* **2017**, *28*, xii33–xii43. [CrossRef] [PubMed]
5. Fishbein, L.; Leshchiner, I.; Walter, V.; Danilova, L.; Robertson, A.G.; Johnson, A.R.; Lichtenberg, T.M.; Murray, B.A.; Ghayee, H.K.; Else, T.; et al. Comprehensive Molecular Characterization of Pheochromocytoma and Paraganglioma. *Cancer Cell* **2017**, *31*, 181–193. [CrossRef] [PubMed]
6. Thorsson, V.; Gibbs, D.L.; Brown, S.D.; Wolf, D.; Bortone, D.S.; Ou Yang, T.H.; Porta-Pardo, E.; Gao, G.F.; Plaisier, C.L.; Eddy, J.A.; et al. The Immune Landscape of Cancer. *Immunity* **2018**, *48*, 812–830. [CrossRef]
7. Wood, M.A.; Paralkar, M.; Paralkar, M.P.; Nguyen, A.; Struck, A.J.; Ellrott, K.; Margolin, A.; Nellore, A.; Thompson, R.F. Population-level distribution and putative immunogenicity of cancer neoepitopes. *BMC Cancer* **2018**, *18*, 414. [CrossRef] [PubMed]
8. Papewalis, C.; Kouatchoua, C.; Ehlers, M.; Jacobs, B.; Porwol, D.; Schinner, S.; Willenberg, H.S.; Anlauf, M.; Raffel, A.; Eisenhofer, G.; et al. Chromogranin A as potential target for immunotherapy of malignant pheochromocytoma. *Mol. Cell. Endocrinol.* **2011**, *335*, 69–77. [CrossRef]
9. Gubin, M.M.; Zhang, X.; Schuster, H.; Caron, E.; Ward, J.P.; Noguchi, T.; Ivanova, Y.; Hundal, J.; Arthur, C.D.; Krebber, W.J.; et al. Checkpoint blockade cancer immunotherapy targets tumour-specific mutant antigens. *Nature* **2014**, *515*, 577–581. [CrossRef]
10. Rosenberg, S.A.; Restifo, N.P. Adoptive cell transfer as personalized immunotherapy for human cancer. *Science* **2015**, *348*, 62–68. [CrossRef]
11. Corrales, L.; Matson, V.; Flood, B.; Spranger, S.; Gajewski, T.F. Innate immune signaling and regulation in cancer immunotherapy. *Cell Res.* **2017**, *27*, 96–108. [CrossRef] [PubMed]
12. Coley, W.B. The treatment of malignant tumors by repeated inoculations of erysipelas. With a report of ten original cases. 1893. *Clin. Orthop. Relat. Res.* **1991**, 3–11.
13. Akira, S.; Uematsu, S.; Takeuchi, O. Pathogen recognition and innate immunity. *Cell* **2006**, *124*, 783–801. [CrossRef]
14. Herr, H.W.; Morales, A. History of bacillus Calmette-Guerin and bladder cancer: An immunotherapy success story. *J. Urol.* **2008**, *179*, 53–56. [CrossRef]
15. Janotova, T.; Jalovecka, M.; Auerova, M.; Svecova, I.; Bruzlova, P.; Maierova, V.; Kumzakova, Z.; Cunatova, S.; Vlckova, Z.; Caisova, V.; et al. The use of anchored agonists of phagocytic receptors for cancer immunotherapy: B16-F10 murine melanoma model. *PLoS ONE* **2014**, *9*, e85222. [CrossRef]
16. Caisova, V.; Vieru, A.; Kumzakova, Z.; Glaserova, S.; Husnikova, H.; Vacova, N.; Krejcova, G.; Padoukova, L.; Jochmanova, I.; Wolf, K.I.; et al. Innate immunity based cancer immunotherapy: B16-F10 murine melanoma model. *BMC Cancer* **2016**, *16*, 940. [CrossRef]
17. Caisova, V.; Uher, O.; Nedbalova, P.; Jochmanova, I.; Kvardova, K.; Masakova, K.; Krejcova, G.; Padoukova, L.; Chmelar, J.; Kopecky, J.; et al. Effective cancer immunotherapy based on combination of TLR agonists with stimulation of phagocytosis. *Int. Immunopharmacol.* **2018**, *59*, 86–96. [CrossRef]
18. Stahl, P.D.; Ezekowitz, R.A. The mannose receptor is a pattern recognition receptor involved in host defense. *Curr. Opin. Immunol.* **1998**, *10*, 50–55. [CrossRef]
19. Freeman, S.A.; Grinstein, S. Phagocytosis: Receptors, signal integration, and the cytoskeleton. *Immunol. Rev.* **2014**, *262*, 193–215. [CrossRef]
20. Garred, P.; Genster, N.; Pilely, K.; Bayarri-Olmos, R.; Rosbjerg, A.; Ma, Y.J.; Skjoedt, M.O. A journey through the lectin pathway of complement-MBL and beyond. *Immunol. Rev.* **2016**, *274*, 74–97. [CrossRef]
21. Fujita, T.; Matsushita, M.; Endo, Y. The lectin-complement pathway-its role in innate immunity and evolution. *Immunol. Rev.* **2004**, *198*, 185–202. [CrossRef] [PubMed]
22. Reis, E.S.; Mastellos, D.C.; Ricklin, D.; Mantovani, A.; Lambris, J.D. Complement in cancer: Untangling an intricate relationship. *Nat. Rev. Immunol.* **2018**, *18*, 5–18. [CrossRef] [PubMed]
23. Medzhitov, R. Toll-like receptors and innate immunity. *Nat. Rev. Immunol.* **2001**, *1*, 135–145. [CrossRef] [PubMed]
24. Takeda, K.; Akira, S. Toll-like receptors in innate immunity. *Int. Immunol.* **2005**, *17*, 1–14. [CrossRef] [PubMed]
25. Kawasaki, T.; Kawai, T. Toll-like receptor signaling pathways. *Front. Immunol.* **2014**, *5*, 461. [CrossRef] [PubMed]

26. Kauffman, E.C.; Liu, H.; Schwartz, M.J.; Scherr, D.S. Toll-like receptor 7 agonist therapy with imidazoquinoline enhances cancer cell death and increases lymphocytic infiltration and proinflammatory cytokine production in established tumors of a renal cell carcinoma mouse model. *J. Oncol.* **2012**, *2012*, 103298. [CrossRef] [PubMed]
27. Wu, J.J.; Huang, D.B.; Tyring, S.K. Resiquimod: A new immune response modifier with potential as a vaccine adjuvant for Th1 immune responses. *Antiviral. Res.* **2004**, *64*, 79–83. [CrossRef]
28. Matsumoto, M.; Seya, T. TLR3: Interferon induction by double-stranded RNA including poly(I:C). *Adv. Drug Deliv. Rev.* **2008**, *60*, 805–812. [CrossRef]
29. Seo, H.S.; Michalek, S.M.; Nahm, M.H. Lipoteichoic acid is important in innate immune responses to gram-positive bacteria. *Infect. Immun.* **2008**, *76*, 206–213. [CrossRef]
30. Martiniova, L.; Lai, E.W.; Elkahloun, A.G.; Abu-Asab, M.; Wickremasinghe, A.; Solis, D.C.; Perera, S.M.; Huynh, T.T.; Lubensky, I.A.; Tischler, A.S.; et al. Characterization of an animal model of aggressive metastatic pheochromocytoma linked to a specific gene signature. *Clin. Exp. Metastasis* **2009**, *26*, 239–250. [CrossRef]
31. Korpershoek, E.; Pacak, K.; Martiniova, L. Murine models and cell lines for the investigation of pheochromocytoma: Applications for future therapies? *Endocr. Pathol.* **2012**, *23*, 43–54. [CrossRef] [PubMed]
32. Cai, Z.; Sanchez, A.; Shi, Z.; Zhang, T.; Liu, M.; Zhang, D. Activation of Toll-like receptor 5 on breast cancer cells by flagellin suppresses cell proliferation and tumor growth. *Cancer Res.* **2011**, *71*, 2466–2475. [CrossRef] [PubMed]
33. Liu, C.Y.; Xu, J.Y.; Shi, X.Y.; Huang, W.; Ruan, T.Y.; Xie, P.; Ding, J.L. M2-polarized tumor-associated macrophages promoted epithelial-mesenchymal transition in pancreatic cancer cells, partially through TLR4/IL-10 signaling pathway. *Lab. Invest.* **2013**, *93*, 844–854. [CrossRef] [PubMed]
34. Sagiv-Barfi, I.; Czerwinski, D.K.; Levy, S.; Alam, I.S.; Mayer, A.T.; Gambhir, S.S.; Levy, R. Eradication of spontaneous malignancy by local immunotherapy. *Sci. Transl. Med.* **2018**, 10. [CrossRef]
35. Johansson, M.; Denardo, D.G.; Coussens, L.M. Polarized immune responses differentially regulate cancer development. *Immunol Rev.* **2008**, *222*, 145–154. [CrossRef] [PubMed]
36. Napolitani, G.; Rinaldi, A.; Bertoni, F.; Sallusto, F.; Lanzavecchia, A. Selected Toll-like receptor agonist combinations synergistically trigger a T helper type 1-polarizing program in dendritic cells. *Nat. Immunol.* **2005**, *6*, 769–776. [CrossRef]
37. Waldmannova, E.; Caisova, V.; Faberova, J.; Svackova, P.; Kovarova, M.; Svackova, D.; Kumzakova, Z.; Jackova, A.; Vacova, N.; Nedbalova, P.; et al. The use of Zymosan A and bacteria anchored to tumor cells for effective cancer immunotherapy: B16-F10 murine melanoma model. *Int. Immunopharmacol.* **2016**, *39*, 295–306. [CrossRef]
38. Vonderheide, R.H.; Glennie, M.J. Agonistic CD40 antibodies and cancer therapy. *Clin. Cancer Res.* **2013**, *19*, 1035–1043. [CrossRef]
39. Elgueta, R.; Benson, M.J.; de Vries, V.C.; Wasiuk, A.; Guo, Y.; Noelle, R.J. Molecular mechanism and function of CD40/CD40L engagement in the immune system. *Immunol. Rev.* **2009**, *229*, 152–172. [CrossRef]
40. Ahonen, C.L.; Doxsee, C.L.; McGurran, S.M.; Riter, T.R.; Wade, W.F.; Barth, R.J.; Vasilakos, J.P.; Noelle, R.J.; Kedl, R.M. Combined TLR and CD40 triggering induces potent CD8+ T cell expansion with variable dependence on type I IFN. *J. Exp. Med.* **2004**, *199*, 775–784. [CrossRef]
41. Scarlett, U.K.; Cubillos-Ruiz, J.R.; Nesbeth, Y.C.; Martinez, D.G.; Engle, X.; Gewirtz, A.T.; Ahonen, C.L.; Conejo-Garcia, J.R. In situ stimulation of CD40 and Toll-like receptor 3 transforms ovarian cancer-infiltrating dendritic cells from immunosuppressive to immunostimulatory cells. *Cancer Res.* **2009**, *69*, 7329–7337. [CrossRef]
42. Lutz, E.; Yeo, C.J.; Lillemoe, K.D.; Biedrzycki, B.; Kobrin, B.; Herman, J.; Sugar, E.; Piantadosi, S.; Cameron, J.L.; Solt, S.; et al. A lethally irradiated allogeneic granulocyte-macrophage colony stimulating factor-secreting tumor vaccine for pancreatic adenocarcinoma. A Phase II trial of safety, efficacy, and immune activation. *Ann. Surg.* **2011**, *253*, 328–335.
43. Srivatsan, S.; Patel, J.M.; Bozeman, E.N.; Imasuen, I.E.; He, S.; Daniels, D.; Selvaraj, P. Allogeneic tumor cell vaccines: The promise and limitations in clinical trials. *Hum. Vaccin. Immunother.* **2014**, *10*, 52–63. [CrossRef]
44. Yu, P.; Lee, Y.; Wang, Y.; Liu, X.; Auh, S.; Gajewski, T.F.; Schreiber, H.; You, Z.; Kaynor, C.; Wang, X.; et al. Targeting the primary tumor to generate CTL for the effective eradication of spontaneous metastases. *J. Immunol.* **2007**, *179*, 1960–1968. [CrossRef]

45. Lengagne, R.; Graff-Dubois, S.; Garcette, M.; Renia, L.; Kato, M.; Guillet, J.G.; Engelhard, V.H.; Avril, M.F.; Abastado, J.P.; Prevost-Blondel, A. Distinct role for CD8 T cells toward cutaneous tumors and visceral metastases. *J. Immunol.* **2008**, *180*, 130–137. [CrossRef] [PubMed]
46. Lubner, M.G.; Brace, C.L.; Hinshaw, J.L.; Lee, F.T., Jr. Microwave tumor ablation: Mechanism of action, clinical results, and devices. *J. Vasc. Interv. Radiol.* **2010**, *21*, S192–S203. [CrossRef] [PubMed]
47. Brody, J.D.; Ai, W.Z.; Czerwinski, D.K.; Torchia, J.A.; Levy, M.; Advani, R.H.; Kim, Y.H.; Hoppe, R.T.; Knox, S.J.; Shin, L.K.; et al. In situ vaccination with a TLR9 agonist induces systemic lymphoma regression: A phase I/II study. *J. Clin. Oncol.* **2010**, *28*, 4324–4332. [CrossRef]
48. Maleki Vareki, S. High and low mutational burden tumors versus immunologically hot and cold tumors and response to immune checkpoint inhibitors. *J. Immunother. Cancer* **2018**, *6*, 157. [CrossRef]
49. Gujar, S.; Pol, J.G.; Kroemer, G. Heating it up: Oncolytic viruses make tumors 'hot' and suitable for checkpoint blockade immunotherapies. *Oncoimmunology* **2018**, *7*, e1442169. [CrossRef]
50. Vonderheide, R.H. The Immune Revolution: A Case for Priming, Not Checkpoint. *Cancer Cell* **2018**, *33*, 563–569. [CrossRef]
51. Pinato, D.J.; Black, J.R.; Trousil, S.; Dina, R.E.; Trivedi, P.; Mauri, F.A.; Sharma, R. Programmed cell death ligands expression in phaeochromocytomas and paragangliomas: Relationship with the hypoxic response, immune evasion and malignant behavior. *Oncoimmunology* **2017**, *6*, e1358332. [CrossRef] [PubMed]
52. Dwary, A.D.; Master, S.; Patel, A.; Cole, C.; Mansour, R.; Mills, G.; Koshy, N.; Peddi, P.; Burton, G.; Hammoud, D.; et al. Excellent response to chemotherapy post immunotherapy. *Oncotarget* **2017**, *8*, 91795–91802. [CrossRef] [PubMed]
53. Ghayee, H.K.; Bhagwandin, V.J.; Stastny, V.; Click, A.; Ding, L.H.; Mizrachi, D.; Zou, Y.S.; Chari, R.; Lam, W.L.; Bachoo, R.M.; et al. Progenitor cell line (hPheo1) derived from a human pheochromocytoma tumor. *PLoS ONE* **2013**, *8*, e65624. [CrossRef]
54. Li, J.; Piao, Y.F.; Jiang, Z.; Chen, L.; Sun, H.B. Silencing of signal transducer and activator of transcription 3 expression by RNA interference suppresses growth of human hepatocellular carcinoma in tumor-bearing nude mice. *World J. Gastroenterol.* **2009**, *15*, 2602–2608. [CrossRef] [PubMed]
55. Eisenhofer, G.; Goldstein, D.S.; Stull, R.; Keiser, H.R.; Sunderland, T.; Murphy, D.L.; Kopin, I.J. Simultaneous liquid-chromatographic determination of 3,4-dihydroxyphenylglycol, catecholamines, and 3,4-dihydroxyphenylalanine in plasma, and their responses to inhibition of monoamine oxidase. *Clin. Chem.* **1986**, *32*, 2030–2033.
56. Stassen, M.; Valeva, A.; Walev, I.; Schmitt, E. Activation of mast cells by streptolysin O and lipopolysaccharide. *Methods Mol. Biol.* **2006**, *315*, 393–403.
57. Dewas, C.; Dang, P.M.; Gougerot-Pocidalo, M.A.; El-Benna, J. TNF-alpha induces phosphorylation of p47(phox) in human neutrophils: Partial phosphorylation of p47phox is a common event of priming of human neutrophils by TNF-alpha and granulocyte-macrophage colony-stimulating factor. *J. Immunol.* **2003**, *171*, 4392–4398. [CrossRef] [PubMed]

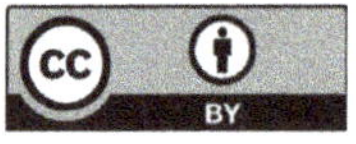

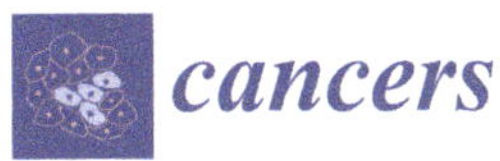 *cancers*

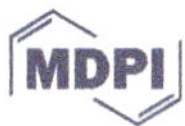

Review

Pheochromocytomas and Paragangliomas: From Genetic Diversity to Targeted Therapies

Ying Pang [1,†], Yang Liu [2,†], Karel Pacak [1] and Chunzhang Yang [2,*]

1 Section on Medical Neuroendocrinology, Eunice Kennedy Shriver National Institute of Child Health and Human Development, National Institutes of Health, Bethesda, MD 20892, USA; ying.pang@nih.gov (Y.P.); karel@mail.nih.gov (K.P.)

2 Neuro-Oncology Branch, Center for Cancer Research, National Cancer Institute, Bethesda, MD 20892, USA; yang.liu5@nih.gov

* Correspondence: yangc2@nih.gov; Tel.: +1-240-760-7083

† These authors contributed equally to the work.

Received: 14 March 2019; Accepted: 26 March 2019; Published: 28 March 2019

Abstract: Pheochromocytoma and paraganglioma (PCPGs) are rare neuroendocrine tumors that arise from the chromaffin tissue of adrenal medulla and sympathetic ganglia. Although metastatic PCPGs account for only 10% of clinical cases, morbidity and mortality are high because of the uncontrollable mass effect and catecholamine level generated by these tumors. Despite our expanding knowledge of PCPG genetics, the clinical options to effectively suppress PCPG progression remain limited. Several recent translational studies revealed that PCPGs with different molecular subtypes exhibit distinctive oncogenic pathways and spectrum of therapy resistance. This suggests that therapeutics can be adjusted based on the signature molecular and metabolic pathways of PCPGs. In this review, we summarized the latest findings on PCPG genetics, novel therapeutic targets, and perspectives for future personalized medicine.

Keywords: pheochromocytoma; paraganglioma; neuroendocrine tumor; targeted therapy; therapy resistance

---

1. Introduction

Pheochromocytomas and paragangliomas (PGPCs) are catecholamine-producing tumors that arise from adrenal medulla, or from extra-adrenal ganglial sympathetic/parasympathetic chains (of chromaffin or non-chromaffin origin), respectively. Tumor-associated secretion of catecholamine causes symptoms of hyperactivity in the sympathetic nervous system including paroxysmal hypertension, headache and diaphoresis. PCPGs result from genetic abnormalities, mostly disruption/mutation in single disease-related genes [1]. Approximately 30–35% of patients with PCPG carry germline mutations in over 20 susceptible genes [2]. In pediatric patients, or in patients who developed the origin tumor in their childhood, approximately 69–87.5% of cases carry germline mutations [3]. Germline mutations may lead to clinical syndromes with symptoms that affect multiple organs, such as von Hippel-Lindau disease, multiple endocrine neoplasia type 2 syndrome, and neurofibromatosis type 1 [4]. On the other hand, somatic mutations in key oncogenic pathways, such as *SDHx, VHL, HIF2A, H-RAS, NF1, RET*, or *MAX*, predispose PCPG formation [5].

Despite our expanding understanding of PCPG genetics and transcriptomics, therapies against this malignancy, especially those against PCPG metastatic lesions, are limited. In addition to surgical resection and radiation therapy, combination chemotherapy that includes cyclophosphamide–vincristine–dacarbazine (CVD) is recommended for advanced PCPG. However, retrospective studies showed that CVD-based treatment provides limited benefit to patient quality of life and overall survival [6]. There is an urgent need to decipher the molecular signature of PCPG for optimized therapeutic regimens, which may result in improved selectivity and efficacy of treatment. In this review, we summarized the latest reports on PCPG genetics, clinical findings and management, and emerging targeted therapies against PCPG subtypes.

2. Genetics of PCPGs

Transcriptomic analysis of patient-derived specimens revealed distinctive gene-expression signatures among histologically similar PCPGs. Based on mRNA-expression signatures, PCPGs can be divided into two main categories: Cluster I and Cluster II diseases (Figure 1). Cluster I disease exhibits metabolic reprogramming and pseudo hypoxic signaling commonly linked to mutations in oxygen-sensing genes or those encoding key enzymes in the Krebs cycle such as *VHL, SDHx, HIF2A, EGLN1/2* and *FH*. Cluster I disease is further stratified into respective subgroups based on differentially-expressed genes. PCPGs showing mutation of *SDHx* and *VHL* are sub-characterized into Cluster IA and Cluster IB, respectively [5]. In contrast, Cluster II PCPGs are commonly related to genetic mutations affecting kinase signaling, gene translation, protein synthesis and neural differentiation; the genes showing mutations include *NF1, RET, KIF1Bβ, TMEM127* and *MAX*. Cluster II disease is further categorized into Cluster 2A (in which patient show mutations in *RET, NF1,* and *TMEM127*), Cluster 2B (sporadic tumors) and Cluster 2C (patients with mutations in 3.7% *VHL* and 11.1% *RET,* and sporadic tumors) [5]. Recent findings show that mutations in the Wnt/Hedgehog pathway are involved in a new molecular subtype of PCPGs [7]. Fishbein et al. discovered that the in-frame RNA fusion transcripts of the *UBTF-MAML3* gene and somatic *CSDE1* mutation may drive activation of the Wnt and Hedgehog pathways, and trigger PCPG oncogenesis [8]. In addition to assessing mutations in coding sequences, analysis of somatic copy-number alterations and miRNA profiling are increasingly used to determine sub-clusters in PCPGs [9].

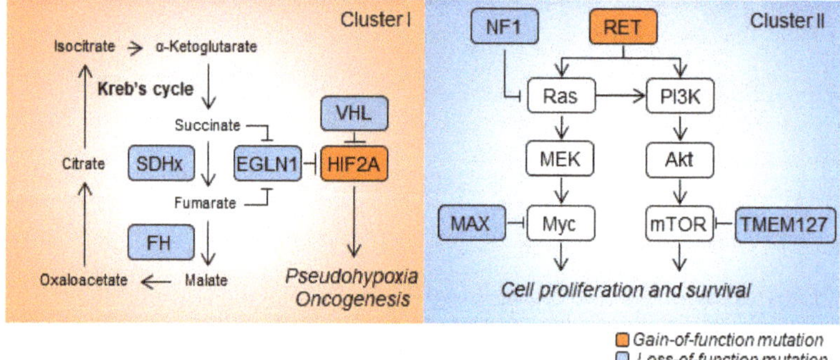

Figure 1. Schematic illustrations of cancer-associated mutations in pheochromocytomas and paragangliomas (PCPGs). Cluster I PCPGs exhibit dysfunction in the Krebs cycle and hypoxia sensing pathways. Loss-of-function mutations in *SDHx, FH, EGLN1* or *VHL* are commonly identified in this disease cluster. *HIF2A* mutations that activate hypoxia signaling are also found in Cluster I disease. Cluster II PCPGs exhibit abnormal kinase activity. This is caused by mutations of major regulators in the feedback loop, such as *NF1, MAX* and *TMEM127*. Gain-of-function mutations in *RET* prompt cellular proliferation and survival by initiating kinase pathways such as Ras/MEK and PI3K/Akt.

2.1. SDHx

Germline mutations in *SDHx* are attributed to approximately half of hereditary PCPGs and are detected in 15% of total patients [10]. Germline mutations in *SDHx* are commonly accompanied by the loss of heterozygosity on the other healthy allele, which leads to substantial loss of SDH catalytic activity [11]. Familial PCPGs, caused by *SDHx* germline mutations, usually show earlier onsets and more severe clinical presentations (including bilateral or multiple tumors) compared with those observed in sporadic cases [12]. In 2000, *SDHC* and *SDHD* were first identified as susceptibility genes for hereditary PCPGs [13,14]. *SDHC* mutations account for 6% of PCPGs, and patients usually present head and neck paragangliomas (HNPGL), while PHEO and PGL occur far less frequently [15]. *SDHD*-mutant PCPGs typically show multiple HNPGL, but PGL and PHEO in other locales have also been described; less than 5% of patients with *SDHD* mutations develop metastatic lesions [15]. Overall, the penetrance of *SDHD*-mutant PCPGs is approximately 71% at age 60 and increases to 90% in the following 10 years [16]. Germline mutations of *SDHD* exhibit 'parent-of-origin' expression phenotype, with tumor onset only when mutations are inherited from the paternal DNA [17,18]. This phenomenon has also been described in other PCPG predisposition genes such as *SDHAF2* and *MAX* [19–21]. In 2001, mutations in *SDHB* were also discovered in patients with familial PCPG [22]. *SDHB*-mutant tumors can occur at adrenal, extra-adrenal and pelvic locations, but mainly develop in the abdomen. Several studies demonstrated that compared with other molecular subtypes, *SDHB*-mutant PCPGs are associated with increased incidence of early onset (25–30 years old), increased metastatic risk and poor prognosis [23]. In 2009, *SDHAF2*, also known as *SDH5*, was identified as the driver gene for HNPGL without PHEO, which occurs via compromised flavination of the SDH complex [19]. In patients with familial PCPGs who carry *SDHAF2* germline mutations, 91% present with more than one HNPGL, and no metastatic tumors have been reported [24]. Mutations in *SDHA* have not been identified as a cancer susceptibility gene in PCPG until recently [20]. Approximately 3% of patients with sporadic PCPG carry *SDHA* germline mutations [25]. Somatic mutations in *SDHx* are rare and occur in approximately 1% of patients with PCPG [5].

SDHx genes encode succinate dehydrogenase (SDH), also known as mitochondrial complex II. SDH consists of four subunits: SDHA, SDHB, SDHC and SDHD. SDHA is a flavoprotein that contains a flavin adenine dinucleotide (FAD) cofactor. SDHB contains three iron-sulfur clusters, which assist electron transfer via the SDH complex. SDHC and SDHD subunits anchor the entire SDH complex to the inner mitochondrial membrane. Mechanistically, SDHA converts succinate into fumarate, which converts FAD to $FADH_2$. The electrons from $FADH_2$ are then transferred via iron-sulfur clusters in SDHB, eventually forming the ubiquinone pool via SDHC/D subunits. SDH complex plays key roles in energy metabolism by participating in both the Krebs cycle and electron transport chain. Deleterious mutations in *SDHx* lead to deficiencies in energy metabolism and accumulation of succinate, which promotes susceptibility to PCPGs, renal cell carcinoma and mitochondrial encephalopathy. Studies using in vivo and in vitro models have shown that loss of succinate dehydrogenase activity results in: (i) abnormal activation of hypoxia-signaling pathway in the presence of oxygen (pseudohypoxia) and angiogenesis [26]; (ii) increased production of reactive oxygen species (ROS) [27]; and (iii) impeded repair and hypermethylation of DNA [28]. The distinctive signatures in tumor biology have supplied valuable clues for developing future molecular-targeted therapeutics against *SDHx*-mutant PCPGs.

2.2. *Von Hippel-Lindau (VHL)*

Germline mutations in the *VHL* gene cause the von Hippel-Lindau syndrome (VHL disease). VHL disease is an autosomal dominant disorder associated with retinal, cerebellar, brainstem and spinal hemangioblastoma, as well as with neuroendocrine tumors, renal cell carcinoma (RCC) and multiple pancreatic cysts [29]. PHEO is present in approximately 7–20% of patients with VHL, who are then diagnosed with VHL syndrome type 2; patients diagnosed with type 1 VHL do not present with PHEO [30]. PHEO usually occurs as bilateral or multifocal tumors in the second decade of life in patients with VHL. Although *VHL* mutations lead to early onset of symptoms, they rarely develop into metastatic disease. In addition to the VHL syndrome, Chuvash polycythemia is a type of inherited hematopoetic disease caused by a specific germline *VHL* mutation (p.R200W). The mutation leads to activation of the hypoxia inducible factors (HIF) signaling pathway under normal oxygen level and increased concentration of erythropoietin, causing overproduction of red blood cells [31]. Germline *VHL* pathogenic mutations are also reported in patients with PHEO and polycythemia, causing by stabilized HIF-2α and elevated production of erythropoietin [32].

Approximately 14% of sporadic PCPGs are found in patients carrying somatic *VHL* mutations, and this is consistently accompanied by the loss of the 3p chromosome [5]. Our previous study has shown that somatic *VHL* gene mutations are also involved in tumorigenesis in hereditary MEN 2A-associatd PHEO [33]. Somatic *VHL* mutations play roles in HNPGL by stimulating the HIF-1α/miR-210 pathway [34]. Although the relationship between somatic *VHL* mutations and prognosis is unclear, different *VHL* variants may contribute to the differential clinical phenotype and prognosis. In our recent study, we established a *VHL* knockout mouse model and found that retinal hemangioblastomas are derived from the hemangioblast cell lineage [35].

VHL is a tumor-suppressor gene that is located on chromosome 3p25.3 and encodes the pVHL protein. The pVHL protein functions as an E3 ligase that ubiquitinates its client proteins. For example, pVHL recognizes the hydroxylated HIF-α oxygen-sensing domains (ODD) domain and recruits other components of the E3 ligase complex such as Elongin B, Elongin C, RBx 1 and Cul2. The VHL-Elongin B/C (VBC) complex processes HIF-α for ubiquitination and subsequent proteasomal degradation. Under hypoxic conditions, VHL recognition of HIF-α is compromised due to reduced ODD hydroxylation. HIF-α is then stabilized and initiates transcription of hypoxia-related genes. Pathogenic *VHL* mutations lead to compromised VBC activity and abnormal oxygen sensing. Consequent transcription of hypoxia-related genes, such as *EPO* and *VEGFA*, serves as oncogenic factors for *VHL*-related symptoms such as hemangioblastomas and PHEO. Moreover, mutations in *VHL* may disrupt the binding of Elongin C and p53, leading to deregulation of cellular apoptosis and consequent tumorigenesis [36].

2.3. *HIF2A*

Hypoxia inducible factors (HIFs), transcriptional factors that govern cellular responses to low oxygen, were first described by Semenza in 1995 [37]. HIFs are composed of α and β subunits. The α subunits are nuclear factors that are sensitive to the oxygen level in the microenvironment, whereas β subunits are constitutively expressed and serve as cofactors for HIF-α. Under normoxia, the ODD in HIF-α are rapidly hydroxylated by prolyl hydroxylase, which alters the conformation of HIF-α. Hydroxylated HIF-α is recognized by the VBC complex and is rapidly degraded via the ubiquitin proteasome pathway [38]. Under hypoxic or pseudohypoxic conditions, the function of prolyl hydroxylase is compromised, leading to stabilization and accumulation of HIF-α. HIF-α is then translocated into the nucleus as a heterodimer HIF-β, initiating transcriptional activation of hypoxia-related genes involved in biological reactions such as angiogenesis, glycolysis and erythropoiesis.

Overexpression of HIF-1/2α is frequently identified in most human cancers, and activation of tumorigenesis and angiogenesis [39]. Low oxygen concentration activates the hypoxia-signaling pathway in tumors, especially in regions with minimal oxygen penetration. On the other hand, the hypoxia pathway can also be activated under normoxia due to genetic abnormalities in key regulatory genes of the oxygen-sensing pathway. Elevated expression of HIF-1α is associated with poor outcomes in multiple human cancers such as those of head and neck, breast and colorectal cancers [40]. HIF-2α overexpression is associated with higher metastatic potential and with metastases-presenting tumors such as melanoma and glioma [41]. HIF-2α overexpression may be preferentially linked with metastatic progression and poor prognosis in patients [41].

Mutations in *HIF2A* have been identified in human diseases such as polycythemia, PCPG and somatostatinoma [42,43]. *HIF2A* mutations present as somatic mutations or somatic mosaicism, affecting multiple lineages of somatic cells [44]. *HIF2A* mutations are mainly located on exon 12, resulting in amino-acid substitutions in the ODD domain of HIF-2α. Alterations in peptide sequences lead to compromised prolyl hydroxylation, VBC recognition and transcription of hypoxia-related genes. Accordingly, *HIF2A*-mutated PHEO/PGLs show increased expression of hypoxia-related genes such as *EPO*, *EDN1* and *VEGFA*, which may be linked to polycythemia and oncogenesis [43].

2.4. Neurofibromin 1 (NF1)

The NF1 syndrome, also known as von Recklinghausen disease, is caused by germline mutations in *NF1*. Mutations in *NF1* are involved in numerous types of tumors such as desmoplastic melanoma, glioblastomas, neuroblastomas, PCPGs, gastrointestinal tumors, ovarian tumors and urinary tract transitional cell carcinoma [45]. Approximately 0.1–6% of patients with NF1 present with PHEO [46]. Patients with NF1 usually develop PHEO after their third decade of life. Approximately 80% of these patients present solitary adrenal tumors, and 10% present with bilateral adrenal tumors. Additionally, over 10% of patients with NF1 and PHEO develop metastatic tumors, and most of these metastatic tumors are distant from the primary location [47]. A common feature observed in patients with *NF1*-related PCPGs is a significantly up-regulated level of catecholamine in plasma and urine [48].

Somatic mutations in *NF1* occur in 20–25% of patients with PCPGs. *NF1* is the most frequently occurring susceptibility gene in all sporadic PCPGs. An integrative genomic study has shown that 26% of sporadically occurring tumors show loss of one allele in *NF1*. Additionally, 91% of tumors in patients with *NF1*-related PCPGs show somatic truncating mutations on the other wild-type allele [48]. However, a genetic-mapping study has shown that only 20% of patients with *NF1*-related PCPGs show deletion of the other allele [5], indicating that other molecular pathways may be involved in NF1-mediated oncogenesis.

NF1 is a tumor-suppressor gene located on chromosome 17q11.2. The *NF1* gene spans approximately 300 kb in genomic DNA, contains 58 coding exons and encodes 2818 amino acids. Currently, genetic detection and characterization of *NF1* mutations in patients is challenging because of the large size of the *NF1* gene, presence of multiple pseudogenes, and a wide spectrum of mutations without obvious hotspots. *NF1* encodes neurofibromin, a GTPase-activating protein (GAP) that negatively regulates the Ras/MAPK pathway. The 20 to 27 exons of *NF1* encode a GAP-associated domain, which hydrolyses Ras-GTP to its inactive GDP-bound form, thereby deactivating the Ras signaling pathway. Loss-of-function mutations in *NF1* lead to uncontrollable activation of kinase and tumorigenesis. Several genetically-engineered *NF1* mouse models have shown pigmentary lesions, skeletal abnormalities, and tumors.

2.5. RET

Germline mutations in *RET* are linked with multiple endocrine neoplasia type 2 (MEN2). MEN2 is a rare autosomal dominant syndrome that is classified into MEN2A (Sipple syndrome), MEN2B (Gorlin syndrome) and familial medullary thyroid carcinoma (FMTC). Patients with MEN2 have a nearly 100% risk for developing medullary thyroid carcinoma (MTC) and 57% risk for developing PHEO [49]. Additionally, patients with MEN2A can also develop primary hyperparathyroidism, while those with MEN2B can develop Marfanoid habitus, mucosal neuromas and ganglioneuromatosis. Although mutations in *RET* have been detected on all exons, 95% of patients with MEN2A carry *RET* mutations on exon 10 (codons 609, 611, 618 and 620) or exon 11 (codon 634). Similarly, most mutations in patients with MEN2B occur on exon 16 (codon 918) [50]. The most common *RET* mutations in PHEO-related syndrome usually occur on exon 10, 11, 13 and 16. However, penetrance and age of onset are not necessarily associated with types of *RET* mutations [51]. Carriers of codon 634 germline mutations present with much younger mean age of onset, and have a higher risk of developing PHEO, than do carriers of other mutations. In patients with MEN2, most PCPG-related PHEOs occur on the adrenal glands, and more than half of these are bilateral; parasympathetic head and neck PGLs have been found, but are very rare [52]. These patients rarely develop metastatic PCPGs, and mean age of onset is approximately 36 years old [53].

The *RET* proto-oncogene is located on chromosome 10q11.2 and contains 21 exons. *RET* encodes transmembrane receptor tyrosine kinase (RTK), which binds to growth factors such as glial derived neurotrophic factor (GDNF). The RET protein contains an extracellular portion, a single transmembrane domain and an intracellular portion. There are 12 autophosphorylation sites on the intracellular portion, and phosphorylated tyrosine may be the docking site for multiple intracellular-signaling pathway proteins, including those involved in cell growth and differentiation [54]. Genetic alterations in *RET* include gain-of-function mutations, which lead to constitutive RTK activation and tumorigenesis such as those observed in patients with MEN2A.

2.6. *MAX*

Germline mutations in *MAX* were first implicated in susceptibility to hereditary PHEO in a whole-exome sequencing study. Loss-of-function mutations in *MAX* are also a risk for metastatic PHEO [21]. Most of the *MAX* mutations occur on the highly-conserved basic helix-loop-helix leucine-zipper (bHLHZ) domain. Loss of heterozygosity on the wild-type allele is also detected in the tumors of patients with germline missense mutations in *MAX*. Although metastatic PHEOs are rare, except in patients carrying *SDHB* mutations, Mendez found that approximately 37% of patients with *MAX* mutations present with metastases at diagnosis [21]; this suggests *MAX* mutations may be risk factors for metastatic disease. Somatic *MAX* mutations are detected in patients with sporadic PCPGs at an incidence of 1.65% [55]. Tumors with *MAX* mutations show substantial upregulation of normetanephrine expression, with almost normal or slighted increased levels of metanephrine.

The *MAX* gene is located on chromosome 14q23, which encodes the transcriptional regulator MAX. MAX belongs to the family of bHLHZ transcriptional factors. It can form heterodimers with MYC or MAX dimerization protein 1 (MXD1), which controls the transcription of numerous downstream genes that regulate cellular proliferation, differentiation and apoptosis [56]. The highly-conserved bHLHZ domain of MAX is vital for the protein-DNA and protein-protein interactions. Furthermore, casein kinase II phosphorylation sites on MAX modulate DNA-binding kinetics of MAX-MAX or Myc-MAX dimerization [57]. Therefore, alteration in MAX, especially mutations on the bHLHZ domain and casein kinase II phosphorylation sites, can induce the dysfunction of the MYC/MAX/MXD1 axis and consequent tumorigenesis.

2.7. *Harvey Rat Sarcoma Viral Oncogene Homologue (HRAS)*

The first somatic mutation in *HRAS* in a patient with pheochromocytoma was reported by Yoshimoto et al. in 1992 [58]. Missense gain-of-function mutations in *HRAS* have been detected in various types of human tumors; the hotspots for *HRAS* mutations are G13R and Q61K [1]. Until now, *HRAS* somatic mutations were found in approximately 5% of sporadic patients with PCPGs and present as mostly benign tumors [1]. No germline HRAS mutation has been discovered in patients with PCPGs thus far. The other two proteins in the RAS family, NRAS and KRAS, have never been described as susceptibility factors for PCPGs.

HRAS is located on the chromosome 11p15.5. *HRAS* encodes GTPase HRas, also known as transforming protein p21. HRas is activated via binding to GTP. The activity of HRas can be inactivated by GTP hydrolysis to GDP [9]. Activation of the HRas signaling pathway stimulates downstream pathways such as Ras/Raf/Erk and PI3K/Akt/mTOR, which are vital for cellular proliferation and oncogenic transformation.

3. Current Therapies and Limitations

The goal of anti-PCPG therapies is to effectively control tumor growth and other disease-related symptoms. Alpha-blockers, calcium channel blockers, or β-blockers are the first line treatment to control hypertension and prevent hypertensive crisis. When β blockers are used without prior alpha blockade, there is a theoretical risk of hypertensive crisis due to alpha adrenergic receptor mediated vasoconstriction without the opposition of the β2-adrenergic receptor mediated vasodilation. For benign and locally invasive PCPGs, surgical intervention, including minimal invasion endoscopic surgery, is considered standard therapy. Laparoscopic surgery can be used for patients with bilateral and extra-adrenal PCPGs, with laparotomy showing similar outcomes. For multifocal and metastatic cases, and for tumors larger than 7 to 8 cm, surgical procedures are usually preferable for ensuring complete removal of all suspected tumors. When surgery is not applicable, radio-and/or chemotherapies are considered alternative approaches. For the metaiodobenzylguanidine (MIBG) scintigraphy-positive patients, ^{131}iodine-meta-iodobenzylguanidine (^{131}I-MIBG) therapy is considered a priority. MIBG positive patients with metastatic PCPG have been demonstrated to benefit from ^{131}I-MIBG-based treatment, showing symptomatic and hormonal responses [59]. However, dose-dependent side effects of this therapy, such as severe thrombocytopenia, hypothyroidism and neutropenia, are also observed [60]. Most importantly, ^{131}I-MIBG-based treatment is less likely to achieve complete response. In a study that included 243 patients, 3% of patients showed complete response, while 27% and 52% of patients showed partial response and stable disease, respectively [61].

Overexpression of somatostatin receptors in PCPGs promotes application of radiolabeled somatostatin agonists, for imaging and treatment of the PCPGs patients. ^{123}I-Tyr-octreotide and ^{111}In-pentetreotide were first introduced as the radiolabeled somatostatin agonists. However, the ^{90}Y and ^{177}Lu peptide-labelled somatostatin radionuclides were recommended by European centers to replace the old ones, due to higher uptake ratio and less side effects [62,63]. Besides, the ^{90}Y is more effective on larger tumors due to higher energy β emission, while the ^{177}Lu is favorable for smaller tumors. Less side effects were also found in ^{177}Lu compared to ^{90}Y, especially in the aspect of renal toxicity [64]. A successful phase III clinical trial NETTER-1 regarding the ^{177}Lu-DOTATATE showed to prolong the median progression-free survival to 40 months in mid-gut neuroendocrine tumors, compared to a long-acting somatostatin analogue, octreotide-LAR (median progression-free survival: 8.4 months) [65]. For inoperable PCPGs patients, the ^{177}Lu-DOTATATE is under a phase II clinical trial to evaluate the safety, tolerability and overall survival (NCT03206060). However, radiolabeled somatostatin agonists are only applied for somatostatin receptor positive patients and side effects still need further evaluation.

Chemotherapy is another valuable treatment modality for controlling tumor growth in patients with metastatic PCPGs. Most traditional chemotherapy regimens, such as those using cyclophosphamide, vincristine and dacarbazine (CVD), have been used to treat patients with PCPGs over the past 30 years. Although clinical studies have shown that 33–57% of patients with PCPGs respond to CVD or similar regimens, a 22 year-long follow-up study found there were no significant differences in patient survival between CVD responders and CVD non-responders. Overall, the present options of chemotherapy do not provide survival benefits for advanced PCPG, and their value remains limited [6].

4. Targeted Molecular Therapies

Current knowledge of signatures involved in the molecular signaling, metabolism and resistance mechanisms of PCPGs suggests that therapeutic regimens can be optimized to each molecular subtype. Profiling of gene expression and methylation can serve as a powerful tool for characterizing disease clusters and for guiding targeted therapy for improved selectivity and efficacy. In the following sections, we introduce the latest advances in targeted therapeutics against PHEO/PGL.

4.1. Antiangiogenic Therapies

Antiangiogenic therapies have been proposed for targeting pseudohypoxic and angiogenic phenotypes in Cluster I PCPGs, which are commonly accompanied by mutations in *SDH* or *VHL* [66]. Humanized VEGF-A monoclonal antibodies (such as bevacizumab) and tyrosine kinase inhibitors (such as sunitinib and sorafenib) are used in current antiangiogenic therapies. These regimens are approved by the FDA for the treatment of patients with advanced renal cell carcinoma, which includes patients with mutations in *SDHB* [67,68]. Interestingly, several case studies on sunitinib have shown partial response or stable disease in patients with Cluster I PCPGs. This indicates that patients with Cluster I PCPGs may show improved responses to antiangiogenic therapies [69–74]. Several ongoing clinical trials are aiming to further validate the efficacy of sunitinib-based therapy in patients with progressive PCPGs. For example, a randomized double-blind phase II clinical trial, called the FIRSTMAPPP (First Randomized STudy in MAlignant Progressive Pheochromocytomas and

Paragangliomas) study (NCT01371201), is currently conducting recruitment to evaluate the efficacy of sunitinib vs placebo in patients with progressive malignant PCPGs. A single arm, nonrandomized phase II study (NCT00843037) aims to evaluate the response and toxicity profile of sunitinib in a cohort of 25 patients with malignant PCPGs. Another tyrosine kinase inhibitor, Axitinib (AG-013736), is currently under evaluation in a phase II nonrandomized clinical trial including 14 patients with PCPGs (NCT01967576). Moreover, a phase II clinical trial is ongoing to determine the efficacy of Lenvatinib, a multiple kinase inhibitor against VEGFR1, VEGFR2 and VEGFR3 in patients with metastatic or advanced PCPGs (NCT03008369).

4.2. Hypoxia-Inducible Factor (HIF) Inhibitors

The abnormal activation of hypoxia signaling is a hallmark of Cluster I PCPGs. HIF inhibitors may potentially be used in therapy against Cluster I PCPGs. HIF inhibitors, such as PX-12 and PX-478, have been studied in various tumor xenograft models [75,76]. Recently, PT2339 and PT2385, two selective HIF-2α antagonists, were developed and evaluated for their anti-tumor effects. PT2399 showed a stronger suppression effect than that of sunitinib in cell lines derived from *VHL*-mutated clear cell renal cell carcinomas (ccRCCs) [77]. An ongoing phase I clinical trial (NCT02293980), designed to evaluate the efficacy of PT2385, indicated that complete response, partial response and stable disease were achieved in 2%, 12% and 52% of patients with ccRCCs [78]. A phase II clinical trial (NCT03108066) is currently ongoing to evaluate the use of PT2385 in patients with *VHL*-associated ccRCCs. These compounds have not been evaluated in patients with PCPGs; however, the tumor-suppressing effects of these compounds on HIF-driven solid tumors are promising, suggesting that HIF-2α inhibitors can be used to treat patients with Cluster I PCPGs in the future. Recently, anthracyclines (daunorubicin, doxorubicin, epirubicin and idarubicin) have been reported to suppress cell growth of metastatic PCPGs by inhibiting both HIF-1 and 2α, indicating a new therapeutic option for patients with metastatic PCPGs, especially those with alterations in HIF pathways [79].

4.3. mTOR Inhibitors

Hyperactivation of kinase activity is commonly detected in the Ras/Raf/Erk or PI3K/Akt/mTOR pathways of patients with Cluster II PCPGs and mutations in *RET*, *NF1*, *TMEM127* and *MAX*, [46,55,80–82]. Inhibitors of pro-survival kinase signaling have been proposed for targeted therapeutics. For example, treatment with mTORC1 inhibitor everolimus (RAD001) has been evaluated in patients with progressive PHEO. However, this therapy showed unfavorable results, with disease progression in all four recruited patients [83]. In another phase II study (NCT01152827), five out of seven patients with PCPGs achieved stable disease [84]. In 2013, a selective ATP-competitive dual mTORC1/2 small molecule inhibitor was evaluated in a mouse model of sporadic PHEO, and PHEO associated with *VHL* or *SDHB* mutations. The results showed promising therapeutic effects of AZD8055, indicated by decreased tumor size and metastatic burden in athymic nude mice [85]. Moreover, combining AZD8055 with an Erk inhibitor AEZS-131 may prevent the compensatory feedback loop and overcome resistance [86].

4.4. DNA Demethylation

Mutations in *SDHx* result in accumulation of succinate, an oncometabolite that inhibits 2-oxoglutarate (2-OG)-dependent dioxygenases, resulting in a global DNA and histone hypermethylation phenotype [87,88]. Demethylating agents may rectify the hypermethylation phenotype in *SDH*- or *FH*-mutated PCPGs. For example, DNA-demethylating agent decitabine suppresses cellular proliferation and metastasis in *SDHB*-knockout chromaffin cells [87]. SGI-110, a DNA methyltransferase inhibitor, is currently under investigation in a phase II non-randomized trial (NCT03165721) for treatment of patients with PCPGs associated with SDH deficiency. Further preclinical studies are needed to assess the safety profile and therapeutic efficacy of these compounds before proceeding to clinical trials.

4.5. DNA-Alkylating Agents

Temozolomide (TMZ) is an FDA-approved DNA-alkylating agent used for treatment of glioblastoma in combination with radiotherapy. TMZ generates DNA alkylation at O6-guanine, N7-guanine and N3-adenine, which causes base-pair mismatch and leads to the death of tumor cells. In some tumor cells, the expression of O6-methylguanine-DNA methyltransferase (MGMT) can directly remove the alkyl group from O6-guanine, resulting in resistance to TMZ. However, tumors with mutations in genes encoding Krebs-cycle enzymes, such as *IDH1/2* and *SDHx*, often show CpG island methylator phenotype (CIMP), which results in hypermethylation of the *MGMT* promoter and reduced expression of MGMT [87,89]. Loss of MGMT expression predisposes patients to a better therapeutic response to TMZ because of reduced methyltransferase activity. Several studies have shown the remarkable sensitivity of *IDH1/2*-mutant glioblastoma to TMZ [90,91]. Similarly, TMZ exerts strong therapeutic effect on metastatic neuroendocrine carcinoma, especially that with mutations in *SDHB* [92]. A phase II clinical trial (NCT00165230) is currently evaluating the efficacy of TMZ combined with thalidomide in therapy against neuroendocrine tumors. Additionally, one out of three patients with PCPGs shows response to radiotherapy [93]. Clinical trials with larger patient cohorts are needed to further evaluate the efficacy of TMZ in patients with PCPGs.

4.6. PARP Inhibitors

Mutations in enzymes encoding Krebs-cycle enzymes, such as *SDHx*, are associated with hereditary PCPGs that are characterized by increased level of succinate. High level of succinate serves as an intrinsic inhibitor of homologous recombination (HR)-based DNA repair; this occurs via inhibition of the lysine demethylases KDM4A and KDM4B [94]. Moreover, SDH deficiency in Cluster I PCPGs is associated with alterations in NAD^+/NADH metabolism and potentiation of the PARP-mediated DNA repair pathways [95]. These findings indicate that SDH-deficient tumor cells are highly sensitive to treatment with PARP inhibitors. Combinations of PARP inhibitors with other genotoxic agents may be a promising approach for treating patients with Cluster I PCPGs. Olaparib, an FDA-proved PARP inhibitor, markedly potentiates the therapeutic effect of TMZ in *SDHB*-mutant preclinical models; this occurs via induction of DNA lesions and inhibition of tumor growth in vitro and in vivo [94,95].

4.7. Histone Deacetylase Inhibitors

Histone deacetylase (HDAC) inhibitors were also reported to have anti-tumor effect in PCPGs. HDAC inhibitors have been shown to induce cell cycle arrest and apoptosis in PCPGs through activation of Notch1 signaling or inhibition of nuclear factor erythroid 2-related factor 2/heme oxygenase 1(Nrf2/HO-1) pathway [96–99]. Additionally, our previous study demonstrated that HDAC inhibitors improved the stability of SDHB protein, and therefore supported the function of mitochondrial complex II, which might limit disease progression of PCPGs with *SDHB* deficiency [100].

4.8. Immunotherapy

The pseudo-hypoxia phenotype may alter the immune system through inactivation of cytotoxic T-cell lymphocytes, activation of immune-suppressive monocytes and increased expression of the immune checkpoint protein programmed death-ligand 1 (PD-L1) and its receptor [101–103]. Thus, immunotherapy has been considered as a candidate therapeutic approach for Cluster I PCPGs. A study of 14 patients with progressive metastatic PCPGs treated with interferon alpha-2b resulted in 12 patients with disease stabilization and two with partial responses [104]. Two phase II clinical trials of checkpoint inhibitors (Nivolumab, ipilimumab and pembrolizumab) are currently ongoing in patients with rare tumors, including metastasis PCPGs (NCT02834013, NCT02721732).

4.9. Other Potential Therapies

Our previously study indicated that cells with high baseline level of reactive oxygen species (ROS), such as *IDH*-mutated glioma, dependency on antioxidative pathways are crucial to maintain ROS homeostasis. Blockade of antioxidative pathways showed promising therapeutic effects in *IDH*-mutated cancers [105]. Similarly, evidence has shown that the deficiency in *SDH* and accumulation of succinate may lead to elevated generation of ROS [27,106]. Our recent data indicated that *SDHB* deficient PCPG cells developed addiction to the Nrf2 antioxidative pathway and Nrf2 blockade might be a novel therapeutic approach to this type of PCPGs.

5. Future Directions

Despite our increased understanding of PCPG biology and advancements in translational medicine, the underlying pathogenetic mechanisms and molecular pathways of PCPG require further investigation. Cell-based and preclinical mouse models do not fully recapitulate the molecular subtypes of human cancers, posing a challenge in studies on PCPG. PCPG cell lines, derived from heterozygous *NF1*-knockout mouse (MTT and MPC cells) and representative rat pheochromocytoma (PC12 cells), are widely accepted and used in molecular biology studies; however, generating cell lines from patient-derived PCPGs remains challenging. Currently, only one progenitor cell line (hPheo1 cells) derived from a human pheochromocytoma tumor has been established successfully [107]. This illustrates an urgent need to develop patient-derived cell lines, especially those for modeling Cluster I PCPG in vitro.

With the rapid development of genomic sequencing platforms, large-scale sequencing projects have illustrated the genomics, methylomics and epigenenomic changes of PCPG. The concept of personalized medicine has been brought into vision to treating individuals based on their specific genetic and micro-environmental background. By altering specific signaling pathways, enzymes and receptors, targeted therapies can be optimized for each individual, with reduced side effects with respect to normal tissues. To this end, tumoral genetic and molecular profiles should be investigated in future clinical studies and trials. On the other hand, continuous investigation of molecular mechanisms involved in PCPG oncogenesis is highly important. Detailed understanding of PCPG genetics and key oncogenic pathways will lead to novel therapeutic targets. Overall, understanding the genetic background, developing effective molecular-targeted agents and optimizing the design of clinical trials will improve prognosis and survival in patients with PCPG.

6. Conclusions

In this review, we briefly summarized the latest knowledge of PCPG molecular subtypes and their implications to clinical management. PCPGs generate tumors with genetic alterations; therefore, detailed genetic analysis should be recommended for all patients with PCPGs to better characterize the potential therapeutic vulnerabilities in each case. Therapeutic regimens with long-term efficacy are needed to improve patient survival and quality of life. Development of patient-derived cell lines and disease-relevant preclinical animal models will generate novel therapeutic targets for future management of PCPGs.

Funding: This study was supported by the Neuro-Oncology Branch, Center for Cancer Research, National Cancer Institute and *Eunice Kennedy Shriver* National Institute of Child Health and Human Development, National Institutes of Health, Bethesda MD USA 20892.

Conflicts of Interest: The authors declare no conflict of interest.

References

1. Crona, J.; Delgado Verdugo, A.; Maharjan, R.; Stalberg, P.; Granberg, D.; Hellman, P.; Bjorklund, P. Somatic mutations in H-RAS in sporadic pheochromocytoma and paraganglioma identified by exome sequencing. *J. Clin. Endocrinol. Metab.* **2013**, *98*, E1266–E1271. [PubMed]

2. Luchetti, A.; Walsh, D.; Rodger, F.; Clark, G.; Martin, T.; Irving, R.; Sanna, M.; Yao, M.; Robledo, M.; Neumann, H.P.; et al. Profiling of somatic mutations in phaeochromocytoma and paraganglioma by targeted next generation sequencing analysis. *Int. J. Endocrinol.* **2015**, *2015*, 138573. [CrossRef] [PubMed]
3. King, K.S.; Prodanov, T.; Kantorovich, V.; Fojo, T.; Hewitt, J.K.; Zacharin, M.; Wesley, R.; Lodish, M.; Raygada, M.; Gimenez-Roqueplo, A.P.; et al. Metastatic pheochromocytoma/paraganglioma related to primary tumor development in childhood or adolescence: Significant link to SDHB mutations. *J. Clin. Oncol.* **2011**, *29*, 4137–4142. [CrossRef] [PubMed]
4. Erlic, Z.; Neumann, H.P. Familial pheochromocytoma. *Hormones (Athens)* **2009**, *8*, 29–38. [CrossRef] [PubMed]
5. Burnichon, N.; Vescovo, L.; Amar, L.; Libe, R.; de Reynies, A.; Venisse, A.; Jouanno, E.; Laurendeau, I.; Parfait, B.; Bertherat, J.; et al. Integrative genomic analysis reveals somatic mutations in pheochromocytoma and paraganglioma. *Hum. Mol. Genet.* **2011**, *20*, 3974–3985. [CrossRef]
6. Huang, H.; Abraham, J.; Hung, E.; Averbuch, S.; Merino, M.; Steinberg, S.M.; Pacak, K.; Fojo, T. Treatment of malignant pheochromocytoma/paraganglioma with cyclophosphamide, vincristine, and dacarbazine: Recommendation from a 22-year follow-up of 18 patients. *Cancer* **2008**, *113*, 2020–2028. [CrossRef]
7. Jochmanova, I.; Pacak, K. Genomic Landscape of Pheochromocytoma and Paraganglioma. *Trends Cancer* **2018**, *4*, 6–9. [CrossRef]
8. Fishbein, L.; Leshchiner, I.; Walter, V.; Danilova, L.; Robertson, A.G.; Johnson, A.R.; Lichtenberg, T.M.; Murray, B.A.; Ghayee, H.K.; Else, T.; et al. Comprehensive Molecular Characterization of Pheochromocytoma and Paraganglioma. *Cancer Cell* **2017**, *31*, 181–193. [CrossRef]
9. Castro-Vega, L.J.; Letouze, E.; Burnichon, N.; Buffet, A.; Disderot, P.H.; Khalifa, E.; Loriot, C.; Elarouci, N.; Morin, A.; Menara, M.; et al. Multi-omics analysis defines core genomic alterations in pheochromocytomas and paragangliomas. *Nat. Commun.* **2015**, *6*, 6044. [CrossRef]
10. Gill, A.J.; Benn, D.E.; Chou, A.; Clarkson, A.; Muljono, A.; Meyer-Rochow, G.Y.; Richardson, A.L.; Sidhu, S.B.; Robinson, B.G.; Clifton-Bligh, R.J. Immunohistochemistry for SDHB triages genetic testing of SDHB, SDHC, and SDHD in paraganglioma-pheochromocytoma syndromes. *Hum. Pathol.* **2010**, *41*, 805–814. [CrossRef]
11. Gottlieb, E.; Tomlinson, I.P. Mitochondrial tumour suppressors: A genetic and biochemical update. *Nat. Rev. Cancer* **2005**, *5*, 857–866. [CrossRef]
12. Vicha, A.; Taieb, D.; Pacak, K. Current views on cell metabolism in SDHx-related pheochromocytoma and paraganglioma. *Endocr. Relat. Cancer* **2014**, *21*, R261–277. [CrossRef]
13. Baysal, B.E.; Ferrell, R.E.; Willett-Brozick, J.E.; Lawrence, E.C.; Myssiorek, D.; Bosch, A.; van der Mey, A.; Taschner, P.E.; Rubinstein, W.S.; Myers, E.N.; et al. Mutations in SDHD, a mitochondrial complex II gene, in hereditary paraganglioma. *Science* **2000**, *287*, 848–851. [CrossRef]
14. Niemann, S.; Muller, U. Mutations in SDHC cause autosomal dominant paraganglioma, type 3. *Nat. Genet.* **2000**, *26*, 268–270. [CrossRef]
15. Jafri, M.; Maher, E.R. The genetics of phaeochromocytoma: Using clinical features to guide genetic testing. *Eur. J. Endocrinol.* **2012**, *166*, 151–158. [CrossRef]
16. Pasini, B.; Stratakis, C.A. SDH mutations in tumorigenesis and inherited endocrine tumours: Lesson from the phaeochromocytoma-paraganglioma syndromes. *J. Intern. Med.* **2009**, *266*, 19–42. [CrossRef]
17. Bayley, J.P.; Oldenburg, R.A.; Nuk, J.; Hoekstra, A.S.; van der Meer, C.A.; Korpershoek, E.; McGillivray, B.; Corssmit, E.P.; Dinjens, W.N.; de Krijger, R.R.; et al. Paraganglioma and pheochromocytoma upon maternal transmission of SDHD mutations. *BMC Med. Genet.* **2014**, *15*, 111. [CrossRef]
18. Van der Mey, A.G.; Maaswinkel-Mooy, P.D.; Cornelisse, C.J.; Schmidt, P.H.; van de Kamp, J.J. Genomic imprinting in hereditary glomus tumours: Evidence for new genetic theory. *Lancet* **1989**, *2*, 1291–1294. [CrossRef]
19. Hao, H.X.; Khalimonchuk, O.; Schraders, M.; Dephoure, N.; Bayley, J.P.; Kunst, H.; Devilee, P.; Cremers, C.W.; Schiffman, J.D.; Bentz, B.G.; et al. SDH5, a gene required for flavination of succinate dehydrogenase, is mutated in paraganglioma. *Science* **2009**, *325*, 1139–1142. [CrossRef]
20. Burnichon, N.; Briere, J.J.; Libe, R.; Vescovo, L.; Riviere, J.; Tissier, F.; Jouanno, E.; Jeunemaitre, X.; Benit, P.; Tzagoloff, A.; et al. SDHA is a tumor suppressor gene causing paraganglioma. *Hum. Mol. Genet.* **2010**, *19*, 3011–3020. [CrossRef]
21. Comino-Mendez, I.; Gracia-Aznarez, F.J.; Schiavi, F.; Landa, I.; Leandro-Garcia, L.J.; Leton, R.; Honrado, E.; Ramos-Medina, R.; Caronia, D.; Pita, G.; et al. Exome sequencing identifies MAX mutations as a cause of hereditary pheochromocytoma. *Nat. Genet.* **2011**, *43*, 663–667. [CrossRef]

22. Astuti, D.; Latif, F.; Dallol, A.; Dahia, P.L.; Douglas, F.; George, E.; Skoldberg, F.; Husebye, E.S.; Eng, C.; Maher, E.R. Gene mutations in the succinate dehydrogenase subunit SDHB cause susceptibility to familial pheochromocytoma and to familial paraganglioma. *Am. J. Hum. Genet.* **2001**, *69*, 49–54. [CrossRef]
23. Timmers, H.J.; Kozupa, A.; Eisenhofer, G.; Raygada, M.; Adams, K.T.; Solis, D.; Lenders, J.W.; Pacak, K. Clinical presentations, biochemical phenotypes, and genotype-phenotype correlations in patients with succinate dehydrogenase subunit B-associated pheochromocytomas and paragangliomas. *J. Clin. Endocrinol. Metab.* **2007**, *92*, 779–786. [CrossRef]
24. Kunst, H.P.; Rutten, M.H.; de Monnink, J.P.; Hoefsloot, L.H.; Timmers, H.J.; Marres, H.A.; Jansen, J.C.; Kremer, H.; Bayley, J.P.; Cremers, C.W. SDHAF2 (PGL2-SDH5) and hereditary head and neck paraganglioma. *Clin. Cancer Res.* **2011**, *17*, 247–254. [CrossRef]
25. Korpershoek, E.; Favier, J.; Gaal, J.; Burnichon, N.; van Gessel, B.; Oudijk, L.; Badoual, C.; Gadessaud, N.; Venisse, A.; Bayley, J.P.; et al. SDHA immunohistochemistry detects germline SDHA gene mutations in apparently sporadic paragangliomas and pheochromocytomas. *J. Clin. Endocrinol. Metab.* **2011**, *96*, E1472–1476. [CrossRef]
26. Saxena, N.; Maio, N.; Crooks, D.R.; Ricketts, C.J.; Yang, Y.; Wei, M.H.; Fan, T.W.; Lane, A.N.; Sourbier, C.; Singh, A.; et al. SDHB-Deficient Cancers: The Role of Mutations That Impair Iron Sulfur Cluster Delivery. *J. Natl. Cancer Inst.* **2016**, *108*. [CrossRef]
27. Guzy, R.D.; Sharma, B.; Bell, E.; Chandel, N.S.; Schumacker, P.T. Loss of the SdhB, but Not the SdhA, subunit of complex II triggers reactive oxygen species-dependent hypoxia-inducible factor activation and tumorigenesis. *Mol. Cell Biol.* **2008**, *28*, 718–731. [CrossRef]
28. de Cubas, A.A.; Korpershoek, E.; Inglada-Perez, L.; Letouze, E.; Curras-Freixes, M.; Fernandez, A.F.; Comino-Mendez, I.; Schiavi, F.; Mancikova, V.; Eisenhofer, G.; et al. DNA Methylation Profiling in Pheochromocytoma and Paraganglioma Reveals Diagnostic and Prognostic Markers. *Clin. Cancer Res.* **2015**, *21*, 3020–3030. [CrossRef]
29. Lonser, R.R.; Glenn, G.M.; Walther, M.; Chew, E.Y.; Libutti, S.K.; Linehan, W.M.; Oldfield, E.H. von Hippel-Lindau disease. *Lancet* **2003**, *361*, 2059–2067. [CrossRef]
30. Friedrich, C.A. Genotype-phenotype correlation in von Hippel-Lindau syndrome. *Hum. Mol. Genet.* **2001**, *10*, 763–767. [CrossRef]
31. Semenza, G.L. Involvement of oxygen-sensing pathways in physiologic and pathologic erythropoiesis. *Blood* **2009**, *114*, 2015–2019. [CrossRef] [PubMed]
32. Capodimonti, S.; Teofili, L.; Martini, M.; Cenci, T.; Iachininoto, M.G.; Nuzzolo, E.R.; Bianchi, M.; Murdolo, M.; Leone, G.; Larocca, L.M. Von hippel-lindau disease and erythrocytosis. *J. Clin. Oncol.* **2012**, *30*, e137–e139. [CrossRef]
33. Koch, C.A.; Huang, S.C.; Zhuang, Z.; Stolle, C.; Stolle, C.; Azumi, N.; Chrousos, G.P.; Vortmeyer, A.O.; Pacak, K. Somatic VHL gene deletion and point mutation in MEN 2A-associated pheochromocytoma. *Oncogene* **2002**, *17*, 479–482. [CrossRef] [PubMed]
34. Merlo, A.; de Quiros, S.B.; de Santa-Maria, I.S.; Pitiot, A.S.; Balbin, M.; Astudillo, A.; Scola, B.; Aristegui, M.; Quer, M.; Suarez, C.; et al. Identification of somatic VHL gene mutations in sporadic head and neck paragangliomas in association with activation of the HIF-1alpha/miR-210 signaling pathway. *J. Clin. Endocrinol. Metab.* **2013**, *98*, E1661–E1666. [CrossRef] [PubMed]
35. Wang, H.; Shepard, M.J.; Zhang, C.; Dong, L.; Walker, D.; Guedez, L.; Park, S.; Wang, Y.; Chen, S.; Pang, Y.; et al. Deletion of the von Hippel-Lindau Gene in Hemangioblasts Causes Hemangioblastoma-like Lesions in Murine Retina. *Cancer Res.* **2018**, *78*, 1266–1274. [CrossRef]
36. Roe, J.S.; Kim, H.; Lee, S.M.; Kim, S.T.; Cho, E.J.; Youn, H.D. p53 stabilization and transactivation by a von Hippel-Lindau protein. *Mol. Cell* **2006**, *22*, 395–405. [CrossRef]
37. Semenza, G.L.; Rue, E.A.; Iyer, N.V.; Pang, M.G.; Kearns, W.G. Assignment of the hypoxia-inducible factor 1alpha gene to a region of conserved synteny on mouse chromosome 12 and human chromosome 14q. *Genomics* **1996**, *34*, 437–439. [CrossRef]
38. Semenza, G.L. Hypoxia-inducible factor 1 (HIF-1) pathway. *Sci. STKE* **2007**, *2007*, cm8. [CrossRef]
39. Zhong, H.; De Marzo, A.M.; Laughner, E.; Lim, M.; Hilton, D.A.; Zagzag, D.; Buechler, P.; Isaacs, W.B.; Semenza, G.L.; Simons, J.W. Overexpression of hypoxia-inducible factor 1alpha in common human cancers and their metastases. *Cancer Res.* **1999**, *59*, 5830–5835.

40. Amar, L.; Baudin, E.; Burnichon, N.; Peyrard, S.; Silvera, S.; Bertherat, J.; Bertagna, X.; Schlumberger, M.; Jeunemaitre, X.; Gimenez-Roqueplo, A.P.; et al. Succinate dehydrogenase B gene mutations predict survival in patients with malignant pheochromocytomas or paragangliomas. *J. Clin. Endocrinol. Metab.* **2007**, *92*, 3822–3828. [CrossRef] [PubMed]
41. Keith, B.; Johnson, R.S.; Simon, M.C. HIF1alpha and HIF2alpha: Sibling rivalry in hypoxic tumour growth and progression. *Nat. Rev. Cancer* **2011**, *12*, 9–22. [CrossRef]
42. Percy, M.J.; Furlow, P.W.; Lucas, G.S.; Li, X.; Lappin, T.R.; McMullin, M.F.; Lee, F.S. A gain-of-function mutation in the HIF2A gene in familial erythrocytosis. *N. Engl. J. Med.* **2008**, *358*, 162–168. [CrossRef]
43. Zhuang, Z.; Yang, C.; Lorenzo, F.; Merino, M.; Fojo, T.; Kebebew, E.; Popovic, V.; Stratakis, C.A.; Prchal, J.T.; Pacak, K. Somatic HIF2A gain-of-function mutations in paraganglioma with polycythemia. *N. Engl. J. Med.* **2012**, *367*, 922–930. [CrossRef]
44. Yang, C.; Hong, C.S.; Prchal, J.T.; Balint, M.T.; Pacak, K.; Zhuang, Z. Somatic mosaicism of EPAS1 mutations in the syndrome of paraganglioma and somatostatinoma associated with polycythemia. *Hum. Genome. Var.* **2015**, *2*, 15053. [CrossRef] [PubMed]
45. Ratner, N.; Miller, S.J. A RASopathy gene commonly mutated in cancer: The neurofibromatosis type 1 tumour suppressor. *Nat. Rev. Cancer* **2015**, *15*, 290–301. [CrossRef]
46. Bausch, B.; Borozdin, W.; Mautner, V.F.; Hoffmann, M.M.; Boehm, D.; Robledo, M.; Cascon, A.; Harenberg, T.; Schiavi, F.; Pawlu, C.; et al. Germline NF1 mutational spectra and loss-of-heterozygosity analyses in patients with pheochromocytoma and neurofibromatosis type 1. *J. Clin. Endocrinol. Metab.* **2007**, *92*, 2784–2792. [CrossRef]
47. Gutmann, D.H.; Ferner, R.E.; Listernick, R.H.; Korf, B.R.; Wolters, P.L.; Johnson, K.J. Neurofibromatosis type 1. *Nat. Rev. Dis. Primers* **2017**, *3*, 17004. [CrossRef]
48. Welander, J.; Larsson, C.; Backdahl, M.; Hareni, N.; Sivler, T.; Sivler, T.; Brauckhoff, M.; Soderkvist, P.; Gimm, O. Integrative genomics reveals frequent somatic NF1 mutations in sporadic pheochromocytomas. *Hum. Mol. Genet.* **2012**, *21*, 5406–5416. [CrossRef]
49. Correia, M.J.; Lopes, L.O.; Bugalho, M.J.; Cristina, L.; Santos, A.I.; Bordalo, A.D.; Pinho, B.; da Silva, H.L.; Goncalves, M.D.; Ribeiro, C.; et al. Multiple endocrine neoplasia type 2A. Study of a family. *Rev. Port. Cardiol.* **2000**, *19*, 11–31.
50. Bergsland, E.K. The evolving landscape of neuroendocrine tumors. *Semin. Oncol.* **2013**, *40*, 4–22. [CrossRef]
51. Machens, A.; Brauckhoff, M.; Holzhausen, H.J.; Thanh, P.N.; Lehnert, H.; Dralle, H. Codon-specific development of pheochromocytoma in multiple endocrine neoplasia type 2. *J. Clin. Endocrinol. Metab.* **2005**, *90*, 3999–4003. [CrossRef]
52. Boedeker, C.C.; Erlic, Z.; Richard, S.; Kontny, U.; Gimenez-Roqueplo, A.P.; Cascon, A.; Robledo, M.; de Campos, J.M.; van Nederveen, F.H.; de Krijger, R.R.; et al. Head and neck paragangliomas in von Hippel-Lindau disease and multiple endocrine neoplasia type 2. *J. Clin. Endocrinol. Metab.* **2009**, *94*, 1938–1944. [CrossRef]
53. Fishbein, L.; Nathanson, K.L. Pheochromocytoma and paraganglioma: Understanding the complexities of the genetic background. *Cancer Genet.* **2012**, *205*, 1–11. [CrossRef]
54. Plaza-Menacho, I.; Barnouin, K.; Goodman, K.; Martinez-Torres, R.J.; Borg, A.; Murray-Rust, J.; Mouilleron, S.; Knowles, P.; McDonald, N.Q. Oncogenic RET kinase domain mutations perturb the autophosphorylation trajectory by enhancing substrate presentation in trans. *Mol. Cell* **2014**, *53*, 738–751. [CrossRef]
55. Burnichon, N.; Cascon, A.; Schiavi, F.; Morales, N.P.; Comino-Mendez, I.; Abermil, N.; Inglada-Perez, L.; de Cubas, A.A.; Amar, L.; Barontini, M.; et al. MAX mutations cause hereditary and sporadic pheochromocytoma and paraganglioma. *Clin. Cancer Res.* **2012**, *18*, 2828–2837. [CrossRef]
56. Blackwood, E.M.; Eisenman, R.N. Max: A helix-loop-helix zipper protein that forms a sequence-specific DNA-binding complex with Myc. *Science* **1991**, *251*, 1211–1217. [CrossRef]
57. Bousset, K.; Henriksson, M.; Luscher-Firzlaff, J.M.; Litchfield, D.W.; Luscher, B. Identification of casein kinase II phosphorylation sites in Max: Effects on DNA-binding kinetics of Max homo- and Myc/Max heterodimers. *Oncogene* **1993**, *8*, 3211–3220.
58. Yoshimoto, K.; Iwahana, H.; Fukuda, A.; Sano, T.; Katsuragi, K.; Kinoshita, M.; Saito, S.; Itakura, M. ras mutations in endocrine tumors: Mutation detection by polymerase chain reaction-single strand conformation polymorphism. *Jpn. J. Cancer Res.* **1992**, *83*, 1057–1062. [CrossRef]

59. Safford, S.D.; Coleman, R.E.; Gockerman, J.P.; Moore, J.; Feldman, J.M.; Leight, G.S., Jr.; Tyler, D.S.; Olson, J.A., Jr. Iodine -131 metaiodobenzylguanidine is an effective treatment for malignant pheochromocytoma and paraganglioma. *Surgery* **2003**, *134*, 956–962. [CrossRef]
60. Fitzgerald, P.A.; Goldsby, R.E.; Huberty, J.P.; Price, D.C.; Hawkins, R.A.; Veatch, J.J.; Dela Cruz, F.; Jahan, T.M.; Linker, C.A.; Damon, L.; et al. Malignant pheochromocytomas and paragangliomas: A phase II study of therapy with high-dose 131I-metaiodobenzylguanidine (131I-MIBG). *Ann. NY Acad. Sci.* **2006**, *1073*, 465–490. [CrossRef]
61. van Hulsteijn, L.T.; Niemeijer, N.D.; Dekkers, O.M.; Corssmit, E.P. (131)I-MIBG therapy for malignant paraganglioma and phaeochromocytoma: Systematic review and meta-analysis. *Clin. Endocrinol. (Oxf)* **2014**, *80*, 487–501. [CrossRef] [PubMed]
62. Otte, A.; Jermann, E.; Behe, M.; Goetze, M.; Bucher, H.C.; Roser, H.W.; Heppeler, A.; Mueller-Brand, J.; Maecke, H.R. DOTATOC: A powerful new tool for receptor-mediated radionuclide therapy. *Eur. J. Nucl. Med.* **1997**, *24*, 792–795. [PubMed]
63. Kwekkeboom, D.J.; Bakker, W.H.; Kam, B.L.; Teunissen, J.J.; Kooij, P.P.; de Herder, W.W.; Feelders, R.A.; van Eijck, C.H.; de Jong, M.; Srinivasan, A.; et al. Treatment of patients with gastro-entero-pancreatic (GEP) tumours with the novel radiolabelled somatostatin analogue [177Lu-DOTA(0),Tyr3]octreotate. *Eur. J. Nucl. Med. Mol. Imaging* **2003**, *30*, 417–422. [CrossRef] [PubMed]
64. Bodei, L.; Mueller-Brand, J.; Baum, R.P.; Pavel, M.E.; Horsch, D.; O–Dorisio, M.S.; O–Dorisio, T.M.; Howe, J.R.; Cremonesi, M.; Kwekkeboom, D.J.; et al. The joint IAEA, EANM, and SNMMI practical guidance on peptide receptor radionuclide therapy (PRRNT) in neuroendocrine tumours. *Eur. J. Nucl. Med. Mol. Imaging* **2013**, *40*, 800–816. [CrossRef]
65. Strosberg, J.; El-Haddad, G.; Wolin, E.; Hendifar, A.; Yao, J.; Chasen, B.; Mittra, E.; Kunz, P.L.; Kulke, M.H.; Jacene, H.; et al. Phase 3 Trial of (177)Lu-Dotatate for Midgut Neuroendocrine Tumors. *N. Engl. J. Med.* **2017**, *376*, 125–135. [CrossRef] [PubMed]
66. Favier, J.; Igaz, P.; Burnichon, N.; Amar, L.; Libe, R.; Badoual, C.; Tissier, F.; Bertherat, J.; Plouin, P.F.; Jeunemaitre, X.; et al. Rationale for anti-angiogenic therapy in pheochromocytoma and paraganglioma. *Endocr. Pathol.* **2012**, *23*, 34–42. [CrossRef] [PubMed]
67. Janeway, K.A.; Kim, S.Y.; Lodish, M.; Nose, V.; Rustin, P.; Gaal, J.; Dahia, P.L.; Liegl, B.; Ball, E.R.; Raygada, M.; et al. Defects in succinate dehydrogenase in gastrointestinal stromal tumors lacking KIT and PDGFRA mutations. *Proc. Natl. Acad. Sci. USA* **2011**, *108*, 314–318. [CrossRef]
68. Ricketts, C.; Woodward, E.R.; Killick, P.; Morris, M.R.; Astuti, D.; Latif, F.; Maher, E.R. Germline SDHB mutations and familial renal cell carcinoma. *J. Natl. Cancer Inst.* **2008**, *100*, 1260–1262. [CrossRef]
69. Tuthill, M.; Barod, R.; Pyle, L.; Cook, T.; Chew, S.; Gore, M.; Maxwell, P.; Eisen, T. A report of succinate dehydrogenase B deficiency associated with metastatic papillary renal cell carcinoma: Successful treatment with the multi-targeted tyrosine kinase inhibitor sunitinib. *BMJ Case Rep.* **2009**, *2009*. [CrossRef]
70. Joshua, A.M.; Ezzat, S.; Asa, S.L.; Evans, A.; Broom, R.; Freeman, M.; Knox, J.J. Rationale and evidence for sunitinib in the treatment of malignant paraganglioma/pheochromocytoma. *J. Clin. Endocrinol. Metab.* **2009**, *94*, 5–9. [CrossRef] [PubMed]
71. Hahn, N.M.; Reckova, M.; Cheng, L.; Baldridge, L.A.; Cummings, O.W.; Sweeney, C.J. Patient with malignant paraganglioma responding to the multikinase inhibitor sunitinib malate. *J. Clin. Oncol.* **2009**, *27*, 460–463. [CrossRef] [PubMed]
72. Jimenez, C.; Cabanillas, M.E.; Santarpia, L.; Jonasch, E.; Kyle, K.L.; Lano, E.A.; Matin, S.F.; Nunez, R.F.; Perrier, N.D.; Phan, A.; et al. Use of the tyrosine kinase inhibitor sunitinib in a patient with von Hippel-Lindau disease: Targeting angiogenic factors in pheochromocytoma and other von Hippel-Lindau disease-related tumors. *J. Clin. Endocrinol. Metab.* **2009**, *94*, 386–391. [CrossRef] [PubMed]
73. Nemoto, K.; Miura, T.; Shioji, G.; Tsuboi, N. Sunitinib treatment for refractory malignant pheochromocytoma. *Neuro. Endocrinol. Lett.* **2012**, *33*, 260–264. [PubMed]
74. Ayala-Ramirez, M.; Chougnet, C.N.; Habra, M.A.; Palmer, J.L.; Leboulleux, S.; Cabanillas, M.E.; Caramella, C.; Anderson, P.; Al Ghuzlan, A.; Waguespack, S.G.; et al. Treatment with sunitinib for patients with progressive metastatic pheochromocytomas and sympathetic paragangliomas. *J. Clin. Endocrinol. Metab.* **2012**, *97*, 4040–4050. [CrossRef]

75. Welsh, S.J.; Williams, R.R.; Birmingham, A.; Newman, D.J.; Kirkpatrick, D.L.; Powis, G. The thioredoxin redox inhibitors 1-methylpropyl 2-imidazolyl disulfide and pleurotin inhibit hypoxia-induced factor 1alpha and vascular endothelial growth factor formation. *Mol. Cancer Ther.* **2003**, *2*, 235–243. [PubMed]
76. Welsh, S.; Williams, R.; Kirkpatrick, L.; Paine-Murrieta, G.; Powis, G. Antitumor activity and pharmacodynamic properties of PX-478, an inhibitor of hypoxia-inducible factor-1alpha. *Mol. Cancer Ther.* **2004**, *3*, 233–244.
77. Chen, W.; Hill, H.; Christie, A.; Kim, M.S.; Holloman, E.; Pavia-Jimenez, A.; Homayoun, F.; Ma, Y.; Patel, N.; Yell, P.; et al. Targeting renal cell carcinoma with a HIF-2 antagonist. *Nature* **2016**, *539*, 112–117. [CrossRef]
78. Courtney, K.D.; Infante, J.R.; Lam, E.T.; Figlin, R.A.; Rini, B.I.; Brugarolas, J.; Zojwalla, N.J.; Lowe, A.M.; Wang, K.; Wallace, E.M.; et al. Phase I Dose-Escalation Trial of PT2385, a First-in-Class Hypoxia-Inducible Factor-2alpha Antagonist in Patients With Previously Treated Advanced Clear Cell Renal Cell Carcinoma. *J. Clin. Oncol.* **2018**, *36*, 867–874. [CrossRef]
79. Pang, Y.; Yang, C.; Schovanek, J.; Wang, H.; Bullova, P.; Caisova, V.; Gupta, G.; Wolf, K.I.; Semenza, G.L.; Zhuang, Z.; et al. Anthracyclines suppress pheochromocytoma cell characteristics, including metastasis, through inhibition of the hypoxia signaling pathway. *Oncotarget* **2017**, *8*, 22313–22324. [CrossRef]
80. Burnichon, N.; Lepoutre-Lussey, C.; Laffaire, J.; Gadessaud, N.; Molinie, V.; Hernigou, A.; Plouin, P.F.; Jeunemaitre, X.; Favier, J.; Gimenez-Roqueplo, A.P. A novel TMEM127 mutation in a patient with familial bilateral pheochromocytoma. *Eur. J. Endocrinol.* **2011**, *164*, 141–145. [CrossRef]
81. Attie, T.; Pelet, A.; Edery, P.; Eng, C.; Mulligan, L.M.; Amiel, J.; Boutrand, L.; Beldjord, C.; Nihoul-Fekete, C.; Munnich, A.; et al. Diversity of RET proto-oncogene mutations in familial and sporadic Hirschsprung disease. *Hum. Mol. Genet.* **1995**, *4*, 1381–1386. [CrossRef] [PubMed]
82. Ma, X.M.; Blenis, J. Molecular mechanisms of mTOR-mediated translational control. *Nat. Rev. Mol. Cell. Biol.* **2009**, *10*, 307–318. [CrossRef] [PubMed]
83. Druce, M.R.; Kaltsas, G.A.; Fraenkel, M.; Gross, D.J.; Grossman, A.B. Novel and evolving therapies in the treatment of malignant phaeochromocytoma: Experience with the mTOR inhibitor everolimus (RAD001). *Horm. Metab. Res.* **2009**, *41*, 697–702. [CrossRef] [PubMed]
84. Oh, D.Y.; Kim, T.W.; Park, Y.S.; Shin, S.J.; Shin, S.H.; Song, E.K.; Lee, H.J.; Lee, K.W.; Bang, Y.J. Phase 2 study of everolimus monotherapy in patients with nonfunctioning neuroendocrine tumors or pheochromocytomas/paragangliomas. *Cancer* **2012**, *118*, 6162–6170. [CrossRef] [PubMed]
85. Giubellino, A.; Bullova, P.; Nolting, S.; Turkova, H.; Powers, J.F.; Liu, Q.; Guichard, S.; Tischler, A.S.; Grossman, A.B.; Pacak, K. Combined inhibition of mTORC1 and mTORC2 signaling pathways is a promising therapeutic option in inhibiting pheochromocytoma tumor growth: In vitro and in vivo studies in female athymic nude mice. *Endocrinology* **2013**, *154*, 646–655. [CrossRef]
86. Matro, J.; Giubellino, A.; Pacak, K. Current and future therapeutic approaches for metastatic pheochromocytoma and paraganglioma: Focus on SDHB tumors. *Horm. Metab. Res.* **2013**, *45*, 147–153. [CrossRef]
87. Letouze, E.; Martinelli, C.; Loriot, C.; Burnichon, N.; Abermil, N.; Ottolenghi, C.; Janin, M.; Menara, M.; Nguyen, A.T.; Benit, P.; et al. SDH mutations establish a hypermethylator phenotype in paraganglioma. *Cancer Cell* **2013**, *23*, 739–752. [CrossRef]
88. Killian, J.K.; Kim, S.Y.; Miettinen, M.; Smith, C.; Merino, M.; Tsokos, M.; Quezado, M.; Smith, W.I., Jr.; Jahromi, M.S.; Xekouki, P.; et al. Succinate dehydrogenase mutation underlies global epigenomic divergence in gastrointestinal stromal tumor. *Cancer Discov.* **2013**, *3*, 648–657. [CrossRef]
89. Turcan, S.; Rohle, D.; Goenka, A.; Walsh, L.A.; Fang, F.; Yilmaz, E.; Campos, C.; Fabius, A.W.; Lu, C.; Ward, P.S.; et al. IDH1 mutation is sufficient to establish the glioma hypermethylator phenotype. *Nature* **2012**, *483*, 479–483. [CrossRef]
90. SongTao, Q.; Lei, Y.; Si, G.; YanQing, D.; HuiXia, H.; XueLin, Z.; LanXiao, W.; Fei, Y. IDH mutations predict longer survival and response to temozolomide in secondary glioblastoma. *Cancer Sci.* **2012**, *103*, 269–273. [CrossRef]
91. Lu, Y.; Kwintkiewicz, J.; Liu, Y.; Tech, K.; Frady, L.N.; Su, Y.T.; Bautista, W.; Moon, S.I.; MacDonald, J.; Ewend, M.G.; et al. Chemosensitivity of IDH1-Mutated Gliomas Due to an Impairment in PARP1-Mediated DNA Repair. *Cancer Res.* **2017**, *77*, 1709–1718. [CrossRef] [PubMed]

92. Hadoux, J.; Favier, J.; Scoazec, J.Y.; Leboulleux, S.; Al Ghuzlan, A.; Caramella, C.; Deandreis, D.; Borget, I.; Loriot, C.; Chougnet, C.; et al. SDHB mutations are associated with response to temozolomide in patients with metastatic pheochromocytoma or paraganglioma. *Int. J. Cancer* **2014**, *135*, 2711–2720. [CrossRef] [PubMed]
93. Kulke, M.H.; Stuart, K.; Enzinger, P.C.; Ryan, D.P.; Clark, J.W.; Muzikansky, A.; Vincitore, M.; Michelini, A.; Fuchs, C.S. Phase II study of temozolomide and thalidomide in patients with metastatic neuroendocrine tumors. *J. Clin. Oncol.* **2006**, *24*, 401–406. [CrossRef] [PubMed]
94. Sulkowski, P.L.; Sundaram, R.K.; Oeck, S.; Corso, C.D.; Liu, Y.; Noorbakhsh, S.; Niger, M.; Boeke, M.; Ueno, D.; Kalathil, A.N.; et al. Krebs-cycle-deficient hereditary cancer syndromes are defined by defects in homologous-recombination DNA repair. *Nat. Genet.* **2018**, *50*, 1086–1092. [CrossRef] [PubMed]
95. Pang, Y.; Lu, Y.; Caisova, V.; Liu, Y.; Bullova, P.; Huynh, T.T.; Zhou, Y.; Yu, D.; Frysak, Z.; Hartmann, I.; et al. Targeting NAD(+)/PARP DNA Repair Pathway as a Novel Therapeutic Approach to SDHB-Mutated Cluster I Pheochromocytoma and Paraganglioma. *Clin. Cancer Res.* **2018**, *24*, 3423–3432. [CrossRef]
96. Zhang, Z.; Guo, Z.; Zhan, Y.; Li, H.; Wu, S. Role of histone acetylation in activation of nuclear factor erythroid 2-related factor 2/heme oxygenase 1 pathway by manganese chloride. *Toxicol. Appl. Pharmacol.* **2017**, *336*, 94–100. [CrossRef] [PubMed]
97. Li, Z.Y.; Li, Q.Z.; Chen, L.; Chen, B.D.; Zhang, C.; Wang, X.; Li, W.P. HPOB, an HDAC6 inhibitor, attenuates corticosterone-induced injury in rat adrenal pheochromocytoma PC12 cells by inhibiting mitochondrial GR translocation and the intrinsic apoptosis pathway. *Neurochem. Int.* **2016**, *99*, 239–251. [CrossRef]
98. Cayo, M.A.; Cayo, A.K.; Jarjour, S.M.; Chen, H. Sodium butyrate activates Notch1 signaling, reduces tumor markers, and induces cell cycle arrest and apoptosis in pheochromocytoma. *Am. J. Transl. Res.* **2009**, *1*, 178–183.
99. Adler, J.T.; Hottinger, D.G.; Kunnimalaiyaan, M.; Chen, H. Histone deacetylase inhibitors upregulate Notch-1 and inhibit growth in pheochromocytoma cells. *Surgery* **2008**, *144*, 956–961. [CrossRef]
100. Yang, C.; Matro, J.C.; Huntoon, K.M.; Ye, D.Y.; Huynh, T.T.; Fliedner, S.M.; Breza, J.; Zhuang, Z.; Pacak, K. Missense mutations in the human SDHB gene increase protein degradation without altering intrinsic enzymatic function. *FASEB J.* **2012**, *26*, 4506–4516. [CrossRef] [PubMed]
101. Hatfield, S.M.; Sitkovsky, M. A2A adenosine receptor antagonists to weaken the hypoxia-HIF-1alpha driven immunosuppression and improve immunotherapies of cancer. *Curr. Opin. Pharmacol.* **2016**, *29*, 90–96. [CrossRef]
102. Labiano, S.; Palazon, A.; Bolanos, E.; Azpilikueta, A.; Sanchez-Paulete, A.R.; Morales-Kastresana, A.; Quetglas, J.I.; Perez-Gracia, J.L.; Gurpide, A.; Rodriguez-Ruiz, M.; et al. Hypoxia-induced soluble CD137 in malignant cells blocks CD137L-costimulation as an immune escape mechanism. *Oncoimmunology* **2016**, *5*, e1062967. [CrossRef] [PubMed]
103. Chouaib, S.; Noman, M.Z.; Kosmatopoulos, K.; Curran, M.A. Hypoxic stress: Obstacles and opportunities for innovative immunotherapy of cancer. *Oncogene* **2017**, *36*, 439–445. [CrossRef] [PubMed]
104. Hadoux, J.; Terroir, M.; Leboulleux, S.; Deschamps, F.; Al Ghuzlan, A.; Hescot, S.; Tselikas, L.; Borget, I.; Caramella, C.; Deandreis, D.; et al. Interferon-alpha Treatment for Disease Control in Metastatic Pheochromocytoma/Paraganglioma Patients. *Horm. Cancer* **2017**, *8*, 330–337. [CrossRef]
105. Liu, Y.; Lu, Y.; Celiku, O.; Li, A.; Wu, Q.; Zhou, Y.; Yang, C. Targeting IDH1-Mutated Malignancies with NRF2 Blockade. *J. Natl. Cancer Inst.* **2019**. [CrossRef]
106. Chouchani, E.T.; Pell, V.R.; Gaude, E.; Aksentijevic, D.; Sundier, S.Y.; Robb, E.L.; Logan, A.; Nadtochiy, S.M.; Ord, E.N.J.; Smith, A.C.; et al. Ischaemic accumulation of succinate controls reperfusion injury through mitochondrial ROS. *Nature* **2014**, *515*, 431–435. [CrossRef]
107. Ghayee, H.K.; Bhagwandin, V.J.; Stastny, V.; Click, A.; Ding, L.H.; Mizrachi, D.; Zou, Y.S.; Chari, R.; Lam, W.L.; Bachoo, R.M.; et al. Progenitor cell line (hPheo1) derived from a human pheochromocytoma tumor. *PLoS ONE* **2013**, *8*, e65624. [CrossRef] [PubMed]

MDPI
St. Alban-Anlage 66
4052 Basel
Switzerland
Tel. +41 61 683 77 34
Fax +41 61 302 89 18
www.mdpi.com

Cancers Editorial Office
E-mail: cancers@mdpi.com
www.mdpi.com/journal/cancers

www.ingramcontent.com/pod-product-compliance
Lightning Source LLC
Chambersburg PA
CBHW041214220326
41597CB00032BA/5417
* 9 7 8 3 0 3 9 2 1 6 5 4 3 *